LIPPINCOTT MANUAL
of NURSING PRACTICE
Series

PATHOPHYSIOLOGY

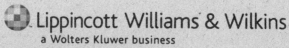
Lippincott Williams & Wilkins
a Wolters Kluwer business

Philadelphia • Baltimore • New York • London
Buenos Aires • Hong Kong • Sydney • Tokyo

STAFF

Executive Publisher
Judith A. Schilling McCann, RN, MSN

Editorial Director
H. Nancy Holmes

Clinical Director
Joan M. Robinson, RN, MSN

Senior Art Director
Arlene Putterman

Clinical Manager
Eileen Cassin Gallen, RN, BSN

Editorial Project Manager
Jennifer Lynn Kowalak

Editor
Julie Munden

Clinical Editors
Joanne M. Bartelmo, RN, MSN
Anita Lockhart, RN, C, MSN

Copy Editors
Kimberly Bilotta (supervisor),
Scotti Cohn, Jen Fielding, Amy Furman,
Shana Harrington, Judith Orioli,
Lisa Stockslager, Pamela Wingrod

Designers
Debra Moloshok (book design),
Linda Jovinelly Franklin (project
manager)

Digital Composition Services
Diane Paluba (manager), Joyce
Rossi Biletz, Donna S. Morris

Manufacturing
Patricia K. Dorshaw (director),
Beth J. Welsh

Editorial Assistants
Megan L. Aldinger, Karen J. Kirk,
Linda K. Ruhf

Design Assistant
Georg Purvis, 4th

Indexer
Barbara Hodgson

LMNPP010206

**Library of Congress
Cataloging-in-Publication Data**

Pathophysiology.
    p.;cm.—(Lippincott manual of nursing
practice series)
    Includes bibliographical references and index.
    1. Nursing —Handbooks, manuals, etc. 2.
Physiology, Pathological—Handbooks, manuals,
etc. I.Lippincott Williams and Wilkins. II. Title.
III. Series.
    [DNLM: 1. Disease—Handbooks.   2. Nursing
Care—Handbooks.   3. Pathology—Handbooks.
WY 49 P2962 2007]
RT51.P32 2007
616.07'5—dc22
    ISBN 1-58255-663-6 (alk.paper)
    ISBN 10: 0-7817-8167-1 (Philippine Edition)
    ISBN 13: 978-0-7817-8167-1
                                        2005030653

CONTENTS

Contributors and consultants   v

1   Cardiovascular system   1
2   Respiratory system   84
3   Nervous system   129
4   Gastrointestinal system   189
5   Renal system   228
6   Endocrine system   262
7   Hematologic system   289
8   Immune system   308
9   Sensory system   336
10   Integumentary system   351
11   Musculoskeletal system   370
12   Reproductive system   402
13   Cancer   417
14   Fluids and electrolytes   447
15   Genetics   481
16   Infection   501

Selected references   523
Index   527

CONTRIBUTORS AND CONSULTANTS

◆

Gary J. Arnold, MD
Associate Professor
College of Nursing and Allied Health
    Professions
University of Louisiana at Lafayette

Cheryl A. Bean, APRN,BC, DSN, ANP,
    AOCN
Associate Professor/Adult Nurse Practitioner
Indiana University School of Nursing
Indianapolis

Mary Ann Boucher, APRN,BC, ND
Assistant Professor of Nursing
University of Massachusetts Dartmouth

Peggy Bozarth, RN, MSN
Professor
Hopkinsville (Ky.) Community College

Janie Choate, PA-C, MAT, BS, BA
Adjunct Faculty
University of the Sciences
Philadelphia

Laura M. Criddle, RN, MS, CCNS, CEN
Doctoral Student
Oregon Health & Science University
Portland

Diane Dixon, PA-C, MA, MMSc
Assistant Professor and Academic Coordinator
University of South Alabama
Department of Physician Assistant Studies
Mobile

Shirley Lyon Garcia, RN, BSN
Nursing Program Director, PNE
McDowell Technical Community Colleg
Marion, N.C.

Charla K. Hollin, RN, BSN
Nursing Program Director
Rich Mountain Community College
Mena, Ark.

Shelley Yerger Huffstutler, RN, DSN,
    CFNP, GNP
Associate Professor and Director, FNP Progran
University of Alabama at Birmingham
    School of Nursing

Mary T. Kowalski, RN, BA, MSN
*Director Vocational Nursing and Health Caree
    Programs*
Cerro Coso Community College
Ridgecrest, Calif.

Grace G. Lewis, RN, MS, BC
Assistant Professor of Nursing
Georgia Baptist College of Nursing of
    Mercer University
Atlanta

Patricia J. McBride, RN, MSN, CIC
Infection Control Manager
Bryn Mawr (Pa.) Hospital

Cynthia A. Prows, RN, MSN, CNS
Clinical Nurse Specialist
Children's Hospital Medical Center
Cincinnati

Betty E. Sims, RN, MSN
Nurse Consultant
Board of Nurse Examiners
Austin, Tex.
Adjunct Instructor
St. Philip's College
San Antonio, Tex.

Sheryl Thomas, RN, MSN
Nurse Instructor
Wayne County Community College
Detroit

Dan Vetrosky, PA-C, MEd, PhD(c)
Assistant Professor
University of South Alabama
Mobile

Colleen R. Walsh, RN, MSN, ACNP-BC,
    CS, ONC
Faculty, Graduate Nursing
University of Southern Indiana School of
    Nursing & Health Professions
Evansville

CARDIOVASCULAR SYSTEM

The cardiovascular system begins its activity when the fetus is barely 1 month old, and it's the last system to cease activity at the end of life. The heart, arteries, veins, and lymphatics make up this system. These structures transport life-supporting oxygen and nutrients to cells, remove metabolic waste products, and carry hormones from one part of the body to another. Circulation requires normal heart function, which propels blood through the system by continuous rhythmic contractions.

Despite advances in disease detection and treatment, cardiovascular disease remains the leading cause of death in the United States. The cardiovascular disorders covered in this chapter include acute coronary syndromes, arterial occlusive disease, atrial septal defect, cardiac arrhythmias, cardiac tamponade, cardiomyopathy, coarctation of the aorta, endocarditis, heart failure, hypertension, patent ductus arteriosus, pericarditis, Raynaud's disease, rheumatic fever and rheumatic heart disease, shock, tetralogy of Fallot, transposition of the great arteries, valvular heart disease, and ventricular septal defect.

✳ Life-threatening

Acute coronary syndromes

Acute myocardial infarction (MI), ST-segment elevation MI (STEMI), non-ST-segment elevation MI (NSTE-MI), and unstable angina are now recognized as a part of a group of clinical disorders known as acute coronary syndromes (ACSs).

In cardiovascular disease, death usually results from cardiac damage or complications of MI — the leading cause of death in the United States and Western Europe. Each year, approximately 900,000 people in the United States experience MI. Mortality is high when treatment is delayed, and almost one-half of sudden deaths due to MI occur before hospitalization, within 1 hour of the onset of symptoms. The prognosis improves if vigorous treatment begins immediately.

CAUSES
- Aging
- Drug use, especially cocaine and amphetamines

- Elevated serum triglyceride, total cholesterol, and low-density lipoprotein levels
- Excessive intake of saturated fats
- Gender (Men and postmenopausal women are more susceptible to MI than premenopausal women, although the incidence is increasing among women, especially those who smoke and take hormonal contraceptives.)
- Hypertension
- Obesity
- Positive family history
- Sedentary lifestyle
- Smoking
- Stress or type A personality

PATHOPHYSIOLOGY

Rupture or erosion of plaque—an unstable and lipid-rich substance—initiates all coronary syndromes. The rupture results in platelet adhesions, fibrin clot formation, and activation of thrombin.

Early thrombus doesn't necessarily block coronary blood flow. When the thrombus progresses and occludes blood flow, an ACS results. The degree of blockage and the time that the affected vessel remains occluded are major determinants for the type of infarction that occurs.

For patients with unstable angina, a thrombus partially occludes a coronary vessel. This thrombus is full of platelets. The partially occluded vessel may have distal microthrombi that cause necrosis in some myocytes. The smaller vessels infarct, and patients are at higher risk for MI. These patients may progress to an NSTEMI.

If a thrombus fully occludes the vessel for a prolonged time, this is known as an STEMI. In this type of MI, there's a greater concentration of thrombin and fibrin.

Three stages occur when a vessel is occluded: ischemia, injury, and infarct.
- Ischemia occurs first. It indicates that blood flow and oxygen demand are out of balance. Ischemia can be resolved by improving flow or reducing oxygen needs. Electrocardiogram (ECG) changes indicate ST-segment depression or T-wave changes.
- Injury is the next stage. This occurs when the ischemia is prolonged enough to damage the area of the heart. ECG changes usually reveal ST-segment elevation (usually in two or more contiguous leads).
- In infarct, the third stage, actual death of the myocardial cells has occurred. ECG changes reveal abnormal Q waves. The Q waves are considered abnormal when they appear greater than or equal to 0.04 second wide and their height is greater than 25% of the R wave in height in that lead. Most patients with ST-segment elevation will develop Q-wave MI. (See *Zones of myocardial infarction*.)

Although ischemia begins immediately, the size of the infarct can be limited if circulation is restored within 6 hours.

Several changes occur after MI. Cardiac enzymes and proteins are released by the infarcted myocardial cells, which are used in the diagnosis of an MI. Within 24 hours, the infarcted muscle becomes edematous and cyanotic. During the next several days, leukocytes infiltrate the necrotic area and begin to remove necrotic cells, thinning the ventricular wall. Scar formation begins by the third week after MI, and by the sixth week, scar tissue is well established.

The scar tissue that forms on the necrotic area inhibits contractility. When this occurs, the compensatory mechanisms (vascular constriction, in-

Focus in

ZONES OF
MYOCARDIAL INFARCTION

Myocardial infarction has a central area of necrosis surrounded by a zone of injury that may recover if revascularization occurs. This zone of injury is surrounded by an outer ring of reversible ischemia. Characteristic electrocardiographic changes are associated with each zone.

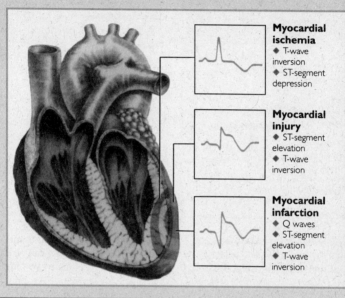

Myocardial ischemia
- T-wave inversion
- ST-segment depression

Myocardial injury
- ST-segment elevation
- T-wave inversion

Myocardial infarction
- Q waves
- ST-segment elevation
- T-wave inversion

creased heart rate, and renal retention of sodium and water) try to maintain cardiac output. Ventricular dilation may also occur in a process called remodeling. Functionally, an MI may cause reduced contractility with abnormal wall motion, altered left ventricular compliance, reduced stroke volume, reduced ejection fraction, and elevated left ventricular end-diastolic pressure.

CLINICAL FINDINGS

- Persistent, crushing substernal chest pain that may radiate to the left arm, jaw, neck, or shoulder blades caused by reduced oxygen supply to the myocardial cells (It may be described as heavy, squeezing, or crushing.)

Alert Women may experience typical chest pain with acute ischemia and MI, but women and occasionally men, elderly people, and patients with diabetes may also experience atypical chest pain. Atypical symptoms include upper back dis-

PINPOINTING MYOCARDIAL INFARCTION

Depending on the location, ischemia or infarction causes changes in specific electrocardiographic leads.

TYPES OF MYOCARDIAL INFARCTION	LEADS
Inferior	II, III, aV$_F$
Anterior	V$_3$, V$_4$
Septal	V$_1$, V$_2$
Lateral	I, aV$_L$ V$_5$, V$_6$
Anterolateral	I, aV$_L$, V$_3$ to V$_6$
Posterior	V$_1$ or V$_2$
Right ventricular	V$_{1R}$ to V$_{4R}$

comfort between the shoulder blades, palpitations, feeling of fullness in the neck, nausea, abdominal discomfort, dizziness, unexplained fatigue, and exhaustion or shortness of breath.
● Cool extremities, perspiration, anxiety, and restlessness due to the release of catecholamines
● Blood pressure and pulse initially elevated resulting from sympathetic nervous system activation (If cardiac output is reduced, blood pressure may fall. Bradycardia may be associated with conduction disturbances, particularly with damage to the inferior wall of the left ventricle.)
● Fatigue and weakness caused by reduced perfusion to skeletal muscles
● Nausea and vomiting as a result of reflex stimulation of vomiting centers by pain fibers or from vasovagal reflexes
● Shortness of breath and crackles reflecting heart failure
● Low-grade temperature in the days following acute MI due to the inflammatory response
● Jugular vein distention reflecting right ventricular dysfunction and pulmonary congestion
● S$_3$ and S$_4$ reflecting ventricular dysfunction
● Loud holosystolic murmur in apex, possibly caused by papillary muscle rupture
● Reduced urine output secondary to reduced renal perfusion and increased aldosterone and antidiuretic hormone

TEST RESULTS
● Serial 12-lead ECG may reveal characteristic changes, such as serial ST-segment depression in NSTEMI (a more limited area of damage insufficient to cause changes in the pattern of ventricular depolarization) and ST-segment elevation in STEMI (a larger area of damage, which causes permanent change in the pattern of ventricular depolarization). An ECG can also identify the location of MI, arrhythmias, hypertrophy, and pericarditis. (See *Pinpointing myocardial infarction.*)
● Serial cardiac enzymes and proteins may show a characteristic rise and fall, specifically CK-MB, the proteins troponin T and I, and myoglobin, to confirm the diagnosis of MI.
● Laboratory testing may reveal elevated white blood cell count, C-reactive protein level, and erythrocyte sedimentation rate due to inflammation, and increased glucose levels following the release of catecholamines.

- Echocardiography may show ventricular wall motion abnormalities and may detect septal or papillary muscle rupture.
- Chest X-rays may show left-sided heart failure or cardiomegaly due to ventricular dilation.
- Nuclear imaging scanning using sestamibi, thallium 201, and technetium 99m can be used to identify areas of infarction and viable muscle cells.
- Cardiac catheterization may be used to identify the involved coronary artery as well as to provide information on ventricular function and pressures and volumes within the heart.

TREATMENT

Treatment of an MI typically involves following the treatment guidelines recommended by the American College of Cardiology/American Heart Association (ACC/AHA) Task Force on Practice Guidelines. These include:
- assessment of the patient with chest pain in the emergency department within 10 minutes of symptom onset because at least 50% of deaths take place within 1 hour of the onset of symptoms (Moreover, thrombolytic therapy is most effective when started within the first 3 hours after the onset of symptoms.)
- oxygen by nasal cannula for 2 to 3 hours to increase blood oxygenation (see *Treating MI,* pages 6 and 7)
- nitroglycerin sublingually or I.V. to relieve chest pain, unless systolic blood pressure is less than 90 mm Hg or heart rate is less than 50 or greater than 100 beats/minute
- morphine for analgesia because pain stimulates the sympathetic nervous system, leading to an increase in heart rate and vasoconstriction

- aspirin every day indefinitely to inhibit platelet aggregation
- continuous cardiac monitoring to detect arrhythmias and ischemia
- I.V. fibrinolytic therapy for the patient with chest pain of at least 30 minutes' duration who reaches the health care facility within 12 hours of the onset of symptoms (unless contraindications exist) and whose ECG shows new left bundle-branch block (LBBB) or ST-segment elevation of at least 1 to 2 mm in two or more ECG leads (The greatest benefit of reperfusion therapy, however, occurs when reperfusion takes place within 3 hours of the onset of chest pain.)
- I.V. heparin for the patient who has received fibrinolytic therapy to increase the chances of patency in the affected coronary artery
- percutaneous transluminal coronary angioplasty (PTCA), which is superior to fibrinolytic therapy if it can be performed in a timely manner in a health care facility with personnel skilled in the procedure
- glycoprotein IIb/IIIa receptor blocking agents, which strongly inhibit platelet aggregation (They're indicated as adjunct therapy with PTCA in acute STEMI and as a primary therapy in NSTEMI; their use in combination with fibrinolytics is controversial.)
- limitation of physical activity for the first 12 hours to reduce cardiac workload, thereby limiting the area of necrosis
- keeping atropine, amiodarone (Cordarone), transcutaneous pacing patches or a transvenous pacemaker, a defibrillator, and epinephrine readily available to treat arrhythmias (The ACC/AHA doesn't recommend the

(Text continues on page 8.)

TREATING MI

This chart shows how treatments can be applied to myocardial infarction (MI) at various stages of its development.

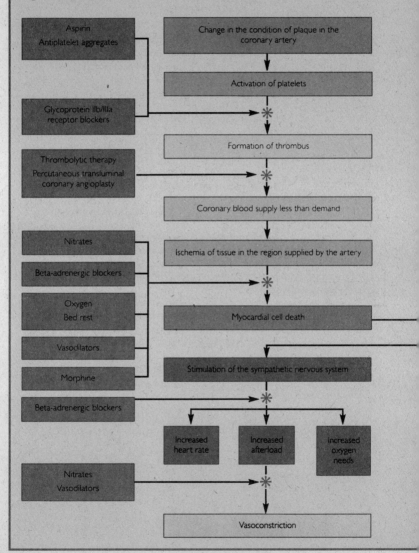

Aspirin Antiplatelet aggregates	→	Change in the condition of plaque in the coronary artery
		↓
		Activation of platelets
Glycoprotein IIb/IIIa receptor blockers	→ ✳	↓
		Formation of thrombus
Thrombolytic therapy Percutaneous transluminal coronary angioplasty	→ ✳	↓
		Coronary blood supply less than demand
		↓
Nitrates	→	Ischemia of tissue in the region supplied by the artery
Beta-adrenergic blockers	→ ✳	↓
Oxygen Bed rest		Myocardial cell death
Vasodilators		↓
Morphine		Stimulation of the sympathetic nervous system
Beta-adrenergic blockers	→ ✳	

Increased heart rate | Increased afterload | increased oxygen needs

| Nitrates
Vasodilators | → ✳ | ↓ |
| | | Vasoconstriction |

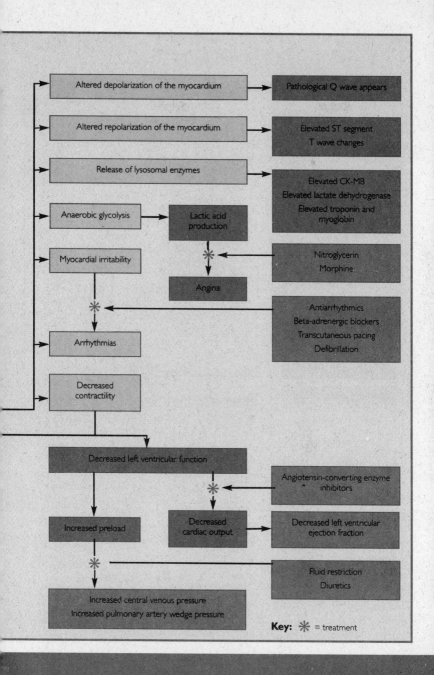

prophylactic use of antiarrhythmic drugs during the first 24 hours.)
● I.V. nitroglycerin for 24 to 48 hours in the patient without hypotension, bradycardia, or excessive tachycardia to reduce afterload and preload and relieve chest pain
● early I.V. beta-adrenergic blockers to the patient with an evolving acute MI followed by oral therapy, as long as there are no contraindications, to reduce heart rate and myocardial contractile force, thereby reducing myocardial oxygen requirements
● angiotensin-converting enzyme inhibitors in the patient with an evolving MI with ST-segment elevation or LBBB but without hypotension or other contraindications, to reduce afterload and preload and prevent remodeling
● magnesium sulfate for 24 hours to correct hypomagnesemia, if needed
● angiography and possible percutaneous or surgical revascularization for the patient with spontaneous or provoked myocardial ischemia following an acute MI
● exercise testing before discharge to determine the adequacy of medical therapy and to obtain baseline information for an appropriate exercise prescription (It can also determine functional capacity and stratify the patient's risk of a subsequent cardiac event.)
● cardiac risk modification program of weight control; a low-fat, low-cholesterol diet; smoking cessation; and regular exercise to reduce cardiac risk
● lipid-lowering drugs as indicated by the fasting lipid profile.

NURSING CONSIDERATIONS
Care for the patient who has suffered an MI is directed toward detecting complications, preventing further myocardial damage, and promoting comfort, rest, and emotional well-being. Commonly, the patient with an MI receives treatment in the intensive care unit (ICU), where he's under constant observation for complications.
● On admission to the ICU, monitor and record the patient's ECG, blood pressure, temperature, and heart and breath sounds.
● Assess and record the severity and duration of pain, and administer analgesics. Avoid I.M. injections; absorption from the muscle is unpredictable and bleeding is likely if the patient is receiving fibrinolytic therapy.
● Check the patient's blood pressure after giving nitroglycerin, especially the first dose.
● Frequently monitor the ECG to detect rate changes or arrhythmias. Place rhythm strips in the patient's chart periodically for evaluation.
● During episodes of chest pain, obtain 12-lead ECG, blood pressure, and pulmonary artery catheter measurements and monitor them for changes.
● Watch for signs and symptoms of fluid retention (crackles, cough, tachypnea, and edema), which may indicate impending heart failure. Carefully monitor daily weight, intake and output, respirations, serum enzyme levels, and blood pressure. Auscultate for adventitious breath sounds periodically (the patient on bed rest commonly has atelectatic crackles, which disappear after coughing), for S_3 or S_4 gallops, and for new-onset heart murmurs.
● Organize patient care and activities to maximize periods of uninterrupted rest.
● Ask the dietary department to provide a clear liquid diet until nausea subsides. A low-cholesterol, low-

sodium, low-fat, high-fiber diet may be prescribed.

● Provide a stool softener to prevent straining during defecation, which causes vagal stimulation and may slow the heart rate. Allow the patient to use a bedside commode, and provide as much privacy as possible.

● Assist the patient with range-of-motion exercises. If he's completely immobilized by a severe MI, turn him often. Antiembolism stockings help prevent venostasis and thrombophlebitis.

● Provide emotional support to the patient, and help reduce stress and anxiety; administer tranquilizers as needed. Explain procedures and answer questions. Explaining the ICU's environment and routine can ease anxiety. Involve the patient's family in his care as much as possible.

Preparing for discharge

● Thoroughly explain dosages and therapy to promote compliance with the prescribed medication regimen and other treatment measures. Warn about drug adverse effects, and advise the patient to watch for and report signs of toxicity (anorexia, nausea, vomiting, and yellow vision, for example, if the patient is receiving digoxin [Lanoxin]).

● Review dietary restrictions with the patient. If he must follow a low-sodium or low-fat and low-cholesterol diet, provide a list of foods that he should avoid. Ask the dietitian to speak to the patient and his family.

● Counsel the patient to resume sexual activity progressively.

● Advise the patient to report typical or atypical chest pain. Postinfarction syndrome may develop, producing chest pain that must be differentiated from recurrent MI, pulmonary infarct, or heart failure.

● If the patient has a Holter monitor in place, explain its purpose and use.

● Stress the need to stop smoking.

● Encourage the patient to participate in a cardiac rehabilitation program.

● Review follow-up procedures, such as office visits and treadmill testing, with the patient.

Arterial occlusive disease

Arterial occlusive disease is the obstruction or narrowing of the lumen of the aorta and its major branches, causing an interruption of blood flow, usually to the legs and feet. This disorder may affect the carotid, vertebral, innominate, subclavian, mesenteric, iliac, and femoral arteries. (See *Possible sites of major artery occlusion,* page 10.)

Arterial occlusive disease is more common in males than in females. The prognosis depends on the occlusion's location, the development of collateral circulation to counteract reduced blood flow and, in acute disease, the time elapsed between occlusion and its removal.

CAUSES

● Atherosclerosis
● Predisposing factors
– Aging
– Diabetes
– Family history of vascular disorders, myocardial infarction, or stroke
– Hyperlipidemia
– Hypertension
– Smoking

POSSIBLE SITES OF
MAJOR ARTERY OCCLUSION

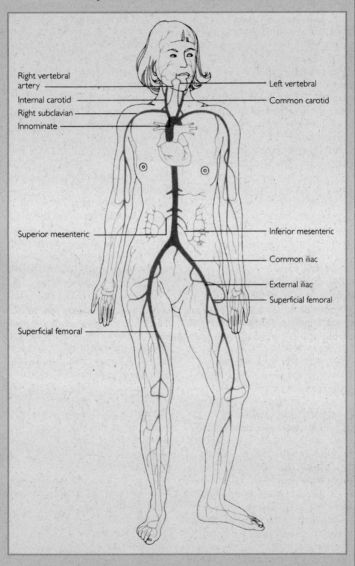

Right vertebral artery

Internal carotid

Right subclavian

Innominate

Superior mesenteric

Superficial femoral

Left vertebral

Common carotid

Inferior mesenteric

Common iliac

External iliac

Superficial femoral

PATHOPHYSIOLOGY

Arterial occlusive disease is almost always the result of atherosclerosis, in which fatty, fibrous plaques narrow the lumen of blood vessels. This occlusion can occur acutely or progressively over 20 to 40 years, with areas of vessel branching, or bifurcation, being the most common sites. The narrowing of the lumens reduces the blood volume that can flow through them, causing arterial insufficiency to the affected area. Ischemia usually occurs after the vessel lumens have narrowed by at least 50%, reducing blood flow to a level at which it no longer meets the needs of tissue and nerves.

CLINICAL FINDINGS

Signs and symptoms of arterial occlusive disease depend on the site of the occlusion. (See *Types of arterial occlusive disease,* page 12.)

TEST RESULTS

Diagnosis of arterial occlusive disease is usually indicated by patient history and physical examination. These pertinent tests support the diagnosis:
● Arteriography demonstrates the type (thrombus or embolus), location, and degree of obstruction and the collateral circulation. Arteriography is particularly useful in chronic disease or for evaluating candidates for reconstructive surgery.
● Doppler ultrasonography and plethysmography are noninvasive tests that show decreased blood flow distal to the occlusion in acute disease.
● Ophthalmodynamometry helps determine the degree of obstruction in the internal carotid artery by comparing ophthalmic artery pressure with brachial artery pressure on the affected side. More than a 20% difference between pressures suggests insufficiency.
● EEG and computed tomography scan may be necessary to rule out brain lesions.

TREATMENT

Treatment of arterial occlusive disease depends on the cause, location, and size of the obstruction, for example:
● for mild chronic disease, supportive measures including smoking cessation, hypertension control, and mild exercise such as walking
● for carotid artery occlusion, antiplatelet therapy beginning with ticlopidine (Ticlid) or clopidogrel (Plavix) and aspirin
● for intermittent claudication of chronic occlusive disease, pentoxifylline (Trental) and cilostazol (Pletal) to improve blood flow through the capillaries, particularly for patients who are poor candidates for surgery.

Acute arterial occlusive disease usually requires surgery to restore circulation to the affected area, for example:
● embolectomy — balloon-tipped Fogarty catheter to remove thrombotic material from the artery; used mainly for mesenteric, femoral, or popliteal artery occlusion
● thromboendarterectomy — opening of the occluded artery and direct removal of the obstructing thrombus and the medial layer of the arterial wall; usually performed after angiography and commonly used with autogenous vein or Dacron bypass surgery (femoral-popliteal or aortofemoral)
● patch grafting — thrombosed arterial segment removed and replaced with an autogenous vein or Dacron graft

Types of arterial occlusive disease

SITE OF OCCLUSION	SIGNS AND SYMPTOMS
Carotid arterial system ♦ Internal carotids ♦ External carotids	Neurologic dysfunction: transient ischemic attacks (TIAs) due to reduced cerebral circulation produce unilateral sensory or motor dysfunction (transient monocular blindness, hemiparesis), possible aphasia or dysarthria, confusion, decreased mentation, and headache; recurrent clinical features usually last 5 to 10 minutes but may persist up to 24 hours and may herald a stroke; absent or decreased pulsation with an auscultatory bruit over the affected vessels
Vertebrobasilar system ♦ Vertebral arteries ♦ Basilar arteries	Neurologic dysfunction: TIAs of brain stem and cerebellum producing binocular visual disturbances, vertigo, dysarthria, and "drop attacks" (falling down without loss of consciousness); less common than carotid TIA
Innominate ♦ Brachiocephalic artery	Neurologic dysfunction: signs and symptoms of vertebrobasilar occlusion; indications of ischemia (claudication) of right arm; possible bruit over right side of neck
Subclavian artery	Subclavian steal syndrome (characterized by blood backflow from the brain through the vertebral artery on the same side as the occlusion, into the subclavian artery distal to the occlusion); clinical effects of vertebrobasilar occlusion and exercise-induced arm claudication; possible gangrene, usually limited to the digits
Mesenteric artery ♦ Superior (most commonly affected) ♦ Celiac axis ♦ Inferior	Bowel ischemia, infarct necrosis, and gangrene; sudden, acute abdominal pain; nausea and vomiting; diarrhea; leukocytosis; and shock due to massive intraluminal fluid and plasma loss
Aortic bifurcation (Saddle block occlusion, a medical emergency associated with cardiac embolization)	Sensory and motor deficits (muscle weakness, numbness, paresthesias, paralysis) and signs of ischemia (sudden pain; cold, pale legs with decreased or absent peripheral pulses) in both legs
Iliac artery (Leriche syndrome)	Intermittent claudication of lower back, buttocks, and thighs, relieved by rest; absent or reduced femoral or distal pulses; possible bruit over femoral arteries; impotence in males
Femoral and popliteal artery (Associated with aneurysm formation)	Intermittent claudication of the calves on exertion; ischemic pain in feet; pretrophic pain (heralds necrosis and ulceration); leg pallor and coolness; blanching of feet on elevation; gangrene; no palpable pulses in ankles and feet

- bypass graft — blood flow diverted through an anastomosed autogenous or Dacron graft past the thrombosed segment
- thrombolytic therapy — urokinase, streptokinase, or alteplase, causing lysis of clot around or in the plaque
- atherectomy — plaque excised using a drill or slicing mechanism
- balloon angioplasty — balloon inflation compressing the obstruction
- laser angioplasty — obstruction excised and vaporized using hot-tip lasers
- stents — mesh of wires that stretch and mold to the arterial wall inserted to prevent reocclusion. (This new adjunct follows laser angioplasty or atherectomy.)

Other treatments
- Combined therapy, using any of the surgical treatments listed above
- Lumbar sympathectomy, as a possible adjunct to surgery depending on the condition of the sympathetic nervous system
- Amputation becoming necessary if arterial reconstructive surgery fails or if gangrene, persistent infection, or intractable pain develops
- Heparin to prevent emboli for embolic occlusion
- Bowel resection after restoration of blood flow for mesenteric artery occlusion

NURSING CONSIDERATIONS
- Provide comprehensive patient teaching such as proper foot care.
- Explain all diagnostic tests and procedures.
- Advise the patient to stop smoking and to follow the prescribed medical regimen.

Preoperatively
During an acute episode:
- assess the patient's circulatory status by checking for the most distal pulses and by inspecting his skin color and temperature
- provide pain relief as needed
- administer heparin by continuous I.V. drip, as ordered, using an infusion pump to ensure the proper flow rate
- wrap the patient's affected foot in soft cotton batting, and reposition it frequently to prevent pressure on any one area
- strictly avoid elevating or applying heat to the affected leg
- watch for signs of fluid and electrolyte imbalance, and monitor intake and output for signs of renal failure (urine output less than 30 ml/hour)
- if the patient has carotid, innominate, vertebral, or subclavian artery occlusion, monitor him for signs of stroke, such as numbness in his arm or leg and intermittent blindness.

Postoperatively
- Monitor the patient's vital signs. Continually assess his circulatory function by inspecting skin color and temperature and by checking for distal pulses. In charting, compare earlier assessments and observations. Watch closely for signs of hemorrhage (tachycardia and hypotension), and check dressings for excessive bleeding.
- In carotid, innominate, vertebral, or subclavian artery occlusion, assess the patient's neurologic status frequently for changes in level of consciousness or muscle strength and pupil size.
- In mesenteric artery occlusion, connect a nasogastric tube to low intermittent suction. Monitor the patient's intake and output (low urine output may indicate damage to renal arteries during surgery). Check bowel

sounds for return of peristalsis. Increased abdominal distention and tenderness may indicate extension of bowel ischemia with resulting gangrene, necessitating further excision, or it may indicate peritonitis.

- In saddle block occlusion, check distal pulses for adequate circulation. Watch for signs of renal failure and mesenteric artery occlusion (severe abdominal pain) as well as cardiac arrhythmias, which may precipitate embolus formation.
- In iliac artery occlusion, monitor urine output for signs of renal failure from decreased perfusion to the kidneys as a result of surgery. Provide meticulous catheter care.
- In femoral and popliteal artery occlusions, assist the patient with early ambulation but discourage prolonged sitting.
- After amputation, check the patient's stump carefully for drainage and record its color and amount and the time. Elevate the stump, as ordered, and administer adequate analgesic medication. Because phantom limb pain is common, explain this phenomenon to the patient.
- When preparing the patient for discharge, instruct him to watch for signs of recurrence (pain, pallor, numbness, paralysis, and absence of pulse) that can result from graft occlusion or occlusion at another site. Warn him against wearing constrictive clothing.

Atrial septal defect

In atrial septal defect (ASD), an acyanotic congenital heart defect, an opening between the left and right atria, allows blood to flow from left to right, resulting in ineffective pumping of the heart and thus increasing the risk of heart failure.

The three types of ASDs are:
- an ostium secundum defect, the most common type, which occurs in the region of the fossa ovalis and, occasionally, extends inferiorly, close to the vena cava
- a sinus venosus defect that occurs in the superior-posterior portion of the atrial septum, sometimes extending into the vena cava, and is almost always associated with abnormal drainage of pulmonary veins into the right atrium
- an ostium primum defect that occurs in the inferior portion of the septum primum and is usually associated with atrioventricular valve abnormalities (cleft mitral valve) and conduction defects.

ASD accounts for about 10% of congenital heart defects and is almost twice as common in females as in males, with a strong familial tendency. Although an ASD is usually a benign defect during infancy and childhood, delayed development of symptoms and complications makes it one of the most common congenital heart defects diagnosed in adults.

The prognosis is excellent in asymptomatic patients and in those with uncomplicated surgical repair, but poor in patients with cyanosis caused by large, untreated defects.

CAUSES
- Unknown
- Ostium primum defects common in patients with Down syndrome

PATHOPHYSIOLOGY
In an ASD, blood shunts from the left atrium to the right atrium because the left atrial pressure is normally slightly higher than the right atrial pressure.

This pressure difference forces large amounts of blood through a defect. This shunt results in right heart volume overload, affecting the right atrium, right ventricle, and pulmonary arteries. Eventually, the right atrium enlarges, and the right ventricle dilates to accommodate the increased blood volume. If pulmonary artery hypertension develops, increased pulmonary vascular resistance and right ventricular hypertrophy follow. In some adults, irreversible pulmonary artery hypertension causes reversal of the shunt direction, which results in unoxygenated blood entering the systemic circulation, causing cyanosis.

CLINICAL FINDINGS

● Fatigue after exertion due to decreased cardiac output from the left ventricle
● Early to midsystolic murmur at the second or third left intercostal space, caused by extra blood passing through the pulmonic valve
● Low-pitched diastolic murmur at the lower left sternal border, more pronounced on inspiration, resulting from increased tricuspid valve flow in patients with large shunts
● Fixed, widely split S_2 due to delayed closure of the pulmonic valve, resulting from an increased volume of blood
● Systolic click or late systolic murmur at the apex, resulting from mitral valve prolapse in older children with an ASD
● Clubbing and cyanosis, if a right-to-left shunt develops

Alert *An infant may be cyanotic because he has a cardiac or pulmonary disorder. Cyanosis that worsens with crying is most likely associated with cardiac causes because crying increases pulmonary resistance to blood flow, resulting in*

an increased right-to-left shunt. Cyanosis that improves with crying is most likely due to pulmonary causes as deep breathing improves tidal volume.

TEST RESULTS

A history of increasing fatigue and characteristic physical features suggest an ASD. These tests confirm the diagnosis:
● Chest X-ray shows an enlarged right atrium and right ventricle, a prominent pulmonary artery, and increased pulmonary vascular markings.
● Electrocardiography results may be normal but commonly show right axis deviation, a prolonged PR interval, varying degrees of right bundle-branch block, right ventricular hypertrophy, atrial fibrillation (particularly in severe cases after age 30) and, in ostium primum defect, left axis deviation.
● Echocardiography measures right ventricular enlargement, may locate the defect, and shows volume overload in the right side of the heart. It may reveal right ventricular and pulmonary artery dilation.
● Two-dimensional echocardiography with color Doppler flow, contrast echocardiography, or both have supplanted cardiac catheterization as the confirming tests for an ASD. Cardiac catheterization is used if the clinical data contain inconsistencies or if significant pulmonary hypertension is suspected.

TREATMENT

● Operative repair is advised for the patient with an uncomplicated ASD with evidence of significant left-to-right shunting and should:
– be performed when the patient is age 2 to 4

– not be performed on a patient with small defects and trivial left-to-right shunts.

● Because an ASD seldom produces complications in an infant or a toddler, surgery can be delayed until preschool or early school age.

● A large defect may need immediate surgical closure with sutures or a patch graft.

● Although experimental, treatment for a small ASD may involve inserting an umbrella-like patch through a cardiac catheter instead of performing open-heart surgery.

NURSING CONSIDERATIONS

● Before cardiac catheterization, explain pretest and posttest procedures to the child and parents. If possible, use drawings or other visual aids to explain it to the child.

● As needed, teach the patient about antibiotic prophylaxis to prevent infective endocarditis.

● If surgery is scheduled, teach the child and parents about the intensive care unit and introduce them to the staff. Show parents where they can wait during the operation. Explain postoperative procedures, tubes, dressings, and monitoring equipment.

● After surgery, closely monitor the patient's vital signs, central venous and intra-arterial pressures, and intake and output. Watch for atrial arrhythmias, which may remain uncorrected.

Cardiac arrhythmias

In arrhythmias, abnormal electrical conduction or automaticity changes the heart's rate and rhythm. Arrhythmias vary in severity, from those that are mild, produce no symptoms, and require no treatment (such as sinus arrhythmia, in which heart rate increases and decreases with respiration) to catastrophic ventricular fibrillation, which requires immediate resuscitation. Arrhythmias are generally classified according to their origin (ventricular or supraventricular). Their effect on cardiac output and blood pressure, partially influenced by the site of origin, determines their clinical significance.

CAUSES

● Acid-base imbalances
● Cellular hypoxia
● Congenital defects
● Connective tissue disorders
● Degeneration of the conductive tissue
● Drug toxicity
● Electrolyte imbalances
● Emotional stress
● Hypertrophy of the heart muscle
● Myocardial ischemia or infarction
● Organic heart disease

However, each arrhythmia may have its own specific causes. (See *Types of cardiac arrhythmias,* pages 18 to 25.)

PATHOPHYSIOLOGY

Arrhythmias may result from enhanced automaticity, reentry, escape beats, or abnormal electrical conduction. (See *Comparing normal and abnormal conduction,* pages 26 and 27.)

CLINICAL FINDINGS

Signs and symptoms of arrhythmias result from reduced cardiac output and altered perfusion to the organs, and may include:
● dyspnea
● hypotension
● dizziness, syncope, and weakness
● chest pain

- cool, clammy skin
- altered level of consciousness (LOC)
- reduced urine output.

TEST RESULTS
- Electrocardiography detects arrhythmias as well as ischemia and infarction that may result in arrhythmias.
- Laboratory testing may reveal electrolyte abnormalities, acid-base abnormalities, or drug toxicities that may cause arrhythmias.
- Holter monitoring, event monitoring, and loop recording can detect arrhythmias and the effectiveness of drug therapy during a patient's daily activities.
- Exercise testing may detect exercise-induced arrhythmias.
- Electrophysiologic testing identifies the mechanism of an arrhythmia and the location of accessory pathways; it also assesses the effectiveness of antiarrhythmic drugs, radiofrequency ablation, and implanted cardioverter-defibrillators.

TREATMENT
Follow the specific treatment guidelines for each arrhythmia. (See *Types of cardiac arrhythmias,* pages 18 to 25.)

NURSING CONSIDERATIONS
- Assess an unmonitored patient for rhythm disturbances.
- If the patient's pulse is abnormally rapid, slow, or irregular, watch for signs of hypoperfusion, such as hypotension and diminished urine output.
- Document arrhythmias in a monitored patient, and assess for possible causes and effects.

- When life-threatening arrhythmias develop, rapidly assess LOC, respirations, and pulse rate.
- Initiate cardiopulmonary resuscitation if indicated.
- Evaluate the patient for altered cardiac output resulting from arrhythmias.
- Administer medications as ordered, and prepare to assist with medical procedures if indicated (for example, cardioversion).
- Monitor for predisposing factors — such as fluid and electrolyte imbalances — and signs of drug toxicity, especially with digoxin (Lanoxin). If you suspect drug toxicity, report such signs to the physician immediately and withhold the next dose.
- To prevent arrhythmias in a postoperative cardiac patient, provide adequate oxygen and reduce the heart's workload while carefully maintaining metabolic, neurologic, respiratory, and hemodynamic status.
- To avoid temporary pacemaker malfunction, install a fresh battery before each insertion. Carefully secure the external catheter wires and the pacemaker box. Assess the threshold daily. Watch closely for premature contractions, a sign of myocardial irritation.
- To avert permanent pacemaker malfunction, restrict the patient's activity after insertion as ordered. Monitor the pulse rate regularly, and watch for signs of decreased cardiac output.
- If the patient has a permanent pacemaker, warn him about environmental hazards, as indicated by the pacemaker's manufacturer. Although hazards may not present a problem, 24-hour Holter monitoring may be

(Text continues on page 24.)

TYPES OF CARDIAC ARRHYTHMIAS

This chart reviews many common cardiac arrhythmias and outlines their features, causes, and treatments. Use a normal electrocardiogram strip, if available, to compare normal cardiac rhythm configurations with the rhythm strips below. Characteristics of normal sinus rhythm include:

◆ ventricular and atrial rates of 60 to 100 beats/minute
◆ regular and uniform QRS complexes and P waves
◆ PR interval of 0.12 to 0.20 second
◆ QRS duration < 0.12 second
◆ identical atrial and ventricular rates, with constant PR intervals.

ARRHYTHMIA   FEATURES

Sinus tachycardia

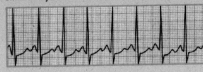

◆ Atrial and ventricular rhythms regular
◆ Rate > 100 beats/minute; rarely
> 160 beats/minute
◆ Normal P wave preceding each QRS complex

Sinus bradycardia

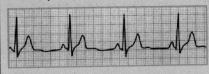

◆ Atrial and ventricular rhythms regular
◆ Rate < 60 beats/minute
◆ Normal P waves preceding each QRS complex

Paroxysmal supraventricular tachycardia

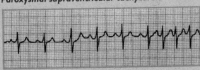

◆ Atrial and ventricular rhythms regular
◆ Heart rate > 160 beats/minute; rarely exceeds 250 beats/minute
◆ P waves regular but aberrant; difficult to differentiate from preceding T wave
◆ P wave preceding each QRS complex
◆ Sudden onset and termination of arrhythmia

CAUSES	TREATMENT
◆ Normal physiologic response to fever, exercise, anxiety, pain, dehydration; may also accompany shock, left ventricular failure, cardiac tamponade, hyperthyroidism, anemia, hypovolemia, pulmonary embolism, and anterior wall myocardial infarction (MI)	◆ Correction of underlying cause
◆ May also occur with atropine, epinephrine, isoproterenol, quinidine, caffeine, alcohol, cocaine, amphetamine, and nicotine use	◆ Beta-adrenergic blocker or calcium channel blocker
◆ Normal, in well-conditioned heart, as in an athlete	◆ Correction of underlying cause
◆ Increased intracranial pressure; increased vagal tone due to straining during defecation, vomiting, intubation, or mechanical ventilation; sick sinus syndrome; hypothyroidism; and inferior wall MI	◆ For low cardiac output, dizziness, weakness, altered level of consciousness, or low blood pressure, follow advanced cardiac life support (ACLS) protocol for administration of atropine
◆ May also occur with anticholinesterase, beta-adrenergic blocker, digoxin, and morphine use	◆ Temporary or permanent pacemaker ◆ Dopamine or epinephrine infusion
◆ Intrinsic abnormality of atrioventricular (AV) conduction system	◆ If patient is unstable, immediate cardioversion
◆ Physical or psychological stress, hypoxia, hypokalemia, cardiomyopathy, congenital heart disease, MI, valvular disease, Wolff-Parkinson-White syndrome, cor pulmonale, hyperthyroidism, and systemic hypertension	◆ If patient is stable, vagal stimulation, Valsalva's maneuver, and carotid sinus massage
◆ Digoxin toxicity; use of caffeine, marijuana, or central nervous system stimulants	◆ If cardiac function is preserved, treatment priority: calcium channel blocker, beta-adrenergic blocker, digoxin (Lanoxin), and cardioversion; then consider procainamide (Pronestyl), amiodarone (Cordarone), or sotalol (Betapace) if each preceding treatment is ineffective in rhythm conversion
	◆ If the ejection fraction is less than 40% or if the patient is in heart failure, treatment order: digoxin, amiodarone, then diltiazem (Cardizem)

(continued)

ARRHYTHMIA	FEATURES
Atrial flutter 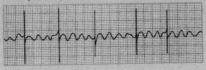	◆ Atrial rhythm regular; rate 250 to 400 beats/minute ◆ Ventricular rate variable, depending on degree of AV block (usually 60 to 100 beats/minute) ◆ No P waves; atrial activity appears as fibrillatory waves (F waves); sawtooth configuration common in lead II ◆ QRS complexes uniform in shape, but usually irregular in rate
Atrial fibrillation 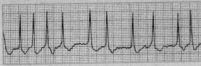	◆ Atrial rhythm grossly irregular; rate > 400 beats/minute ◆ Ventricular rhythm grossly irregular ◆ QRS complexes of uniform configuration and duration ◆ PR interval indiscernible ◆ No P waves; atrial activity appears as erratic, irregular, baseline fibrillatory waves (F waves)
Junctional rhythm 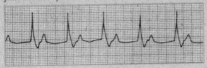	◆ Atrial and ventricular rhythms regular; atrial rate 40 to 60 beats/minute; ventricular rate usually 40 to 60 beats/minute (60 to 100 beats/minute is accelerated junctional rhythm) ◆ P waves preceding, hidden within (absent), or after QRS complex; usually inverted if visible ◆ PR interval (when present) < 0.12 second ◆ QRS complex configuration and duration normal, except in aberrant conduction
First-degree AV block 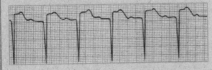	◆ Atrial and ventricular rhythms regular ◆ PR interval > 0.20 second ◆ P wave precedes QRS complex ◆ QRS complex normal

Causes	Treatment
◆ Heart failure, tricuspid or mitral valve disease, pulmonary embolism, cor pulmonale, inferior wall MI, and pericarditis ◆ Digoxin toxicity	◆ If patient is unstable with a ventricular rate > 150 beats/minute, immediate cardioversion ◆ If patient is stable, follow ACLS protocol for cardioversion and drug therapy, which may include calcium channel blockers, beta-adrenergic blockers, or antiarrhythmics ◆ Anticoagulation therapy possibly also needed ◆ Radiofrequency ablation to control rhythm
◆ Heart failure, chronic obstructive pulmonary disease, thyrotoxicosis, constrictive pericarditis, ischemic heart disease, sepsis, pulmonary embolus, rheumatic heart disease, hypertension, mitral stenosis, atrial irritation, or complication of coronary bypass or valve replacement surgery ◆ Nifedipine and digoxin use	◆ If patient is unstable with a ventricular rate > 150 beats/minute, immediate cardioversion ◆ If patient is stable, follow ACLS protocol and drug therapy, which may include calcium channel blockers, beta-adrenergic blockers, or antiarrhythmics ◆ Anticoagulation therapy possibly also needed ◆ In some patients with refractory atrial fibrillation uncontrolled by drugs, radiofrequency catheter ablation
◆ Inferior wall MI or ischemia, hypoxia, vagal stimulation, and sick sinus syndrome ◆ Acute rheumatic fever ◆ Valve surgery ◆ Digoxin toxicity	◆ Correction of underlying cause ◆ Atropine for symptom-producing slow rate ◆ Pacemaker insertion if patient doesn't respond to drugs ◆ Discontinuation of digoxin if appropriate
◆ May be seen in healthy people ◆ Inferior wall MI or ischemia, hypothyroidism, hypokalemia, and hyperkalemia ◆ Digoxin toxicity; use of quinidine, procainamide, beta-adrenergic blockers, calcium channel blockers, or amiodarone	◆ Correction of underlying cause ◆ Possibly atropine if severe symptom-producing bradycardia develops ◆ Cautious use of digoxin, calcium channel blockers, and beta-adrenergic blockers

(continued)

ARRHYTHMIA	FEATURES

Second-degree AV block
Type I (Wenckebach)

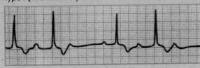

- ◆ Atrial rhythm regular
- ◆ Ventricular rhythm irregular
- ◆ Atrial rate exceeds ventricular rate
- ◆ PR interval progressively, but only slightly, longer with each cycle until QRS complex disappears (dropped beat); PR interval shorter after dropped beat

Second-degree AV block
Type II

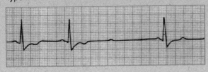

- ◆ Atrial rhythm regular
- ◆ Ventricular rhythm regular or irregular, with varying degree of block
- ◆ P-P interval constant
- ◆ QRS complexes periodically absent

Third-degree AV block
(complete heart block)

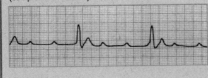

- ◆ Atrial rhythm regular
- ◆ Ventricular rhythm regular and rate slower than atrial rate
- ◆ No relation between P waves and QRS complexes
- ◆ No constant PR interval
- ◆ QRS duration normal (junctional pacemaker) or wide and bizarre (ventricular pacemaker)

Premature ventricular contraction (PVC)

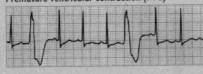

- ◆ Atrial rhythm regular
- ◆ Ventricular rhythm irregular
- ◆ QRS complex premature, usually followed by a complete compensatory pause
- ◆ QRS complex wide and distorted, usually > 0.14 second
- ◆ Premature QRS complexes occurring alone, in pairs, or in threes, alternating with normal beats; focus from one or more sites
- ◆ Ominous when clustered, multifocal, with R wave on T pattern

CAUSES	TREATMENT
◆ Inferior wall MI, cardiac surgery, acute rheumatic fever, and vagal stimulation ◆ Digoxin toxicity; use of propranolol, quinidine, or procainamide	◆ Treatment of underlying cause ◆ Atropine or temporary pacemaker for symptom-producing bradycardia ◆ Discontinuation of digoxin if appropriate
◆ Severe coronary artery disease, anterior wall MI, and acute myocarditis ◆ Digoxin toxicity	◆ Temporary or permanent pacemaker ◆ Atropine, dopamine, or epinephrine for symptom-producing bradycardia ◆ Discontinuation of digoxin if appropriate
◆ Inferior or anterior wall MI, congenital abnormality, rheumatic fever, hypoxia, postoperative complication of mitral valve replacement, postprocedure complication of radiofrequency ablation in or near AV nodal tissue, Lev's disease (fibrosis and calcification that spreads from cardiac structures to the conductive tissue), and Lenègre's disease (conductive tissue fibrosis) ◆ Digoxin toxicity	◆ Atropine, dopamine, or epinephrine for symptom-producing bradycardia ◆ Temporary or permanent pacemaker
◆ Heart failure; old or acute MI, ischemia, or contusion; myocardial irritation by ventricular catheter or a pacemaker; hypercapnia; hypokalemia; hypocalcemia; and hypomagnesemia ◆ Drug toxicity (digoxin, aminophylline, tricyclic antidepressants, beta-adrenergic blockers, isoproterenol, or dopamine) ◆ Caffeine, tobacco, or alcohol use ◆ Psychological stress, anxiety, pain, or exercise	◆ If warranted, procainamide, amiodarone, or lidocaine I.V. ◆ Treatment of underlying cause ◆ Discontinuation of drug causing toxicity ◆ Potassium chloride I.V. if PVC induced by hypokalemia ◆ Magnesium sulfate I.V. if PVC induced by hypomagnesemia

(continued)

ARRHYTHMIA	FEATURES

Ventricular tachycardia

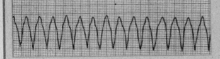

- ◆ Ventricular rate 100 to 220 beats/ minute, rhythm usually regular
- ◆ QRS complexes wide, bizarre, and independent of P waves
- ◆ P waves not discernible
- ◆ May start and stop suddenly

Ventricular fibrillation

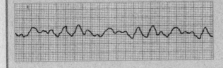

- ◆ Ventricular rhythm and rate chaotic and rapid
- ◆ QRS complexes wide and irregular; no visible P waves

Asystole

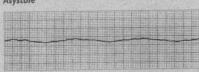

- ◆ No atrial or ventricular rate or rhythm
- ◆ No discernible P waves, QRS complexes, or T waves

helpful. Tell the patient to report light-headedness or syncope, and stress the importance of regular checkups.

☀ Life-threatening
Cardiac tamponade

Cardiac tamponade is a rapid, unchecked increase in pressure in the pericardial sac that compresses the

CAUSES	TREATMENT
◆ Myocardial ischemia, MI, or aneurysm; coronary artery disease; rheumatic heart disease; mitral valve prolapse; heart failure; cardiomyopathy; ventricular catheters; hypokalemia; hypercalcemia; hypomagnesemia; and pulmonary embolism ◆ Digoxin, procainamide, epinephrine, or quinidine toxicity ◆ Anxiety	◆ With pulse: if hemodynamically stable with monomorphic QRS complexes, administration of procainamide, sotalol, amiodarone, or lidocaine (follow ACLS protocol); if drugs are ineffective, cardioversion ◆ If polymorphic QRS complexes and normal QT interval, admnistration of beta-adrenergic blockers, lidocaine, amiodarone, procainamide, or sotalol (follow ACLS protocol); if drug is unsuccessful, cardioversion ◆ If polymorphic QRS and QT interval is prolonged, magnesium I.V., then overdrive pacing if rhythm persists; may also administer isoproterenol, phenytoin, or lidocaine ◆ Pulseless: cardiopulmonary rescusitation (CPR); follow ACLS protocol for defibrillation, endotracheal (ET) intubation, and administration of epinephrine or vasopressin, followed by amiodarone or lidocaine and, if ineffective, magnesium sulfate or procainamide ◆ Implanted cardioverter-defibrillator (ICD) if recurrent ventricular tachycardia
◆ Myocardial ischemia, MI, untreated ventricular tachycardia, R-on-T phenomenon, hypokalemia, hyperkalemia, hypercalcemia, hypoxemia, alkalosis, electric shock, and hypothermia ◆ Digoxin, epinephrine, or quinidine toxicity	◆ CPR; follow ACLS protocol for defibrillation, ET intubation, and administration of epinephrine or vasopressin, amiodarone, or lidocaine and, if ineffective, magnesium sulfate or procainamide ◆ ICD if at risk for recurrent ventricular fibrillation
◆ Myocardial ischemia, MI, aortic valve disease, heart failure, hypoxia, hypokalemia, severe acidosis, electric shock, ventricular arrhythmia, AV block, pulmonary embolism, heart rupture, cardiac tamponade, hyperkalemia, and electromechanical dissociation ◆ Cocaine overdose	◆ Continue CPR; follow ACLS protocol for ET intubation, transcutaneous pacing, and administration of epinephrine and atropine

heart, impairs diastolic filling, and reduces cardiac output. The pressure increase usually results from blood or fluid accumulation in the pericardial sac. Even a small amount of fluid (50 to 100 ml) can cause a serious tamponade if it accumulates rapidly.

Prognosis depends on the rate of fluid accumulation. If it accumulates rapidly, cardiac tamponade requires emergency lifesaving measures to prevent death. A slow accumulation and increase in pressure, as in pericardial effusion associated with malignant tu-

COMPARING NORMAL AND ABNORMAL CONDUCTION

NORMAL CARDIAC CONDUCTION

The heart's conduction system, shown below, begins at the sinoatrial (SA) node — the heart's pacemaker. When an impulse leaves the SA node, it travels through the atria along Bachmann's bundle and the internodal pathways to the atrioventricular (AV) node, and then down the bundle of His, along the bundle branches and, finally, down the Purkinje fibers to the ventricles.

ABNORMAL CARDIAC CONDUCTION

Altered automaticity, reentry, or conduction disturbances may cause cardiac arrhythmias.

ALTERED AUTOMATICITY

Altered automaticity is the result of partial depolarization, which may increase the intrinsic rate of the SA node or latent pacemakers, or may induce ectopic pacemakers to reach threshold and depolarize.

Automaticity may be altered by drugs, such as epinephrine, atropine, and digoxin, and by such conditions as acidosis, alkalosis, hypoxia, myocardial infarction (MI), hypo-

kalemia, and hypocalcemia. Examples of arrhythmias caused by altered automaticity include atrial fibrillation and flutter; supraventricular tachycardia; premature atrial, junctional, and ventricular complexes; ventricular tachycardia and fibrillation; and accelerated idioventricular and junctional rhythms.

REENTRY

Ischemia or a deformity causes an abnormal circuit to develop within conductive fibers. Although current flow is blocked in one direction within the circuit, the descending impulse can travel in the other direction. By the time the impulse completes the circuit, the previously depolarized tissue within the circuit is no longer refractory to stimulation, allowing reentry of the impulse and repetition of this cycle.

Conditions that increase the likelihood of reentry include hyperkalemia, myocardial ischemia, and the use of certain antiarrhythmic drugs. Reentry may be responsible for such arrhythmias as paroxysmal supraventricular tachycardia; premature atrial, junctional, and ventricular complexes; and ventricular tachycardia.

---

mors, may not produce immediate symptoms because the fibrous wall of the pericardial sac can gradually stretch to accommodate as much as 2 L of fluid.

CAUSES

- Acute myocardial infarction
- Chronic renal failure requiring dialysis
- Connective tissue disorders (such as rheumatoid arthritis, systemic lupus erythematosus, rheumatic fever, vasculitis, and scleroderma)

- Drug reaction from procainamide, hydralazine (Apresoline), minoxidil (Loniten), isoniazid (Laniazid)), penicillin, or daunorubicin (Cerubidine)
- Effusion (from cancer, bacterial infections, tuberculosis and, rarely, acute rheumatic fever)
- Hemorrhage from nontraumatic causes (such as anticoagulant therapy in patients with pericarditis or rupture of the heart or great vessels)
- Hemorrhage from trauma (such as gunshot or stab wounds to the chest or perforation by the catheter during

An alternative reentry mechanism depends on the presence of a congenital accessory pathway linking the atria and the ventricles outside the AV junction—for example, Wolff-Parkinson-White syndrome.

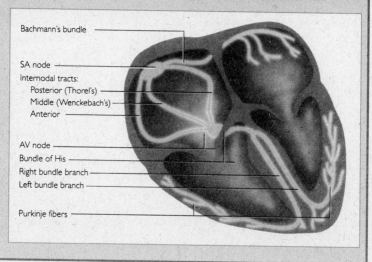

Bachmann's bundle

SA node

Internodal tracts:
    Posterior (Thorel's)
    Middle (Wenckebach's)
    Anterior

AV node
Bundle of His
Right bundle branch
Left bundle branch

Purkinje fibers

cardiac or central venous catheterization or postcardiac surgery)
- Idiopathic causes (Dressler's syndrome)
- Viral or postirradiation pericarditis

PATHOPHYSIOLOGY

In cardiac tamponade, the progressive accumulation of fluid in the pericardial sac causes compression of the heart chambers. This compression obstructs blood flow into the ventricles and reduces the amount of blood that can be pumped out of the heart with each contraction. (See *Understanding cardiac tamponade,* page 28.)

Each time the ventricles contract, more fluid accumulates in the pericardial sac. This further limits the amount of blood that can fill the ventricular chambers—especially the left ventricle—during the next cardiac cycle.

The amount of fluid necessary to cause cardiac tamponade varies greatly; it may be as little as 50 ml when the fluid accumulates rapidly or more than 2 L if the fluid accumulates slow-

UNDERSTANDING
CARDIAC TAMPONADE

The pericardial sac, which surrounds and protects the heart, is composed of several layers. The fibrous pericardium is the tough outermost membrane; the inner membrane, called the serous membrane, consists of the visceral and parietal layers. The visceral layer clings to the heart and is also known as the *epicardial layer* of the heart. The parietal layer lies between the visceral layer and the fibrous pericardium. The pericardial space — between the visceral and parietal layers — contains 10 to 30 ml of pericardial fluid. This fluid lubricates the layers and minimizes friction when the heart contracts.

Normal heart and pericardium

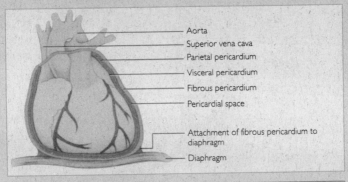

Aorta
Superior vena cava
Parietal pericardium
Visceral pericardium
Fibrous pericardium
Pericardial space

Attachment of fibrous pericardium to diaphragm
Diaphragm

In cardiac tamponade, blood or fluid fills the pericardial space, compressing the heart chambers, increasing intracardiac pressure, and obstructing venous return. As blood flow into the ventricles falls, so does cardiac output. Without prompt treatment, low cardiac output can be fatal.

Cardiac tamponade

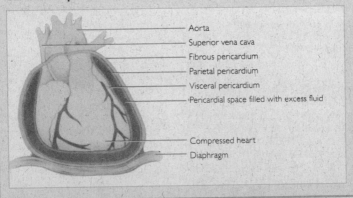

Aorta
Superior vena cava
Fibrous pericardium
Parietal pericardium
Visceral pericardium
Pericardial space filled with excess fluid

Compressed heart
Diaphragm

ly and the pericardium stretches to adapt.

CLINICAL FINDINGS
- Elevated central venous pressure (CVP) with jugular vein distention due to increased jugular venous pressure
- Muffled heart sounds caused by fluid in the pericardial sac
- Pulsus paradoxus (an inspiratory decrease in systemic blood pressure greater than 15 mm Hg) due to impaired diastolic filling
- Diaphoresis and cool clammy skin caused by a decrease in cardiac output
- Anxiety, restlessness, and syncope due to a drop in cardiac output
- Cyanosis due to reduced oxygenation of the tissues
- Weak, rapid pulse in response to a drop in cardiac output
- Cough, dyspnea, orthopnea, and tachypnea due to lung compression by an expanding pericardial sac and the inability to move blood from the pulmonary vasculature into the compromised left ventricle

TEST RESULTS
- Chest X-rays show a slightly widened mediastinum and possible cardiomegaly. The cardiac silhouette may have a goblet-shaped appearance.
- Electrocardiography (ECG) may show a low-amplitude QRS complex and electrical alternans, an alternating beat-to-beat change in amplitude of the P wave, QRS complex, and T wave. Generalized ST-segment elevation is noted in all leads. An ECG is used to rule out other cardiac disorders; it may reveal changes produced by acute pericarditis.
- Pulmonary artery catheterization detects increased right atrial pressure, right ventricular diastolic pressure, and CVP.
- Echocardiography may reveal pericardial effusion with signs of right ventricular and atrial compression.

TREATMENT
- Supplemental oxygen to improve oxygenation
- Continuous ECG and hemodynamic monitoring in an intensive care unit to detect complications and monitor effects of therapy
- Pericardiocentesis (needle aspiration of the pericardial cavity) to reduce fluid in the pericardial sac and improve systemic arterial pressure and cardiac output (A catheter may be left in the pericardial space attached to a drainage container to allow for continuous fluid drainage.)
- Pericardial window (surgical creation of an opening) to remove accumulated fluid from the pericardial sac
- Pericardectomy (resection of a portion or all of the pericardium) to allow full communication with the pleura, if repeated pericardiocentesis fails to prevent recurrence
- Trial volume loading with crystalloids, such as I.V. normal saline solution, to maintain systolic blood pressure
- Inotropic drugs, such as isoproterenol or dopamine, to improve myocardial contractility until fluid in the pericardial sac can be removed
- Blood transfusion or a thoracotomy to drain reaccumulating fluid or to repair bleeding sites possibly needed in traumatic injury
- Administration of a heparin antagonist, such as protamine sulfate, to stop bleeding in heparin-induced tamponade
- Use of vitamin K to stop bleeding in warfarin-induced tamponade

NURSING CONSIDERATIONS
For pericardiocentesis
- Explain the procedure to the patient.
- Keep at the bedside a pericardial aspiration needle attached to a 50-ml syringe by a three-way stopcock, an ECG machine, and an emergency cart with a defibrillator. Make sure the equipment is turned on and ready for immediate use.
- Position the patient at a 45- to 60-degree angle.
- Connect the precordial ECG lead to the hub of the aspiration needle with an alligator clamp and connecting wire, and assist with fluid aspiration.
- When the needle touches the myocardium, you'll see an ST-segment elevation or premature ventricular contractions.
- Monitor blood pressure and CVP during and after pericardiocentesis. Infuse I.V. solutions, as prescribed, to maintain blood pressure. Watch for a decrease in CVP and a concomitant increase in blood pressure, which indicate relief of cardiac compression.
- Watch for complications of pericardiocentesis, such as ventricular fibrillation, vasovagal response, or coronary artery or cardiac chamber puncture. Closely monitor ECG changes, blood pressure, pulse rate, level of consciousness, and urine output.

For thoracotomy
- Explain the procedure to the patient. Tell him what to expect postoperatively (chest tubes, drainage bottles, and administration of oxygen). Teach him how to turn, deep breathe, and cough.
- Give antibiotics, protamine sulfate, or vitamin K, as ordered.

- Postoperatively, monitor critical parameters, such as vital signs and arterial blood gas values, and assess heart and respiratory rates. Give pain medication as ordered. Maintain the chest drainage system, and be alert for complications, such as hemorrhage and arrhythmias.

Life-threatening
Cardiomyopathy

Cardiomyopathy generally applies to disease of the heart muscle fibers, and it occurs in three main forms: dilated, hypertrophic, and restrictive (extremely rare). Cardiomyopathy is the second most common direct cause of sudden death; coronary artery disease (CAD) is first. Approximately 5 to 8 per 100,000 U.S. residents have dilated cardiomyopathy, the most common type. At greatest risk for dilated cardiomyopathy are males and blacks; other risk factors include CAD, hypertension, pregnancy, viral infections, and alcohol or illegal drug use. Because dilated cardiomyopathy usually isn't diagnosed until its advanced stages, the prognosis is generally poor.

There are two types of hypertrophic cardiomyopathy. The more common form is caused by aortic valve stenosis. The second form, hypertrophic obstructive cardiomyopathy (HOCM), is due to a genetic abnormality. The course of hypertrophic cardiomyopathy is variable. Some patients progressively deteriorate, whereas others remain stable for years. It's estimated that almost 50% of all sudden deaths in competitive athletes age 35 or younger are a result of HOCM. If severe, restrictive cardiomyopathy is irreversible.

CAUSES

● Dilated cardiomyopathy usually due to idiopathic, or primary, disease; sometimes secondary to identifiable causes (see *Comparing cardiomyopathies,* pages 32 and 33)

● HOCM usually inherited as a non-sex-linked autosomal dominant trait

PATHOPHYSIOLOGY

Dilated cardiomyopathy results from extensively damaged myocardial muscle fibers. Consequently, there's reduced contractility in the left ventricle. As systolic function declines, stroke volume, ejection fraction, and cardiac output fall. As end-diastolic volumes rise, pulmonary congestion may occur. The elevated end-diastolic volume is a compensatory response to preserve stroke volume despite a reduced ejection fraction. The sympathetic nervous system is also stimulated to increase heart rate and contractility. The kidneys are stimulated to retain sodium and water to maintain cardiac output, and vasoconstriction also occurs as the renin-angiotensin system is stimulated. When these compensatory mechanisms can no longer maintain cardiac output, the heart begins to fail. Left ventricular dilation occurs as venous return and systemic vascular resistance rise. Eventually, the atria also dilate as more work is required to pump blood into the full ventricles. Cardiomegaly occurs as a consequence of dilation of the atria and ventricles. Blood pooling in the ventricles increases the risk of emboli.

Alert *Barth syndrome is a rare genetic disorder that can cause dilated cardiomyopathy in boys. It may be associated with skeletal muscle changes, short stature, neutropenia, and increased susceptibility to bacterial infections. Evidence of dilated cardiomyopathy may appear as early as the first few days or months of life.*

Unlike dilated cardiomyopathy, which affects systolic function, hypertrophic cardiomyopathy primarily affects diastolic function. The hypertrophied ventricle becomes stiff, noncompliant, and unable to relax during ventricular filling. Consequently, ventricular filling is reduced and left ventricular filling pressure rises, causing a rise in left atrial and pulmonary venous pressures and leading to venous congestion and dyspnea. Ventricular filling time is further reduced as a compensatory response to tachycardia leading to low cardiac output. If papillary muscles become hypertrophied and don't close completely during contraction, mitral insufficiency occurs. The features of HOCM include asymmetrical left ventricular hypertrophy; hypertrophy of the intraventricular septum; rapid, forceful contractions of the left ventricle; impaired relaxation; and obstruction of left ventricular outflow. The forceful ejection of blood draws the anterior leaflet of the mitral valve to the intraventricular septum. This causes early closure of the outflow tract, decreasing ejection fraction. Moreover, intramural coronary arteries are abnormally small and may not be sufficient to supply the hypertrophied muscle with enough blood and oxygen to meet the increased needs of the hyperdynamic muscle.

Restrictive cardiomyopathy is characterized by stiffness of the ventricle caused by left ventricular hypertrophy and endocardial fibrosis and thickening, thus reducing the ability of the ventricle to relax and fill during diastole. Moreover, the rigid myocardium fails to contract completely during systole. As a result, cardiac output falls.

(Text continues on page 34.)

COMPARING CARDIOMYOPATHIES

Cardiomyopathies include various structural or functional abnormalities of the ventricles. They're grouped into three main pathophysiologic types: dilated, hypertrophic, and restrictive. These conditions may lead to heart failure by impairing myocardial structure and function.

NORMAL HEART	DILATED CARDIOMYOPATHY
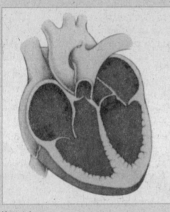	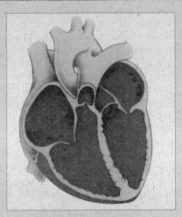
Ventricles	◆ Greatly increased chamber size ◆ Thinning of left ventricular muscle
Atrial chamber size	◆ Increased
Myocardial mass	◆ Increased
Ventricular inflow resistance	◆ Normal
Contractility	◆ Decreased
Possible causes	◆ Viral or bacterial infection ◆ Hypertension ◆ Peripartum syndrome related to toxemia ◆ Ischemic heart disease ◆ Valvular disease ◆ Drug hypersensitivity ◆ Chemotherapy ◆ Cardiotoxic effects of drugs or alcohol

HYPERTROPHIC CARDIOMYOPATHY

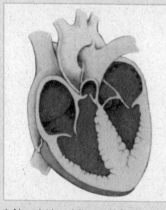

- Normal right and decreased left chamber size
- Left ventricular hypertrophy
- Thickened interventricular septum (hypertrophic obstructive cardiomyopathy [HOCM])

- Increased on left

- Increased

- Increased

- Increased or decreased

- Autosomal dominant trait (HOCM)
- Hypertension
- Obstructive valvular disease
- Thyroid disease

RESTRICTIVE CARDIOMYOPATHY

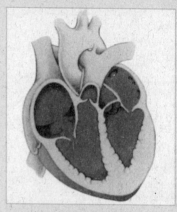

- Decreased ventricular chamber size
- Left ventricular hypertrophy

- Increased

- Normal

- Increased

- Decreased

- Amyloidosis
- Sarcoidosis
- Hemochromatosis
- Infiltrative neoplastic disease

CLINICAL FINDINGS

Dilated cardiomyopathy

- Shortness of breath, orthopnea, dyspnea on exertion, paroxysmal nocturnal dyspnea, fatigue, and a dry cough at night due to left-sided heart failure
- Peripheral edema, hepatomegaly, jugular vein distention, and weight gain caused by right-sided heart failure
- Peripheral cyanosis associated with a low cardiac output
- Tachycardia as a compensatory response to low cardiac output
- Pansystolic murmur associated with mitral and tricuspid insufficiency secondary to cardiomegaly and weak papillary muscles
- S_3 and S_4 gallop rhythms associated with heart failure
- Irregular pulse if atrial fibrillation exists
- Worsening renal function as decreased cardiac output produces decreased renal perfusion

Hypertrophic cardiomyopathy

- Dyspnea due to elevated left ventricular filling pressure
- Fatigue associated with a reduced cardiac output
- Angina caused by the inability of the intramural coronary arteries to supply enough blood to meet the increased oxygen demands of the hypertrophied heart
- Peripheral pulse with a characteristic double impulse (pulsus biferiens) caused by powerful left ventricular contractions and rapid ejection of blood during systole
- Abrupt arterial pulse secondary to vigorous left ventricular contractions
- Irregular pulse if an enlarged atrium causes atrial fibrillation

HOCM

- Systolic ejection murmur along the left sternal border and at the apex caused by mitral insufficiency
- Angina caused by the inability of the intramural coronary arteries to supply enough blood to meet the increased oxygen demands of the hypertrophied heart
- Syncope resulting from arrhythmias or reduced ventricular filling leading to a reduced cardiac output
- Activity intolerance due to worsening of outflow tract obstruction from exercise-induced catecholamine release
- Abrupt arterial pulse secondary to vigorous left ventricular contractions and early termination of left ventricular ejection
- Irregular pulse if an enlarged atrium causes atrial fibrillation

Restrictive cardiomyopathy

- Fatigue, dyspnea, orthopnea, chest pain, edema, liver engorgement, peripheral cyanosis, pallor, and S_3 or S_4 gallop rhythms due to heart failure
- Systolic murmurs caused by mitral and tricuspid insufficiency

TEST RESULTS

- Echocardiography confirms dilated cardiomyopathy.
- Chest X-ray may reveal cardiomegaly associated with any of the cardiomyopathies.
- Cardiac catheterization with possible heart biopsy can be definitive with HOCM.
- Diagnosis requires elimination of other possible causes of heart failure and arrhythmias. (See *Comparing diagnostic tests in cardiomyopathy,* pages 36 and 37.)

TREATMENT
Dilated cardiomyopathy
- Treatment of the underlying cause if identifiable
- Angiotensin-converting enzyme (ACE) inhibitors, as first-line therapy, to reduce afterload through vasodilation
- Diuretics, taken with ACE inhibitors, to reduce fluid retention
- Digoxin, for the patient who doesn't respond to ACE inhibitor and diuretic therapy, to improve myocardial contractility
- Hydralazine and isosorbide dinitrate in combination, to produce vasodilation
- Beta-adrenergic blockers for the patient with New York Heart Association (NYHA) class II or III heart failure (see *Classifying heart failure,* page 38)
- Antiarrhythmics such as amiodarone, used cautiously, to control arrhythmias
- Implantable cardioverter-defibrillator (ICD) to treat ventricular arrhythmias and for prophylaxis (due to the high incidence of sudden death in the patient with NYHA class III or IV heart failure)
- Cardioversion to convert atrial fibrillation to sinus rhythm
- Pacemaker insertion to correct arrhythmias
- Anticoagulants (controversial) to reduce the risk of emboli
- Biventricular pacemaker for cardiac resynchronization therapy if symptoms continue despite optimal drug therapy, the patient is classified as NYHA class III or IV heart failure, the QRS duration is 0.13 second or more, or ejection fraction is 35% or less
- Revascularization, such as coronary artery bypass graft surgery, if dilated cardiomyopathy is due to ischemia

- Valvular repair or replacement, if dilated cardiomyopathy is due to valve dysfunction
- Heart transplantation in the patient refractory to medical therapy
- Lifestyle modifications, such as smoking cessation; low-fat, low-sodium diet; physical activity; and abstinence from alcohol

Hypertrophic cardiomyopathy
- Optimal control of hypertension
- Aortic valve replacement if valve is stenotic
- Verapamil or diltiazem to reduce ventricular stiffness and elevated diastolic pressures
- Cardioversion to treat atrial fibrillation
- Anticoagulation to reduce the risk of systemic embolism with atrial fibrillation

HOCM
- Beta-adrenergic blockers to slow the heart rate, reduce myocardial oxygen demands, and increase ventricular filling by relaxing the obstructing muscle, thereby increasing cardiac output
- Antiarrhythmic drugs, such as amiodarone, to reduce arrhythmias
- Cardioversion to treat atrial fibrillation
- Anticoagulation to reduce the risk of systemic embolism with atrial fibrillation
- Verapamil or diltiazem to reduce septal stiffness and elevated diastolic pressures
- Ablation of the atrioventricular node and implantation of a dual-chamber pacemaker (controversial), in the patient with HOCM and ventricular tachycardia, to reduce the outflow gradient by altering the pattern of ventricular contractions

COMPARING DIAGNOSTIC TESTS IN CARDIOMYOPATHY

Cardiomyopathies include various structural or functional abnormalities of the ventricles. They're grouped into three main pathophysiologic types: dilated, hypertrophic, and restrictive. These conditions may lead to heart failure by impairing myocardial structure and function.

DILATED CARDIOMYOPATHY	HYPERTROPHIC CARDIOMYOPATHY
Electrocardiography	
Biventricular hypertrophy, sinus tachycardia, atrial enlargement, atrial and ventricular arrhythmias, bundle-branch block, and ST-segment and T-wave abnormalities	Left ventricular hypertrophy, ST-segment and T-wave abnormalities, left anterior hemiblock, Q waves in precordial and inferior leads, ventricular arrhythmias and, possibly, atrial fibrillation
Echocardiography	
Left ventricular thrombi, global hypokinesia, enlarged atria, left ventricular dilation and, possibly, valvular abnormalities	Symmetrical thickening of the left ventricular wall and intraventricular septum and left atrial dilation
Chest X-ray	
Cardiomegaly, pulmonary congestion, pulmonary hypertension, and pleural or pericardial effusions	Cardiomegaly
Cardiac catheterization	
Elevated left atrial and left ventricular end-diastolic pressures, left ventricular enlargement, and mitral and tricuspid incompetence; may identify coronary artery disease as a cause	Elevated ventricular end-diastolic pressure and, possibly, mitral insufficiency, hyperdynamic systolic function, and aortic valve pressure gradient if aortic valve is stenotic
Radionuclide studies	
Left ventricular dilation and hypokinesis; reduced ejection fraction	Reduced left ventricular volume, increased muscle mass, and ischemia

- ICD to treat ventricular arrhythmias
- Ventricular myotomy or myectomy (resection of the hypertrophied septum) to ease outflow tract obstruction and relieve symptoms
- Mitral valve replacement to treat mitral insufficiency (controversial)
- Heart transplantation for intractable symptoms

Restrictive cardiomyopathy
- Treatment of the underlying cause, such as administering deferoxamine (Desferal) to bind iron in restrictive cardiomyopathy due to hemochromatosis
- Although no therapy exists for restricted ventricular filling, digoxin (Lanoxin), diuretics, and a restricted sodium diet to ease the symptoms of heart failure

HYPERTROPHIC OBSTRUCTIVE CARDIOMYOPATHY	RESTRICTIVE CARDIOMYOPATHY
Left ventricular hypertrophy with QRS complexes tallest across midprecordium, ST-segment and T-wave abnormalities, left axis deviation, left atrial abnormality, supraventricular tachycardia, and ventricular tachycardia	Low voltage, hypertrophy, atrioventricular conduction defects, and arrhythmias
Asymmetrical septal hypertrophy; anterior movement of the anterior mitral leaflet during systole, early termination of left ventricular ejection that worsens with dobutamine (Dobutrex) or nitrate provocation, mitral insufficiency, and atrial dilation	Increased left ventricular muscle mass, normal or reduced left ventricular cavity size, and decreased systolic function; rules out constrictive pericarditis
Normal or mild cardiomegaly	Cardiomegaly, pericardial effusion, and pulmonary congestion
Asymmetrical septal hypertrophy, early termination of systole with decreased ejection fraction, outflow tract pressure gradient increasing from the apex to just below the aortic valve, and mitral insufficiency	Reduced systolic function and myocardial infiltration; increased left ventricular end-diastolic pressure; rules out constrictive pericarditis
Reduced left ventricular volume, increased septal muscle mass, septal ischemia	Left ventricular hypertrophy with restricted ventricular filling and reduced ejection fraction

- Oral vasodilators to decrease afterload and facilitate ventricular ejection

NURSING CONSIDERATIONS
Dilated cardiomyopathy in acute failure

- Monitor the patient for signs of progressive failure (increasing crackles and dyspnea and increased jugular vein distention) and compromised renal perfusion (oliguria, elevated blood urea nitrogen and creatinine levels, and electrolyte imbalances). Weigh the patient daily.
- If the patient is receiving vasodilators, check blood pressure and heart rate. If he becomes hypotensive, stop the infusion and place him in a supine position with legs elevated to increase venous return and to ensure cerebral blood flow.

● If the patient is receiving diuretics, monitor for signs of resolving congestion (decreased crackles and dyspnea) or too vigorous diuresis. Check serum potassium level for hypokalemia, especially if therapy includes digoxin.

● Therapeutic restrictions and an uncertain prognosis usually cause profound anxiety and depression, so offer support and let the patient express his feelings. Be flexible with visiting hours.

● Before discharge, teach the patient about his illness and its treatment. Emphasize the need to avoid alcohol, to restrict sodium intake, to watch for weight gain, and to take digoxin as prescribed and watch for its adverse effects (anorexia, nausea, vomiting, and yellow vision).

● Encourage family members to learn cardiopulmonary resuscitation (CPR).

Hypertrophic cardiomyopathy

● Warn the patient against strenuous physical activity, such as running, because syncope or sudden death may follow well-tolerated exercise.

● Administer medications as prescribed. Avoid nitroglycerin, digoxin, and diuretics because they can worsen obstruction. Warn the patient not to stop taking propranolol abruptly because doing so may increase myocardial demands. To determine the patient's tolerance for an increased dosage of propranolol, take his pulse to check for bradycardia. Also, take his blood pressure while he's in a supine position and while he's standing (a drop in blood pressure [greater than 10 mm Hg] when standing may indicate orthostatic hypotension).

● Administer prophylaxis for subacute infective endocarditis before dental work or surgery.

● Provide psychological support. If the patient is hospitalized for a long time, be flexible with visiting hours and encourage occasional weekends away from the hospital, if possible. Refer the patient for psychosocial counseling to help him and his family accept his restricted lifestyle and poor prognosis.

● If the patient is a child, have his parents arrange for him to continue his studies in the health care facility.

● Urge the patient's family to learn CPR because sudden cardiac arrest is possible.

Restrictive cardiomyopathy

● In the acute phase, monitor heart rate and rhythm, blood pressure, urine output, and pulmonary artery pressure readings to help guide treatment.

● Give psychological support. Provide appropriate diversionary activities for the patient restricted to prolonged bed rest. Because a poor prognosis may cause profound anxiety and depression, be especially supportive and understanding and encourage the patient to express his fears. Refer him for psychosocial counseling, as necessary, for assistance in coping with his restricted lifestyle. Be flexible with visiting hours whenever possible.

● Before discharge, teach the patient to watch for and report signs of digoxin toxicity (anorexia, nausea, vomiting, and yellow vision); to record and report weight gain; and, if sodium restriction is ordered, to avoid canned foods, pickles, smoked meats, and use of table salt.

Coarctation of the aorta

Coarctation is a narrowing of the aorta, usually just below the left subclavian artery, near the site where the ligamentum arteriosum (the remnant of the ductus arteriosus, a fetal blood vessel) joins the pulmonary artery to the aorta. Coarctation may occur with aortic valve stenosis (usually of a bicuspid aortic valve) and with severe cases of hypoplasia of the aortic arch, patent ductus arteriosus (PDA), and ventricular septal defect (VSD). The obstruction to blood flow results in ineffective pumping of the heart and increases the risk of heart failure.

This acyanotic condition accounts for about 7% of congenital heart defects in children and is twice as common in males as in females. When coarctation of the aorta occurs in females, it's commonly associated with Turner's syndrome, a chromosomal disorder that causes ovarian dysgenesis.

The prognosis depends on the severity of associated cardiac anomalies. If corrective surgery is performed before isolated coarctation induces severe systemic hypertension or degenerative changes in the aorta, the prognosis is good.

CAUSES

Although the cause of this defect is unknown, it may be associated with Turner's syndrome.

PATHOPHYSIOLOGY

Coarctation of the aorta may develop as a result of spasm and constriction of the smooth muscle in the ductus arteriosus as it closes. Possibly, this contractile tissue extends into the aortic wall, causing narrowing. The obstructive process causes hypertension in the aortic branches above the constriction (arteries that supply the arms, neck, and head) and diminished pressure in the vessel below the constriction.

Restricted blood flow through the narrowed aorta increases the pressure load on the left ventricle and causes dilation of the proximal aorta and ventricular hypertrophy.

As oxygenated blood leaves the left ventricle, a portion travels through the arteries that branch off the aorta proximal to the coarctation. If PDA is present, the rest of the blood travels through the coarctation, mixes with deoxygenated blood from the PDA, and travels to the legs. If the PDA is closed, the legs and lower portion of the body must rely solely on the blood that gets through the coarctation.

Untreated, this condition may lead to left-sided heart failure and, rarely, to cerebral hemorrhage and aortic rupture. If VSD accompanies coarctation, blood shunts from left to right, straining the right side of the heart. This leads to pulmonary hypertension and, eventually, right-sided heart hypertrophy and failure.

If coarctation doesn't produce symptoms in infancy, it usually produces no symptoms throughout adolescence as collateral circulation develops to bypass the narrowed segment.

CLINICAL FINDINGS

- Tachypnea, dyspnea, pulmonary edema, pallor, tachycardia, failure to thrive, cardiomegaly, and hepatomegaly due to heart failure during an infant's first year of life
- Claudication due to reduced blood flow to the legs
- Hypertension in the upper body due to increased pressure in the arteries proximal to the coarctation
- Headache, vertigo, and epistaxis secondary to hypertension
- Upper extremity blood pressure greater than lower extremity blood pressure because blood flow through the coarctation is greater to the upper body than to the lower body
- Pink upper extremities and cyanotic lower extremities due to reduced oxygenated blood reaching the legs
- Absent or diminished femoral pulses due to restricted blood flow to the lower extremities through the constricted aorta

- In most cases, normal heart sounds unless a coexisting cardiac defect is present
- Chest and arms possibly more developed than the legs because circulation to the legs is restricted

TEST RESULTS

- Physical examination reveals the cardinal signs — resting systolic hypertension in the upper body, absent or diminished femoral pulses, and a wide pulse pressure.
- Chest X-rays may demonstrate left ventricular hypertrophy, heart failure, a wide ascending and descending aorta, and notching of the undersurfaces of the ribs due to erosion by collateral circulation.
- Electrocardiography may reveal left ventricular hypertrophy.
- Echocardiography may show increased left ventricular muscle thickness, coexisting aortic valve abnormalities, and the coarctation site.
- Cardiac catheterization evaluates collateral circulation and measures pressure in the right and left ventricles and in the ascending and descending aortas (on both sides of the obstruction). Aortography locates the site and extent of coarctation.

TREATMENT

- Digoxin, diuretics, oxygen, and sedatives in infants with heart failure
- Prostaglandin infusion to keep the ductus open
- Antibiotic prophylaxis against infective endocarditis before and after surgery
- Antihypertensive therapy for children with previous undetected coarctation until surgery is performed
- Preparation of the infant with heart failure or hypertension for early surgery, or else surgery delayed until the

preschool-age years (A flap of the left subclavian artery may be used to reconstruct the aorta. Balloon angioplasty or resection with end-to-end anastomosis or use of a tubular graft may also be performed.)

NURSING CONSIDERATIONS

● When coarctation in an infant requires rapid digitalization, monitor vital signs closely and watch for digoxin toxicity (poor feeding and vomiting).
● Balance intake and output carefully, especially if the infant is receiving diuretics with fluid restriction.
● Because the infant may not be able to maintain proper body temperature, regulate environmental temperature with an overbed warmer if needed.
● Monitor blood glucose levels to detect possible hypoglycemia, which may occur as glycogen stores become depleted.
● Offer the parents emotional support and an explanation of the disorder. Also explain diagnostic procedures, surgery, and drug therapy. Tell parents what to expect postoperatively.
● For an older child, assess the blood pressure in his extremities regularly, explain exercise restrictions, stress the need to take medications properly and to watch for adverse effects, and teach him about tests and other procedures.

After corrective surgery
● Monitor blood pressure closely using an intra-arterial line. Take blood pressure in all extremities. Monitor intake and output.
● If the patient develops hypertension and requires nitroprusside, administer by continuous I.V. infusion using an infusion pump. Watch for severe hypotension, and regulate the dosage carefully.

● Provide pain relief, and encourage a gradual increase in activity.
● Promote adequate respiratory functioning through turning, coughing, and deep breathing.
● Watch for abdominal pain or rigidity and signs of GI or urinary bleeding.
● If an older child needs to continue antihypertensives after surgery, teach him and his parents about them.
● Stress the importance of continued endocarditis prophylaxis.

Endocarditis

Endocarditis (also known as *infective* or *bacterial endocarditis*) is an infection of the endocardium, heart valves, or cardiac prosthesis resulting from bacterial or fungal invasion.

Untreated endocarditis is usually fatal but, with proper treatment, 70% of patients recover. The prognosis is worst when endocarditis causes severe valvular damage, leading to insufficiency and heart failure, or when it involves a prosthetic valve.

CAUSES
● Bacterial or fungal infection (rare)
Most cases of endocarditis occur in patients:
● who are I.V. drug abusers
● with mitral valve prolapse (especially males with a systolic murmur)
● with prosthetic heart valves
● with rheumatic heart disease.
Other predisposing conditions include:
● a syphilitic aortic valve.
● coarctation of the aorta
● degenerative heart disease, especially calcific aortic stenosis
● Marfan syndrome
● pulmonary stenosis

DEGENERATIVE CHANGES IN ENDOCARDITIS

This illustration shows typical growths on the endocardium produced by fibrin and platelet deposits on infection sites.

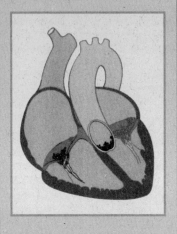

- subaortic and valvular aortic stenosis
- tetralogy of Fallot
- ventricular septal defects.

Some patients with endocarditis have no underlying heart disease.

Infecting organisms differ among these groups:

- In patients with native valve endocarditis who aren't I.V. drug abusers, causative organisms usually include (in order of frequency) streptococci, especially *Streptococcus viridans;* staphylococci; or enterococci. Although other bacteria occasionally cause the disorder, fungal causes are rare in this group. The mitral valve is involved most commonly, followed by the aortic valve.

- In patients who are I.V. drug abusers, *Staphylococcus aureus* is the most common infecting organism. Less commonly, streptococci, enterococci, gram-negative bacilli, or fungi cause the disorder. The tricuspid valve is involved most commonly, followed by the aortic and then the mitral valve.

- In patients with prosthetic valve endocarditis, early cases (those that develop within 60 days of valve insertion) are usually due to staphylococcal infection. However, gram-negative aerobic organisms, fungi, streptococci, enterococci, or diphtheroids may also cause the disorder. The course is usually fulminant and is associated with high mortality. Late cases (occurring after 60 days) show signs and symptoms similar to native valve endocarditis.

PATHOPHYSIOLOGY

In endocarditis, bacteremia — even transient bacteremia following dental or urogenital procedures — introduces the pathogen into the bloodstream. This infection causes fibrin and platelets to aggregate on the valve tissue and engulf circulating bacteria or fungi that flourish and form friable wartlike vegetative growths on the heart valves, the endocardial lining of a heart chamber, or the epithelium of a blood vessel. (See *Degenerative changes in endocarditis.*) Such growths may cover the valve surfaces, causing ulceration and necrosis; they may also extend to the chordae tendineae, leading to rupture and subsequent valvular insufficiency. Ultimately, they may embolize to the spleen, kidneys, central nervous system, and lungs.

CLINICAL FINDINGS

Early clinical features of endocarditis are usually nonspecific and include:

- malaise, weakness, fatigue
- weight loss, anorexia, arthralgia
- night sweats, chills
- valvular insufficiency
- in 90% of patients, an intermittent fever that may recur for weeks.

A more acute onset is associated with organisms of high pathogenicity such as *S. aureus*. Endocarditis commonly causes a loud, regurgitant murmur typical of the underlying heart lesion. A suddenly changing murmur or the discovery of a new murmur in the presence of fever is a classic physical sign of endocarditis.

In about 30% of patients, embolization from growing lesions or diseased valvular tissue may produce:
- splenic infarction — pain in the left upper quadrant, radiating to the left shoulder, and abdominal rigidity
- renal infarction — hematuria, pyuria, flank pain, and decreased urine output
- cerebral infarction — hemiparesis, aphasia, or other neurologic deficits
- pulmonary infarction (most common in right-sided endocarditis, which commonly occurs among I.V. drug abusers and after cardiac surgery) — cough, pleuritic pain, pleural friction rub, dyspnea, and hemoptysis
- peripheral vascular occlusion — numbness and tingling in an arm, leg, finger, or toe or signs of impending peripheral gangrene.

Other signs may include:
- splenomegaly
- petechiae of the skin (especially common on the upper anterior trunk) and buccal, pharyngeal, or conjunctival mucosa
- splinter hemorrhages under the nails.

Rarely, endocarditis produces:
- Osler's nodes (tender, raised, subcutaneous lesions on the fingers or toes)
- Roth's spots (hemorrhagic areas with white centers on the retina)
- Janeway lesions (purplish macules on the palms or soles).

TEST RESULTS
- Three or more blood cultures in a 24- to 48-hour period (each from a separate venipuncture) identify the causative organism in up to 90% of patients. Blood cultures should be drawn from three different sites, with 1 hour between each venipuncture.
- The remaining 10% of patients may have negative blood cultures, possibly suggesting fungal infection or infections that are difficult to diagnose such as *Haemophilus parainfluenzae*.

Other abnormal but nonspecific laboratory test results may include:
- normal or elevated white blood cell count
- abnormal histiocytes (macrophages)
- elevated erythrocyte sedimentation rate
- normocytic, normochromic anemia (in 70% to 90% of patients)
- proteinuria and microscopic hematuria (in about 50% of patients)
- positive serum rheumatoid factor (in about one-half of all patients after endocarditis is present for 3 to 6 weeks)
- valvular damage, identified by echocardiogram — particularly transesophageal echocardiogram
- atrial fibrillation and other arrhythmias that accompany valvular disease, identified by electrocardiogram.

TREATMENT
- Treatment goal to eradicate the infecting organism; first-line therapy

usually a combination of penicillin and an aminoglycoside, typically gentamicin
- Antimicrobial therapy usually starting promptly and continuing over 4 to 6 weeks
- Selection of an antibiotic based on identification of the infecting organism and on sensitivity studies (While awaiting results, or if blood cultures are negative, empiric antimicrobial therapy is based on the likely infecting organism.)
- Supportive treatment, including bed rest, aspirin for fever and aches, and sufficient fluid intake
- Severe valvular damage, especially aortic or mitral insufficiency, requires corrective surgery if refractory heart failure develops or in cases requiring that an infected prosthetic valve be replaced

NURSING CONSIDERATIONS

- Before giving antibiotics, obtain a patient history of allergies. Administer antibiotics on time to maintain consistent antibiotic blood levels.
- Observe for signs of infiltration or inflammation at the venipuncture site, possible complications of long-term I.V. drug administration. To reduce the risk of these complications, rotate venous access sites.
- Watch for signs of embolization (hematuria, pleuritic chest pain, left upper quadrant pain, or paresis), a common occurrence during the first 3 months of treatment. Tell the patient to watch for and report these signs, which may indicate impending peripheral vascular occlusion or splenic, renal, cerebral, or pulmonary infarction.
- Monitor the patient's renal status (blood urea nitrogen levels, creatinine clearance, and urine output) to check

for signs of renal emboli or evidence of drug toxicity.
- Observe for signs of heart failure, such as dyspnea, tachypnea, tachycardia, crackles, jugular vein distention, edema, and weight gain.
- Teach the patient about antibiotic prophylaxis against endocarditis.
- Provide reassurance by teaching the patient and his family about this disease and the need for prolonged treatment. Tell them to watch closely for fever, anorexia, and other signs of relapse about 2 weeks after treatment stops. Suggest quiet diversionary activities to prevent excessive physical exertion.
- Make sure that the patient who's susceptible to endocarditis understands the need for prophylactic antibiotics before, during, and after dental work, childbirth, and genitourinary, GI, or gynecologic procedures.
- Teach the patient how to recognize symptoms of endocarditis, and tell him to notify the physician immediately if such symptoms occur.

Heart failure

A syndrome rather than a disease, heart failure occurs when the heart can't pump enough blood to meet the body's metabolic needs. Heart failure results in intravascular and interstitial volume overload and poor tissue perfusion. An individual with heart failure experiences reduced exercise tolerance, a reduced quality of life, and a shortened life span.

Although the most common cause of heart failure is coronary artery disease (CAD), it also occurs in infants, children, and adults with congenital and acquired heart defects. The inci-

CAUSES OF HEART FAILURE

CAUSE	EXAMPLES
Abnormal cardiac muscle function	◆ Myocardial infarction ◆ Cardiomyopathy
Abnormal left ventricular volume	◆ Valvular insufficiency ◆ High-output states: – Chronic anemia – Arteriovenous fistula – Thyrotoxicosis – Pregnancy – Septicemia – Beriberi – Infusion of a large volume of I.V. fluids in a short period
Abnormal left ventricular pressure	◆ Hypertension ◆ Pulmonary hypertension ◆ Chronic obstructive pulmonary disease ◆ Aortic or pulmonic valve stenosis
Abnormal left ventricular filling	◆ Mitral valve stenosis ◆ Tricuspid valve stenosis ◆ Atrial myxoma ◆ Constrictive pericarditis ◆ Atrial fibrillation ◆ Impaired ventricular relaxation: – Hypertension – Myocardial hibernation – Myocardial stunning

dence of heart failure increases with age. Approximately 1% of people older than age 50 experience heart failure; it occurs in 10% of people older than age 80. About 700,000 U.S. residents die of heart failure each year. Mortality from heart failure is greater for males, blacks, and elderly people.

Although advances in diagnostic and therapeutic techniques have greatly improved the outlook for patients with heart failure, the prognosis still depends on the underlying cause and its response to treatment.

CAUSES

Causes of heart failure may be divided into four general categories. (See *Causes of heart failure*.)

PATHOPHYSIOLOGY

Heart failure may be classified according to the side of the heart affected (left- or right-sided heart failure) or by the cardiac cycle involved (systolic or diastolic dysfunction).

Left-sided heart failure

Left-sided heart failure occurs as a result of ineffective left ventricular contractile function. As the pumping ability of the left ventricle fails, cardiac output falls. Blood is no longer effectively pumped out into the body; it backs up into the left atrium and then into the lungs, causing pulmonary congestion, dyspnea, and activity intolerance. If the condition persists, pulmonary edema and right-sided heart failure may result. Common causes include left ventricular infarction, hypertension, and aortic and mitral valve stenosis.

Right-sided heart failure

Right-sided heart failure results from ineffective right ventricular contractile function. Consequently, blood isn't pumped effectively through the right ventricle to the lungs, causing blood to back up into the right atrium and the peripheral circulation. The patient gains weight and develops peripheral edema and engorgement of the kidney and other organs. It may be due to an acute right ventricular infarction, pulmonary hypertension, or a pulmonary embolus. However, the most common cause is profound backward blood flow due to left-sided heart failure.

Systolic dysfunction

Systolic dysfunction occurs when the left ventricle can't pump enough blood out to the systemic circulation during systole and the ejection fraction falls. Consequently, blood backs up into the pulmonary circulation and pressure increases in the pulmonary venous system. Cardiac output falls; weakness, fatigue, and shortness of breath may occur. Causes of systolic dysfunction include myocardial infarction and dilated cardiomyopathy.

Diastolic dysfunction

Diastolic dysfunction occurs when the ability of the left ventricle to relax and fill during diastole is reduced and the stroke volume falls. Therefore, higher volumes are needed in the ventricles to maintain cardiac output. Consequently, pulmonary congestion and peripheral edema develop. Diastolic dysfunction may occur as a result of left ventricular hypertrophy, hypertension, or restrictive cardiomyopathy. This type of heart failure is less common than systolic dysfunction, and its treatment isn't as clear.

All causes of heart failure eventually lead to reduced cardiac output, which triggers compensatory mechanisms, such as increased sympathetic activity, activation of the renin-angiotensin-aldosterone system, ventricular dilation, and hypertrophy. These mechanisms improve cardiac output at the expense of increased ventricular work.

Increased sympathetic activity — a response to decreased cardiac output and blood pressure — enhances peripheral vascular resistance, contractility, heart rate, and venous return. Signs of increased sympathetic activity, such as cool extremities and clamminess, may indicate impending heart failure.

Increased sympathetic activity also restricts blood flow to the kidneys, causing them to secrete renin, which in turn converts angiotensinogen to angiotensin I, which then becomes angiotensin II — a potent vasoconstrictor. Angiotensin causes the adrenal cortex to release aldosterone, leading to sodium and water retention and an increase in circulating blood volume. This renal mechanism is initially helpful; however, if it persists unchecked, it can aggravate heart failure as the heart struggles to pump against the increased volume.

In ventricular dilation, an increase in end-diastolic ventricular volume (preload) causes increased stroke work and stroke volume during contraction, stretching cardiac muscle fibers so that the ventricle can accept the increased intravascular volume. Eventually, the muscle becomes stretched beyond optimum limits and contractility declines.

In ventricular hypertrophy, an increase in ventricular muscle mass allows the heart to pump against increased resistance to the outflow of blood, improving cardiac output. However, this increased muscle mass also increases myocardial oxygen requirements. An increase in the ventricular diastolic pressure necessary to fill the enlarged ventricle may compromise diastolic coronary blood flow, limiting the oxygen supply to the ventricle and causing ischemia and impaired muscle contractility.

In heart failure, counterregulatory substances — prostaglandins and atrial natriuretic factor — are produced in an attempt to reduce the negative effects of volume overload and vasoconstriction caused by the compensatory mechanisms.

The kidneys release the prostaglandins prostacyclin and prostaglandin E2, which are potent vasodilators. These vasodilators also act to reduce volume overload produced by the renin-angiotensin-aldosterone system by inhibiting sodium and water reabsorption by the kidneys.

Atrial natriuretic factor is a hormone secreted mainly by the atria in response to stimulation of the stretch receptors in the atria caused by excess fluid volume. B-type natriuretic factor is secreted by the ventricles because of fluid volume overload. These natriuretic factors work to counteract the negative effects of sympathetic nervous system stimulation and the renin-angiotensin-aldosterone system by producing vasodilation and diuresis.

CLINICAL FINDINGS
Left-sided heart failure (early stages)
- Dyspnea caused by pulmonary congestion
- Orthopnea as blood is redistributed from the legs to the central circulation when the patient lies down
- Paroxysmal nocturnal dyspnea due to the reabsorption of interstitial fluid when lying down and reduced sympathetic stimulation while sleeping
- Fatigue associated with reduced oxygenation and an inability to increase cardiac output in response to physical activity
- Nonproductive cough associated with pulmonary congestion

Left-sided heart failure (late stages)
- Crackles due to pulmonary congestion
- Hemoptysis resulting from bleeding veins in the bronchial system caused by venous distention
- Point of maximal impulse displaced toward the left anterior axillary line caused by left ventricular hypertrophy
- Tachycardia due to sympathetic stimulation
- S_3 caused by rapid ventricular filling
- S_4 resulting from atrial contraction against a noncompliant ventricle
- Cool, pale skin resulting from peripheral vasoconstriction
- Restlessness and confusion due to reduced cardiac output

Right-sided heart failure
- Elevated jugular vein distention due to venous congestion
- Positive hepatojugular reflux and hepatomegaly secondary to venous congestion

- Right upper quadrant pain caused by liver engorgement
- Anorexia, fullness, and nausea, which may be due to congestion of the liver and intestines
- Nocturia as fluid is redistributed at night and reabsorbed
- Weight gain due to sodium and water retention
- Edema associated with fluid volume excess
- Ascites or anasarca caused by fluid retention

TEST RESULTS
- Chest X-rays show increased pulmonary vascular markings, interstitial edema, or pleural effusion and cardiomegaly.
- Electrocardiography may indicate hypertrophy, ischemic changes, or infarction and may also reveal tachycardia and extrasystoles.
- Laboratory testing may reveal abnormal liver function tests and elevated blood urea nitrogen (BUN) and creatinine levels. Prothrombin time may be prolonged as congestion impairs the liver's ability to synthesize procoagulants.
- Brain natriuretic peptide (BNP) assay levels may be elevated. Along with such clinical signs as edematous ankles, elevated BNP levels strongly indicate heart failure.
- Echocardiography may reveal left ventricular hypertrophy, dilation, and abnormal contractility.
- Pulmonary artery monitoring typically demonstrates elevated pulmonary artery and pulmonary artery wedge pressures, left ventricular end-diastolic pressure in left-sided heart failure, and elevated right atrial pressure or central venous pressure in right-sided heart failure.

- Radionuclide ventriculography may reveal an ejection fraction less than 40%; in diastolic dysfunction, the ejection fraction may be normal.

TREATMENT
- Treatment of the underlying cause, if known
- Angiotensin-converting enzyme (ACE) inhibitors for patients with left ventricular dysfunction to reduce production of angiotensin II, resulting in preload and afterload reduction

Alert *An elderly patient may require lower doses of ACE inhibitors because of impaired renal clearance. Monitor him for severe hypotension, signifying a toxic effect.*
- Digoxin for the patient with heart failure due to left ventricular systolic dysfunction to increase myocardial contractility, improve cardiac output, reduce the volume of the ventricle, and decrease ventricular stretch
- Diuretics to reduce fluid volume overload and venous return
- Beta-adrenergic blockers in the patient with New York Heart Association (NYHA) class II or III heart failure caused by left ventricular systolic dysfunction to prevent remodeling (see *Classifying heart failure,* page 38)
- Inotropic therapy with dobutamine or milrinone for acute treatment of heart failure exacerbation
- Chronic or chronic intermittent inotropic therapy to augment ventricular contractility to avoid exacerbations of heart failure in the patient with NYHA class IV heart failure
- Nesiritide, a human B-type natriuretic peptide, to augment diuresis and to decrease afterload in acute management of heart failure exacerbation
- Diuretics, nitrates, morphine, and oxygen to treat pulmonary edema

- Lifestyle modifications (to reduce symptoms of heart failure), such as weight loss (if overweight), limited sodium (3 g/day) and alcohol intake, reduced fat intake, smoking cessation, stress reduction, and development of an exercise program (Heart failure isn't a contraindication to exercise and cardiac rehabilitation.)
- Coronary artery bypass surgery or angioplasty for heart failure due to CAD
- Heart transplantation in the patient receiving aggressive medical treatment but still experiencing limitations or repeated hospitalizations
- Other surgery or invasive procedures possibly recommended in the patient having severe limitations or repeated hospitalizations despite maximal medical therapy (Some procedures are controversial and may include cardiomyoplasty, insertion of an intra-aortic balloon pump, use of a mechanical ventricular assist device, and implanting an internal cardioverter-defibrillator.)

Alert *Heart failure in children occurs mainly as a result of congenital heart defects. Therefore, treatment guidelines are directed toward the specific cause.*

NURSING CONSIDERATIONS
During acute phase
- Place the patient in Fowler's position and give him supplemental oxygen to help him breathe more easily.
- Weigh the patient daily, and check for peripheral edema. Carefully monitor I.V. intake and urine output, vital signs, and mental status. Auscultate the heart for abnormal sounds (S_3 gallop) and the lungs for crackles or rhonchi. Report changes at once.
- Frequently monitor BUN, creatinine, and serum potassium, sodium, chloride, and magnesium levels.

- Make sure the patient has continuous cardiac monitoring during acute and advanced stages to identify and treat arrhythmias promptly.
- To prevent deep vein thrombosis due to vascular congestion, assist the patient with range-of-motion exercises. Enforce bed rest, and apply antiembolism stockings. Check the patient regularly for calf pain and tenderness.
- Allow adequate rest periods.

Preparing for discharge
- Advise the patient to avoid foods high in sodium, such as canned or commercially prepared foods and dairy products, to curb fluid overload.
- Encourage the patient to participate in an outpatient cardiac rehabilitation program.
- Explain to the patient that the potassium he loses through diuretic therapy may need to be replaced by taking a prescribed potassium supplement and eating high-potassium foods, such as bananas and apricots.
- Stress the need for regular checkups.
- Stress the importance of taking digoxin exactly as prescribed. Tell the patient to watch for and immediately report signs of toxicity, such as anorexia, vomiting, and yellow vision.
- Tell the patient to notify the physician promptly if his pulse is unusually irregular or measures less than 60 beats/minute; if he experiences dizziness, blurred vision, shortness of breath, a persistent dry cough, palpitations, increased fatigue, paroxysmal nocturnal dyspnea, swollen ankles, or decreased urine output; or if he notices rapid weight gain (3 to 5 lb [1.5 to 2 kg] in 1 week).

Hypertension

Hypertension, an elevation in diastolic or systolic blood pressure, occurs as two major types: essential (primary) hypertension, the most common, and secondary hypertension, which results from renal disease or another identifiable cause. Malignant hypertension is a severe, fulminant form of hypertension common to both types. Hypertension is a major cause of stroke, cardiac disease, and renal failure.

Hypertension affects 15% to 20% of adults in the United States. The risk of hypertension increases with age and is higher for Blacks than Whites and in those with less education and lower income. Men have a higher incidence of hypertension in young and early middle adulthood; thereafter, women have a higher incidence.

Essential hypertension usually begins insidiously as a benign disease, slowly progressing to a malignant state. If untreated, even mild cases can cause major complications and death. Carefully managed treatment, which may include lifestyle modifications and drug therapy, improves the prognosis. Untreated, it carries a high mortality. Severely elevated blood pressure (hypertensive crisis) may be fatal.

CAUSES
Primary hypertension
- Advancing age

Alert Elderly people may have isolated systolic hypertension (ISH), in which just the systolic blood pressure is elevated, as atherosclerosis causes a loss of elasticity in large arteries. Previously, it was believed that ISH was a normal part of the aging process and shouldn't be treated. Results of the Systolic Hypertension in the Elderly Program, however, found that treating ISH with antihypertensive drugs lowered the incidence of stroke, coronary artery disease, and left-sided heart failure.

- Diabetes mellitus
- Excess renin
- Excessive alcohol consumption
- Family history
- High intake of saturated fat
- High intake of sodium
- Mineral deficiencies (calcium, potassium, and magnesium)
- Obesity
- Race (most common in blacks)

Alert Blacks are at an increased risk for primary hypertension when predisposition to low plasma renin levels diminishes the ability to excrete excess sodium. Hypertension develops at an earlier age and is more severe than in Whites.

- Sedentary lifestyle
- Sleep apnea
- Stress
- Tobacco use

Secondary hypertension
- Brain tumor, quadriplegia, and head injury
- Coarctation of the aorta
- Excessive alcohol consumption
- Gestational hypertension
- Hormonal contraceptives, cocaine, epoetin alfa, sympathetic stimulants, monoamine oxidase inhibitors taken with tyramine, estrogen replacement therapy, and nonsteroidal anti-inflammatory drugs
- Pheochromocytoma, Cushing's syndrome, hyperaldosteronism, and thyroid, pituitary, or parathyroid dysfunction
- Renal artery stenosis and parenchymal disease

PATHOPHYSIOLOGY
Arterial blood pressure is a product of total peripheral resistance and cardiac output. Cardiac output is increased by

conditions that increase heart rate, stroke volume, or both. Peripheral resistance is increased by factors that increase blood viscosity or reduce the lumen size of vessels, especially the arterioles.

Several theories help to explain the development of hypertension, including:

- changes in the arteriolar bed, causing increased peripheral vascular resistance
- abnormally increased tone in the sympathetic nervous system that originates in the vasomotor system centers, causing increased peripheral vascular resistance
- increased blood volume resulting from renal or hormonal dysfunction
- an increase in arteriolar thickening caused by genetic factors, leading to increased peripheral vascular resistance
- abnormal renin release, resulting in the formation of angiotensin II, which constricts the arteriole and increases blood volume. (See *Understanding blood pressure regulation,* page 52.)

Prolonged hypertension increases the heart's workload as resistance to left ventricular ejection increases. To increase contractile force, the left ventricle hypertrophies, raising the heart's oxygen demands and workload. Cardiac dilation and failure may occur when hypertrophy can no longer maintain sufficient cardiac output. Because hypertension promotes coronary atherosclerosis, the heart may be further compromised by reduced blood flow to the myocardium, resulting in angina or myocardial infarction (MI). Hypertension also causes vascular damage, leading to accelerated atherosclerosis and target organ damage, such as retinal injury, renal failure, stroke, and aortic aneurysm and dis-

section. (See *What happens in hypertensive crisis,* page 53.)

The pathophysiology of secondary hypertension is related to the underlying disease. For example:

- The most common cause of secondary hypertension is chronic renal disease. Insult to the kidney from chronic glomerulonephritis or renal artery stenosis interferes with sodium excretion, the renin-angiotensin-aldosterone system, or renal perfusion, causing blood pressure to increase.
- In Cushing's syndrome, increased cortisol levels raise blood pressure by increasing renal sodium retention, angiotensin II levels, and vascular response to norepinephrine.
- In primary aldosteronism, increased intravascular volume, altered sodium concentrations in vessel walls, or very high aldosterone levels cause vasoconstriction and increased resistance.
- Pheochromocytoma is a chromaffin cell tumor of the adrenal medulla that secretes epinephrine and norepinephrine. Epinephrine increases cardiac contractility and rate, whereas norepinephrine increases peripheral vascular resistance.

CLINICAL FINDINGS

Although hypertension usually produces no symptoms, these signs and symptoms may occur:

- elevated blood pressure readings on at least two consecutive occasions after initial screening

Alert Because many older adults have a wide auscultatory gap — the hiatus between the first Korotkoff sound and the next sound — failure to pump the blood pressure cuff up high enough can lead to missing the first beat and underestimating systolic blood pressure. To avoid missing the

UNDERSTANDING BLOOD PRESSURE REGULATION

Hypertension may result from a disturbance in one of these intrinsic mechanisms.

RENIN-ANGIOTENSIN SYSTEM

The renin-angiotensin system acts to increase blood pressure through these mechanisms:
◆ sodium depletion, reduced blood pressure, and dehydration, which stimulates renin release
◆ renin reacts with angiotensin, a liver enzyme, converting it to angiotensin I, which increases preload and afterload
◆ angiotensin I converts to angiotensin II in the lungs; angiotensin II is a potent vasoconstrictor that targets the arterioles
◆ angiotensin II works to increase preload and afterload by stimulating the adrenal cortex to secrete aldosterone; this increases blood volume by conserving sodium and water.

AUTOREGULATION

Several intrinsic mechanisms work to change an artery's diameter to maintain tissue and organ perfusion despite fluctuations in systemic blood pressure. These mechanisms include stress relaxation and capillary fluid shifts:
◆ In stress relaxation, blood vessels gradually dilate when blood pressure increases to reduce peripheral resistance.
◆ In capillary fluid shift, plasma moves between vessels and extravascular spaces to maintain intravascular volume.

SYMPATHETIC NERVOUS SYSTEM

When blood pressure drops, baroreceptors in the aortic arch and carotid sinuses decrease their inhibition of the medulla's vasomotor center. The consequent increases in sympathetic stimulation of the heart by norepinephrine increases cardiac output by strengthening the contractile force, raising the heart rate, and augmenting peripheral resistance by vasoconstriction. Stress can also stimulate the sympathetic nervous system to increase cardiac output and peripheral vascular resistance.

ANTIDIURETIC HORMONE

The release of antidiuretic hormone can regulate hypotension by increasing reabsorption of water by the kidney. With reabsorption, blood plasma volume increases, thus raising blood pressure.

first Korotkoff sound, palpate the radial artery and inflate the cuff to a point approximately 20 mm Hg beyond which the pulse beat disappears.

● occipital headache (may worsen on rising in the morning as a result of increased intracranial pressure); nausea and vomiting may also occur
● bruits (which may be heard over the abdominal aorta or carotid, renal, and femoral arteries) caused by stenosis or aneurysm
● dizziness, confusion, and fatigue caused by decreased tissue perfusion due to vasoconstriction of blood vessels
● blurry vision as a result of retinal damage
● nocturia caused by an increase in blood flow to the kidneys and an increase in glomerular filtration
● edema caused by increased capillary pressure.

If secondary hypertension exists, other signs and symptoms may be related to the cause. For example:
● Cushing's syndrome may cause truncal obesity and purple striae

Focus in

WHAT HAPPENS IN HYPERTENSIVE CRISIS

Hypertensive crisis is a severe increase in arterial blood pressure caused by a disturbance in one or more of the regulating mechanisms. If untreated, hypertensive crisis may result in renal, cardiac, or cerebral complications and, possibly, death.

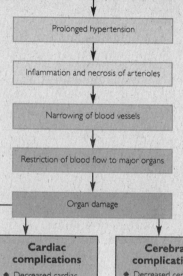

Causes of hypertensive crisis
- Abnormal renal function
- Hypertensive encephalopathy
- Intracerebral hemorrhage
- Withdrawal of antihypertensive drugs (abrupt)
- Myocardial ischemia
- Eclampsia
- Pheochromocytoma
- Monoamine oxidase inhibitor interactions

↓

Prolonged hypertension

↓

Inflammation and necrosis of arterioles

↓

Narrowing of blood vessels

↓

Restriction of blood flow to major organs

↓

Organ damage

Renal complications
- Decreased renal perfusion
- Progressive deterioration of nephrons
- Decreased ability to concentrate urine
- Increased serum creatinine and blood urea nitrogen levels
- Increased renal tubule permeability with protein leakage into tubules
- Renal insufficiency
- Uremia
- Renal failure

Cardiac complications
- Decreased cardiac perfusion
- Coronary artery disease
- Angina or myocardial infarction
- Increased cardiac workload
- Left ventricular hypertrophy
- Heart failure

Cerebral complications
- Decreased cerebral perfusion
- Increased stress on vessel wall
- Arterial spasm
- Ischemia
- Transient ischemic attacks
- Weakening of vessel intima
- Aneurysm formation
- Intracranial hemorrhage

In 2003, the National Institutes of Health issued *The Seventh Report of the Joint National Committee on Prevention, Detection, Evaluation, and Treatment of High Blood Pressure (The JNC 7 Report)*. Updates since *The JNC 6* report include a new category, prehypertension, and the combining of stages 2 and 3 hypertension. Categories now are normal, prehypertension, and stages 1 and 2 hypertension.

The revised categories are based on the average of two or more readings taken on separate visits after an initial screening. They apply to adults ages 18 and older. (If the systolic and diastolic pressures fall into different categories, use the higher of the two pressures to classify the reading. For example, a reading of 160/92 mm Hg should be classified as stage 2.)

Normal blood pressure with respect to cardiovascular risk is a systolic reading below 120 mm Hg and a diastolic reading below 80 mm Hg. Patients with prehypertension are at increased risk for developing hypertension and should follow health-promoting lifestyle modifications to prevent cardiovascular disease.

In addition to classifying stages of hypertension based on average blood pressure readings, health care providers should also take note of target organ disease and additional risk factors, such as a patient with diabetes, left ventricular hypertrophy, or chronic renal disease. This additional information is important to obtain a true picture of the patient's cardiovascular health.

Category	Systolic		Diastolic
Normal	< 120 mm Hg	AND	< 80 mm Hg
Prehypertension	120 to 139 mm Hg	OR	80 to 89 mm Hg
Hypertension Stage 1	140 to 159 mm Hg	OR	90 to 99 mm Hg
Stage 2	≥ 160 mm Hg	OR	≥ 100 mm Hg

● pheochromocytoma may cause headache, nausea, vomiting, palpitations, pallor, and profuse perspiration.

TEST RESULTS

● Serial blood pressure measurements may be useful. (See *Classifying blood pressure readings*.)
● Urinalysis may show protein, casts, red blood cells, or white blood cells, suggesting renal disease; presence of catecholamines associated with pheochromocytoma; or glucose, suggesting diabetes.
● Laboratory testing may reveal elevated blood urea nitrogen and serum creatinine levels suggestive of renal disease, or hypokalemia indicating adrenal dysfunction (primary hyperaldosteronism).
● Complete blood count may reveal other causes of hypertension, such as polycythemia or anemia.
● Excretory urography may reveal renal atrophy, indicating chronic renal disease. One kidney smaller than the other suggests unilateral renal disease.
● Electrocardiography may show left ventricular hypertrophy or ischemia.
● Chest X-rays may show cardiomegaly.
● Echocardiography may reveal left ventricular hypertrophy.

TREATMENT

The Seventh Report of the Joint National Committee on Prevention, Detection, Evaluation, and Treatment of High Blood Pressure of the National Institutes of Health, National Heart, Lung, and Blood Institute recommends:

- Lifestyle modification including weight reduction, use of a Dietary Approaches to Stop Hypertension diet (involves consumption of a diet rich in fruits, vegetables, and low-fat dairy products with a reduced content of saturated and total fat), reduction of dietary sodium intake, physical activity (regular aerobic activity such as brisk walking), and moderation of alcohol intake.
- If the patient fails to achieve the desired blood pressure or make significant progress, continue lifestyle modifications and begin drug therapy.
- For stage 1 hypertension in the absence of compelling indications (heart failure, postmyocardial infarction, high coronary disease risk, diabetes, chronic kidney disease, or recurrent stroke prevention), give most patients thiazide-type diuretics. Consider using an angiotensin-converting enzyme (ACE) inhibitor, angiotensin receptor blocker (ARB), beta-adrenergic blocker (BB), calcium channel blocker (CCB), or a combination.
- For stage 2 hypertension in the absence of compelling indications, give most patients a two-drug combination (usually a thiazide-type diuretic and an ACE inhibitor, ARB, BB, or CCB).
- If the patient has one or more compelling indications, base drug treatment on benefits from outcome studies or existing clinical guidelines. Treatment may include the following, depending on indication:

- Heart failure—diuretic, BB, ACE inhibitor, ARB, or aldosterone antagonist
- Postmyocardial infarction—BB, ACE inhibitor, or aldosterone antagonist
- High coronary disease risk—diuretic, BB, ACE inhibitor, or CCB
- Diabetes—diuretic, BB, ACE inhibitor, ARB, or CCB
- Chronic kidney disease—ACE inhibitor or ARB
- Recurrent stroke prevention—diuretic or ACE inhibitor.
- Give other antihypertensive drugs as needed.

Other treatments

- For secondary hypertension, focus on correcting the underlying cause and controlling hypertensive effects.
- Hypertensive emergencies require parenteral administration of a vasodilator or an adrenergic inhibitor or oral administration of a selected drug, such as nifedipine, captopril, clonidine, or labetalol, to rapidly reduce blood pressure. (Examples of hypertensive emergencies include hypertensive encephalopathy, intracranial hemorrhage, acute left-sided heart failure with pulmonary edema, and dissecting aortic aneurysm. They're also associated with eclampsia or severe gestational hypertension, unstable angina, and acute MI.)
- Initial goal requires reducing mean arterial blood pressure by no more than 25% (within minutes to hours) then to 160/110 mm Hg within 2 hours while avoiding excessive decreases in blood pressure that can precipitate renal, cerebral, or myocardial ischemia.
- Hypertension without accompanying symptoms or target-organ disease

seldom requires emergency drug therapy.

NURSING CONSIDERATIONS

● To encourage adherence to antihypertensive therapy, suggest that the patient establish a daily routine for taking his medication. Warn that uncontrolled hypertension may cause stroke and heart attack. Tell him to report adverse drug effects. Also, advise him to avoid high-sodium antacids and over-the-counter cold and sinus medications, which contain harmful vasoconstrictors.

● Encourage a change in dietary habits. Help the obese patient plan a weight-reduction diet; tell him to avoid high-sodium foods (pickles, potato chips, canned soups, and cold cuts) and table salt.

● Help the patient examine and modify his lifestyle (for example, by reducing stress and exercising regularly).

● If a patient is hospitalized with hypertension, find out if he was taking his prescribed medication. If he wasn't, ask why. If the patient can't afford the medication, refer him to an appropriate social service agency. Tell the patient and his family to keep a record of drugs used in the past, noting especially which ones were or weren't effective. Suggest recording this information on a card so that the patient can show it to his physician.

● When routine blood pressure screening reveals elevated pressure, make sure the cuff size is appropriate for the patient's upper arm circumference. Take the pressure in both arms in lying, sitting, and standing positions. Ask the patient whether he smoked, drank a beverage containing caffeine, or was emotionally upset before the test. Advise the patient to return for blood pressure testing at frequent, regular intervals.

● To help identify hypertension and prevent untreated hypertension, participate in public education programs dealing with hypertension and ways to reduce risk factors. Encourage public participation in blood pressure screening programs. Routinely screen all patients, especially those at risk (blacks and people with family histories of hypertension, stroke, or heart attack).

Patent ductus arteriosus

The ductus arteriosus is a fetal blood vessel that connects the pulmonary artery to the descending aorta, just distal to the left subclavian artery. Normally, the ductus closes within days to weeks after birth. In patent ductus arteriosus (PDA), the lumen of the ductus remains open after birth. This creates a left-to-right shunt of blood from the aorta to the pulmonary artery and results in recirculation of arterial blood through the lungs. Initially, PDA may produce no clinical effects, but over time it can precipitate pulmonary vascular disease, causing symptoms to appear by age 40. PDA affects twice as many females as males and is the most common acyanotic congenital heart defect found in adults.

The prognosis is good if the shunt is small or if surgical repair is effective. Otherwise, PDA may advance to intractable heart failure, which may be fatal.

CAUSES
● Coarctation of the aorta
● Living at high altitudes

- Premature birth, probably as a result of abnormalities in oxygenation or the relaxant action of prostaglandin E, which prevents ductal spasm and contracture necessary for closure
- Pulmonic and aortic stenosis
- Rubella syndrome
- Ventricular septal defect

PATHOPHYSIOLOGY

The ductus arteriosus normally closes as prostaglandin levels from the placenta fall and oxygen levels rise. This process should begin as soon as the neonate takes its first breath but may take as long as 3 months in some children.

In PDA, relative resistances in pulmonary and systemic vasculature and the size of the ductus determine the quantity of blood that's shunted from left to right. Because of increased aortic pressure, oxygenated blood is shunted from the aorta through the ductus arteriosus to the pulmonary artery. The blood returns to the left side of the heart and is pumped out to the aorta once more.

The left atrium and left ventricle must accommodate the increased pulmonary venous return, increasing filling pressure and workload on the left side of the heart and causing left ventricular hypertrophy and, possibly, heart failure. In the final stages of untreated PDA, the left-to-right shunt leads to chronic pulmonary artery hypertension that becomes fixed and unreactive. This causes the shunt to reverse so that unoxygenated blood enters systemic circulation, causing cyanosis.

CLINICAL FINDINGS

- Respiratory distress with signs of heart failure in infants, especially those who are premature, due to the tremendous volume of blood shunted to the lungs through a patent ductus and the increased workload on the left side of the heart
- Classic machinery murmur (Gibson murmur), a continuous murmur heard throughout systole and diastole in older children and adults as a result of shunting of blood from the aorta to the pulmonary artery throughout systole and diastole (It's best heard at the base of the heart, at the second left intercostal space under the left clavicle. The murmur may obscure S_2. However, in a right-to-left shunt, this murmur may be absent.)
- Thrill palpated at the left sternal border caused by the shunting of blood from the aorta to the pulmonary artery
- Prominent left ventricular impulse due to left ventricular hypertrophy
- Bounding peripheral pulses (Corrigan's pulse) due to the high-flow state
- Widened pulse pressure because of an elevated systolic blood pressure and, primarily, a drop in diastolic blood pressure as blood is shunted through the PDA, thus reducing peripheral resistance
- Slow motor development caused by heart failure
- Failure to thrive as a result of heart failure
- Fatigue and dyspnea on exertion, which may develop in adults with undetected PDA

TEST RESULTS

- Chest X-rays may show increased pulmonary vascular markings, prominent pulmonary arteries, and enlargement of the left ventricle and aorta.
- Electrocardiography (ECG) may be normal or may indicate left atrial or ventricular hypertrophy and, in pul-

monary vascular disease, biventricular hypertrophy.

- Echocardiography detects and estimates the size of a PDA. It also reveals an enlarged left atrium and left ventricle, or right ventricular hypertrophy from pulmonary vascular disease.
- Cardiac catheterization shows higher pulmonary arterial oxygen content than right ventricular content because of the influx of aortic blood. Increased pulmonary artery pressure indicates a large shunt or, if it exceeds systemic arterial pressure, severe pulmonary vascular disease. Cardiac catheterization allows for the calculation of blood volume crossing the ductus and can rule out associated cardiac defects. Injection of a contrast agent can conclusively demonstrate PDA.

TREATMENT

- Surgery to ligate the ductus if medical management can't control heart failure (Asymptomatic infants with PDA don't require immediate treatment. If symptoms are mild, surgical ligation of the PDA is usually delayed until age 1.)
- Indomethacin (a prostaglandin inhibitor) to induce ductus spasm and closure in premature infants
- Prophylactic antibiotics to protect against infective endocarditis
- Treatment of heart failure with fluid restriction, diuretics, and digoxin
- Other therapy, including cardiac catheterization, to deposit a plug or umbrella in the ductus to stop shunting

NURSING CONSIDERATIONS

- PDA necessitates careful monitoring, patient and family teaching, and emotional support.
- Watch carefully for signs of PDA in all premature neonates.

- Be alert for respiratory distress symptoms resulting from heart failure, which may develop rapidly in a premature infant. Frequently assess vital signs, ECG, electrolyte levels, and intake and output. Record response to diuretics and other therapy.
- If the infant receives indomethacin for ductus closure, watch for possible adverse effects, such as diarrhea, jaundice, bleeding, and renal dysfunction.
- Before surgery, carefully explain all treatments and tests to parents. Include the child in your explanations. Arrange for the child and parents to meet the intensive care unit staff. Tell them about expected I.V. lines, monitoring equipment, and postoperative procedures.
- Immediately after surgery, the child may have a central venous pressure catheter and an arterial line in place. Carefully assess vital signs, intake and output, and arterial and venous pressures. Provide pain relief as needed.
- Before discharge, review instructions to the parents about activity restrictions based on the child's tolerance and energy levels. Advise parents not to become overprotective as their child's tolerance for physical activity increases.
- Stress the need for regular medical follow-up examinations. Advise parents to inform any physician who treats their child about his history of surgery for PDA — even if the child is being treated for an unrelated medical problem.

Pericarditis

Pericarditis is an inflammation of the pericardium — the fibroserous sac that envelops, supports, and protects the heart. It occurs in acute and chronic forms. Acute pericarditis can be fibrinous or effusive, with purulent, serous, or hemorrhagic exudate. Chronic constrictive pericarditis is characterized by dense fibrous pericardial thickening.

The prognosis depends on the underlying cause but is generally good in acute pericarditis, unless constriction occurs.

CAUSES
- Aortic aneurysm with pericardial leakage (less common)
- Bacterial, fungal, or viral infection (infectious pericarditis)
- Drugs, such as hydralazine (Apresoline) or procainamide
- High-dose radiation to the chest
- Hypersensitivity or autoimmune disease, such as acute rheumatic fever (most common cause of pericarditis in children), systemic lupus erythematosus, and rheumatoid arthritis
- Idiopathic factors (most common in acute pericarditis)
- Myxedema with cholesterol deposits in the pericardium (less common)
- Neoplasms (primary, or metastasis from lungs, breasts, or other organs)
- Previous cardiac injury, such as myocardial infarction (Dressler's syndrome), trauma, or surgery (postcardiotomy syndrome), that leaves the pericardium intact but causes blood to leak into the pericardial cavity
- Uremia

PATHOPHYSIOLOGY
Pericardial tissue damaged by bacteria or other substances results in the release of chemical mediators of inflammation (prostaglandins, histamines, bradykinins, and serotonin) into the surrounding tissue, thereby initiating the inflammatory process. Friction occurs as the inflamed pericardial layers rub against one another. Histamines and other chemical mediators dilate vessels and increase vessel permeability. Vessel walls then leak fluids and protein (including fibrinogen) into tissues, causing extracellular edema. Macrophages already present in the tissue begin to phagocytize the invading bacteria and are joined by neutrophils and monocytes. After several days, the area fills with an exudate composed of necrotic tissue and dead and dying bacteria, neutrophils, and macrophages. Eventually, the contents of the cavity autolyze and are gradually reabsorbed into healthy tissue.

A pericardial effusion develops if fluid accumulates in the pericardial cavity. Cardiac tamponade results when there's a rapid accumulation of fluid in the pericardial space, compressing the heart and preventing it from filling during diastole and resulting in a drop in cardiac output. (See *Understanding cardiac tamponade*, page 28.)

Chronic constrictive pericarditis develops if the pericardium becomes thick and stiff from chronic or recurrent pericarditis, encasing the heart in a stiff shell and preventing it from properly filling during diastole. This causes an increase in left- and right-sided filling pressures, leading to a drop in stroke volume and cardiac output.

CLINICAL FINDINGS
- Pericardial friction rub caused by the roughened pericardial membranes rubbing against one another (Although rub may be heard intermittently, it's best heard when the patient leans forward and exhales.)

- Sharp and typically sudden pain, usually starting over the sternum and radiating to the neck (especially the left trapezius ridge), shoulders, back, and arms due to inflammation and irritation of the pericardial membranes (The pain is typically pleuritic, increasing with deep inspiration and decreasing when the patient sits up and leans forward, pulling the heart away from the diaphragmatic pleurae of the lungs.)
- Shallow, rapid respirations to reduce pleuritic pain
- Mild fever caused by the inflammatory process
- Dyspnea, orthopnea, and tachycardia as well as other signs of heart failure may occur as fluid builds up in the pericardial space, causing pericardial effusion, a major complication of acute pericarditis
- Muffled and distant heart sounds due to fluid buildup
- Pallor, clammy skin, hypotension, pulsus paradoxus, jugular vein distention and, eventually, cardiovascular collapse may occur with the rapid fluid accumulation of cardiac tamponade
- Fluid retention, ascites, hepatomegaly, jugular vein distention, and other signs of chronic right-sided heart failure may occur with chronic constrictive pericarditis as the systemic venous pressure gradually increases
- Pericardial knock in early diastole along the left sternal border produced by restricted ventricular filling
- Kussmaul's sign (increased jugular vein distention on inspiration) due to restricted right-sided filling

TEST RESULTS
- Electrocardiography may reveal diffuse ST-segment elevation in the limb leads and most precordial leads that reflects the inflammatory process.

Downsloping PR segments and upright T waves are present in most leads. QRS segments may be diminished when pericardial effusion exists. Arrhythmias, such as atrial fibrillation and sinus arrhythmias, may occur. In chronic constrictive pericarditis, there may be low-voltage QRS complexes, T-wave inversion or flattening, and P mitrale (wide P waves) in leads I, II, and V_6.
- Laboratory testing may reveal an elevated erythrocyte sedimentation rate as a result of the inflammatory process, or a normal or elevated white blood cell count, especially in infectious pericarditis; blood urea nitrogen tests may detect uremia as a cause of pericarditis.
- Blood cultures may identify an infectious cause.
- Antistreptolysin-O titers may be positive if pericarditis is due to rheumatic fever.
- Purified protein derivative skin test may be positive if pericarditis is due to tuberculosis.
- Echocardiography may show an echo-free space between the ventricular wall and the pericardium and reduced pumping action of the heart.
- Chest X-rays may be normal with acute pericarditis. The cardiac silhouette may be enlarged with a water bottle shape caused by fluid accumulation if pleural effusion is present.

TREATMENT
- Bed rest as long as fever and pain persist, to reduce metabolic needs
- Treatment of the underlying cause if it can be identified
- Nonsteroidal anti-inflammatory drugs (NSAIDs), such as aspirin and indomethacin (Indocin), to relieve pain and reduce inflammation

- Corticosteroids, if NSAIDs are ineffective and no infection exists (Corticosteroids must be administered cautiously because episodes may recur when therapy is discontinued.)
- Antibacterial, antifungal, or antiviral therapy if an infectious cause is suspected
- Pericardiocentesis to remove excess fluid from the pericardial space
- Partial pericardectomy, for recurrent pericarditis, to create a window that allows fluid to drain into the pleural space
- Total pericardectomy, for constrictive pericarditis, to permit adequate filling and contraction of the heart
- Idiopathic pericarditis possibly benign and self-limiting

NURSING CONSIDERATIONS

A patient with pericarditis needs complete bed rest. In addition, health care includes:
- assessing pain in relation to respiration and body position to distinguish pericardial pain from myocardial ischemic pain
- placing the patient in an upright position to relieve dyspnea and chest pain, providing analgesics and oxygen, and reassuring the patient with acute pericarditis that his condition is temporary and treatable
- monitoring for signs of cardiac compression or cardiac tamponade and possible complications of pericardial effusion, which include decreased blood pressure, increased central venous pressure, and pulsus paradoxus (Because cardiac tamponade requires immediate treatment, keep a pericardiocentesis set handy whenever pericardial effusion is suspected.)
- explaining tests and treatments to the patient. If surgery is necessary, he should learn deep-breathing and

coughing exercises before the procedure. Postoperative care is similar to that given after cardiothoracic surgery.

Raynaud's disease

Raynaud's disease is one of several primary arteriospastic disorders characterized by episodic vasospasm in the small peripheral arteries and arterioles, precipitated by exposure to cold or stress. This condition occurs bilaterally and usually affects the hands or, less commonly, the feet. Raynaud's disease is most prevalent in females, particularly between puberty and age 40. It's a benign condition, requiring no specific treatment and causing no serious sequelae.

Raynaud's phenomenon, however, a condition usually associated with several connective disorders — such as scleroderma, systemic lupus erythematosus (SLE), or polymyositis — has a progressive course, leading to ischemia, gangrene, and amputation. Distinguishing between the two disorders is difficult because some patients who experience mild symptoms of Raynaud's disease for several years may later develop overt connective tissue disease, especially scleroderma.

CAUSES

Although family history is a risk factor, the cause of Raynaud's disease is unknown.

Raynaud's phenomenon may develop secondary to:
- arterio-occlusive disease
- connective tissue disorders, such as scleroderma, rheumatoid arthritis, SLE, or polymyositis
- exposure to heavy metals

- long-term exposure to cold, vibrating machinery (such as operating a jackhammer), or pressure to the fingertips (such as in typists and pianists)
- myxedema
- previous damage from cold exposure
- pulmonary hypertension
- serum sickness
- thoracic outlet syndrome
- trauma.

PATHOPHYSIOLOGY

Although the cause is unknown, several theories account for reduced digital blood flow, including:
- intrinsic vascular wall hyperactivity to cold
- increased vasomotor tone due to sympathetic stimulation
- antigen-antibody immune response (the most likely theory because abnormal immunologic test results accompany Raynaud's phenomenon).

CLINICAL FINDINGS

- Blanching of the fingers bilaterally after exposure to cold or stress as vasoconstriction or vasospasm reduces blood flow (This is followed by cyanosis due to increased oxygen extraction resulting from sluggish blood flow. As the spasm resolves, the fingers turn red as blood rushes back into the arterioles.)
- Cold and numbness, possibly occurring during the vasoconstrictive phase because of ischemia
- Throbbing, aching pain, swelling, and tingling, possibly occurring during the hyperemic phase
- Trophic changes, such as sclerodactyly, ulcerations, or chronic paronychia, possibly occurring as a result of ischemia in long-standing disease
- Normal arterial pulses

- History of symptoms for at least 2 years

TEST RESULTS

- Antinuclear antibody (ANA) titer is used to identify autoimmune disease as an underlying cause of Raynaud's phenomenon; further tests must be performed if ANA titer is positive.
- Arteriography rules out arterial occlusive disease.
- Doppler ultrasonography may show reduced blood flow if symptoms result from arterial occlusive disease.

TREATMENT

- Teaching the patient to avoid triggers, such as cold and mechanical or chemical injury
- Encouraging the patient to stop smoking and to avoid decongestants and caffeine to reduce vasoconstriction
- Keeping fingers and toes warm to reduce vasoconstriction
- Calcium channel blockers, such as nifedipine, diltiazem (Cardizem), and nicardipine (Cardene), to produce vasodilation and prevent vasospasm
- Beta-adrenergic blockers, such as phenoxybenzamine (Dibenzyline) or reserpine, which may improve blood flow to fingers or toes
- Biofeedback and relaxation exercises to reduce stress and improve circulation
- Sympathectomy to prevent ischemic ulcers by promoting vasodilation (necessary in less than 25% of patients)
- Amputation, if ischemia causes ulceration and gangrene

NURSING CONSIDERATIONS

- Warn the patient against exposure to the cold. Tell her to wear mittens or gloves in cold weather or when handling cold items or defrosting the freezer.

● Advise the patient to avoid stressful situations and to stop smoking.

● Instruct the patient to inspect her skin frequently and to seek immediate care for signs of skin breakdown or infection.

● Teach the patient about drugs, their use, and their adverse effects.

● Provide psychological support and reassurance to allay the patient's fear of amputation and disfigurement.

Rheumatic fever and rheumatic heart disease

A systemic inflammatory disease of childhood, acute rheumatic fever develops after infection of the upper respiratory tract with group A beta-hemolytic streptococci. It mainly involves the heart, joints, central nervous system, skin, and subcutaneous tissues and commonly recurs. *Rheumatic heart disease* refers to the cardiac manifestations of rheumatic fever and includes pancarditis (myocarditis, pericarditis, and endocarditis) during the early acute phase and chronic valvular disease later. Cardiac involvement develops in up to 50% of patients.

Worldwide, 15 to 20 million new cases of rheumatic fever are reported each year. The disease typically strikes during cool, damp weather in the winter and early spring. In the United States, it's most common in the North.

Rheumatic fever tends to run in families, lending support to the existence of genetic predisposition. Environmental factors also seem to be significant in the development of the disorder. For example, in lower socioeconomic groups, the incidence is highest in children between ages 5 and 15, probably because of malnutrition and crowded living conditions.

Patients without carditis or with mild carditis have a good long-term prognosis. Severe pancarditis occasionally produces fatal heart failure during the acute phase. Of patients who survive this complication, about 20% die within 10 years. Antibiotic therapy has greatly reduced the mortality of rheumatic heart disease.

CAUSES

● Group A beta-hemolytic streptococcal pharyngitis

PATHOPHYSIOLOGY

Rheumatic fever appears to be a hypersensitivity reaction to group A beta-hemolytic streptococcal infection. Because very few persons (3%) with streptococcal infections contract rheumatic fever, altered host resistance must be involved in its development or recurrence. The antigens of group A streptococci bind to receptors in the heart, muscle, brain, and synovial joints, causing an autoimmune response. Because of a similarity between the antigens of the streptococcus bacteria and the antigens of the body's own cells, antibodies may attack healthy body cells by mistake.

Carditis may affect the endocardium, myocardium, or pericardium during the early acute phase. Later, the heart valves may be damaged, causing chronic valvular disease.

Pericarditis produces a serofibrinous effusion. Myocarditis produces characteristic lesions called Aschoff bodies (fibrin deposits surrounded by necrosis) in the interstitial tissue of the heart as well as cellular swelling and fragmentation of interstitial collagen. These lesions lead to progressively fibrotic nodule and interstitial scar formation.

Endocarditis causes valve leaflet swelling, erosion along the lines of leaflet closure, and blood, platelet, and fibrin deposits, which form beadlike growths. Eventually, the valve leaflets become scarred, lose their elasticity, and begin to adhere to one another. Endocarditis strikes the mitral valve most commonly in females and the aortic valve in males. In both sexes, it occasionally affects the tricuspid valve and, rarely, the pulmonic valve.

CLINICAL FINDINGS

The classic signs and symptoms of rheumatic fever and rheumatic heart disease include:

- polyarthritis or migratory joint pain, caused by inflammation, occurring in most patients (Swelling, redness, and signs of effusion usually accompany such pain, which most commonly affects the knees, ankles, elbows, and hips.)
- erythema marginatum, a nonpruritic, macular, transient rash on the trunk or inner aspects of the upper arms or thighs, that gives rise to red lesions with blanched centers
- subcutaneous nodules — firm, movable, and nontender, about 3 mm to 2 cm in diameter, usually near tendons or bony prominences of joints, especially the elbows, knuckles, wrists, and knees (They commonly accompany carditis and may last a few days to several weeks.)
- chorea — rapid jerky movements — possibly developing up to 6 months after the original streptococcal infec-

tion. (Mild chorea may produce hyperirritability, a deterioration in handwriting, or inability to concentrate. Severe chorea causes purposeless, nonrepetitive, involuntary muscle spasms; poor muscle coordination; and weakness.)

Other signs and symptoms of rheumatic fever and rheumatic heart disease include:

- a streptococcal infection a few days to 6 weeks earlier, occurring in 95% of those with rheumatic fever
- temperature of at least 100.4° F (38° C) due to infection and inflammation
- a new mitral or aortic heart murmur, or a worsening murmur in a person with a preexisting murmur
- pericardial friction rub caused by inflamed pericardial membranes rubbing against one another, if pericarditis exists
- chest pain, typically pleuritic, due to inflammation and irritation of the pericardial membranes (Pain may increase with deep inspiration and decrease when the patient sits up and leans forward, pulling the heart away from the diaphragmatic pleurae of the lungs.)
- dyspnea, tachypnea, nonproductive cough, bibasilar crackles, and edema due to heart failure in severe rheumatic carditis.

TEST RESULTS

- Jones criteria revealing either two major criteria, or one major criterion and two minor criteria, plus evidence of a previous group A streptococcal infection are necessary for diagnosis. (See *Jones criteria for diagnosing rheumatic fever.*)
- White blood cell count and erythrocyte sedimentation rate may be elevated during the acute phase.

- Hemoglobin analysis and hematocrit may show slight anemia due to suppressed erythropoiesis during inflammation.
- C-reactive protein may be positive, especially during the acute phase.
- Cardiac enzyme levels may be increased in severe carditis.
- Antistreptolysin-O titer may be elevated in 95% of patients within 2 months of onset.
- Throat cultures may continue to show the presence of group A beta-hemolytic streptococci; however, they usually occur in small numbers.
- Electrocardiography may show changes that aren't diagnostic, but the PR interval is prolonged in 20% of patients.
- Chest X-rays may show normal heart size or cardiomegaly, pericardial effusion, or heart failure.
- Echocardiography can detect valvular damage and pericardial effusion and can measure chamber size and provide information on ventricular function.
- Cardiac catheterization provides information on valvular damage and left ventricular function.

TREATMENT
- Prompt treatment of all group A beta-hemolytic streptococcal pharyngitis with oral penicillin V or I.M. penicillin G benzathine, or erythromycin for patients with penicillin hypersensitivity
- Salicylates to relieve fever and pain and minimize joint swelling
- Corticosteroids if the patient has carditis or if salicylates fail to relieve pain and inflammation
- Strict bed rest for about 5 weeks for the patient with active carditis to reduce cardiac demands

---

JONES CRITERIA FOR DIAGNOSING RHEUMATIC FEVER

The Jones criteria are used to standardize the diagnosis of rheumatic fever. Diagnosis requires that the patient have either two major criteria, or one major criterion and two minor criteria, plus evidence of a previous streptococcal infection.

MAJOR CRITERIA
- Carditis
- Migratory polyarthritis
- Sydenham's chorea
- Subcutaneous nodules
- Erythema marginatum

MINOR CRITERIA
- Fever
- Arthralgia
- Elevated acute phase reactants
- Prolonged PR interval

- Bed rest, sodium restriction, angiotensin-converting enzyme inhibitors, digoxin, and diuretics to treat heart failure
- Corrective surgery, such as commissurotomy (separation of adherent, thickened valve leaflets of the mitral valve), valvuloplasty (inflation of a balloon within a valve), or valve replacement (with a prosthetic valve) for severe mitral or aortic valvular dysfunction that causes persistent heart failure
- Secondary prevention of rheumatic fever, which begins after the acute phase subsides, with monthly I.M. injections of penicillin G benzathine or daily doses of oral penicillin V or sulfadiazine (Treatment usually continues for at least 5 years or until age 21, whichever is longer.)

- Prophylactic antibiotics for dental work and other invasive or surgical procedures to prevent endocarditis

NURSING CONSIDERATIONS

- Because rheumatic fever and rheumatic heart disease require prolonged treatment, your care plan should include comprehensive patient teaching to promote compliance with the prescribed therapy.
- Before giving penicillin, ask the patient or (if the patient is a child) his parents whether he has ever had a hypersensitivity reaction to it. Even if the patient has never had a reaction, warn that such a reaction is possible. Tell him to stop the drug and call the physician immediately if he develops a rash, fever, chills, or other signs of allergy at any time during penicillin therapy.
- Instruct the patient and his family to watch for and report early signs of heart failure, such as dyspnea and a hacking, nonproductive cough.
- Stress the need for bed rest during the acute phase and suggest appropriate, physically undemanding diversions. After the acute phase, encourage family members and friends to spend as much time as possible with the patient to minimize boredom. Advise parents to secure tutorial services to help their child keep up with schoolwork during the long convalescence.
- Help parents overcome guilty feelings they may have about their child's illness. Tell them that failure to seek treatment for streptococcal infection is common because this illness typically seems no worse than a cold. Encourage the parents and the child to vent their frustrations during the long, tedious recovery. If the child has severe carditis, help the parents prepare for permanent changes in the child's lifestyle.
- Teach the patient and his family about this disease and its treatment. Warn parents to watch for and immediately report signs of recurrent streptococcal infection — sudden sore throat, diffuse throat redness and oropharyngeal exudate, swollen and tender cervical lymph glands, pain on swallowing, temperature of 101° to 104° F (38.3° to 40° C), headache, and nausea. Urge them to keep the child away from people with respiratory tract infections.
- Promote good dental hygiene to prevent infection. Make sure the patient and his family understand the need to comply with prolonged antibiotic therapy and follow-up care and the need for additional antibiotics during dental surgery or other invasive procedures. Arrange for a home health nurse to oversee care if necessary.
- Teach the patient to follow current recommendations of the American Heart Association for prevention of bacterial endocarditis. Antibiotic regimens used to prevent recurrence of acute rheumatic fever are inadequate for preventing bacterial endocarditis.

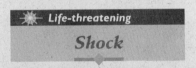

☀ Life-threatening

Shock

Shock isn't a disease but, rather, is a clinical syndrome leading to reduced tissue and organ perfusion and, eventually, organ dysfunction and failure. Shock can be classified into three major categories based on the precipitating factors: distributive (neurogenic, septic, and anaphylactic), cardiogenic, and hypovolemic shock. Even with treatment, shock has a high mortality after the body's compensatory mechanisms fail. (See *Types of shock,* pages 68 and 69.)

CAUSES
Anaphylactic shock
- ABO-incompatible blood
- Contrast media
- Foods
- Medications, vaccines
- Venom

Cardiogenic shock
- Arrhythmias
- Cardiomyopathy
- Heart failure
- Myocardial infarction (MI) (most common cause)
- Obstruction
- Pericardial tamponade
- Pulmonary embolism
- Tension pneumothorax

Hypovolemic shock
- Ascites
- Blood loss (most common cause)
- Burns
- Fluid shifts
- GI fluid loss
- Hemothorax
- Peritonitis
- Renal loss (diabetic ketoacidosis, diabetes insipidus, adrenal insufficiency)

Neurogenic shock
- Hypoglycemia
- Medications
- Severe pain
- Spinal anesthesia
- Spinal cord injury
- Vasomotor center depression

Septic shock
- Gram-negative bacteria (most common cause)
- Gram-positive bacteria
- Viruses, fungi, Rickettsiae, parasites, yeast, protozoa, or mycobacteria

Alert The immature immune system of neonates and infants and the weakened immune system of older adults, commonly accompanied by chronic illness, make these populations more susceptible to septic shock.

PATHOPHYSIOLOGY
There are three basic stages common to each type of shock: compensatory, progressive, and irreversible, or refractory, stages.

Compensatory stage
When arterial pressure and tissue perfusion are reduced, compensatory mechanisms are activated to maintain perfusion to the heart and brain. As the baroreceptors in the carotid sinus and aortic arch sense a decrease in blood pressure, epinephrine and norepinephrine are secreted to increase peripheral resistance, blood pressure, and myocardial contractility. Reduced blood flow to the kidneys activates the renin-angiotensin-aldosterone system, causing vasoconstriction and sodium and water retention, leading to increased blood volume and venous return. As a result of these compensatory mechanisms, cardiac output and tissue perfusion are maintained.

Progressive stage
The progressive stage of shock begins as compensatory mechanisms fail to maintain cardiac output. Tissues become hypoxic because of poor perfusion. As cells switch to anaerobic metabolism, lactic acid builds up, producing metabolic acidosis. This acidotic state depresses myocardial function. Tissue hypoxia also promotes the release of endothelial mediators, which produce vasodilation and

TYPES OF SHOCK

DISTRIBUTIVE SHOCK

In this type of shock, vasodilation causes a state of hypovolemia. There are three types of distributive shock.

NEUROGENIC SHOCK

A loss of sympathetic vasoconstrictor tone in the vascular smooth muscle and reduced autonomic function lead to widespread arterial and venous vasodilation. Venous return is reduced as blood pools in the venous system, leading to a drop in cardiac output and hypotension.

SEPTIC SHOCK

An immune response is triggered when bacteria release endotoxins. In response, macrophages secrete tumor necrosis factor (TNF) and interleukins. These mediators, in turn, are responsible for an increased release of platelet-activating factor (PAF), prostaglandins, leukotrienes, thromboxane A_2, kinins, and complement. The consequences are vasodilation and vasoconstriction, increased capillary permeability, reduced systemic vascular resistance, microemboli, and an elevated cardiac output. Endotoxins also stimulate the release of histamine, further increasing capillary per-

meability. Moreover, myocardial depressant factor, TNF, PAF, and other factors depress myocardial function. Cardiac output falls, resulting in multiple-organ-dysfunction syndrome (MODS).

ANAPHYLACTIC SHOCK

Triggered by an allergic reaction, anaphylactic shock occurs when a person is exposed to an antigen to which he has already been sensitized. Exposure results in the production of specific immuno-globulin (Ig) E antibodies by plasma cells that bind to membrane receptors on mast cells and basophils. On reexposure, the antigen binds to IgE antibodies or cross-linked IgE receptors, triggering the release of powerful chemical mediators from mast cells. IgG or IgM enters into the reaction and activates the release of complement factors. At the same time, the chemical mediators bradykinin and leukotrienes induce vascular collapse by stimulating contraction of certain groups of smooth muscles and by increasing vascular permeability, leading to decreased peripheral resistance and plasma leakage into the extravascular tissues, thereby reducing blood volume and causing hypotension, hypovolemic shock, and cardiac dysfunc-

---

endothelial abnormalities, leading to venous pooling and increased capillary permeability. Sluggish blood flow increases the risk of disseminated intravascular coagulation (DIC).

Irreversible (refractory) stage

As the shock syndrome progresses, permanent organ damage occurs as compensatory mechanisms can no longer maintain cardiac output. Reduced perfusion damages cell membranes, lysosomal enzymes are released, and energy stores are depleted, possibly leading to cell death. As cells use anaerobic metabolism, lactic acid accumulates, increasing capillary per-

meability and the movement of fluid out of the vascular space. This loss of intravascular fluid further contributes to hypotension. Perfusion to the coronary arteries is reduced, causing myocardial depression and a further reduction in cardiac output. Eventually, circulatory and respiratory failure occurs. Death is inevitable.

CLINICAL FINDINGS
Compensatory stage

● Tachycardia and bounding pulse due to sympathetic stimulation
● Restlessness and irritability related to cerebral hypoxia

tion. Bronchospasm and laryngeal edema also occur.

CARDIOGENIC SHOCK

In cardiogenic shock, the left ventricle can't maintain an adequate cardiac output. Compensatory mechanisms increase heart rate, strengthen myocardial contractions, promote sodium and water retention, and cause selective vasoconstriction. However, these mechanisms increase myocardial workload and oxygen consumption, which reduces the heart's ability to pump blood, especially if the patient has myocardial ischemia. Consequently, blood backs up, resulting in pulmonary edema. Eventually, cardiac output falls and MODS develops as the compensatory mechanisms fail to maintain perfusion.

HYPOVOLEMIC SHOCK

When fluid is lost from the intravascular space through external losses or the shift of fluid from the vessels to the interstitial or intracellular spaces, venous return to the heart is reduced. This reduction in preload decreases ventricular filling, leading to a drop in stroke volume. Then, cardiac output falls, causing reduced perfusion of the tissues and organs.

● Tachypnea to compensate for hypoxia
● Reduced urine output secondary to vasoconstriction
● Cool, pale skin associated with vasoconstriction; warm, dry skin in septic shock due to vasodilation

Progressive stage
● Hypotension as compensatory mechanisms begin to fail
● Narrowed pulse pressure associated with reduced stroke volume; weak, rapid, thready pulse caused by decreased cardiac output; shallow respirations as the patient weakens; re-

duced urine output as poor renal perfusion continues
● Cold, clammy skin caused by vasoconstriction
● Cyanosis related to hypoxia

Alert Hypotension, an altered level of consciousness, and hyperventilation may be the only signs of septic shock in infants and elderly people.

Irreversible (refractory) stage
● Unconsciousness and absent reflexes caused by reduced cerebral perfusion, acid-base imbalance, or electrolyte abnormalities
● Rapidly falling blood pressure as decompensation occurs
● Weak pulse caused by reduced cardiac output
● Slow, shallow, or Cheyne-Stokes respirations secondary to respiratory center depression
● Anuria related to renal failure

TEST RESULTS
● Hematocrit may be reduced in hemorrhage or elevated in other types of shock caused by hypovolemia.
● Blood, urine, and sputum cultures may identify the organism responsible for septic shock.
● Coagulation studies may detect coagulopathy from DIC.
● Laboratory testing may reveal increased white blood cell count and erythrocyte sedimentation rate due to injury and inflammation; elevated blood urea nitrogen and creatinine levels due to reduced renal perfusion; increased serum lactate secondary to anaerobic metabolism; and increased serum glucose in early stages of shock as liver releases glycogen stores in response to sympathetic stimulation.
● Cardiac enzymes and proteins may be elevated, indicating MI as a cause of cardiogenic shock.

- Arterial blood gas (ABG) analysis may reveal respiratory alkalosis in early shock associated with tachypnea, respiratory acidosis in later stages associated with respiratory depression, and metabolic acidosis in later stages secondary to anaerobic metabolism.
- Urine specific gravity may be high in response to effects of antidiuretic hormone.
- Chest X-rays may be normal in early stages; pulmonary congestion may be seen in later stages.
- Hemodynamic monitoring may reveal characteristic patterns of intracardiac pressures and cardiac output, which are used to guide fluid and drug management. (See *Putting hemodynamic monitoring to use.*)
- Electrocardiography (ECG) determines the heart rate and detects arrhythmias, ischemic changes, and MI.
- Echocardiography determines left ventricular function and reveals valvular abnormalities.

TREATMENT
- Identification and treatment of the underlying cause, if possible
- Maintaining a patent airway; preparing for intubation and mechanical ventilation if the patient develops respiratory distress
- Supplemental oxygen to increase oxygenation
- Continuous cardiac monitoring to detect changes in heart rate and rhythm; administration of antiarrhythmics as necessary
- Initiating and maintaining at least two I.V. lines with large-gauge needles for fluid and drug administration
- I.V. fluids, crystalloids, colloids, or blood products, as necessary, to maintain intravascular volume

Anaphylactic shock
- In addition to the above measures, give epinephrine I.M. or subcutaneously to open airways and increase blood pressure
- H_1 and H_2 antihistamines to block histamine response
- Inhaled beta-agonists to treat bronchospasm

Cardiogenic shock
- Inotropic drugs, such as dopamine (Intropin), dobutamine (Dobutrex), inamrinone, and epinephrine, to increase heart contractility and cardiac output
- Vasodilators, such as nitroglycerin or nitroprusside, given with a vasopressor to reduce the left ventricle's workload
- Diuretics to reduce preload, if the patient has fluid volume overload
- Intra-aortic balloon pump (IABP) therapy to reduce the work of the left ventricle by decreasing systemic vascular resistance (Diastolic pressure is increased, resulting in improved coronary artery perfusion.)
- Thrombolytic therapy or coronary artery revascularization to restore coronary artery blood flow, if cardiogenic shock is due to acute MI
- Emergency surgery to repair papillary muscle rupture or ventricular septal defect, if either is the cause of cardiogenic shock
- Ventricular assist device to assist the pumping action of the heart when IABP and drug therapy fail
- Heart transplantation, which may be considered when other medical and surgical therapeutic measures fail

Hypovolemic shock
- Pneumatic antishock garment, which may be applied to control inter-

PUTTING HEMODYNAMIC MONITORING TO USE

Hemodynamic monitoring provides information on intracardiac pressures and cardiac output. To understand intracardiac pressures, picture the cardiovascular system as a continuous loop with constantly changing pressure gradients that keep the blood moving.

RIGHT ATRIAL PRESSURE, OR CENTRAL VENOUS PRESSURE

The right atrial pressure (RAP) reflects right atrial, or right heart, function and end-diastolic pressure.

◆ **Normal:** 1 to 6 mm Hg (1.34 to 8 cm H_2O). (To convert mm Hg to cm H_2O, multiply mm Hg by 1.34.)

◆ **Elevated value suggests:** right-sided heart failure, volume overload, tricuspid valve stenosis or insufficiency, constrictive pericarditis, pulmonary hypertension, cardiac tamponade, or right ventricular (RV) infarction.

◆ **Low value suggests:** reduced circulating blood volume.

RV PRESSURE

RV systolic pressure normally equals pulmonary artery systolic pressure; RV end-diastolic pressure, which equals RAP, reflects RV function.

◆ **Normal:** systolic, 15 to 25 mm Hg; diastolic, 0 to 8 mm Hg.

◆ **Elevated value suggests:** mitral stenosis or insufficiency, pulmonary disease, hypoxemia, constrictive pericarditis, chronic heart failure, atrial and ventricular septal defects, and patent ductus arteriosus.

PULMONARY ARTERY PRESSURE

Pulmonary artery systolic pressure reflects RV function and pulmonary circulation pressures. Pulmonary artery diastolic pressure reflects left ventricular (LV) pressures, specifically LV end-diastolic pressure.

◆ **Normal:** systolic, 15 to 25 mm Hg; diastolic, 8 to 15 mm Hg; mean, 10 to 20 mm Hg.

◆ **Elevated value suggests:** left-sided heart failure, increased pulmonary blood flow (left or right shunting, as in atrial or ventricular septal defects), mitral stenosis or insuffiency, and in any condition causing increased pulmonary arteriolar resistance.

PULMONARY ARTERY WEDGE PRESSURE

Pulmonary artery wedge pressure (PAWP) reflects left atrial and LV pressures unless the patient has mitral stenosis. Changes in PAWP reflect changes in LV filling pressure. The heart momentarily relaxes during diastole as it fills with blood from the pulmonary veins; this permits the pulmonary vasculature, left atrium, and left ventricle to act as a single chamber.

◆ **Normal:** mean pressure, 6 to 12 mm Hg.

◆ **Elevated value suggests:** left-sided heart failure, mitral stenosis or insufficiency, and pericardial tamponade.

◆ **Low value suggests:** hypovolemia.

LEFT ATRIAL PRESSURE

Left atrial pressure reflects LV end-diastolic pressure in patients without mitral valve disease.

◆ Normal: 6 to 12 mm Hg.

CARDIAC OUTPUT

Cardiac output is the amount of blood ejected by the heart each minute.

◆ **Normal:** 4 to 8 L; varies with a patient's weight, height, and body surface area. Adjusting the cardiac output to the patient's size yields a measurement called the cardiac index.

---

nal and external hemorrhage by direct pressure

● Fluids, such as normal saline solution or lactated Ringer's solution, initially, to restore filling pressures

● Packed red blood cells in hemorrhagic shock to restore blood loss and improve the blood's oxygen-carrying capacity

Neurogenic shock
● Vasopressor drugs to raise blood pressure by vasoconstriction
● Fluid replacement to maintain blood pressure and cardiac output

Septic shock
● Antibiotic therapy to eradicate the causative organism
● Inotropic and vasopressor drugs, such as dopamine, dobutamine, and norepinephrine, to improve perfusion and maintain blood pressure
● Monoclonal antibodies to tumor necrosis factor, endotoxin, and interleukin-1 to counteract septic shock mediators

NURSING CONSIDERATIONS
Management of shock necessitates prompt, aggressive supportive measures and careful assessment and monitoring of vital signs. Follow these priorities:
● Check for a patent airway and adequate circulation. If blood pressure and heart rate are absent, start cardiopulmonary resuscitation.
● Record blood pressure, pulse rate, peripheral pulses, respiratory rate, and other vital signs every 15 minutes and the ECG continuously. Systolic blood pressure lower than 80 mm Hg usually results in inadequate coronary artery blood flow, cardiac ischemia, arrhythmias, and further complications of low cardiac output. When blood pressure drops below 80 mm Hg, increase the oxygen flow rate and notify the physician immediately. A progressive decrease in blood pressure accompanied by a thready pulse generally signals inadequate cardiac output from reduced intravascular volume. Notify the physician, and increase the infusion rate.

● Start I.V. lines with normal saline or lactated Ringer's solution, using a large-bore catheter (14G), which allows easier administration of later blood transfusions.

Alert Don't start I.V. administration in the legs of a patient in shock who has suffered abdominal trauma because the infused fluid may escape through the ruptured vessel into the abdomen.

● An indwelling urinary catheter may be inserted to measure hourly urine output. If output is less than 30 ml/hour in adults, increase the fluid infusion rate but watch for signs of fluid overload, such as an increase in pulmonary artery wedge pressure (PAWP). Notify the physician if urine output doesn't improve. An osmotic diuretic, such as mannitol, may be ordered to increase renal blood flow and urine output. Determine how much fluid to give by checking blood pressure, urine output, central venous pressure (CVP), or PAWP. (To increase accuracy, CVP should be measured at the level of the right atrium, using the same reference point on the chest each time.)
● Draw an arterial blood sample to measure ABG levels. Administer oxygen by face mask or airway to ensure adequate tissue oxygenation. Adjust the oxygen flow rate to a higher or lower level, as ABG measurements indicate.
● Draw venous blood for complete blood count and electrolyte, type and crossmatch, and coagulation studies.
● During therapy, assess skin color and temperature, and note changes. Cold, clammy skin may be a sign of continuing peripheral vascular constriction, indicating progressive shock.
● Watch for signs of impending coagulopathy (petechiae, bruising, and

bleeding or oozing from gums or venipuncture sites).
- Explain all procedures and their purpose to the patient, and provide emotional support to the patient and his family.

Tetralogy of Fallot

Tetralogy of Fallot is a combination of four cardiac defects: ventricular septal defect (VSD), right ventricular outflow tract obstruction (pulmonic stenosis), right ventricular hypertrophy, and dextroposition of the aorta, with overriding of the VSD. Blood shunts from right to left through the VSD, allowing unoxygenated blood to mix with oxygenated blood and resulting in cyanosis. This cyanotic heart defect sometimes coexists with other congenital acyanotic heart defects, such as patent ductus arteriosus or atrial septal defect. It accounts for about 10% of all congenital defects and occurs equally in males and females. Before surgical advances made correction possible, about one-third of these children died in infancy.

CAUSES
The cause of tetralogy of Fallot is unknown but may be associated with:
- fetal alcohol syndrome
- thalidomide use during pregnancy.

PATHOPHYSIOLOGY
In tetralogy of Fallot, unoxygenated venous blood returning to the right side of the heart may pass through the VSD to the left ventricle, bypassing the lungs, or it may enter the pulmonary artery, depending on the extent of the pulmonic stenosis. Rather

than originating from the left ventricle, the aorta overrides both ventricles.

The VSD usually lies in the outflow tract of the right ventricle and is generally large enough to permit equalization of right and left ventricular pressures. However, the ratio of systemic vascular resistance to pulmonic stenosis affects the direction and magnitude of shunt flow across the VSD. Severe obstruction of right ventricular outflow produces a right-to-left shunt, causing decreased systemic arterial oxygen saturation, cyanosis, reduced pulmonary blood flow, and hypoplasia of the entire pulmonary vasculature. Right ventricular hypertrophy develops in response to the extra force needed to push blood into the stenotic pulmonary artery. Milder forms of pulmonic stenosis result in a left-to-right shunt or no shunt at all.

CLINICAL FINDINGS
- Cyanosis, the hallmark of tetralogy of Fallot, caused by a right-to-left shunt
- Cyanotic or "blue" spells (tet spells), characterized by dyspnea; deep, sighing respirations; bradycardia; fainting; seizures; and loss of consciousness following exercise, crying, straining, infection, or fever (It may result from reduced oxygen to the brain because of increased right-to-left shunting, possibly caused by spasm of the right ventricular outflow tract, increased systemic venous return, or decreased systemic arterial resistance.)
- Clubbing, diminished exercise tolerance, increasing dyspnea on exertion, growth retardation, and eating difficulties in older children due to poor oxygenation
- Squatting with shortness of breath to reduce venous return of unoxy-

genated blood from the legs and to increase systemic arterial resistance
- Loud systolic murmur best heard along the left sternal border, which may diminish or obscure the pulmonic component of S_2
- Continuous murmur of the ductus in a patient with a large patent ductus, which may obscure systolic murmur
- Thrill at the left sternal border caused by abnormal blood flow through the heart
- Obvious right ventricular impulse and prominent inferior sternum associated with right ventricular hypertrophy

TEST RESULTS
- Chest X-rays may demonstrate decreased pulmonary vascular marking (depending on the severity of the pulmonary obstruction), an enlarged right ventricle, and a boot-shaped cardiac silhouette.
- Electrocardiography shows right ventricular hypertrophy, right axis deviation and, possibly, right atrial hypertrophy.
- Echocardiography identifies septal overriding of the aorta, the VSD, and pulmonic stenosis and detects the hypertrophied walls of the right ventricle.
- Laboratory testing reveals diminished oxygen saturation and polycythemia (hematocrit may be more than 60%) if the cyanosis is severe and longstanding, predisposing the patient to thrombosis.
- Cardiac catheterization confirms the diagnosis by providing visualization of pulmonic stenosis, the VSD, and the overriding aorta and ruling out other cyanotic heart defects. This test also measures the degree of oxygen saturation in aortic blood.

TREATMENT
- Knee-chest position and administration of oxygen and morphine to improve oxygenation
- Palliative surgery with a Blalock-Taussig operation, which joins the subclavian artery to the pulmonary artery to enhance blood flow to the lungs to reduce hypoxia
- Propranolol to prevent "tet" spells and prophylactic antibiotics to prevent infective endocarditis or cerebral abscesses
- Corrective surgery to relieve pulmonic stenosis and close the VSD, directing left ventricular outflow to the aorta

NURSING CONSIDERATIONS
- Explain tetralogy of Fallot to the parents. Inform them that their child will set his own exercise limits and will know when to rest. Make sure they understand that their child can engage in physical activity, and advise them not to be overprotective.
- Teach parents to recognize serious hypoxic spells, which can cause dramatically increased cyanosis; deep, sighing respirations; and loss of consciousness. Tell them to place their child in the knee-chest position and to report such spells immediately. Emergency treatment may be necessary.
- To prevent infective endocarditis and other infections, warn parents to keep their child away from people with infections. Urge them to encourage good dental hygiene, and tell them to watch for ear, nose, and throat infections and dental caries, all of which necessitate immediate treatment. When dental care, infections, or surgery requires prophylactic antibiotics, tell parents to make sure the child completes the prescribed regimen.

- If the child requires medical attention for an unrelated problem, advise the parents to inform the physician immediately of the child's history of tetralogy of Fallot because any treatment must take this serious heart defect into consideration.
- During hospitalization, alert the staff to the child's condition. Because of the right-to-left shunt through the VSD, treat I.V. lines like arterial lines. Remember, a clot dislodged from a catheter tip in a vein can cross the VSD and cause cerebral embolism. The same thing can happen if air enters the venous lines.

After palliative surgery
- Monitor oxygenation and arterial blood gas (ABG) values closely in the intensive care unit.
- If the child has undergone the Blalock-Taussig operation, don't use the arm on the operative side for measuring blood pressure, inserting I.V. lines, or drawing blood samples because blood perfusion on this side diminishes greatly until collateral circulation develops. Note this on the child's chart and at his bedside.

After corrective surgery
- Watch for right bundle-branch block or more serious disturbances of atrioventricular conduction and for ventricular ectopic beats.
- Be alert for other postoperative complications, such as bleeding, right-sided heart failure, and respiratory failure. After surgery, transient heart failure is common and may require treatment with digoxin and diuretics.
- Monitor left atrial pressure directly. A pulmonary artery catheter may also be used to check central venous and pulmonary artery pressures.

- Frequently check color and vital signs. Obtain ABG measurements regularly to assess oxygenation. As needed, suction to prevent atelectasis and pneumonia. Monitor mechanical ventilation.
- Monitor and record intake and output accurately.
- If atrioventricular block develops with a low heart rate, a temporary external pacemaker may be necessary.
- If blood pressure or cardiac output is inadequate, catecholamines may be ordered by continuous I.V. infusion. To decrease left ventricular workload, administer nitroprusside, if ordered. Provide analgesics as needed.
- Keep the parents informed about their child's progress.
- After discharge, the child may require digoxin (Lanoxin), diuretics, and other drugs. Stress the importance of complying with the prescribed regimen, and make sure the parents know how and when to administer these medications. Teach parents to watch for signs of digoxin toxicity (anorexia, nausea, and vomiting). Prophylactic antibiotics to prevent infective endocarditis will still be required.
- Advise the parents to avoid becoming overprotective as the child's tolerance for physical activity increases.

Transposition of the great arteries

Transposition of the great arteries is a cyanotic congenital heart defect in which the great arteries are reversed such that the aorta arises from the right ventricle and the pulmonary artery from the left ventricle, producing two noncommunicating circulatory systems (pulmonic and systemic). The right-to-left shunting of blood leads to an increased risk of heart failure and anoxia. Transposition accounts for about 5% of all congenital heart defects and commonly coexists with other congenital heart defects, such as ventricular septal defect (VSD), VSD with pulmonic stenosis, atrial septal defect (ASD), and patent ductus arteriosus (PDA). It affects two to three times more males than females.

CAUSES
• Unknown

PATHOPHYSIOLOGY
Transposition of the great arteries results from faulty embryonic development. Oxygenated blood returning to the left side of the heart is carried back to the lungs by a transposed pulmonary artery. Unoxygenated blood returning to the right side of the heart is carried to the systemic circulation by a transposed aorta.

Communication between the pulmonary and systemic circulations is necessary for survival. In infants with isolated transposition, blood mixes only at the patent foramen ovale and at the PDA, resulting in slight mixing of unoxygenated systemic blood and oxygenated pulmonary blood. In infants with concurrent cardiac defects, greater mixing of blood occurs.

CLINICAL FINDINGS
• Cyanosis and tachypnea that worsens with crying within the first few hours after birth, when no other heart defects exist that allow mixing of systemic and pulmonary blood (Cyanosis may be minimized with associated defects, such as ASD, VSD, or PDA.)
• Gallop rhythm, tachycardia, dyspnea, hepatomegaly, and cardiomegaly within days to weeks as a result of heart failure
• Loud S_2 because the anteriorly transposed aorta is directly behind the sternum
• Murmurs of ASD, VSD, or PDA
• Diminished exercise tolerance, fatigability, and clubbing due to reduced oxygenation

TEST RESULTS
• Chest X-rays are normal in the first days after birth. Within days to weeks, right atrial and right ventricular enlargement characteristically cause the heart to appear oblong. X-ray may also show increased pulmonary vascular markings, except when pulmonic stenosis exists.
• Electrocardiography typically reveals right axis deviation and right ventricular hypertrophy, but these may be normal in a neonate.
• Echocardiography demonstrates the reversed position of the aorta and pulmonary artery and records echoes from both semilunar valves simultaneously because of aortic valve displacement. It also detects other cardiac defects.
• Cardiac catheterization reveals decreased oxygen saturation in left ventricular blood and aortic blood; increased right atrial, right ventricular, and pulmonary artery oxygen saturation; and right ventricular systolic pressure equal to systemic pressure. Dye injection reveals the transposed vessels and the presence of other cardiac defects.
• Arterial blood gas (ABG) analysis indicates hypoxia and secondary metabolic acidosis.

TREATMENT
The immediate management of the infant is to establish safe oxygen levels

while stabilizing cardiopulmonary function.

Treatment of this disorder may involve:

● prostaglandin infusion to keep the ductus arteriosus patent until surgical correction

● Rashkind balloon atrial septostomy during cardiac catheterization, if needed as a palliative measure until surgery can be performed (It enlarges the patent foramen ovale and thereby improves oxygenation and alleviates hypoxia by allowing greater mixing of blood from the pulmonary and systemic circulations.)

● digoxin (Lanoxin) and diuretics after atrial balloon septostomy to lessen heart failure until the infant is ready to withstand corrective surgery

● surgery to correct transposition (commonly in the first week of life), although the procedure depends on the physiology of the defect.

NURSING CONSIDERATIONS

● Explain cardiac catheterization and all necessary procedures to the parents. Offer emotional support.

● Monitor vital signs, ABG values, urine output, and central venous pressure, watching for signs of heart failure. Give digoxin and I.V. fluids, being careful to avoid fluid overload.

● Teach parents to recognize signs of heart failure and digoxin toxicity (poor feeding and vomiting). Stress the importance of regular checkups to monitor cardiovascular status.

● Teach parents to protect their infant from infection and to give antibiotics.

● Tell the parents to let their child develop normally. They need not restrict activities; he'll set his own limits.

● If the patient is scheduled for surgery, explain the procedure to the parents and child, if old enough. Teach them about the intensive care unit, and introduce them to the staff. Also explain postoperative care.

● Preoperatively, monitor ABG values, acid-base balance, intake and output, and vital signs.

After corrective surgery

● Monitor cardiac output by checking blood pressure, skin color, heart rate, urine output, central venous and left atrial pressures, and level of consciousness. Report abnormalities or changes.

● Carefully measure ABG levels.

● To detect supraventricular conduction blocks and arrhythmias, monitor the patient closely. Watch for signs of atrioventricular block, atrial arrhythmia, and faulty sinoatrial function.

● After a Mustard or Senning operation, watch for signs of baffle obstruction such as marked facial edema.

● Encourage parents to help their child assume new activity levels and independence. Teach them about postoperative antibiotic prophylaxis for endocarditis.

Valvular heart disease

In valvular heart disease, three types of mechanical disruption can occur: stenosis, or narrowing, of the valve opening; incomplete closure of the valve; or valve prolapse. Valvular disorders in children and adolescents most commonly occur as a result of congenital heart defects. In adults, rheumatic heart disease is a common cause.

(Text continues on page 80.)

TYPES OF VALVULAR HEART DISEASE

CAUSES AND INCIDENCE

CLINICAL FINDINGS

Mitral insufficiency
- Results from rheumatic fever, hypertrophic obstructive cardiomyopathy, mitral valve prolapse, myocardial infarction, severe left ventricular dilation or left-sided heart failure, or ruptured chordae tendineae
- Associated with other congenital anomalies such as transposition of the great arteries
- Rare in children without other congenital anomalies

- Orthopnea, dyspnea, fatigue, angina, and palpitations
- Peripheral edema, jugular vein distention, and hepatomegaly (right-sided heart failure)
- Tachycardia, crackles, and pulmonary edema
- Auscultation revealing a holosystolic murmur at apex, a possible split S_2, and an S_3

Mitral stenosis
- Results from rheumatic fever (most common cause) or endocarditis
- Most common in females
- May be associated with other congenital anomalies

- Dyspnea on exertion, paroxysmal nocturnal dyspnea, orthopnea, weakness, fatigue, and palpitations
- Peripheral edema, jugular vein distention, ascites, and hepatomegaly (right-sided heart failure)
- Crackles, atrial fibrillation, and signs of systemic emboli
- Auscultation revealing a loud S_1 or opening snap and a diastolic murmur at the apex

Aortic insufficiency
- Results from rheumatic fever, syphilis, hypertension, or endocarditis or may be idiopathic
- Associated with Marfan syndrome
- Most common in males
- Associated with ventricular septal defect, even after surgical closure

- Dyspnea, cough, fatigue, palpitations, angina, and syncope
- Pulmonary congestion, left-sided heart failure, and "pulsating" nail beds (Quincke's sign)
- Rapidly rising and collapsing pulses (pulsus biferiens), cardiac arrhythmias, and widened pulse pressure
- Auscultation revealing an S_3 and a diastolic blowing murmur at left sternal border
- Palpation and visualization of apical impulse in chronic disease

Aortic stenosis
- Results from congenital aortic bicuspid valve (associated with coarctation of the aorta), congenital stenosis of valve cusps, rheumatic fever, or atherosclerosis in elderly patients
- Most common in males

- Dyspnea on exertion, paroxysmal nocturnal dyspnea, fatigue, syncope, angina, and palpitations
- Pulmonary congestion and left-sided heart failure
- Diminished carotid pulses, decreased cardiac output, and cardiac arrhythmias; may have pulsus alternans
- Auscultation revealing systolic murmur heard at base or in carotids and, possibly, an S_4

Pulmonic stenosis
- Results from congenital stenosis of valve cusp or rheumatic heart disease (uncommon)
- Associated with tetralogy of Fallot

- May produce symptoms with dyspnea on exertion, fatigue, chest pain, and syncope
- May cause jugular vein distention or right-sided heart failure
- Auscultation revealing a systolic murmur at the left sternal border and a split S_2 with a delayed or absent pulmonic component

DIAGNOSTIC MEASURES

◆ *Cardiac catheterization:* mitral insufficiency with increased left ventricular end-diastolic volume and pressure, increased atrial pressure and pulmonary artery wedge pressure (PAWP), and decreased cardiac output
◆ *Chest X-rays:* left atrial and ventricular enlargement and pulmonary venous congestion
◆ *Echocardiography:* abnormal valve leaflet motion and left atrial enlargement
◆ *Electrocardiogram (ECG):* may show left atrial and ventricular hypertrophy, sinus tachycardia, and atrial fibrillation

---

◆ *Cardiac catheterization:* diastolic pressure gradient across valve; elevated left atrial pressure and PAWP > 15 mm Hg with severe pulmonary hypertension; elevated right-sided heart pressure with decreased cardiac output; and abnormal contraction of the left ventricle
◆ *Chest X-rays:* left atrial and ventricular enlargement, enlarged pulmonary arteries, and mitral valve calcification
◆ *Echocardiography:* thickened mitral valve leaflets and left atrial enlargement
◆ *ECG:* left atrial hypertrophy, atrial fibrillation, right ventricular hypertrophy, and right axis deviation

---

◆ *Cardiac catheterization:* reduction in arterial diastolic pressures, aortic insufficiency, other valvular abnormalities, and increased left ventricular end-diastolic pressure
◆ *Chest X-rays:* left ventricular enlargement and pulmonary venous congestion
◆ *Echocardiography:* left ventricular enlargement, alterations in mitral valve movement (indirect indication of aortic valve disease), and mitral thickening
◆ *ECG:* sinus tachycardia, left ventricular hypertrophy, and left atrial hypertrophy in severe disease

---

◆ *Cardiac catheterization:* pressure gradient across valve (indicating obstruction) and increased left ventricular end-diastolic pressures
◆ *Chest X-rays:* valvular calcification, left ventricular enlargement, and pulmonary vein congestion
◆ *Echocardiography:* thickened aortic valve and left ventricular wall, possibly coexistent with mitral valve stenosis
◆ *ECG:* left ventricular hypertrophy

◆ *Cardiac catheterization:* increased right ventricular pressure, decreased pulmonary artery pressure, and abnormal valve orifice
◆ *ECG:* may show right ventricular hypertrophy, right axis deviation, right atrial hypertrophy, and atrial fibrillation

CAUSES

The causes of valvular heart disease are varied and differ for each type of valve disorder. (See *Types of valvular heart disease,* pages 78 and 79.)

PATHOPHYSIOLOGY

Pathophysiology of valvular heart disease varies according to the valve and the disorder.

Mitral insufficiency

An abnormality of the mitral leaflets, mitral annulus, chordae tendineae, papillary muscles, left atrium, or left ventricle can lead to mitral insufficiency. Blood from the left ventricle flows back into the left atrium during systole, causing the atrium to enlarge to accommodate the backflow. As a result, the left ventricle also dilates to accommodate the increased blood volume from the atrium and to compensate for diminishing cardiac output. Ventricular hypertrophy and increased end-diastolic pressure result in increased pulmonary artery pressure, eventually leading to left-sided and right-sided heart failure.

Mitral stenosis

Narrowing of the valve by valvular abnormalities, fibrosis, or calcification obstructs blood flow from the left atrium to the left ventricle. Consequently, left atrial volume and pressure rise and the chamber dilates. Greater resistance to blood flow causes pulmonary hypertension, right ventricular hypertrophy, and right-sided heart failure. Also, inadequate filling of the left ventricle produces low cardiac output.

Aortic insufficiency

Blood flows back into the left ventricle during diastole, causing fluid overload in the ventricle, which dilates and hy-

pertrophies. The excess volume causes fluid overload in the left atrium and, finally, the pulmonary system. Left-sided heart failure and pulmonary edema eventually result.

Aortic stenosis

Increased left ventricular pressure tries to overcome the resistance of the narrowed valvular opening. The added workload increases the demand for oxygen, and diminished cardiac output causes poor coronary artery perfusion, ischemia of the left ventricle, and left-sided heart failure.

Pulmonic stenosis

Obstructed right ventricular outflow causes right ventricular hypertrophy, eventually resulting in right-sided heart failure.

CLINICAL FINDINGS

The clinical manifestations vary according to the type of valvular defects. (See *Types of valvular heart disease,* pages 78 and 79, for specific clinical features of each valve disorder.)

TEST RESULTS

The diagnosis of valvular heart disease can be made through cardiac catheterization, chest X-rays, echocardiography, or electrocardiography. (See *Types of valvular heart disease*, pages 78 and 79.)

TREATMENT

● Digoxin (Lanoxin), a low-sodium diet, diuretics, vasodilators, and especially angiotensin-converting enzyme inhibitors to treat left-sided heart failure
● Oxygen in acute situations to increase oxygenation

- Anticoagulants to prevent thrombus formation around diseased or replaced valves
- Prophylactic antibiotics before and after surgery or dental care to prevent endocarditis
- Nitroglycerin to relieve angina in conditions such as aortic stenosis
- Beta-adrenergic blockers or digoxin to slow the ventricular rate in atrial fibrillation or atrial flutter
- Cardioversion to convert atrial fibrillation to sinus rhythm
- Open or closed commissurotomy to separate thick or adherent mitral valve leaflets
- Balloon valvuloplasty to enlarge the orifice of a stenotic mitral, aortic, or pulmonic valve
- Annuloplasty or valvuloplasty to reconstruct or repair the valve in mitral insufficiency
- Valve replacement with a prosthetic valve for mitral and aortic valve disease

NURSING CONSIDERATIONS
- Watch closely for signs of heart failure or pulmonary edema and for adverse effects of drug therapy.
- Teach the patient about diet restrictions, medications, and the importance of consistent follow-up care.
- If the patient has had surgery, watch for hypotension, arrhythmias, and thrombus formation. Monitor vital signs, arterial blood gas values, intake, output, daily weight, blood chemistries, chest X-rays, and pulmonary artery catheter readings.

Ventricular septal defect

In ventricular septal defect (VSD), the most common acyanotic congenital heart disorder, an opening in the septum between the ventricles allows blood to shunt between the left and right ventricles. This results in ineffective pumping of the heart and increases the risk of heart failure.

VSDs account for up to 30% of all congenital heart defects. The prognosis is good for defects that close spontaneously or are correctable surgically, but poor for untreated defects, which are sometimes fatal in children by age 1, usually from secondary complications.

CAUSES
VSD may be associated with these conditions:
- Down syndrome and other autosomal trisomies
- Patent ductus arteriosus and coarctation of the aorta
- Prematurity
- Renal anomalies

PATHOPHYSIOLOGY
In infants with VSD, the ventricular septum fails to close completely by 8 weeks' gestation. VSDs are located in the membranous or muscular portion of the ventricular septum and vary in size. Some defects close spontaneously; in other defects, the septum is entirely absent, creating a single ventricle. Small VSDs are likely to close spontaneously. Large VSDs should be surgically repaired before pulmonary vascular disease occurs or while it's still reversible.

VSD isn't readily apparent at birth because right and left pressures are approximately equal and pulmonary artery resistance is elevated. Alveoli aren't yet completely opened, so blood doesn't shunt through the defect. As the pulmonary vasculature gradually relaxes, between 4 and 8 weeks after birth, right ventricular pressure decreases, allowing blood to shunt from the left to the right ventricle. Initially, large VSD shunts cause left atrial and left ventricular hypertrophy. Later, uncorrected VSD causes right ventricular hypertrophy due to increasing pulmonary resistance. Eventually, right- and left-sided heart failure and cyanosis (from reversal of the shunt direction) occur. Fixed pulmonary hypertension may occur much later in life with right-to-left shunting (Eisenmenger's syndrome), causing cyanosis and clubbing of the nail beds.

CLINICAL FINDINGS

● Thin, small infants who gain weight slowly when a large VSD is present secondary to heart failure
● Loud, harsh, widely transmitted systolic murmur heard best along the left sternal border at the third or fourth intercostal space, caused by abnormal blood flow through the VSD
● Palpable thrill caused by turbulent blood flow between the ventricles through a small VSD
● Loud, widely split pulmonic component of S_2 caused by increased pressure gradient across the VSD
● Displacement of point of maximal impulse to the left due to hypertrophy of the heart

Alert Typically, in infants the apical impulse is palpated over the fourth intercostal space, just to the left of the midclavicular line. In children older than age 7, it's palpated over the fifth intercostal space. When the heart is enlarged, the apical beat is displaced to the left or downward.

● Prominent anterior chest secondary to cardiac hypertrophy
● Liver, heart, and spleen enlargement because of systemic congestion
● Feeding difficulties associated with heart failure
● Diaphoresis, tachycardia, and rapid, grunting respirations secondary to heart failure
● Cyanosis and clubbing if right-to-left shunting occurs later in life secondary to pulmonary hypertension

TEST RESULTS

● Chest X-rays appear normal in small defects. In large VSDs, the X-ray may show cardiomegaly, left atrial and left ventricular enlargement, and prominent vascular markings.
● Electrocardiography may be normal with small VSDs, whereas in large VSDs it may show left and right ventricular hypertrophy, suggestive of pulmonary hypertension.
● Echocardiography can detect VSD in the septum, estimate the size of the left-to-right shunt, suggest pulmonary hypertension, and identify associated lesions and complications.
● Cardiac catheterization determines the size and exact location of the VSD and the extent of pulmonary hypertension; it also detects associated defects. It calculates the degree of shunting by comparing the blood oxygen saturation in each ventricle. The oxygen saturation of the right ventricle is greater than normal because oxygenated blood is shunted from the left to the right ventricle.

TREATMENT

Many VSDs (20% to 60%), especially small ones, may close spontaneously during the first year of life. Correction of a VSD may involve:

• early surgical correction for a large VSD, usually performed using a patch graft, before heart failure and irreversible pulmonary vascular disease develop

• placement of a permanent pacemaker, which may be necessary after VSD repair if complete heart block develops from interference with the bundle of His during surgery

• surgical closure of small defects using sutures (They may not be surgically repaired if the patient has normal pulmonary artery pressure and a small shunt.)

• pulmonary artery banding to normalize pressures and flow distal to the band and to prevent pulmonary vascular disease if the child has other defects and will benefit from delaying surgery

• digoxin (Lanoxin), sodium restriction, and diuretics before surgery to prevent heart failure

• prophylactic antibiotics before and after surgery to prevent infective endocarditis.

NURSING CONSIDERATIONS

• Although the parents of an infant with VSD commonly suspect something is wrong with their child before diagnosis, they need psychological support to help them accept the reality of a serious cardiac disorder.

• Because surgery may take place months after diagnosis, parent teaching is vital to prevent complications until the child is scheduled for surgery or the defect closes. Thorough explanations of all tests are also essential.

• Instruct the parents to watch for signs of heart failure, such as poor feeding, sweating, and heavy breathing.

• If the child is receiving digoxin or other medications, tell the parents how to give it and how to recognize adverse effects. Caution them to keep medications out of the reach of all children.

• Teach parents to recognize and report early signs of infection and to avoid exposing the child to people with obvious infections.

• Encourage parents to let the child engage in normal activities.

• Stress the importance of prophylactic antibiotics before and after surgery.

After surgery

• Monitor vital signs and intake and output. Maintain the infant's body temperature with an overbed warmer. Give catecholamines, nitroprusside, and diuretics, as ordered, and analgesics as needed.

• Monitor central venous pressure, intra-arterial blood pressure, and left atrial or pulmonary artery pressure readings. Assess heart rate and rhythm for signs of conduction block.

• Check oxygenation, particularly in a child who requires mechanical ventilation. Suction as needed to maintain a patent airway and to prevent atelectasis and pneumonia.

• Monitor pacemaker effectiveness if needed. Watch for signs of failure, such as bradycardia and hypotension.

• Reassure parents, and allow them to participate in their child's care.

2

RESPIRATORY SYSTEM

The respiratory system's major function is gas exchange, in which air enters the body on inhalation; travels throughout the respiratory passages, exchanging oxygen for carbon dioxide at the tissue level; and expels carbon dioxide on exhalation.

The upper airway — composed of the nose, mouth, pharynx, and larynx — allows airflow into the lungs. This area is responsible for warming, humidifying, and filtering the air, thereby protecting the lower airway from foreign matter.

The lower airway consists of the trachea, mainstem bronchi, secondary bronchi, bronchioles, and terminal bronchioles. These structures are anatomic dead spaces and function only as passageways for moving air into and out of the lungs. Distal to each terminal bronchiole is the acinus, which consists of respiratory bronchioles, alveolar ducts, and alveolar sacs. The bronchioles and ducts function as conduits, and the alveoli are the chief units of gas exchange. These final subdivisions of the bronchial tree make up the lobules — the functional units of the lungs.

Respiratory disorders can be acute or chronic. The disorders described here include examples from each type.

☀ Life-threatening

Acute respiratory distress syndrome

Acute respiratory distress syndrome (ARDS) is a form of pulmonary edema that can quickly lead to acute respiratory failure. Also known as *shock lung, stiff lung, white lung,* or *wet lung,* ARDS may follow direct or indirect injury to the lung. However, its diagnosis is difficult, and death can occur within 48 hours of onset if it isn't promptly diagnosed and treated. A differential diagnosis needs to rule out cardiogenic pulmonary edema, pulmonary vasculitis, and diffuse pulmonary hemorrhage. Patients who recover may have little or no permanent lung damage.

CAUSES
- Acute miliary tuberculosis
- Anaphylaxis
- Aspiration of gastric contents
- Coronary artery bypass grafting
- Diffuse pneumonia, especially viral pneumonia
- Drug overdose, such as aspirin, ethchlorvynol, or heroin
- Hemodialysis

- Idiosyncratic drug reaction to ampicillin or hydrochlorothiazide
- Inhalation of noxious gases, such as ammonia, chlorine, or nitrous oxide
- Injury to the lung from trauma (most common cause) such as airway contusion
- Leukemia
- Near drowning
- Oxygen toxicity
- Pancreatitis
- Sepsis
- Thrombotic thrombocytopenic purpura
- Trauma-related factors, such as fat emboli, sepsis, shock, pulmonary contusions, and multiple transfusions, which increase the likelihood that microemboli will develop
- Uremia
- Venous air embolism

PATHOPHYSIOLOGY

Injury in ARDS involves the alveolar and pulmonary capillary epithelium. A cascade of cellular and biochemical changes is triggered by the specific causative agent. When initiated, this injury triggers neutrophils, macrophages, monocytes, and lymphocytes to produce various cytokines. The cytokines promote cellular activation, chemotaxis, and adhesion. The activated cells produce inflammatory mediators, including oxidants, proteases, kinins, growth factors, and neuropeptides, which initiate the complement cascade, intravascular coagulation, and fibrinolysis.

These cellular triggers result in increased vascular permeability to proteins, affecting the hydrostatic pressure gradient of the capillary. Elevated capillary pressure — such as resulting from insults of fluid overload or cardiac dysfunction in sepsis — greatly increases interstitial and alveolar edema, which is evident in dependent lung areas and can be visualized as whitened areas on chest X-rays. Alveolar closing pressure then exceeds pulmonary pressures, and alveolar closure and collapse begin.

In ARDS, fluid accumulation in the lung interstitium, the alveolar spaces, and the small airways causes the lungs to stiffen, thus impairing ventilation and reducing oxygenation of the pulmonary capillary blood. The resulting injury reduces normal blood flow to the lungs. Damage can occur directly — by aspiration of gastric contents and inhalation of noxious gases — or indirectly — from chemical mediators released in response to systemic disease.

Platelets begin to aggregate and release substances, such as serotonin, bradykinin, and histamine, which attract and activate neutrophils. These substances inflame and damage the alveolar membrane and later increase capillary permeability. In the early stages of ARDS, signs and symptoms may be undetectable.

Additional chemotactic factors released include endotoxins (such as those present in septic states), tumor necrosis factor, and interleukin-1. The activated neutrophils release several inflammatory mediators and platelet aggravating factors that damage the alveolar capillary membrane and increase capillary permeability.

Histamines and other inflammatory substances increase capillary permeability, allowing fluids to move into the interstitial space. Consequently, the patient experiences tachypnea, dyspnea, and tachycardia. As capillary permeability increases, proteins, blood cells, and more fluid leak out, increasing interstitial osmotic pressure and causing pulmonary edema. Tachycardia, dyspnea, and cyanosis may occur. Hypoxia (usually unresponsive to increasing fraction of inspired oxygen), decreased pulmonary compliance, crackles, and rhonchi develop. The resulting pulmonary edema and hemorrhage significantly reduce lung compliance and impair alveolar ventilation.

The fluid in the alveoli and decreased blood flow damage surfactant in the alveoli. This reduces the ability of alveolar cells to produce more surfactant. Without surfactant, alveoli and bronchioles fill with fluid or collapse, gas exchange is impaired, and the lungs are much less compliant. Ventilation of the alveoli is further decreased. The burden of ventilation and gas exchange shifts to uninvolved areas of the lung, and pulmonary blood flow is shunted from right to left. The work of breathing is increased, and the patient may develop thick, frothy sputum and marked hypoxemia with increasing respiratory distress.

Mediators released by neutrophils and macrophages also cause varying degrees of pulmonary vasoconstriction, resulting in pulmonary hypertension. The result of these changes is a ventilation-perfusion mismatch. Although the patient responds with an increased respiratory rate, sufficient oxygen can't cross the alveolar capillary membrane. Carbon dioxide continues to cross easily and is lost with every exhalation. As oxygen and carbon dioxide levels in the blood decrease, the patient develops increasing tachypnea, hypoxemia, and hypocapnia (low partial pressure of arterial carbon dioxide [$PaCO_2$]).

Pulmonary edema worsens, and hyaline membranes form. Inflammation leads to fibrosis, which further impedes gas exchange. Fibrosis progressively obliterates alveoli, respiratory bronchioles, and the interstitium. Functional residual capacity decreases, and shunting becomes more serious. Hypoxemia leads to metabolic acidosis. At this stage, the patient develops increasing $PaCO_2$, decreasing pH and partial pressure of arterial oxygen (PaO_2), decreasing bicarbonate (HCO_3^-) levels, and mental confusion. (*See Looking at ARDS.*)

The end result is respiratory failure. Systemically, neutrophils and inflammatory mediators cause generalized endothelial damage and increased capillary permeability throughout the body. Multiple-organ-dysfunction syndrome (MODS) occurs as the cascade of mediators affects each system. Death may occur from the influence of ARDS and MODS.

CLINICAL FINDINGS

- Rapid, shallow breathing and dyspnea, which occur hours to days after the initial injury in response to decreasing oxygen levels in the blood
- Increased rate of ventilation due to hypoxemia and its effects on the pneumotaxic center
- Intercostal and suprasternal retractions due to the increased effort required to expand the stiff lung
- Crackles and rhonchi, which are audible and result from fluid accumulation in the lungs
- Restlessness, apprehension, and mental sluggishness, which occur as a result of hypoxic brain cells
- Motor dysfunction, which occurs as hypoxia progresses
- Tachycardia, which signals the heart's effort to deliver more oxygen to the cells and vital organs
- Respiratory acidosis, which occurs as carbon dioxide accumulates in the blood and oxygen levels decrease

Focus in

LOOKING AT ARDS

These diagrams show the process and progress of acute respiratory distress syndrome (ARDS).

In phase 1, injury reduces normal blood flow to the lungs. Platelets aggregate and release histamine (H), serotonin (S), and bradykinin (B).

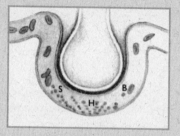

In phase 4, decreased blood flow and fluids in the alveoli damage surfactant and impair the cell's ability to produce more. The alveoli then collapse, thus impairing gas exchange.

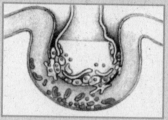

In phase 2, the released substances inflame and damage the alveolar capillary membrane, increasing capillary permeability. Fluids then shift into the interstitial space.

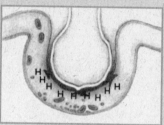

In phase 5, oxygenation is impaired, but carbon dioxide (CO_2) easily crosses the alveolar capillary membrane and is expired. Blood oxygen (O_2) and CO_2 levels are low.

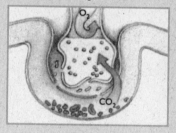

In phase 3, capillary permeability increases and proteins and fluids leak out, increasing interstitial osmotic pressure and causing pulmonary edema.

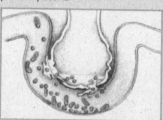

In phase 6, pulmonary edema worsens and inflammation leads to fibrosis. Gas exchange is further impeded.

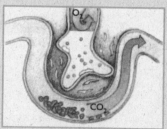

- Metabolic acidosis, which eventually results from failure of compensatory mechanisms

TEST RESULTS

- Arterial blood gas (ABG) analysis with the patient breathing room air initially reveals a reduced PaO_2 (less than 60 mm Hg) and a decreased $PaCO_2$ (less than 35 mm Hg). Hypoxemia, despite increased supplemental oxygen, is the hallmark of ARDS; the resulting blood pH reflects respiratory alkalosis. As ARDS worsens, ABG values show respiratory acidosis evident by an increasing $PaCO_2$ (over 45 mm Hg), metabolic acidosis evident by a decreasing HCO_3^- (less than 22 mEq/L), and a declining PaO_2 despite oxygen therapy.
- Pulmonary artery catheterization helps identify the cause of pulmonary edema (cardiac versus noncardiac) by measuring pulmonary artery wedge pressure (PAWP); allows collection of pulmonary artery blood, which shows decreased oxygen saturation, reflecting tissue hypoxia; measures pulmonary artery pressure; measures cardiac output by thermodilution techniques; and provides information to allow calculation of the percentages of blood shunted though the lungs.
- Serial chest X-rays in early stages show bilateral infiltrates; in later stages, lung fields with a ground-glass appearance and "whiteouts" of both lung fields (with irreversible hypoxemia) may be observed. To differentiate ARDS from heart failure, note that the normal cardiac silhouette appears diffuse; bilateral infiltrates tend to be more peripheral and patchy, as opposed to the usual perihilar "bat wing" appearance of cardiogenic pulmonary edema; and there are fewer pleural effusions.
- Sputum analysis, including Gram stain and culture and sensitivity, identifies causative organisms.
- Blood cultures identify infectious organisms.
- Toxicology testing screens for drug ingestion.
- Serum amylase rules out pancreatitis.

TREATMENT

Therapy is focused on correcting the causes of ARDS and preventing progression of hypoxemia and respiratory acidosis. It may involve:

- administration of humidified oxygen by a tight-fitting mask, which allows for the use of continuous positive airway pressure
- for hypoxemia that doesn't respond adequately to the above measures, ventilatory support with intubation, volume ventilation, and positive end-expiratory pressure (PEEP)
- pressure-controlled inverse ratio ventilation to reverse the conventional inspiration-to-expiration ratio and minimize the risk of barotrauma (Mechanical breaths are pressure-limited to prevent increased damage to the alveoli.)
- permissive hypercapnia to limit peak inspiratory pressure (Although carbon dioxide removal is compromised, treatment isn't given for subsequent changes in blood hydrogen and oxygen concentration.)
- sedatives, opioids, or neuromuscular blockers such as pancuronium, which may be given during mechanical ventilation to minimize restlessness, oxygen consumption, and carbon dioxide production and to facilitate ventilation
- sodium bicarbonate, which may reverse severe metabolic acidosis

- I.V. fluid administration to maintain blood pressure by treating hypovolemia
- vasopressors to maintain blood pressure
- antimicrobial drugs to treat nonviral infections
- diuretics to reduce interstitial and pulmonary edema
- correction of electrolyte and acid-base imbalances to maintain cellular integrity, particularly the sodium-potassium pump
- fluid restriction to prevent increase of interstitial and alveolar edema.

NURSING CONSIDERATIONS

Caring for the patient with ARDS requires careful monitoring and supportive care.

- Frequently assess the patient's respiratory status. Be alert for retractions on inspiration. Note the rate, rhythm, and depth of respirations; watch for dyspnea and the use of accessory muscles of respiration. On auscultation, listen for adventitious or diminished breath sounds. Check for clear, frothy sputum, which may indicate pulmonary edema.
- Observe and document the hypoxemic patient's neurologic status (level of consciousness and mental sluggishness).
- Maintain a patent airway by suctioning, using sterile, nontraumatic technique. Ensure adequate humidification to help liquefy tenacious secretions.
- Closely monitor the patient's heart rate and blood pressure. Watch for arrhythmias that may result from hypoxemia, acid-base disturbances, or electrolyte imbalances. With pulmonary artery catheterization, know the desired PAWP level. Check readings often, and watch for decreasing mixed venous oxygen saturation.
- Monitor serum electrolytes, and correct imbalances. Measure intake and output; weigh the patient daily.
- Check ventilator settings frequently, and empty condensate from tubing promptly to ensure maximum oxygen delivery. Monitor ABG studies; check for metabolic and respiratory acidosis and PaO_2 changes. The patient with severe hypoxemia may need controlled mechanical ventilation with positive pressure. Give sedatives, as needed, to reduce restlessness.
- Because PEEP may decrease cardiac output, check for hypotension, tachycardia, and decreased urine output. Suction only as needed to maintain PEEP, or use an in-line suctioning apparatus. Reposition the patient often, and record an increase in secretions, temperature, or hypotension that may indicate a deteriorating condition. Monitor peak pressures during ventilation. Because of stiff, noncompliant lungs, the patient is at high risk for barotrauma (pneumothorax), evidenced by increased peak pressures, decreased breath sounds on one side, and restlessness.
- Monitor nutrition, maintain joint mobility, and prevent skin breakdown. Accurately record caloric intake. Give tube feedings and parenteral nutrition, as ordered. Perform passive range-of-motion exercises, or help the patient perform active exercises if possible. Provide meticulous skin care. Plan patient care to allow periods of uninterrupted sleep.
- Provide emotional support. Warn the patient who's recovering from ARDS that recovery will take some time and that he'll feel weak for a while.

- Watch for and immediately report all respiratory changes in the patient with injuries that may adversely affect the lungs (especially during the 2- to 3-day period after the injury, when the patient may appear to be improving).

- cor pulmonale
- pneumonia
- pneumothorax
- pulmonary edema
- pulmonary emboli
- ventilatory failure.

Acute respiratory failure

When the lungs can't adequately maintain arterial oxygenation or eliminate carbon dioxide, acute respiratory failure (ARF) results, which can lead to tissue hypoxia. In patients with essentially normal lung tissue, ARF usually means partial pressure of arterial carbon dioxide ($PaCO_2$) above 50 mm Hg and partial pressure of arterial oxygen (PaO_2) below 50 mm Hg. These limits, however, don't apply to patients with chronic obstructive pulmonary disease (COPD), who usually have a consistently high $PaCO_2$ and low PaO_2. In patients with COPD, only acute deterioration in arterial blood gas (ABG) values, with corresponding clinical deterioration, indicates ARF.

CAUSES

Conditions that can result in alveolar hypoventilation, ventilation-perfusion ($\dot{V}/\dot{Q}$) mismatch, or right-to-left shunting can lead to respiratory failure. Such conditions include:
- atelectasis
- bronchitis
- bronchospasm
- central nervous system (CNS) disease
- CNS depression — head trauma or injudicious use of sedatives, opioids, tranquilizers, or oxygen
- COPD

PATHOPHYSIOLOGY

Respiratory failure results from impaired gas exchange. Conditions associated with alveolar hypoventilation, $\dot{V}/\dot{Q}$ mismatch, and intrapulmonary (right-to-left) shunting can cause ARF if left untreated.

Decreased oxygen saturation may result from alveolar hypoventilation, in which chronic airway obstruction reduces alveolar minute ventilation. PaO_2 levels fall and $PaCO_2$ levels rise, resulting in hypoxemia.

Hypoventilation can occur from a decrease in the rate or duration of inspiratory signal from the respiratory center, such as with CNS conditions or trauma or CNS-depressant drugs. Neuromuscular diseases, such as poliomyelitis or amyotrophic lateral sclerosis, can result in alveolar hypoventilation if the condition affects normal contraction of the respiratory muscles. The most common cause of alveolar hypoventilation is airway obstruction, commonly seen with COPD (emphysema or bronchitis).

The most common cause of hypoxemia — $\dot{V}/\dot{Q}$ imbalance — occurs when such conditions as pulmonary embolism or acute respiratory distress syndrome interrupt normal gas exchange in a specific lung region. Too little ventilation with normal blood flow or too little blood flow with normal ventilation may cause the imbalance, resulting in decreased PaO_2 levels and, thus, hypoxemia.

Decreased fraction of inspired oxygen (FIO_2) is also a cause of respiratory failure, although it's uncommon. Hypoxemia results from inspired air that doesn't contain adequate oxygen to establish an adequate gradient for diffusion into the blood — for example, at high altitudes or in confined spaces.

The hypoxemia and hypercapnia characteristics of respiratory failure stimulate strong compensatory responses by all of the body systems, including the respiratory, cardiovascular, and central nervous systems. In response to hypoxemia, for example, the sympathetic nervous system triggers vasoconstriction, increases peripheral resistance, and increases the heart rate. Untreated $\dot{V}/\dot{Q}$ imbalances can lead to right-to-left shunting, in which blood passes from the heart's right side to its left without being oxygenated.

Tissue hypoxemia occurs, resulting in anaerobic metabolism and lactic acidosis. Respiratory acidosis occurs from hypercapnia. Heart rate increases, stroke volume increases, and heart failure may occur. Cyanosis occurs because of increased amounts of unoxygenated blood. Hypoxia of the kidneys results in the release of erythropoietin from renal cells, which causes the bone marrow to increase red blood cell production — an attempt by the body to increase the blood's oxygen-carrying capacity.

The body responds to hypercapnia with cerebral depression, hypotension, circulatory failure, and increased heart rate and cardiac output. Hypoxemia, hypercapnia, or both cause the brain's respiratory control center first to increase respiratory depth (tidal volume) and then to increase the respiratory rate. As respiratory failure worsens, intercostal, supraclavicular, and suprasternal retractions may also occur.

CLINICAL FINDINGS

Specific symptoms vary with the underlying cause of ARF but may include these systems:

● Respiratory — Rate may be increased, decreased, or normal depending on the cause; respirations may be shallow or deep, or may alternate between the two; air hunger may occur. Cyanosis may be present, depending on the hemoglobin level and arterial oxygenation. Auscultation of the chest may reveal crackles, rhonchi, wheezing, or diminished breath sounds.

● CNS — When hypoxemia and hypercapnia occur, the patient may show evidence of restlessness, confusion, loss of concentration, irritability, tremulousness, diminished tendon reflexes, papilledema, and coma.

● Cardiovascular — Tachycardia, with increased cardiac output and mildly elevated blood pressure secondary to adrenal release of catecholamine, occurs early in response to low PaO_2. With myocardial hypoxia, arrhythmias may develop. Pulmonary hypertension, secondary to pulmonary capillary vasoconstriction, may cause increased pressures on the right side of the heart, distended jugular veins, an enlarged liver, and peripheral edema.

TEST RESULTS

● ABG analysis indicates respiratory failure by deteriorating values and a pH below 7.35. Patients with COPD may have a lower than normal pH compared with previous levels.

● Chest X-rays identify pulmonary diseases or conditions, such as emphysema, atelectasis, lesions, pneumothorax, infiltrates, and effusions.

- Electrocardiography can demonstrate ventricular arrhythmias (indicating myocardial hypoxia) or right ventricular hypertrophy (indicating cor pulmonale).
- Pulse oximetry reveals decreasing arterial oxygen saturation.
- White blood cell count increases if there's an underlying infection.
- Hemoglobin level and hematocrit are abnormally low in the presence of excessive blood loss.
- Potassium and chloride levels may be decreased.
- Blood cultures may identify pathogens.
- Pulmonary artery catheterization helps to distinguish pulmonary and cardiovascular causes of ARF and monitors hemodynamic pressures.

TREATMENT

- Oxygen therapy to promote oxygenation and raise PaO_2
- Mechanical ventilation with an endotracheal or a tracheostomy tube, if needed, to provide adequate oxygenation and reverse acidosis
- High-frequency ventilation, if the patient doesn't respond to treatment, to force the airways open, promoting oxygenation and preventing alveoli collapse
- Antibiotics to treat infection
- Bronchodilators to maintain airway patency
- Corticosteroids to decrease inflammation
- Fluid restrictions in cor pulmonale to reduce volume and cardiac workload
- Positive inotropic agents to increase cardiac output
- Vasopressors to maintain blood pressure
- Diuretics to reduce edema and fluid overload

- Deep breathing with pursed lips if patient isn't intubated and mechanically ventilated to help keep airway patent
- Incentive spirometry to increase lung volume

NURSING CONSIDERATIONS

- Because the patient with ARF is usually treated in an intensive care unit (ICU), orient him to the environment, procedures, and routines to minimize his anxiety.
- To reverse hypoxemia, administer oxygen at appropriate concentrations to maintain PaO_2 at a minimum of 50 to 60 mm Hg. Patients with COPD usually require only small amounts of supplemental oxygen. Watch for a positive response such as improvement in the patient's breathing, color, and ABG results.
- Maintain a patent airway. If the patient is retaining carbon dioxide, encourage him to cough and to breathe deeply. Teach him to use pursed-lip and diaphragmatic breathing to control dyspnea. If the patient is alert, have him use an incentive spirometer; if he's intubated and lethargic, turn him every 1 to 2 hours. Use postural drainage and chest physiotherapy to help clear secretions.
- In an intubated patient, suction the trachea as needed after hyperoxygenation. Observe for change in quantity, consistency, and color of sputum. Provide humidification to liquefy secretions.
- Observe the patient closely for respiratory arrest. Auscultate for chest sounds. Monitor ABG levels, and report changes immediately.
- Monitor and record serum electrolyte levels carefully, and correct imbalances; monitor fluid balance by

recording intake and output or daily weight.

- Check the cardiac monitor for arrhythmias.

If the patient requires mechanical ventilation:

- Check ventilator settings, cuff pressures, and ABG values often because the FIO_2 setting depends on ABG levels. Draw samples for ABG analysis 20 to 30 minutes after every FIO_2 change or check with oximetry.
- Prevent infection by using sterile technique while suctioning.
- Stress ulcers are common in intubated ICU patients. Check gastric secretions for evidence of bleeding if the patient has a nasogastric tube or complains of epigastric tenderness, nausea, or vomiting. Monitor hemoglobin level and hematocrit; check stools for occult blood. Administer antacids, histamine-2 receptor antagonists, or sucralfate, as ordered.
- Prevent tracheal erosion, which can result from artificial airway cuff overinflation. Use the minimal leak technique and a cuffed tube with high residual volume (low-pressure cuff), a foam cuff, or a pressure-regulating valve on the cuff.
- To prevent oral or vocal cord trauma, make sure the endotracheal tube is positioned midline.
- To prevent nasal necrosis, keep the nasotracheal tube midline within the nostrils and provide good hygiene. Loosen the tape periodically to prevent skin breakdown. Avoid excessive movement of any tubes; make sure the ventilator tubing is adequately supported.

Asbestosis

Considered a form of pneumoconiosis, asbestosis is characterized by diffuse interstitial pulmonary fibrosis. Prolonged exposure to airborne particles causes pleural plaques and tumors of the pleura and peritoneum. Asbestosis may develop 15 to 20 years after regular exposure to asbestos has ended. It's a potent cocarcinogen and increases a smoker's risk of lung cancer. An asbestos worker who smokes is 90 times more likely to develop lung cancer than a smoker who has never worked with asbestos.

CAUSES

- Exposure to asbestos used in paints, plastics, and brake and clutch linings
- Exposure to fibrous asbestos dust in deteriorating buildings or in waste piles from asbestos plants
- Family members of asbestos workers who may be exposed to stray fibers from the worker's clothing
- Prolonged inhalation of asbestos fibers; people at high risk including workers in the mining, milling, construction, fireproofing, and textile industries

PATHOPHYSIOLOGY

Asbestosis occurs when lung spaces become filled with asbestos fibers. The inhaled asbestos fibers (50 microns or more in length and 0.5 microns or less in diameter) travel down the airway and penetrate respiratory bronchioles and alveolar walls. Coughing attempts to expel the foreign matter. Mucus production and goblet cells are stimulated to protect the airway from the debris and aid in expectoration. Fibers then become encased in a brown, iron-rich, protein-like sheath in sputum or lung tissue, called asbestosis bodies. Chronic irritation by the fibers continues to affect the lower bronchioles and alveoli. The foreign material and inflammation swell airways, and fibrosis develops in response to the chronic irritation. Interstitial fibrosis may develop in lower lung zones, affecting lung parenchyma and the pleurae. Raised hyaline plaques may form in the parietal pleura, the diaphragm, and the pleura adjacent to the pericardium. Hypoxia develops as more alveoli and lower airways are affected.

CLINICAL FINDINGS

- Dyspnea on exertion
- Dyspnea at rest with extensive fibrosis
- Severe, nonproductive cough in nonsmokers
- Productive cough in smokers
- Clubbed fingers due to chronic hypoxia
- Chest pain (commonly pleuritic) due to pleural irritation
- Recurrent respiratory tract infections as pulmonary defense mechanisms begin to fail
- Pleural friction rub due to fibrosis
- Decreased lung inflation due to lung stiffness
- Recurrent pleural effusions due to fibrosis
- Decreased forced expiratory volume due to diminished alveoli
- Decreased vital capacity due to fibrotic changes

TEST RESULTS

- Chest X-rays may show fine, irregular, linear, and diffuse infiltrates. Extensive fibrosis is revealed by a honeycomb or ground-glass appearance. Chest X-rays may also show pleural thickening and calcification, bilateral obliteration of the costophrenic angles and, in later stages, an enlarged heart with a classic "shaggy" border.
- Pulmonary function studies may identify decreased vital capacity, forced vital capacity (FVC), and total lung capacity; decreased or normal forced expiratory volume in 1 second (FEV_1); a normal ratio, or FEV_1 to FVC; and reduced diffusing capacity for carbon monoxide when fibrosis destroys alveolar walls and thickens the alveolar capillary membrane.
- Arterial blood gas analysis may reveal decreased partial pressure of arterial oxygen and partial pressure of arterial carbon dioxide from hyperventilation.

TREATMENT

Asbestosis can't be cured. The goal of treatment is to relieve symptoms and control complications. Treatment may involve:

- chest physiotherapy (controlled coughing and postural drainage with chest percussion and vibration) to help relieve respiratory signs and symptoms and manage hypoxia and cor pulmonale
- aerosol therapy to liquefy mucus
- inhaled mucolytics to liquefy and mobilize secretions
- increased fluid intake to 3 qt (3 L) daily
- antibiotics to treat respiratory tract infections
- oxygen administration to relieve hypoxia
- possibly, diuretics to decrease edema, digoxin to enhance cardiac output, and salt restriction to prevent fluid retention for patients with cor pulmonale.

NURSING CONSIDERATIONS

● Teach the patient to prevent infections by avoiding crowds and persons with infections and by receiving influenza and pneumococcal vaccines.

● Improve the patient's ventilatory efficiency by encouraging physical reconditioning, energy conservation in daily activities, and relaxation techniques.

Asthma

Asthma is a chronic inflammatory airway disorder characterized by airflow obstruction and airway hyperresponsiveness to multiple stimuli. This widespread but variable airflow obstruction is caused by bronchospasm, edema of the airway mucosa, and increased mucus production with plugging and airway remodeling. It's a type of chronic obstructive pulmonary disease (COPD), a long-term pulmonary disease characterized by increased airflow resistance; other types of COPD include chronic bronchitis and emphysema.

Alert *Although asthma strikes at any age, about 50% of patients are younger than age 10; twice as many boys as girls are affected in this age-group. One-third of patients develop asthma between ages 10 and 30, and the incidence is the same in both sexes in this age-group. Moreover, approximately one-third of all patients share the disease with at least one immediate family member.*

Asthma may result from sensitivity to extrinsic or intrinsic allergens. Extrinsic, or atopic, asthma begins in childhood; typically, patients are sensitive to specific external allergens.

Alert *In children, extrinsic asthma is commonly accompanied by other hereditary allergies, such as eczema and allergic rhinitis.*

Intrinsic, or nonatopic, patients with asthma react to internal, hypoallergenic factors; external substances can't be implicated in patients with intrinsic asthma. Most episodes occur after a severe respiratory tract infection, especially in adults. However, many patients with asthma, especially children, have intrinsic and extrinsic asthma.

A significant number of adults acquire an allergic form of asthma or exacerbation of existing asthma from exposure to agents in the workplace. Irritants, such as chemicals in flour, acid anhydrides, toluene diisocyanates, screw flies, river flies, and excreta of dust mites in carpet, have been identified as agents that trigger asthma.

CAUSES
Extrinsic allergens

● Animal dander
● Food additives containing sulfites
● House dust or mold
● Kapok or feather pillows
● Other sensitizing substances
● Pollen

Intrinsic allergens

● Anxiety
● Coughing or laughing
● Emotional stress
● Endocrine changes
● Exposure to noxious fumes
● Fatigue
● Genetic factors (see "Pathophysiology")
● Humidity variations
● Irritants
● Temperature variations

PATHOPHYSIOLOGY

Two genetic influences are identified with asthma—namely, the ability of an individual to develop asthma (atopy) and the tendency to develop hyperresponsiveness of the airways independent of atopy. A locus of chromosome 11 associated with atopy contains an abnormal gene that encodes a part of the immunoglobulin (Ig) E receptor. Environmental factors interact with inherited factors to cause asthmatic reactions with associated bronchospasms.

In asthma, bronchial linings overreact to various stimuli, causing episodic smooth-muscle spasms that severely constrict the airways. (See *Pathophysiology of asthma.*) IgE antibodies, attached to histamine-containing mast cells and receptors on cell membranes, initiate intrinsic asthma attacks. When exposed to an antigen such as pollen, the IgE antibody combines with the antigen.

On subsequent exposure to the antigen, mast cells degranulate and release mediators. Mast cells in the lung interstitium are stimulated to release histamine and leukotrienes. Histamine attaches to receptor sites in the larger bronchi, where it causes swelling in smooth muscles. Mucous membranes become inflamed, irritated, and swollen. The patient may experience dyspnea, prolonged expiration, and an increased respiratory rate.

Leukotrienes attach to receptor sites in the smaller bronchi and cause local swelling of the smooth muscle. Leukotrienes also cause prostaglandins to travel through the bloodstream to the lungs, where they enhance histamine's effect. A wheeze may be audible during coughing — the higher the pitch, the narrower the bronchial lumen. Histamine stimulates the mucous membranes to secrete excessive mucus, further narrowing the bronchial lumen. Goblet cells secrete viscous mucus that's difficult to cough up, resulting in coughing, rhonchi, increased-pitch wheezing, and increased respiratory distress. Mucosal edema and thickened secretions further block the airways. (See *Looking at a bronchiole in asthma,* page 98.)

On inhalation, the narrowed bronchial lumen can still expand slightly, allowing air to reach the alveoli. On exhalation, increased intrathoracic pressure closes the bronchial lumen completely. Air enters but can't escape. The patient develops a barrel chest and hyperresonance to percussion.

Mucus fills the lung bases, inhibiting alveolar ventilation. Blood is shunted to alveoli in other lung parts but still can't compensate for diminished ventilation.

Hyperventilation is triggered by lung receptors to increase lung volume because of trapped air and obstructions. Intrapleural and alveolar gas pressures rise, causing a decreased perfusion of alveoli. Increased alveolar gas pressure, decreased ventilation, and decreased perfusion result in uneven ventilation-perfusion ratios and mismatching within different lung segments.

Hypoxia triggers hyperventilation by respiratory center stimulation, which in turn decreases partial pressure of arterial carbon dioxide ($PaCO_2$) and increases pH, resulting in respiratory alkalosis. As the airway obstruction increases in severity, more alveoli are affected. Ventilation and perfusion remain inadequate, and carbon dioxide retention develops. Respiratory acidosis results, and respiratory failure occurs.

If status asthmaticus occurs, hypoxia worsens and expiratory flows and volumes decrease even further. If

PATHOPHYSIOLOGY OF ASTHMA

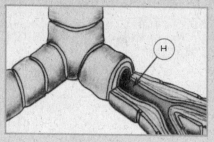

In asthma, hyperresponsiveness of the airways and broncho-spasms occur. These illustrations show the progression of an asthma attack.

◆ Histamine (H) attaches to receptor sites in larger bronchi, causing swelling of the smooth muscles.

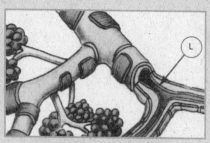

◆ Leukotrienes (L) attach to receptor sites in the smaller bronchi and cause swelling of smooth muscle there. Leuko-trienes also cause prostaglandins to travel through the blood-stream to the lungs, where they enhance histamine's effects.

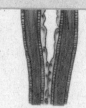
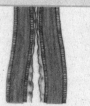

Bronchial lumen on inhalation

Bronchial lumen on exhalation

◆ Histamine stimulates the mu-cous membranes to secrete ex-cessive mucus, further narrow-ing the bronchial lumen. On in-halation, the narrowed bronchial lumen can still expand slightly; however, on exhalation, the in-creased intrathoracic pressure closes the bronchial lumen completely.

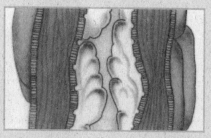

◆ Mucus fills lung bases, inhibit-ing alveolar ventilation. Blood is shunted to alveoli in other parts of the lungs, but it still can't compensate for diminished ven-tilation.

LOOKING AT
A BRONCHIOLE IN ASTHMA

Asthma is characterized by bronchospasms, increased mucus secretion, and mucosal edema, which contribute to airway narrowing and obstruction. Shown here is a normal bronchiole in cross section and an obstructed bronchiole, as it occurs in asthma.

Normal bronchiole

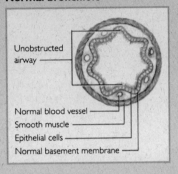

Unobstructed airway

Normal blood vessel
Smooth muscle
Epithelial cells
Normal basement membrane

Obstructed bronchiole

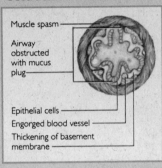

Muscle spasm

Airway obstructed with mucus plug

Epithelial cells
Engorged blood vessel
Thickening of basement membrane

treatment isn't initiated, the patient begins to tire out. (See *Averting an asthma attack*.) Acidosis develops as arterial carbon dioxide increases. The situation becomes life-threatening as no air becomes audible upon auscultation (a silent chest) and $PaCO_2$ rises to greater than 70 mm Hg.

CLINICAL FINDINGS

● Extrinsic asthma is usually accompanied by signs and symptoms of atopy (type I IgE-mediated allergy), such as eczema and allergic rhinitis. It commonly follows a severe respiratory tract infection, especially in adults.
● An acute asthma attack begins dramatically, with simultaneous onset of severe multiple symptoms, or insidiously, with gradually increasing respiratory distress.

● Asthma that occurs with cyanosis, confusion, and lethargy indicates the onset of life-threatening status asthmaticus and respiratory failure.

Other signs and symptoms of asthma include:
● sudden dyspnea, wheezing, and tightness in the chest
● coughing that produces thick, clear, or yellow sputum
● tachypnea, along with use of accessory respiratory muscles
● rapid pulse
● profuse perspiration
● hyperresonant lung fields
● diminished breath sounds.

The National Heart, Lung, and Blood Institute of the National Institutes of Health identified four levels of asthma severity based on the frequency of symptoms and exacerbations,

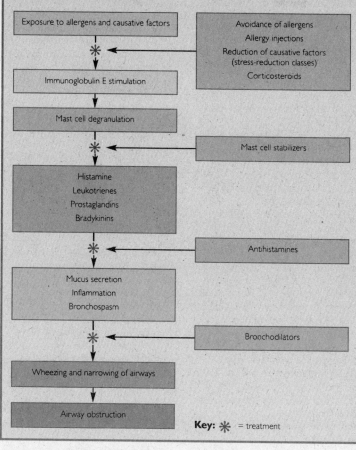

AVERTING AN ASTHMA ATTACK

This flowchart shows pathophysiologic changes that occur with asthma. Treatments and interventions (shaded boxes) show where the physiologic cascade would be altered to stop an asthma attack.

Exposure to allergens and causative factors	Avoidance of allergens Allergy injections Reduction of causative factors (stress-reduction classes) Corticosteroids
Immunoglobulin E stimulation	
Mast cell degranulation	
	Mast cell stabilizers
Histamine Leukotrienes Prostaglandins Bradykinins	
	Antihistamines
Mucus secretion Inflammation Bronchospasm	
	Bronchodilators
Wheezing and narrowing of airways	
Airway obstruction	

Key: ✳ = treatment

effects on activity level, and lung function study results: mild intermittent, mild persistent, moderate persistent, and severe persistent.

Mild intermittent asthma
- Symptoms occur fewer than two times per week.
- The patient is asymptomatic with normal peak expiratory flow (PEF) between exacerbations.

- Brief exacerbations (from a few hours to a few days) vary in intensity.
- Nighttime symptoms occur fewer than two times per month.
- Lung function studies show forced expiratory volume in 1 second (FEV_1) or PEF greater than 80% of normal values; PEF may vary by less than 20%.

Mild persistent asthma

- Symptoms occur more than two times per week but less than once per day; exacerbations may affect activity.
- Nighttime symptoms occur more than two times per month.
- Lung function studies show FEV_1 or PEF greater than 80% of normal values; PEF may vary by 20% to 30%.

Moderate persistent asthma

- Symptoms occur daily.
- Exacerbations occur more than two times per week and may last for days; exacerbations affect activity.
- Bronchodilator therapy is used daily.
- Nighttime symptoms occur more than once per week.
- Lung function studies show FEV_1 or PEF 60% to 80% of normal values; PEF may vary by greater than 30%.

Severe persistent asthma

- Symptoms occur on a continuous basis.
- Exacerbations occur frequently and limit physical activity.
- Nighttime symptoms occur frequently.
- Lung function studies show FEV_1 or PEF less than 60% of normal values; PEF may vary by greater than 30%.

TEST RESULTS

- Pulmonary function studies reveal signs of airway obstructive disease, low-normal or decreased vital capacity, and increased total lung and residual capacities. Pulmonary function may be normal between attacks. Partial pressure of arterial oxygen (PaO_2) and $PaCO_2$ are usually decreased, except in severe asthma, when $PaCO_2$ may be normal or increased, indicating severe bronchial obstruction.
- Serum IgE levels may increase from an allergic reaction.
- Sputum analysis may indicate the presence of Curschmann's spirals (casts of airways), Charcot-Leyden crystals, and eosinophils.
- Complete blood count with differential reveals an increased eosinophil count.
- Chest X-rays can be used to diagnose or monitor the progress of asthma and may show hyperinflation with areas of atelectasis.
- Arterial blood gas (ABG) analysis detects hypoxemia (decreased PaO_2; decreased, normal, or increasing $PaCO_2$) and guides treatment.
- Skin testing may identify specific allergens. Results read in 1 or 2 days detect an early reaction; after 4 or 5 days, a late reaction.
- Bronchial challenge testing evaluates the clinical significance of allergens identified by skin testing.
- Electrocardiography shows sinus tachycardia during an asthma attack; a severe attack may show signs of cor pulmonale (right axis deviation, peaked P wave) that resolve after the attack.

TREATMENT

Drug therapy for the patient with asthma is typically based on the severity of disease. Correcting asthma typically involves:

- prevention, by identifying and avoiding precipitating factors, such as environmental allergens or irritants, which is the best treatment
- desensitization to specific antigens — helpful if the stimuli can't be removed entirely — which decreases the severity of attacks of asthma with future exposure
- bronchodilators — including the methylxanthines (theophylline and aminophylline) and the beta$_2$-adrenergic agonists (albuterol [Proventil] and terbutaline [Brethine]) — to decrease bronchoconstriction, reduce bronchial airway edema, and increase pulmonary ventilation
- corticosteroids (such as hydrocortisone sodium succinate, prednisone, methylprednisolone [Medrol], and beclomethasone [QVAR]) for their anti-inflammatory and immunosuppressive effects, which decrease inflammation and edema of the airways
- mast cell stabilizers (cromolyn sodium [Nasalcrom] and nedocromil [Tilade]), effective in patients with atopic asthma who have seasonal disease (When given prophylactically, they block the acute obstructive effects of antigen exposure by inhibiting the degranulation of mast cells, thereby preventing the release of chemical mediators responsible for anaphylaxis.)
- leukotriene modifiers, such as zileuton (Zyflo), and leukotriene receptor antagonists (LTRAs), such as montelukast (Singulair) and zafirlukast (Accolate), which inhibit the potent bronchoconstriction and inflammatory effects of the cysteinyl leukotrienes (LTRAs can be used as adjunctive therapy to avoid high-dose inhaled corticosteroids. Although this class of medications doesn't replace inhaled corticosteroids as first-line anti-inflammatory treatment, it can be used successfully in cases where poor compliance with inhaled corticosteroid use is suspected.)
- anticholinergic bronchodilators, such as ipratropium (Atrovent), which block acetylcholine, another chemical mediator
- low-flow humidified oxygen, which may be needed to treat dyspnea, cyanosis, and hypoxemia (However, the amount delivered should maintain Pao$_2$ between 65 and 85 mm Hg, as determined by ABG analysis.)
- mechanical ventilation — necessary if the patient doesn't respond to initial ventilatory support and drugs or if he develops respiratory failure
- relaxation exercises, such as yoga, to help increase circulation and to help a patient recover from an asthma attack.

NURSING CONSIDERATIONS
During acute attack
- First, assess the severity of asthma.
- Administer the prescribed treatments, and assess the patient's response.
- Place the patient in high Fowler's position. Encourage pursed-lip and diaphragmatic breathing. Help him to relax.
- Monitor the patient's vital signs. Keep in mind that developing or increasing tachypnea may indicate worsening asthma or drug toxicity. Hypertension may indicate asthma-related hypoxemia.
- Administer prescribed humidified oxygen by nasal cannula at 2 L/minute to ease breathing and to increase arterial oxygen saturation (Sao$_2$). Later, adjust oxygen according

to the patient's vital signs and ABG levels.

• Anticipate intubation and mechanical ventilation if the patient fails to maintain adequate oxygenation.

• Monitor serum theophylline levels to ensure they're in the therapeutic range. Observe the patient for signs and symptoms of theophylline toxicity (vomiting, diarrhea, and headache) as well as for signs of a subtherapeutic dosage (respiratory distress and increased wheezing).

• Observe the frequency and severity of the patient's cough, and note whether it's productive. Then auscultate his lungs, noting adventitious or absent breath sounds. If his cough isn't productive and rhonchi are present, teach him effective coughing techniques. If he can tolerate postural drainage and chest percussion, perform these procedures to clear secretions. Suction an intubated patient as needed.

• Treat dehydration with I.V. fluids until the patient can tolerate oral fluids, which will help loosen secretions.

• If conservative treatment fails to improve the airway obstruction, anticipate bronchoscopy or bronchial lavage when a lobe or larger area collapses.

During long-term care

• Monitor the patient's respiratory status to detect baseline changes, to assess response to treatment, and to prevent or detect complications.

• Auscultate the lungs frequently, noting the degree of wheezing and quality of air movement.

• Review ABG levels, pulmonary function test results, and SaO_2 readings.

• If the patient is taking systemic corticosteroids, observe for complications, such as elevated blood glucose levels and friable skin and bruising. Cushingoid effects resulting from long-term use of corticosteroids may be minimized by alternate-day dosage or use of prescribed inhaled corticosteroids.

• If the patient is taking corticosteroids by inhaler, watch for signs of candidal infection in the mouth and pharynx. Using an extender device and rinsing the mouth afterward may prevent this.

• Observe the patient's anxiety level. Keep in mind that measures that reduce hypoxemia and breathlessness should help relieve anxiety.

• Keep the room temperature comfortable, and use an air conditioner or a fan in hot, humid weather.

• Control exercise-induced asthma by instructing the patient to use a bronchodilator or cromolyn sodium 30 minutes before exercise. Also instruct him to use pursed-lip breathing while exercising.

During patient education

• Teach the patient and his family to avoid known allergens and irritants.

• Describe prescribed drugs, including their names, dosages, actions, adverse effects, and special instructions.

• Teach the patient how to use a metered-dose inhaler. If he has difficulty using an inhaler, he may need an extender device to optimize drug delivery and lower the risk of candidal infection with orally inhaled corticosteroids.

• Explain how to use a peak flow meter to measure the degree of airway obstruction. Tell him to keep a record of peak flow readings and to bring it to medical appointments. Explain the importance of calling the physician immediately if the peak flow drops suddenly (may signal severe respiratory problems).

● Tell the patient to notify the physician if he develops a fever above 100° F (37.8° C), chest pain, shortness of breath without coughing or exercising, or uncontrollable coughing. An uncontrollable asthma attack requires immediate attention.

● Teach the patient diaphragmatic and pursed-lip breathing as well as effective coughing techniques.

● Urge the patient to drink at least 3 qt (3 L) of fluids daily to help loosen secretions and maintain hydration.

Chronic obstructive pulmonary disease

Chronic obstructive pulmonary disease (COPD), also called *chronic obstructive lung disease,* results from emphysema, chronic bronchitis, asthma, or a combination of these disorders. Usually, more than one of these underlying conditions coexist; bronchitis and emphysema commonly occur together.

COPD is the most common lung disease and affects an estimated 17 million U.S. residents; the incidence is increasing. The disease doesn't always produce symptoms and may cause only minimal disability. However, COPD worsens with time.

CAUSES
● Air pollution
● Allergies
● Cigarette smoking
● Familial and hereditary factors such as an alpha$_1$-antitrypsin deficiency
● Recurrent or chronic respiratory tract infections

PATHOPHYSIOLOGY
Smoking, one of the major causes of COPD, impairs ciliary action and macrophage function and causes inflammation in the airways, increased mucus production, destruction of alveolar septa, and peribronchiolar fibrosis. Early inflammatory changes may reverse if the patient stops smoking before lung disease becomes extensive.

The mucus plugs and narrowed airways cause air trapping, as in chronic bronchitis and emphysema. Hyperinflation occurs to the alveoli on expiration. On inspiration, airways enlarge, allowing air to pass beyond the obstruction; on expiration, airways narrow and gas flow is prevented. Air trapping (also called *ball valving*) occurs commonly in asthma and chronic bronchitis. (See *Air trapping in COPD,* page 104.)

CLINICAL FINDINGS
● Reduced ability to perform exercises or do strenuous work because of diminished pulmonary reserve
● Productive cough due to stimulation of the reflex by mucus
● Dyspnea on minimal exertion
● Frequent respiratory tract infections
● Intermittent or continuous hypoxemia
● Grossly abnormal pulmonary function studies
● Thoracic deformities

TEST RESULTS
● Arterial blood gas (ABG) analysis indicates the degree of hypoxia and elevation of carbon dioxide levels.
● Chest X-rays may show an overexpanded lung (hyperinflation).
● Pulmonary function studies may show reduced carbon dioxide re-

AIR TRAPPING IN COPD

In chronic obstructive pulmonary disease (COPD), mucus plugs and narrowed airways trap air (also called *ball valving*). During inspiration, the airways enlarge and gas enters; on expiration, the airways narrow and air can't escape. This commonly occurs in asthma and chronic bronchitis.

Inspiration:
Air is allowed to flow freely in.

Expiration:
Air is trapped.

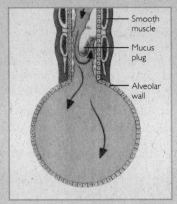

- Smooth muscle
- Mucus plug
- Alveolar wall

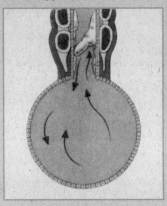

sponse, increased residual volume, increased thoracic gas volume and functional residual capacity; and decreased total lung capacity, forced vital capacity, flow-volume curve, and forced expiratory volume and flow.

- Electrocardiography may show arrhythmias consistent with hypoxemia.

TREATMENT

- Bronchodilators to alleviate bronchospasms and enhance mucociliary clearance of secretions
- Effective coughing to remove secretions
- Postural drainage to help mobilize secretions
- Chest physiotherapy to mobilize secretions
- Low oxygen concentrations as needed (High flow rates of oxygen can lead to narcosis.)
- Antibiotics to allow treatment of respiratory tract infections
- Smoking cessation
- Increased fluid intake to thin mucus
- Use of a humidifier to thin secretions

NURSING CONSIDERATIONS

- Urge the patient to stop smoking. Provide smoking-cessation counseling or refer him to a program. Advise him to avoid other respiratory irritants, such as secondhand smoke, aerosol spray products, and outdoor air pollution. An air conditioner with an air filter in his home may be helpful.

The patient is usually treated with beta-adrenergic agonist bronchodilators (albuterol [Proventil] or salmeterol [Serevent]), anticholinergic bronchodilators (ipratropium [Atrovent]), and corticosteroids (beclomethasone [QVAR] or triamcinolone [Azmacort]). These are usually given by metered-dose inhaler, requiring that the patient be taught the correct administration technique.

● Administer antibiotics, as ordered, to treat respiratory infections. Stress the need to complete the prescribed course of antibiotic therapy. Teach the patient and his family how to recognize early signs of infection; warn him to avoid contact with people with respiratory infections. Encourage good oral hygiene to help prevent infection. Pneumococcal and annual influenza vaccinations are important preventive measures.

● To strengthen the muscles of respiration, teach the patient to take slow, deep breaths and exhale through pursed lips.

● To help mobilize secretions, teach the patient how to cough effectively. If the patient with copious secretions has difficulty mobilizing secretions, teach his family how to perform postural drainage and chest physiotherapy. If secretions are thick, urge the patient to drink 12 to 15 glasses of fluid per day. A home humidifier may be beneficial, particularly in the winter.

● Perform ABG analysis to determine the patient's oxygen needs and to avoid carbon dioxide narcosis. If the patient is to continue oxygen therapy at home, teach him how to use the equipment correctly. The patient with COPD rarely requires more than 2 to 3 L/minute to maintain adequate oxygenation. Higher flow rates can further increase partial pressure of arterial oxygen, but the patient whose ventilatory drive is largely based on hypoxemia commonly develops markedly increased partial pressure of arterial carbon dioxide tensions. In this patient, chemoreceptors in the brain are relatively insensitive to the increase in carbon dioxide. Teach the patient and his family that excessive oxygen therapy may eliminate the hypoxic respiratory drive, causing confusion and drowsiness, signs of carbon dioxide narcosis.

● Emphasize the importance of a balanced diet. Because the patient may tire easily when eating, suggest that he eat frequent, small meals and consider using oxygen, administered by nasal cannula, during meals.

● Help the patient and his family adjust their lifestyles to accommodate the limitations imposed by this debilitating chronic disease. Instruct the patient to allow for daily rest periods and to exercise daily as his physician directs.

● As COPD progresses, encourage the patient to discuss his fears.

● To help prevent COPD, advise the patient not to smoke, especially if he has a family history of COPD or if his disease is in its early stages.

● Assist in the early detection of COPD by urging the patient to have periodic physical examinations, including spirometry and medical evaluation of a chronic cough, and to seek treatment for recurring respiratory infections promptly.

Cor pulmonale

Cor pulmonale (also called *right-sided heart failure*) is a condition in which hypertrophy and dilation of the right ventricle develop secondary to disease affecting the structure or function of the lungs or their vasculature. It can occur at the end stage of various chronic disorders of the lungs, pulmonary vessels, chest wall, and respiratory control center. Cor pulmonale doesn't occur with disorders stemming from congenital heart disease or with those affecting the left side of the heart.

About 85% of patients with cor pulmonale also have chronic obstructive pulmonary disease (COPD), and about 25% of patients with bronchial COPD eventually develop cor pulmonale. The disorder is most common in smokers and in middle-age and elderly males; however, its incidence in females is increasing. Because cor pulmonale occurs late in the course of the individual's underlying condition and with other irreversible diseases, the prognosis is poor.

Alert In children, cor pulmonale may be a complication of cystic fibrosis, hemosiderosis, upper airway obstruction, scleroderma, extensive bronchiectasis, neuromuscular diseases that affect respiratory muscles, or abnormalities of the respiratory control area.

CAUSES
- Bronchial asthma
- COPD
- Disorders that affect the pulmonary parenchyma
- External vascular obstruction resulting from a tumor or aneurysm
- High altitude
- Kyphoscoliosis
- Muscular dystrophy
- Obesity
- Pectus excavatum (funnel chest)
- Poliomyelitis
- Primary pulmonary hypertension
- Pulmonary emboli
- Vasculitis

PATHOPHYSIOLOGY
In cor pulmonale, pulmonary hypertension increases the heart's workload. To compensate, the right ventricle hypertrophies to force blood through the lungs. As long as the heart can compensate for the increased pulmonary vascular resistance, signs and symptoms reflect only the underlying disorder.

Severity of right ventricular enlargement in cor pulmonale is due to increased afterload. An occluded vessel impairs the heart's ability to generate enough pressure. Pulmonary hypertension results from the increased blood flow needed to oxygenate the tissues.

In response to hypoxia, the bone marrow produces more red blood cells (RBCs), causing polycythemia. The blood's viscosity increases, which further aggravates pulmonary hypertension. This increases the right ventricle's workload, causing heart failure. (See *Cor pulmonale: An overview.*)

In COPD, increased airway obstruction makes airflow worse. The resulting hypoxia and hypercarbia can have vasodilatory effects on systemic arterioles. However, hypoxia increases pulmonary vasoconstriction. The liver becomes palpable and tender because it's engorged and displaced downward by the low diaphragm. Hepatojugular reflux may occur.

Compensatory mechanisms begin to fail, and larger amounts of blood remain in the right ventricle at the end of diastole, causing ventricular dilation. Increasing intrathoracic pressures impede venous return and raise jugular vein pressure. Peripheral edema can occur, and right ventricular hypertrophy increases progressively. The main pulmonary arteries enlarge, pulmonary hypertension increases, and heart failure occurs.

CLINICAL FINDINGS
Early stages
- Chronic productive cough to clear secretions from the lungs
- Exertional dyspnea due to hypoxia
- Wheezing respirations as airways narrow
- Fatigue and weakness due to hypoxemia

Progressive stage
- Dyspnea at rest due to hypoxemia
- Tachypnea due to decreased oxygenation to the tissues
- Orthopnea due to pulmonary edema
- Dependent edema due to right-sided heart failure
- Distended jugular veins due to pulmonary hypertension
- Enlarged, tender liver related to polycythemia and decreased cardiac output
- Hepatojugular reflux (distention of the jugular vein induced by pressing over the liver) due to right-sided heart failure
- Right upper quadrant discomfort due to liver involvement
- Tachycardia due to decreased cardiac output and increasing hypoxia
- Weakened pulses due to decreased cardiac output
- Decreased cardiac output
- Pansystolic murmur at the lower left sternal border with tricuspid insufficiency, which increases in intensity when the patient inhales

TEST RESULTS
- Pulmonary artery catheterization shows increased right ventricular and pulmonary artery pressures, resulting

Focus in

COR PULMONALE: AN OVERVIEW

Although pulmonary restrictive disorders (such as fibrosis or obesity), obstructive disorders (such as bronchitis), or primary vascular disorders (such as recurrent pulmonary emboli) may cause cor pulmonale, these disorders share this common pathway.

Pulmonary disorder

↓

Anatomic alterations in the pulmonary blood vessels and functional alterations in the lung

↓

Increased pulmonary vascular resistance

↓

Pulmonary hypertension

↓

Right ventricular hypertrophy (cor pulmonale)

↓

Heart failure

from increased pulmonary vascular resistance. Right ventricular systolic and pulmonary artery systolic pressures are greater than 30 mm Hg, and pulmonary artery diastolic pressure is higher than 15 mm Hg.
- Echocardiography demonstrates right ventricular enlargement.
- Angiography shows right ventricular enlargement.

- Chest X-rays reveal large central pulmonary arteries and right ventricular enlargement.
- Arterial blood gas (ABG) analysis detects decreased partial pressure of arterial oxygen (usually less than 70 mm Hg and rarely more than 90 mm Hg).
- Electrocardiography shows arrhythmias, such as premature atrial and ventricular contractions and atrial fibrillation during severe hypoxia, and right bundle-branch block, right axis deviation, prominent P waves, and an inverted T wave in right precordial leads.
- Pulmonary function studies reflect underlying pulmonary disease.
- Magnetic resonance imaging may show increased right ventricular mass and wall thickness and decreased ejection fraction.
- Cardiac catheterization may reveal increased pulmonary vascular pressures.
- Laboratory testing may reveal hematocrit typically over 50%; serum hepatic tests may show an elevated level of aspartate aminotransferase levels with hepatic congestion and decreased liver function, and serum bilirubin levels may be elevated if liver dysfunction and hepatomegaly exist.

TREATMENT

Therapy of cor pulmonale has three aims: reducing hypoxemia and pulmonary vasoconstriction, increasing exercise tolerance, and correcting the underlying condition when possible. Treatment may involve:
- bed rest to reduce myocardial oxygen demands
- digoxin to increase the strength of contraction of the myocardium
- antibiotics to treat an underlying respiratory tract infection

- a potent pulmonary artery vasodilator, such as diazoxide, nitroprusside, hydralazine, angiotensin-converting enzyme inhibitors, calcium channel blockers, or prostaglandins, to reduce primary pulmonary hypertension
- continuous administration of low concentrations of oxygen to decrease pulmonary hypertension, polycythemia, and tachycardia
- mechanical ventilation to reduce the workload of breathing in acute disease
- a low-sodium diet with restricted fluid to reduce edema
- phlebotomy to decrease excess RBC mass that occurs with polycythemia
- small doses of heparin to decrease the risk of thromboembolism
- tracheotomy, which may be required if the patient has an upper airway obstruction
- corticosteroids to treat vasculitis or an underlying autoimmune disorder.

NURSING CONSIDERATIONS

- Plan the patient's diet carefully with the patient and the staff dietitian. Because the patient may lack energy and tire easily when eating, provide small, frequent feedings rather than three heavy meals.
- Prevent fluid retention by limiting the patient's fluid intake to 1 to 2 qt (1 to 2 L)/day and providing a low-sodium diet.
- Monitor serum potassium levels closely if the patient is receiving diuretics. Low serum potassium levels can increase the risk of arrhythmias associated with cardiac glycosides.
- Watch the patient for signs of digoxin (Lanoxin) toxicity, such as complaints of anorexia, nausea, vomiting, and yellow halos around visual

images; monitor him for cardiac arrhythmias. Teach the patient to check his radial pulse before taking digoxin or other cardiac glycoside. He should be instructed to notify the physician if he detects changes in his pulse rate.
● Reposition the bedridden patient often to prevent atelectasis.
● Provide meticulous respiratory care, including oxygen therapy and, for the patient with COPD, pursed-lip breathing exercises. Periodically measure ABG levels, and watch for such signs of respiratory failure as change in pulse rate; deep, labored respirations; and increased fatigue after exertion.

Before discharge, maintain this protocol:
● Make sure the patient understands the importance of maintaining a low-salt diet, weighing himself daily, and watching for and immediately reporting edema. Teach him to detect edema by pressing the skin over his shins with one finger, holding it for a second or two, then checking for a finger impression.
● Instruct the patient to allow himself frequent rest periods and to do his breathing exercises regularly.
● If the patient needs supplemental oxygen therapy at home, refer him to an agency that can help him obtain the necessary equipment and, as necessary, arrange for follow-up examinations.
● If the patient has been placed on anticoagulant therapy, emphasize the need to watch for bleeding (epistaxis, hematuria, bruising) and to report signs to the physician. Also, encourage him to return for periodic laboratory tests to monitor partial thromboplastin time, fibrinogen level, platelet count, hematocrit and hemoglobin levels, and prothrombin time.

● Because pulmonary infection commonly exacerbates COPD and cor pulmonale, tell the patient to watch for and immediately report early signs of infection, such as increased sputum production, change in sputum color, increased coughing or wheezing, chest pain, fever, and tightness in the chest. Tell the patient to avoid crowds and persons known to have pulmonary infections, especially during the flu season.
● Warn the patient to avoid nonprescribed medications (such as sedatives) that may depress the ventilatory drive.

Pneumonia

Pneumonia is an acute infection of the lung parenchyma that commonly impairs gas exchange. The prognosis is good for patients with normal lungs and adequate immune systems. However, bacterial pneumonia is the leading cause of death in debilitated patients. Pneumonia is classified three ways:
● Origin — Pneumonia may be viral, bacterial, fungal, or protozoal in origin.
● Location — Bronchopneumonia involves distal airways and alveoli; lobular pneumonia, part of a lobe; and lobar pneumonia, an entire lobe.
● Type — Primary pneumonia results from inhalation or aspiration of a pathogen, such as bacteria or a virus, and includes pneumococcal and viral pneumonia. Secondary pneumonia may follow lung damage from a noxious chemical or other insult or may result from hematogenous spread of bacteria. Aspiration pneumonia results from inhalation of foreign matter,

such as vomitus or food particles, into the bronchi.

CAUSES

Pneumonia is caused by exposure to pathogens. After they get into the lower respiratory tract, they colonize and infection develops. Exposure can be by:
- aspiration
- direct contact with contaminated equipment such as suction catheters
- inhalation
- vascular dissemination.

Certain predisposing factors increase the risk of pneumonia. For bacterial and viral pneumonia, these factors include:
- abdominal and thoracic surgery
- alcoholism
- aspiration
- atelectasis
- cancer (particularly lung cancer)
- chronic illness and debilitation
- colds or other viral respiratory infections
- chronic respiratory disease, such as chronic obstructive pulmonary disease, bronchiectasis, or cystic fibrosis
- exposure to noxious gases
- immunosuppressive therapy
- influenza
- malnutrition
- premature birth
- sickle cell disease
- smoking
- tracheostomy.

PATHOPHYSIOLOGY

In bacterial pneumonia, which can occur in any part of the lungs, an infection initially triggers alveolar inflammation and edema. This condition produces an area of low ventilation with normal perfusion. Capillaries become engorged with blood, causing stasis. As the alveolocapillary membrane breaks down, alveoli fill with blood and exudate, resulting in atelectasis (lung collapse).

In severe bacterial infections, the lungs look heavy and liverlike — reminiscent of acute respiratory distress syndrome (ARDS).

In viral pneumonia, the virus first attacks bronchiolar epithelial cells. This attack causes interstitial inflammation and desquamation. The virus also invades bronchial mucous glands and goblet cells. It then spreads to the alveoli, which fill with blood and fluid. In advanced infection, a hyaline membrane may form. Like bacterial infections, viral pneumonia clinically resembles ARDS.

In aspiration pneumonia, inhalation of gastric juices or hydrocarbons triggers inflammatory changes and inactivates surfactant over a large area. Decreased surfactant leads to alveolar collapse. Acidic gastric juices may damage the airways and alveoli. Particles containing aspirated gastric juices may obstruct the airways and reduce airflow, leading to secondary bacterial pneumonia.

CLINICAL FINDINGS

The clinical manifestations of different types of pneumonia vary. (See *Distinguishing among types of pneumonia*.)

TEST RESULTS

- Chest X-rays confirm the diagnosis by disclosing infiltrates.
- Sputum specimen, Gram stain, and culture and sensitivity tests help differentiate the type of infection and the drugs that are effective in treatment.
- White blood cell count indicates leukocytosis in bacterial pneumonia and a normal or low count in viral or mycoplasmal pneumonia.

DISTINGUISHING AMONG TYPES OF PNEUMONIA

The characteristics and prognosis of the different types of pneumonia vary.

TYPE	CHARACTERISTICS
VIRAL	
Influenza	◆ Prognosis poor even with treatment ◆ 50% mortality from cardiopulmonary collapse ◆ Cough (initially nonproductive; later, purulent sputum), marked cyanosis, dyspnea, high fever, chills, substernal pain and discomfort, moist crackles, frontal headache, myalgia
Adenovirus	◆ Insidious onset ◆ Generally affects young adults ◆ Good prognosis; usually clears with no residual effects ◆ Sore throat, fever, cough, chills, malaise, small amounts of mucoid sputum, retrosternal chest pain, anorexia, rhinitis, adenopathy, scattered crackles, and rhonchi
Respiratory syncytial virus	◆ Most prevalent in infants and children ◆ Complete recovery in 1 to 3 weeks; may cause death in premature infants younger than age 6 months ◆ Listlessness, irritability, tachypnea with retraction of intercostal muscles, slight sputum production, fever, severe malaise, possible cough or croup, and fine, moist crackles
Measles (rubeola)	◆ Typically more severe in adults than in children ◆ Fever, dyspnea, cough, small amounts of sputum, rash, cervical adenopathy, and profusely runny nose
Chickenpox (varicella pneumonia)	◆ Uncommon in children but present in 30% of adults with varicella ◆ Characteristic rash, cough, dyspnea, cyanosis, tachypnea, pleuritic chest pain, and hemoptysis and rhonchi 1 to 6 days after onset of rash
Cytomegalovirus	◆ Difficult to distinguish from other nonbacterial pneumonias ◆ In adults with healthy lung tissue, resembles mononucleosis and is generally benign; in neonates, occurs as devastating multisystemic infection; in immunocompromised hosts, varies from clinically inapparent to fatal infection ◆ Fever, cough, shaking chills, dyspnea, cyanosis, weakness, and diffuse crackles
BACTERIAL	
Streptococcus	◆ Sudden onset of a single, shaking chill, and sustained temperature of 102° to 104° F (38.9° to 40° C); commonly preceded by upper respiratory tract infection

(continued)

DISTINGUISHING AMONG
TYPES OF PNEUMONIA *(continued)*

TYPE	CHARACTERISTICS
BACTERIAL *(continued)*	
Klebsiella	◆ More likely in patients with chronic alcoholism, pulmonary disease, and diabetes ◆ Fever and recurrent chills; cough producing rusty, bloody, viscous sputum (currant jelly); cyanosis of lips and nail beds from hypoxemia; shallow, grunting respirations
Staphylococcus	◆ Commonly occurs in patients with viral illness, such as influenza or measles, and in those with cystic fibrosis ◆ Temperature of 102° to 104° F (38.9° to 40° C), recurrent shaking chills, bloody sputum, dyspnea, tachypnea, and hypoxemia
ASPIRATION	
	◆ Results from vomiting and aspiration of gastric or oropharyngeal contents into trachea and lungs ◆ Noncardiogenic pulmonary edema possible with damage to respiratory epithelium from contact with gastric acid ◆ Subacute pneumonia possible with cavity formation ◆ Lung abscess possible if foreign body present ◆ Crackles, dyspnea, cyanosis, hypotension, and tachycardia

● Blood cultures reflect bacteremia and determine the causative organism.
● Arterial blood gas (ABG) levels vary, depending on the severity of pneumonia and the underlying lung state.
● Bronchoscopy or transtracheal aspiration allows the collection of material for culture.
● Pulse oximetry may show a reduced arterial oxygen saturation level.

TREATMENT
The patient with pneumonia needs antimicrobial therapy based on the causative agent. Reevaluation should be done early in treatment. Supportive measures include:
● humidified oxygen therapy for hypoxia
● bronchodilator therapy
● antitussives
● mechanical ventilation for respiratory failure
● positive end-expiratory pressure ventilation to maintain adequate oxygenation for patients with severe pneumonia on mechanical ventilation
● high-calorie diet and adequate fluid intake
● bed rest
● analgesic to relieve pleuritic chest pain.

NURSING CONSIDERATIONS
● Maintain a patent airway and adequate oxygenation. Measure ABG levels, especially if the patient is hypoxic, and monitor his response to oxygen therapy.
● For severe pneumonia that requires endotracheal intubation or a tracheostomy with or without mechanical ventilation, provide thorough res-

piratory care and suction often using
sterile technique to remove secretions.
- Administer I.V. fluids and electrolyte replacement, if needed, for
fever and dehydration.
- Administer antibiotics and pain
medication, as needed.
- Provide a high-calorie, high-protein
diet of soft foods to offset the calories
the patient uses to fight the infection.
If necessary, supplement oral feedings
with nasogastric (NG) tube feedings
or parenteral nutrition. Monitor fluid
intake and output.
- To prevent aspiration during NG
tube feedings, elevate the patient's
head, check the tube position, and administer the feeding slowly. Don't
give large volumes at one time because this can cause vomiting.
- To help prevent the spread of infection, encourage the patient to
sneeze and cough into a disposable
tissue, and tape a waxed bag to the
side of the bed for disposal of used
tissues.
- Provide a quiet, calm environment,
and encourage frequent rest periods.
- Explain all procedures to the patient and family members.
- Teach the patient coughing and
deep-breathing exercises as well as
home oxygen therapy, and chest
physiotherapy if needed.
- Encourage the patient to avoid irritants that stimulate secretions, such as
cigarette smoke, dust, and significant
environmental pollution.
- Encourage annual influenza vaccination for high-risk patients.

☀ Life-threatening
Pneumothorax

Pneumothorax is an accumulation of
air in the pleural cavity that leads to
partial or complete lung collapse.
When the air between the visceral and
parietal pleurae collects and accumulates, increasing tension in the pleural
cavity can cause the lung to progressively collapse. Air is trapped in the
intrapleural space and determines the
degree of lung collapse. Venous return
to the heart may be impeded to cause
a life-threatening condition called tension pneumothorax.

The most common types of pneumothorax are open, closed, and tension.

CAUSES
Open pneumothorax
- Chest surgery
- Insertion of a central venous
catheter
- Penetrating chest injury (gunshot
or stab wound)
- Thoracentesis or closed pleural
biopsy
- Transbronchial biopsy

Closed pneumothorax
- Air leakage from ruptured blebs
- Blunt chest trauma
- Interstitial lung disease such as
eosinophilic granuloma
- Rupture resulting from barotrauma
caused by high intrathoracic pressures
during mechanical ventilation
- Tubercular or cancerous lesions
that erode into the pleural space

Tension pneumothorax
- Chest tube occlusion or malfunction

- Fractured ribs
- High-level positive end-expiratory pressure that causes alveolar blebs to rupture
- Mechanical ventilation
- Penetrating chest wound treated with an air-tight dressing

PATHOPHYSIOLOGY

A rupture in the visceral or parietal pleura and chest wall causes air to accumulate and separate the visceral and parietal pleurae. Negative pressure is destroyed, and the elastic recoil forces are affected. The lung recoils by collapsing toward the hilus.

Open pneumothorax (also called a *sucking chest wound, traumatic pneumothorax,* or *communicating pneumothorax*) results when atmospheric air (positive pressure) flows directly into the pleural cavity (negative pressure). As the air pressure in the pleural cavity becomes positive, the lung collapses on the affected side, resulting in decreased total lung capacity, vital capacity, and lung compliance. Ventilation-perfusion imbalances lead to hypoxia.

Closed (spontaneous) pneumothorax occurs when air enters the pleural space from within the lung, causing increased pleural pressure, which prevents lung expansion during normal inspiration. Spontaneous pneumothorax is another type of closed pneumothorax.

Alert Spontaneous pneumothorax is common in older patients with chronic pulmonary disease, but it may also occur in healthy, tall, young adults due to the increase of shear force at the apex of the lung.

Both types of closed pneumothorax can result in a collapsed lung with hypoxia and decreased total lung capacity, vital capacity, and lung compli-

ance. The range of lung collapse is between 5% and 95%.

Tension pneumothorax results when air in the pleural space is under higher pressure than air in the adjacent lung. The air enters the pleural space from the site of pleural rupture, which acts as a one-way valve. Air is allowed to enter into the pleural space on inspiration but can't escape as the rupture site closes on expiration. More air enters on inspiration, and air pressure begins to exceed barometric pressure. Increasing air pressure pushes against the recoiled lung, causing compression atelectasis. Air also presses against the mediastinum, compressing and displacing the heart and great vessels. The air can't escape, and the accumulating pressure causes the lung to collapse. As air continues to accumulate and intrapleural pressures increase, the mediastinum shifts away from the affected side and decreases venous return. This forces the heart, trachea, esophagus, and great vessels to the unaffected side, compressing the heart and the contralateral lung. Without immediate treatment, this emergency can rapidly become fatal. (See *Understanding tension pneumothorax.*)

CLINICAL FINDINGS

Open and closed pneumothorax produces such symptoms as:
- sudden, sharp pleuritic pain exacerbated by chest movement, breathing, and coughing
- asymmetrical chest wall movement due to lung collapse
- shortness of breath due to hypoxia
- cyanosis due to hypoxia
- respiratory distress
- decreased vocal fremitus related to lung collapse

UNDERSTANDING
TENSION PNEUMOTHORAX

In tension pneumothorax, air accumulates intrapleurally and can't escape. As intrapleural pressure increases, the ipsilateral lung is affected and also collapses.

On inspiration, the mediastinum shifts toward the unaffected lung, impairing ventilation.

On expiration, the mediastinal shift distorts the vena cava and reduces venous return.

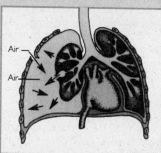

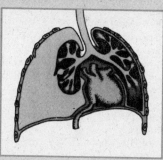

• absent breath sounds on the affected side due to lung collapse
• chest rigidity on the affected side due to decreased expansion
• tachycardia due to hypoxia
• crackling beneath the skin on palpation (subcutaneous emphysema), which is due to air leaking into the tissues.

Tension pneumothorax produces the most severe respiratory symptoms, including:
• decreased cardiac output
• hypotension due to decreased cardiac output
• compensatory tachycardia
• tachypnea due to hypoxia
• lung collapse due to air or blood in the intrapleural space
• mediastinal shift due to increasing tension
• tracheal deviation to the opposite side

• distended jugular veins due to intrapleural pressure, mediastinal shift, and increased cardiovascular pressure
• pallor related to decreased cardiac output
• anxiety related to hypoxia
• weak and rapid pulse due to decreased cardiac output.

TEST RESULTS
• Chest X-rays confirm the diagnosis by revealing air in the pleural space and, possibly, a mediastinal shift.
• Arterial blood gas analysis may reveal hypoxemia, possibly with respiratory acidosis and hypercapnia. Partial pressure of arterial oxygen levels may decrease at first but typically return to normal within 24 hours.

TREATMENT
Treatment depends on the type of pneumothorax.

Open (traumatic) pneumothorax
may be corrected with:
• chest tube drainage to reexpand
the lung
• surgical repair of the lung.
Closed (spontaneous) pneumothorax with less than 30% of lung collapse, no signs of increased pleural
pressure, and no dyspnea or indications of physiologic compromise may
be corrected with:
• bed rest to conserve energy and reduce oxygenation demands
• monitoring of blood pressure and
pulse for early detection of physiologic compromise
• monitoring of respiratory rate to
detect early signs of respiratory compromise
• oxygen administration to enhance
oxygenation and improve hypoxia
• aspiration of air with a large-bore
needle attached to a syringe to restore
negative pressure within the pleural
space.
Correction of pneumothorax with
more than 30% of lung collapse may
include:
• thoracostomy tube placed in the
second or third intercostal space in the
midclavicular line with connection to
underwater-seal and low-pressure suction to try to reexpand the lung by
restoring negative intrapleural pressure
• if recurrent spontaneous pneumothorax, thoracotomy and pleurec-
tomy may be performed, which causes the lung to adhere to the parietal
pleura.
Correction of tension pneumothorax typically involves:
• immediate treatment with large-
bore needle insertion into the pleural
space through the second intercostal
space to reexpand the lung
• insertion of a thoracostomy tube

• analgesics to promote comfort and
encourage deep breathing and coughing.

NURSING CONSIDERATIONS

• Watch for pallor, gasping respirations, and sudden chest pain. Carefully monitor vital signs at least every
hour for indications of shock, increasing respiratory distress, and mediastinal shift. Listen for breath sounds over
both lungs. Falling blood pressure and
rising pulse and respiratory rates may
indicate tension pneumothorax,
which could be fatal without prompt
treatment.
• Urge the patient to control coughing and gasping during thoracotomy.
However, after the chest tube is in
place, encourage him to cough and
breathe deeply (at least once per hour)
to facilitate lung expansion.
• If the patient is undergoing chest
tube drainage, watch for continuing
air leakage (bubbling), indicating the
lung defect has failed to close; this
may require surgery. Also watch for
increasing subcutaneous emphysema
by checking around the neck or at the
tube insertion site for crackling beneath the skin. If the patient is on a
ventilator, watch for difficulty in
breathing in time with the ventilator
as well as pressure changes on ventilator gauges.
• Change dressings around the chest
tube insertion site as necessary. Be
careful not to reposition or dislodge
the tube. If the tube dislodges, place a
petroleum gauze dressing over the
opening immediately to prevent rapid
lung collapse.
• Monitor vital signs frequently after
thoracotomy. Also, for the first 24
hours, assess respiratory status by
checking breath sounds hourly. Observe the chest tube site for leakage,

noting the amount and color of drainage. Help the patient walk, as ordered (usually on the first postoperative day), to facilitate deep inspiration and lung expansion.

● To reassure the patient, explain what pneumothorax is, what causes it, and all diagnostic tests and procedures. Make him as comfortable as possible. (The patient with pneumothorax is usually most comfortable sitting upright.)

✹ Life-threatening
Pulmonary edema

Pulmonary edema is an accumulation of fluid in the extravascular spaces of the lungs. It's a common complication of cardiac disorders and may occur as a chronic condition or may develop quickly and rapidly become fatal.

CAUSES
Pulmonary edema is caused by left-sided heart failure due to:
● arteriosclerosis
● cardiomyopathy
● hypertension
● valvular heart disease.

Factors that predispose the patient to pulmonary edema include:
● barbiturate or opiate poisoning
● cardiac failure
● excess infusion of I.V. fluids or overly rapid infusion
● impaired pulmonary lymphatic drainage (from Hodgkin's disease or obliterative lymphangitis after radiation)
● inhalation of irritating gases
● mitral stenosis and left atrial myxoma (which impairs left atrial emptying)
● pneumonia

● pulmonary veno-occlusive disease.

PATHOPHYSIOLOGY
Normally, pulmonary capillary hydrostatic pressure, capillary oncotic pressure, capillary permeability, and lymphatic drainage are in balance. When this balance changes or the lymphatic drainage system is obstructed, fluid infiltrates into the lung and pulmonary edema results. If pulmonary capillary hydrostatic pressure increases, the compromised left ventricle requires increased filling pressures to maintain adequate cardiac output. These pressures are transmitted to the left atrium, pulmonary veins, and pulmonary capillary bed, forcing fluids and solutes from the intravascular compartment into the interstitium of the lungs. As the interstitium overloads with fluid, fluid floods the peripheral alveoli and impairs gas exchange.

If colloid osmotic pressure decreases, the hydrostatic force that regulates intravascular fluids (the natural pulling force) is lost because there's no opposition. Fluid flows freely into the interstitium and alveoli, impairing gas exchange and leading to pulmonary edema. (See *Understanding pulmonary edema,* pages 118 and 119.)

A blockage of the lymph vessels can result from compression by edema or tumor fibrotic tissue and by increased systemic venous pressure. Hydrostatic pressure in the large pulmonary veins increases, the pulmonary lymphatic system can't drain correctly into the pulmonary veins, and excess fluid moves into the interstitial space. Pulmonary edema then results from fluid accumulation.

Capillary injury, such as occurs in acute respiratory distress syndrome (ARDS) or with inhalation of toxic

UNDERSTANDING
PULMONARY EDEMA

In pulmonary edema, diminished function of the left ventricle causes blood to back up into pulmonary veins and capillaries. The increasing capillary hydrostatic pressure pushes fluid into the interstitial spaces and alveoli. These illustrations show a normal alveolus and an alveolus affected by pulmonary edema.

Normal alveolus

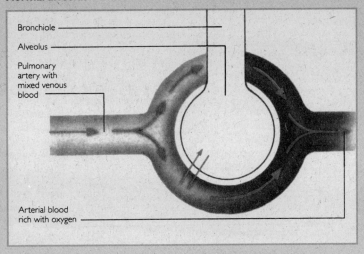

Bronchiole

Alveolus

Pulmonary artery with mixed venous blood

Arterial blood rich with oxygen

gases, increases capillary permeability. The injury causes plasma proteins and water to leak out of the capillary and move into the interstitium, increasing the interstitial oncotic pressure, which is normally low. As interstitial oncotic pressure begins to equal capillary oncotic pressure, the water begins to move out of the capillary and into the lungs, resulting in pulmonary edema.

CLINICAL FINDINGS
Early stages
● Dyspnea on exertion due to hypoxia

● Paroxysmal nocturnal dyspnea due to decreased lung expansion
● Orthopnea due to decreased ability of the diaphragm to expand
● Cough due to stimulation of cough reflex by excessive fluid
● Mild tachypnea due to hypoxia
● Increased blood pressure due to increased pulmonary pressures and decreased oxygenation
● Dependent crackles as air moves through fluid in the lungs
● Jugular vein distention due to decreased cardiac output and increased pulmonary vascular resistance

Alveolus in pulmonary edema

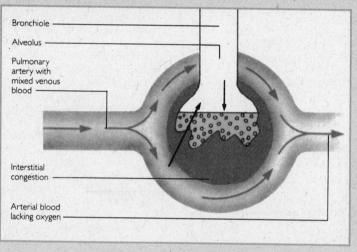

Bronchiole

Alveolus

Pulmonary artery with mixed venous blood

Interstitial congestion

Arterial blood lacking oxygen

- Tachycardia due to hypoxia

Late stages
- Labored, rapid respiration due to hypoxia
- More diffuse crackles as air moves through fluid in the lungs
- Cough producing frothy, bloody sputum
- Increased tachycardia due to hypoxemia
- Arrhythmias due to hypoxic myocardium
- Cold, clammy skin due to peripheral vasoconstriction

- Diaphoresis due to decreased cardiac output and shock
- Cyanosis due to hypoxia
- Decreased blood pressure due to decreased cardiac output and shock
- Thready pulse due to decreased cardiac output and shock

TEST RESULTS
- Arterial blood gas (ABG) analysis usually reveals hypoxia with variable partial pressure of arterial carbon dioxide, depending on the patient's degree of fatigue. Respiratory acidosis may occur.

- Chest X-rays show diffuse haziness of the lung fields and, usually, cardiomegaly and pleural effusion.
- Pulse oximetry may reveal decreasing arterial oxygen saturation levels.
- Pulmonary artery catheterization identifies left-sided heart failure and helps rule out ARDS.
- Electrocardiography may show previous or current myocardial infarction.

TREATMENT

Treatment measures for pulmonary edema are designed to reduce extravascular fluid, to improve gas exchange and myocardial function and, if possible, to correct underlying pathologic conditions. Correcting this disorder typically involves:

- high concentrations of oxygen administered by nasal cannula to enhance gas exchange and improve oxygenation
- assisted ventilation to improve oxygen delivery to the tissues and promote acid-base balance
- diuretics, such as furosemide (Lasix) and bumetanide (Bumex), to increase urination, which helps mobilize extravascular fluid
- positive inotropic agents, such as digoxin (Lanoxin) and inamrinone, to enhance contractility in myocardial dysfunction
- pressor agents to enhance contractility and promote vasoconstriction in peripheral vessels
- antiarrhythmics for arrhythmias related to decreased cardiac output
- arterial vasodilators, such as nitroprusside, to decrease peripheral vascular resistance, preload, and afterload
- morphine to reduce anxiety and dyspnea and to dilate the systemic venous bed, promoting blood flow from pulmonary circulation to the periphery.

NURSING CONSIDERATIONS

- Carefully monitor the vulnerable patient for early signs of pulmonary edema, especially tachypnea, tachycardia, and abnormal breath sounds. Report abnormalities. Check for peripheral edema, which may also indicate that fluid level is accumulating in pulmonary tissue.
- Administer oxygen as ordered.
- Monitor vital signs every 15 to 30 minutes while administering nitroprusside in dextrose 5% in water by I.V. drip. Protect the nitroprusside solution from light by wrapping the bottle or bag with aluminum foil, and discard unused solution after 4 hours. Watch for arrhythmias in the patient receiving cardiac glycosides and for marked respiratory depression in the patient receiving morphine.
- Assess the patient's condition frequently, and record his response to treatment. Monitor ABG levels, oral and I.V. fluid intake, urine output and, in the patient with a pulmonary artery catheter, pulmonary end-diastolic and wedge pressures. Check cardiac monitoring often. Report changes immediately.
- Carefully record the time and amount of morphine given.
- Reassure the patient, who will be frightened by decreased respiratory capability, in a calm voice, and explain all procedures. Provide emotional support to his family as well.

Life-threatening

Pulmonary embolism

The most common pulmonary complication in hospitalized patients, pulmonary embolism is an obstruction of the pulmonary arterial bed by a dislodged thrombus, heart-valve growths, or a foreign substance. It strikes an estimated 6 million adults each year in the United States, resulting in 100,000 deaths. Although pulmonary infarction that results from embolism may be so mild that it produces no symptoms, massive embolism (more than 50% obstruction of pulmonary arterial circulation) and the accompanying infarction can be rapidly fatal.

CAUSES

- Pulmonary embolism generally results from dislodged thrombi originating in the leg veins or pelvis. More than one-half of such thrombi arise in the deep veins of the legs.

Other less common sources of thrombi are:
- hepatic vein
- pelvic veins
- renal veins
- right side of the heart
- upper extremities.

Predisposing factors for pulmonary embolism include:
- advanced age
- autoimmune hemolytic anemia
- burns
- cancer
- chronic pulmonary disease
- heart failure or atrial fibrillation
- hormonal contraceptives.
- I.V. drug abuse
- long-term immobility

- lower-extremity fractures or surgery
- obesity
- polycythemia vera
- pregnancy
- previous deep vein thrombosis, and pulmonary emboli
- recent surgery
- sickle cell disease
- thrombocytosis
- thrombophlebitis
- varicose veins
- vascular injury.

PATHOPHYSIOLOGY

Thrombus formation results directly from vascular wall damage, venostasis, or hypercoagulability of the blood. Trauma, clot dissolution, sudden muscle spasm, intravascular pressure changes, or a change in peripheral blood flow can cause the thrombus to loosen or fragment. Then the thrombus — now called an embolus — floats to the heart's right side and enters the lung through the pulmonary artery. There, the embolus may dissolve, continue to fragment, or grow.

By occluding the pulmonary artery, the embolus prevents alveoli from producing enough surfactant to maintain alveolar integrity. As a result, alveoli collapse and atelectasis develops. If the embolus enlarges, it may clog most or all of the pulmonary vessels and cause death.

Rarely, the emboli contain air, fat, bacteria, amniotic fluid, talc (from drugs intended for oral administration that are injected I.V. by addicts), or tumor cells.

CLINICAL FINDINGS

Total occlusion of the main pulmonary artery is rapidly fatal; smaller or fragmented emboli produce symptoms that vary with the size, number, and location. Usually, the first symptoms are:

- dyspnea
- anginal or pleuritic chest pain.
  Other clinical features may include:
- tachycardia
- productive cough (sputum may be blood-tinged)
- low-grade fever
- pleural effusion
- massive hemoptysis
- splinting of the chest
- leg edema
- with a large embolus, cyanosis, syncope, and distended jugular veins
- pleural friction rub
- signs of circulatory collapse (weak, rapid pulse and hypotension)
- signs of hypoxia (restlessness and anxiety)
- right ventricular S_3 gallop, an increased intensity of a pulmonic component of S_2, crackles.

TEST RESULTS

- Chest X-ray helps to rule out other pulmonary diseases; areas of atelectasis, elevated diaphragm and pleural effusion, prominent pulmonary artery and, occasionally, the characteristic wedge-shaped infiltrate suggestive of pulmonary infarction, or focal oligemia of blood vessels, are apparent.
- Lung scan shows perfusion defects in areas beyond occluded vessels; however, it doesn't rule out microemboli.
- Pulmonary angiography is the most definitive test but requires a skilled angiographer and radiologic equipment; it also poses some risk to the patient. Its use depends on the uncertainty of the diagnosis and the need to avoid unnecessary anticoagulant therapy in a high-risk patient.

- Electrocardiography (ECG) is inconclusive but helps distinguish pulmonary embolism from myocardial infarction. In extensive embolism, the ECG may show right axis deviation; right bundle-branch block; tall, peaked P waves; depression of ST segments and T-wave inversions (indicative of right-sided heart strain); and supraventricular tachyarrhythmias. A pattern sometimes observed is S1, Q3, and T3 (S wave in lead I, Q wave in lead III, and inverted T wave in lead III).
- Arterial blood gas (ABG) measurements showing decreased partial pressure of arterial oxygen and partial pressure of arterial carbon dioxide are characteristic but don't always occur.
- If pleural effusion is present, thoracentesis may rule out empyema, which indicates pneumonia.

TREATMENT

- Treatment is designed to maintain adequate cardiovascular and pulmonary function during resolution of the obstruction and to prevent embolus recurrence.
- Because most emboli resolve within 10 to 14 days, treatment consists of oxygen therapy, as needed, and anticoagulation with heparin to inhibit new thrombus formation.
- Heparin therapy is monitored by daily coagulation studies (partial thromboplastin time [PTT]).
- Patients with massive pulmonary embolism and shock may need fibrinolytic therapy with urokinase (Abbokinase), streptokinase (Streptase), or alteplase (Activase) to enhance fibrinolysis of the pulmonary emboli and remaining thrombi.
- Emboli that cause hypotension may require the use of vasopressors.
- Treatment of septic emboli requires antibiotics, not anticoagulants, and

evaluation for the infection's source, particularly endocarditis.

- Surgery is performed on patients who can't take anticoagulants (because of recent surgery or blood dyscrasia) or who have recurrent emboli during anticoagulant therapy. Surgery (which shouldn't be performed without angiographic evidence of pulmonary embolism) consists of vena caval ligation, plication, or insertion of a device (umbrella filter) to filter blood returning to the heart and lungs.
- To prevent postoperative venous thromboembolism, a combination of heparin and dihydroergotamine may be given.

NURSING CONSIDERATIONS

- Give oxygen by nasal cannula or mask. Check ABG levels if the patient develops fresh emboli or worsening dyspnea. Be prepared to provide endotracheal intubation with assisted ventilation if breathing is severely compromised.
- Administer heparin, as ordered, through I.V. push or continuous drip. Monitor coagulation studies daily. Effective heparin therapy raises the PTT to more than 1¼ times normal. Watch closely for nosebleed, petechiae, and other signs of abnormal bleeding; check stools for occult blood. Tell the patient to prevent bleeding by shaving with an electric razor and by brushing his teeth with a soft toothbrush.
- After the patient is stable, encourage him to move about often, and assist with isometric and range-of-motion exercises. Check the pedal pulses, temperature, and color of his feet to detect venostasis. Never vigorously massage the patient's legs. Offer diversional activities to promote rest and relieve restlessness.

- Help the patient walk as soon as possible after surgery to prevent venostasis.
- Maintain adequate nutrition and fluid balance to promote healing.
- Report frequent pleuritic chest pain so that analgesics can be prescribed. Also, incentive spirometry can assist in deep breathing.
- Warn the patient not to cross his legs or sit with his legs in a dependent position for prolonged periods; this promotes thrombus formation.
- To relieve anxiety, explain procedures and treatments. Encourage the patient's family to participate in his care.
- The patient usually takes an oral anticoagulant (warfarin) for 3 to 6 months after a pulmonary embolism. Advise him to watch for signs of bleeding (bloody stools, blood in urine, and large ecchymoses), to take the prescribed medication exactly as ordered, not to change dosages without consulting his physician, and to avoid taking additional medication (even for headaches or colds). Stress the importance of follow-up laboratory tests (prothrombin time) to monitor anticoagulant therapy.
- To prevent pulmonary emboli, encourage early ambulation in the patient predisposed to this condition. With close medical supervision, low-dose heparin may be used prophylactically.
- Low-molecular-weight heparin may be given to prevent pulmonary embolism in the high-risk patient.

Respiratory distress syndrome of the newborn

Respiratory distress syndrome (RDS) of the newborn, also known as *hyaline membrane disease,* is the most common cause of neonatal death; in the United States alone, it kills about 40,000 neonates every year.

Alert RDS occurs most exclusively in neonates born before 37 weeks' gestation; it occurs in about 60% of those born before 28 weeks' gestation.

RDS of the newborn is marked by widespread alveolar collapse. Occurring mainly in premature neonates and in sudden infant death syndrome, it strikes apparently healthy neonates. It's most common in neonates of mothers who have diabetes and in those delivered by cesarean birth; it may also occur suddenly after antepartum hemorrhage.

In RDS of the newborn, premature neonates develop a widespread alveolar collapse due to surfactant deficiency. If untreated, the syndrome causes death within 72 hours of birth in up to 14% of neonates weighing less than 2,500 g (5.5 lb). Aggressive management and mechanical ventilation can improve the prognosis, although some surviving neonates are left with bronchopulmonary dysplasia. Mild cases of the syndrome subside after about 3 days.

CAUSES
- Lack of surfactant
- Premature birth

PATHOPHYSIOLOGY

Surfactant, a lipoprotein present in alveoli and respiratory bronchioles, helps to lower surface tension, maintain alveolar patency, and prevent alveolar collapse, particularly at the end of expiration.

Although the neonatal airways are developed by 27 weeks' gestation, the intercostal muscles are weak and the alveoli and capillary blood supply are immature. Surfactant deficiency causes a higher surface tension. Unable to maintain patency, the alveoli begin to collapse.

With alveolar collapse, ventilation is decreased and hypoxia develops. The resulting pulmonary injury and inflammatory reaction lead to edema and swelling of the interstitial space, thus impeding gas exchange between the capillaries and the functional alveoli. The inflammation also stimulates production of hyaline membranes composed of white fibrin accumulation in the alveoli. These deposits further reduce gas exchange in the lung and decrease lung compliance, resulting in increased work of breathing.

Decreased alveolar ventilation results in decreased ventilation-perfusion ratio and pulmonary arteriolar vasoconstriction. The pulmonary vasoconstriction can result in increased right cardiac volume and pressure, causing blood to be shunted from the right atrium through a patent foramen ovale to the left atrium. Increased pulmonary resistance also results in deoxygenated blood passing through the ductus arteriosus, totally bypassing the lungs, and causing a right-to-left shunt. The shunt further increases hypoxia.

Because of immature lungs and an already increased metabolic rate, the neonate must expend more energy to ventilate collapsed alveoli. This further increases oxygen demand and contributes to cyanosis. The infant attempts to compensate with rapid shallow breathing, causing an initial respiratory alkalosis as carbon dioxide is expelled. The increased effort at lung expansion causes respirations to slow and respiratory acidosis to occur, leading to respiratory failure.

CLINICAL FINDINGS

Alert *Suspect RDS of the newborn in a patient with a history that includes preterm birth (before 28 weeks' gestation), cesarean delivery, maternal history of diabetes, or antepartum hemorrhage.*

- Rapid, shallow respirations due to hypoxia
- Intercostal, subcostal, or sternal retractions due to hypoxia
- Nasal flaring due to hypoxia
- Audible expiratory grunting (The grunting is a natural compensatory mechanism that produces positive end-expiratory pressure [PEEP] to prevent further alveolar collapse.)
- Hypotension due to cardiac failure
- Peripheral edema due to cardiac failure
- Oliguria due to vasoconstriction of the kidneys

In severe cases

- Apnea due to respiratory failure
- Bradycardia due to cardiac failure
- Cyanosis from hypoxemia, right-to-left shunting through the foramen ovale, or right-to-left shunting through the atelectatic lung areas
- Pallor due to decreased circulation
- Frothy sputum due to pulmonary edema and atelectasis
- Low body temperature, resulting from an immature nervous system and inadequate subcutaneous fat

- Diminished air entry and crackles on auscultation because of atelectasis

TEST RESULTS

- Chest X-rays may be normal for the first 6 to 12 hours in 50% of patients, although later films show a fine reticulonodular pattern and dark streaks, indicating air-filled, dilated bronchioles.
- Arterial blood gas (ABG) analysis reveals a diminished partial pressure of arterial oxygen level; a normal, decreased, or increased partial pressure of arterial carbon dioxide level; and a reduced pH, indicating a combination of respiratory and metabolic acidosis.
- Lecithin/sphingomyelin ratio helps to assess prenatal lung development and infants at risk for this syndrome; this test is usually ordered if a cesarean delivery will be performed before 36 weeks' gestation.

TREATMENT

- Warm, humidified, oxygen-enriched gases administered by oxygen hood or, if such treatment fails, by mechanical ventilation to promote adequate oxygenation and reverse hypoxia
- Administration of surfactant by an endotracheal tube to prevent atelectasis
- Mechanical ventilation with PEEP or continuous positive airway pressure (CPAP) administered by nasal prongs (This forces the alveoli to remain open on expiration and promotes increased surface area for exchange of oxygen and carbon dioxide.)
- High-frequency oscillation ventilation if the neonate can't maintain adequate gas exchange (This provides satisfactory minute volume [the total air

breathed in 1 minute] with lower airway pressures.)

- Radiant warmer or an Isolette to help maintain thermoregulation and reduce metabolic demands
- I.V. fluids to promote adequate hydration and maintain circulation with capillary refill of less than 2 seconds (Fluid and electrolyte balance is also maintained.)
- Sodium bicarbonate to control acidosis
- Tube feedings or total parenteral nutrition
- Prophylactic antibiotics for underlying infections
- Diuretics to reduce pulmonary edema

Alert Corticosteroids may be administered to the mother to stimulate surfactant production in a fetus at high risk for preterm birth.

- Delayed delivery of a neonate (if premature labor) to possibly prevent RDS

NURSING CONSIDERATIONS

Neonates with RDS require continual assessment and monitoring in a neonatal intensive care unit.

- Closely monitor blood gases as well as fluid intake and output. If the infant has an umbilical catheter (arterial or venous), check for arterial hypotension or abnormal central venous pressure. Watch for complications, such as infection, thrombosis, or decreased circulation to the legs. If the neonate has a transcutaneous oxygen monitor, change the site of the lead placement every 2 to 4 hours to avoid burning the skin.
- Weigh the infant once or twice daily. To evaluate his progress, assess skin color, rate and depth of respirations, severity of retractions, nostril flaring, frequency of expiratory grunt-

ing, frothing at the lips, and restlessness.

- Regularly assess the effectiveness of oxygen or ventilator therapy. Evaluate every change in fraction of inspired oxygen and PEEP or CPAP by monitoring arterial oxygen saturation or ABG levels. Be sure to adjust PEEP or CPAP as indicated, based on findings.
- Mechanical ventilation in infants is usually done in a pressure-limited mode rather than the volume-limited mode used in adults.
- When the infant is on mechanical ventilation, watch carefully for signs of barotrauma (increase in respiratory distress and subcutaneous emphysema) and accidental disconnection from the ventilator. Check ventilator settings frequently. Be alert for signs of complications of PEEP or CPAP therapy, such as decreased cardiac output, pneumothorax, and pneumomediastinum. Mechanical ventilation increases the risk of infection in premature infants, so preventive measures are essential.
- As needed, arrange for follow-up care with a neonatal ophthalmologist to check for retinal damage. Premature infants in an oxygen-rich environment are at increased risk for developing retinopathy of prematurity.
- Teach the parents about their neonate's condition and, if possible, let them participate in his care, to encourage normal parent-infant bonding. Advise parents that full recovery may take up to 12 months. When the prognosis is poor, prepare the parents for the infant's impending death, and offer emotional support.
- Help reduce mortality in RDS by detecting respiratory distress early. Recognize intercostal retractions and grunting, especially in a premature in-

fant, as signs of RDS; make sure the infant receives immediate treatment.

Tuberculosis

Tuberculosis is an infectious disease that primarily affects the lungs but can invade other body systems as well. In tuberculosis, pulmonary infiltrates accumulate, cavities develop, and masses of granulated tissue form within the lungs. Tuberculosis may occur as an acute or a chronic infection.

Incidence is highest in people who live in crowded, poorly ventilated, unsanitary conditions, such as prisons, tenement houses, and homeless shelters. Others at high risk for tuberculosis include alcoholics, I.V. drug abusers, elderly people, and those who are immunocompromised.

CAUSES
- Exposure to *Mycobacterium tuberculosis*
- Exposure to other strains of mycobacteria (sometimes)

PATHOPHYSIOLOGY
Transmission occurs when an infected person coughs or sneezes, spreading infected droplets. When someone without immunity inhales these droplets, the bacilli are deposited in the lungs. The immune system responds by sending leukocytes, and inflammation results. After a few days, leukocytes are replaced by macrophages. Bacilli are then ingested by the macrophages and carried off by the lymphatics to the lymph nodes. Macrophages that ingest the bacilli fuse to form epithelioid cell tubercles, tiny nodules surrounded by lymphocytes. Within the lesion, caseous

necrosis develops and scar tissue encapsulates the tubercle. The organism may be killed in the process.

If the tubercles and inflamed nodes rupture, the infection contaminates the surrounding tissue and may spread through the blood and lymphatic circulation to distant sites. This process is called hematogenous dissemination.

Tuberculosis can cause massive pulmonary tissue damage, with inflammation and tissue necrosis eventually leading to respiratory failure. Bronchopleural fistulas can develop from lung tissue damage, resulting in pneumothorax. The disease can also lead to hemorrhage, pleural effusion, and pneumonia. Small mycobacterial foci can infect other body organs, including the kidneys, skeleton, and central nervous system.

In other infected people, microorganisms cause a latent infection. The host's immunologic defense system may destroy the bacillus. Alternatively, the encapsulated bacilli may live within the tubercle. It may lie dormant for years, reactivating later to cause active infection.

CLINICAL FINDINGS
After exposure to *M. tuberculosis,* roughly 5% of infected people develop active tuberculosis within 1 year. They may complain of the following:
- a low-grade fever at night
- a productive cough that lasts longer than 3 weeks
- symptoms of airway obstruction from lymph node involvement.

TEST RESULTS
- Chest X-rays show nodular lesions, patchy infiltrates (mainly in upper lobes), cavity formation, scar tissue, and calcium deposits.

- A tuberculin skin test reveals infection at some point but doesn't indicate active disease.
- Stains and cultures of sputum, cerebrospinal fluid, urine, drainage from abscesses, or pleural fluid show heat-sensitive, nonmotile, aerobic, acid-fast bacilli.
- Computed tomography or magnetic resonance imaging scans show the extent of lung damage and may confirm a difficult diagnosis.
- Bronchoscopy shows inflammation and altered lung tissue. It may also be performed to obtain sputum if the patient can't produce an adequate sputum specimen.

TREATMENT
- The usual treatment for tuberculosis is daily oral doses of isoniazid (Laniazid) or rifampin (Rifadin), with ethambutol (Myambutol) added in some cases, for at least 9 months.
- After 2 to 4 weeks, the disease is no longer infectious, and the patient can resume normal activities while continuing to take medication.
- The patient with atypical mycobacterial disease or drug-resistant tuberculosis may require second-line drugs, such as capreomycin (Capastat), streptomycin, pyrazinamide, and cycloserine (Seromycin).
- Many patients find it difficult to follow this lengthy treatment regimen. Therefore, the incidence of noncompliance is high. This noncompliance has led to the development of resistant strains of tuberculosis in recent years.

NURSING CONSIDERATIONS
- Isolate the infectious patient in a quiet, properly ventilated room, as per guidelines from the Centers for Disease Control and Prevention, and maintain proper precautions.
- Tell the patient to wear a mask when outside his room, to prevent spreading of the infection. Visitors and health care personnel should also take proper precautions while in the patient's room.
- Provide a well-balanced, high-calorie diet, preferably in small, frequent meals to conserve energy. Record weight weekly.
- Perform chest physiotherapy including postural drainage and chest percussion several times per day.
- Teach the patient and family members coughing and deep breathing, postural drainage and chest percussion techniques.
- Emphasize the importance of scheduling follow-up examinations and following long-term treatment.
- Warn the patient taking rifampin that it causes body secretions to appear orange. Reassure him that this is harmless.
- If the patient is a woman, advise her that hormonal contraceptives may be less effective while she's taking rifampin.
- Instruct the patient to inform others of his disorder, such as dentists and other health care providers.

3
NERVOUS SYSTEM

The nervous system coordinates and organizes the functions of all body systems. This intricate network of interlocking receptors and transmitters is a dynamic system that controls and regulates every mental and physical function. It has three main divisions:
- central nervous system (CNS) — the brain and spinal cord
- peripheral nervous system — the motor and sensory nerves, which carry messages between the CNS and remote parts of the body
- autonomic nervous system — actually part of the peripheral nervous system, regulates involuntary functions of the internal organs.

The fundamental unit that participates in all nervous system activity is the neuron, a highly specialized cell that receives and transmits electrochemical nerve impulses through delicate, threadlike fibers that extend from the central cell body. Axons carry impulses away from the cell body; dendrites carry impulses to it. Most neurons have several dendrites but only one axon. Neurons include:
- sensory (or afferent) neurons that transmit impulses from receptors to the spinal cord or the brain
- motor (or efferent) neurons that transmit impulses from the CNS to

regulate the activity of muscles or glands
- interneurons, also known as *connecting* or *association neurons,* that carry signals through complex pathways between sensory and motor neurons; they account for 99% of all the neurons in the nervous system.

From birth to death, the nervous system efficiently organizes and controls the smallest action, thought, or feeling; monitors communication and the instinct for survival; and allows introspection, wonder, abstract thought, and self-awareness. Together, the CNS and peripheral nervous system keep a person alert, awake, oriented, and able to move about freely without discomfort and with all body systems working to maintain homeostasis.

Thus, any disorder affecting the nervous system can cause signs and symptoms in any and all body systems. Patients with nervous system disorders commonly have signs and symptoms that are elusive, subtle, and sometimes latent.

Alzheimer's disease

Alzheimer's disease is a degenerative disorder of the cerebral cortex, especially the frontal lobe, which accounts for more than one-half of all cases of dementia. Although primarily found in the elderly population, 1% to 10% of cases have their onset in middle age. Because this is a primary progressive dementia, the prognosis for a patient with this disease is poor.

CAUSES

The exact cause of Alzheimer's disease is unknown. Factors that have been associated with its development include:

- environmental — repeated head trauma; exposure to aluminum or manganese
- genetic — autosomal dominant form of Alzheimer's disease associated with early onset and death and the established risk factors of a family history of the disease or the presence of Down syndrome in the patient
- neurochemical — deficiencies in the neurotransmitters acetylcholine, somatostatin, substance P, and norepinephrine.

PATHOPHYSIOLOGY

The brain tissue of patients with Alzheimer's disease exhibits three distinct and characteristic features:

- Neurofibrillatory tangles (fibrous proteins) are found; they are bundles of filaments inside the neuron that abnormally twist around one another. Numerous neurofibrillary tangles appear in areas of the brain associated with memory and learning (hippocampus), fear and aggression (amygdala), and thinking (cerebral cortex). These tangles play a role in the memory loss and personality changes that the patient with Alzheimer's disease suffers.
- Neuritic plaques (composed of degenerating axons and dendrites) or amyloid plaques (senile plaques) are found outside neurons in the extracellular space of the cerebral cortex and hippocampus. They contain a core of beta amyloid protein that's surrounded by abnormal nerve endings, or neurites. The plaques also occur in the walls of cerebral blood vessels, causing the condition called *amyloid angiopathy.*
- Granulovascular degeneration is found inside the neurons of the hippocampus. An abnormally high number of fluid-filled spaces, called *vacuoles,* enlarge the cell's body, possibly causing the cell to malfunction or die.

Additional structural changes include cortical atrophy, ventricular dilation, deposition of amyloid (a glycoprotein) around the cortical blood vessels, and reduced brain volume. Also found is a selective loss of cholinergic neurons in the pathways to the frontal lobes and hippocampus, areas that are important for memory and cognitive functions. Examination of the brain after death commonly reveals an atrophic brain, often weighing less than 1,000 g (normal, 1,380 g).

CLINICAL FINDINGS

The typical signs and symptoms reflect neurologic abnormalities associated with the disease.

- Gradual loss of recent and remote memory, loss of sense of smell and coordination, and flattening of affect and personality; loss of eye contact and fearful look
- Difficulty with learning new information
- Deterioration in personal hygiene
- Inability to concentrate, write, or speak
- Increasing difficulty with abstraction and judgment
- Impaired communication

- Severe deterioration in memory, language, and motor function
- Personality changes, wanderings, disorientation, and emotional lability
- Nocturnal awakenings
- Signs of anxiety such as wringing of hands; acute confusion, agitation, compulsiveness or fearfulness when overwhelmed with anxiety
- Progressive deterioration of physical and intellectual ability

Alert The most common complications of Alzheimer's disease include injury secondary to violent behavior or wandering; aspiration pneumonia and other infections; and malnutrition and dehydration.

TEST RESULTS

Alzheimer's disease is diagnosed by exclusion; that is, by ruling out other disorders as the cause for the patient's signs and symptoms. The only true way to confirm Alzheimer's disease is by finding pathological changes in the brain at autopsy. However, these diagnostic tests may be useful:
- Positron-emission tomography shows changes in metabolism of the cerebral cortex.
- Computed tomography scan shows evidence of early brain atrophy in excess of that which occurs in normal aging.
- Magnetic resonance imaging shows no lesion as the cause of dementia.
- EEG shows evidence of slowed brain waves in later stages of disease.
- Cerebral blood flow studies show abnormalities in blood flow.

TREATMENT

No cure or definitive treatment exists for Alzheimer's disease. Therapy may include:

- rivastigmine (Exelon) or tacrine (Cognex), cholinesterase inhibitors, to help improve memory deficits
- acetylcholinesterase inhibitors, donepezil (Aricept) or galantamine (Razadyne), or N-methyl-D-aspartate–receptor antagonist, memantine (Namenda), to ease the symptoms of dementia
- psychostimulants such as methylphenidate (Ritalin) to enhance the patient's mood
- antidepressants, if depression appears to exacerbate the dementia
- physostigmine, used alone or with lecithin, may help improve cognitive or behavioral function in some patients
- hyperbaric oxygen to increase oxygenation to the brain.

NURSING CONSIDERATIONS

Overall care is focused on supporting the patient's remaining abilities and compensating for those he has lost.
- Establish an effective communication system with the patient and family to help them adjust to the patient's altered cognitive abilities.
- Offer emotional support to the patient and family members. Behavior problems may be worsened by excess stimulation or change in established routine. Teach them about the disease, and refer them to social service and community resources for legal and financial advice and support.
- Anxiety may cause the patient to become agitated or fearful. Intervene by helping him focus on another activity.
- Provide the patient with a safe environment. Encourage him to exercise, as ordered, to help maintain mobility.

Amyotrophic lateral sclerosis

Commonly called *Lou Gehrig disease,* amyotrophic lateral sclerosis (ALS) is the most common of the motor neuron diseases causing muscular atrophy. Other motor neuron diseases include progressive muscular atrophy and progressive bulbar palsy. Onset usually occurs between ages 40 and 70. A chronic, progressively debilitating disease, ALS may be fatal in less than 1 year or continue for 10 years or more, depending on the muscles affected. More than 30,000 Americans have ALS; about 5,000 new cases are diagnosed each year; and the disease affects three times as many men as women.

CAUSES

The exact cause of ALS is unknown, but 5% to 10% of cases have a genetic component—an autosomal dominant trait that affects men and women equally. Several mechanisms have been postulated, including:
● a metabolic interference in nucleic acid production by the nerve fibers
● a nutritional deficiency related to a disturbance in enzyme metabolism
● a slow-acting virus
● autoimmune disorders that affect immune complexes in the renal glomerulus and basement membrane.

Precipitating factors for acute deterioration include severe stress, such as myocardial infarction, trauma, viral infections, and physical exhaustion.

PATHOPHYSIOLOGY

ALS progressively destroys the upper and lower motor neurons. It doesn't affect cranial nerves III, IV, and VI and, therefore, some facial movements, such as blinking, persist. Intellectual and sensory functions aren't affected.

Some believe that glutamate—the primary excitatory neurotransmitter of the central nervous system—accumulates to toxic levels at the synapses. The affected motor units are no longer innervated and progressive degeneration of axons causes loss of myelin. Some nearby motor nerves may sprout axons in an attempt to maintain function but, ultimately, nonfunctional scar tissue replaces normal neuronal tissue.

CLINICAL FINDINGS

● Fasciculations accompanied by spasticity, atrophy, and weakness, due to degeneration of the upper and lower motor neurons, and loss of functioning motor units, especially in the muscles of the forearms and the hands
● Impaired speech, difficulty chewing and swallowing, choking, and excessive drooling from degeneration of cranial nerves V, IX, X, and XII
● Difficulty breathing, especially if brain stem affected
● Muscle atrophy due to loss of innervation
● Mental deterioration doesn't usually occur, but patients possibly experience depression as a reaction to the disease; progressive bulbar palsy possibly causes crying spells or inappropriate laughter

Alert The most common complications of ALS include respiratory infections, respiratory failure, and aspiration.

TEST RESULTS

Although no tests are specific to ALS, these may aid in the diagnosis:
● Electromyography shows abnormalities of electrical activity in involved muscles.

- Muscle biopsy shows atrophic fibers interspersed between normal fibers.
- Nerve conduction studies show normal results.
- Computed tomography scan and EEG show normal results and thus rule out multiple sclerosis, spinal cord neoplasm, polyarteritis, syringomyelia, myasthenia gravis, progressive muscular dystrophy, and progressive stroke.

TREATMENT

ALS has no cure. Treatment is supportive and may include:
- diazepam (Valium), dantrolene (Dantrium), or baclofen (Kemstro) for decreasing spasticity
- quinidine to relieve painful muscle cramps
- thyrotropin-releasing hormone (I.V. or intrathecally) to temporarily improve motor function (successful only in some patients)
- riluzole (Rilutek) to modulate glutamate activity and slow disease progression
- respiratory, speech, and physical therapy to maintain function as much as possible
- psychological support to assist with coping with this progressive, fatal illness.

NURSING CONSIDERATIONS

Remember that because mental status remains intact while progressive physical degeneration takes place, the patient acutely perceives every change. This threatens the patient's relationships, career, income, muscle coordination, sexuality, and energy.
- Implement a rehabilitation program designed to maintain independence as long as possible.

- Help the patient obtain assistive equipment, such as a walker and a wheelchair. Arrange for a visiting nurse to oversee the patient's status, provide support, and teach the family about the illness.
- Depending on the patient's muscular capacity, assist with bathing, personal hygiene, and transfers from wheelchair to bed. Help establish a regular bowel and bladder routine.
- To help the patient handle an increased accumulation of secretions and dysphagia, teach him to suction himself. He should have a suction machine handy at home to reduce the fear of choking.
- To prevent skin breakdown, provide good skin care when the patient is bedridden. Turn him often, keep his skin clean and dry, and use pressure-reducing devices such as an alternating air mattress.
- If the patient has trouble swallowing, give him soft, solid foods and position him upright during meals. Gastrostomy or nasogastric tube feedings may be necessary if he can no longer swallow. Teach the family (or the patient if he's still able to feed himself) how to administer gastrostomy feedings.
- Provide emotional support. A discussion of directives regarding health care decisions should be instituted before the patient becomes unable to communicate his wishes. Prepare the patient and family members for his eventual death, and encourage the start of the grieving process. Patients with ALS may benefit from a hospice program or the local ALS support group chapter.

Arteriovenous malformations

Arteriovenous malformations (AVMs) are tangled masses of thin-walled, dilated blood vessels between arteries and veins that don't connect by capillaries. AVMs are common in the brain, primarily in the posterior portion of the cerebral hemispheres. Abnormal channels between the arterial and venous system mix oxygenated and unoxygenated blood and, thereby, prevent adequate perfusion of brain tissue.

AVMs range in size from a few millimeters to large malformations extending from the cerebral cortex to the ventricles. Commonly more than one AVM is present. Males and females are affected equally, and some evidence exists that AVMs occur in families. Most AVMs are present at birth; however, symptoms typically don't occur until the person is age 10 to 20.

CAUSES
- Acquired from penetrating injuries such as trauma
- Congenital, due to a hereditary defect

PATHOPHYSIOLOGY
AVMs lack the typical structural characteristics of the blood vessels. The vessels of an AVM are very thin; one or more arteries feed into the AVM, causing it to appear dilated and torturous. The typically high-pressured arterial flow moves into the venous system through the connecting channels to increase venous pressure, engorging and dilating the venous structures. An aneurysm may develop. If the AVM is large enough, the shunting can deprive the surrounding tissue of adequate blood flow. Additionally, the thin-walled vessels may ooze small amounts of blood or actually rupture, causing hemorrhage into the brain or subarachnoid space.

CLINICAL FINDINGS
Typically the patient experiences few, if any, signs and symptoms unless the AVM is large, leaks, or ruptures. Possible signs and symptoms include:
- chronic mild headache and confusion from AVM dilation, vessel engorgement, and increased pressure
- seizures secondary to compression of the surrounding tissues by the engorged vessels
- systolic bruit over carotid artery, mastoid process, or orbit, indicating turbulent blood flow
- focal neurologic deficits (depending on the location of the AVM) resulting from compression and diminished perfusion
- symptoms of intracranial (intracerebral, subarachnoid, or subdural) hemorrhage, including sudden severe headache, seizures, confusion, lethargy, and meningeal irritation from bleeding into the brain tissue or subarachnoid space
- hydrocephalus from AVM extension into the ventricular lining.

Alert Complications depend on the severity (location and size) of the AVM. This includes aneurysm development and subsequent rupture, hemorrhage (intracerebral, subarachnoid, or subdural, depending on the location of the AVM), and hydrocephalus.

TEST RESULTS
A definitive diagnosis depends on these diagnostic tests:

- Cerebral arteriogram confirms the presence of AVMs and evaluates blood flow.
- Doppler ultrasonography of cerebrovascular system indicates abnormal, turbulent blood flow.

TREATMENT

Treatment can be supportive, corrective, or both, and includes:
- support measures, along with aneurysm precautions to prevent possible rupture
- surgery (block dissection, laser, or ligation) to repair the communicating channels and remove the feeding vessels
- embolization or radiation therapy if surgery isn't possible, to close the communicating channels and feeder vessels and thus reduce blood flow to the AVM.

NURSING CONSIDERATIONS

- Monitor vital signs frequently.
- Control hypertension and seizure activity as well as other activity or stress that could elevate the patient's systemic blood pressure. Administer drug therapy as ordered, conduct ongoing neurologic assessments, and maintain a quiet, therapeutic environment.
- Control elevated intracranial pressure as ordered. Promote a quiet environment, administer medications as ordered, and monitor neurologic status.

Cerebral palsy

The most common cause of crippling in children, cerebral palsy (CP) is a group of neuromuscular disorders caused by prenatal, perinatal, or post-natal damage to the upper motor neurons. Although nonprogressive, these disorders may become more obvious as an affected infant grows.

The three major types of CP — spastic, athetoid, and ataxic — may occur alone or in combination. Motor impairment may be minimal (sometimes apparent only during physical activities such as running) or severely disabling. Common associated defects are seizures, speech disorders, and mental retardation.

CP occurs in an estimated 7,000 live births every year. Incidence is highest in premature infants (anoxia plays the greatest role in contributing to the disease) and in those who are small for gestational age. Almost one-half of children with CP are mentally retarded, approximately one-fourth have seizure disorders, and more than three-fourths have impaired speech. Additionally, children with CP typically have dental abnormalities, vision and hearing defects, and reading disabilities.

The prognosis varies. Treatment may make a near-normal life possible for children with mild impairment; those with severe impairment require special services and schooling.

CAUSES

The exact cause of CP is unknown; however, conditions resulting in cerebral anoxia, hemorrhage, or other CNS damage are probably responsible. Potential causes vary with time of damage.
- Perinatal and birth factors may include forceps delivery, breech presentation, placenta previa, abruptio placentae, depressed maternal vital signs from general or spinal anesthesia, prolapsed cord with delay in blood delivery to the head; premature birth, pro-

longed or unusually rapid labor, multiple births (especially infants born last), and infection or trauma during infancy.

● Postnatal causes include kernicterus resulting from erythroblastosis fetalis, brain infection or tumor, head trauma, prolonged anoxia, cerebral circulatory anomalies causing blood vessel rupture, and systemic disease resulting in cerebral thrombosis or embolus.

● Prenatal causes include maternal infection (especially rubella), exposure to radiation, anoxia, toxemia, maternal diabetes, abnormal placental attachment, malnutrition, and isoimmunization.

PATHOPHYSIOLOGY

In the early stages of brain development, a lesion or abnormality causes structural and functional defects that in turn cause impaired motor function or cognition. Even though the defects are present at birth, problems may not be apparent until months later, when the axons have become myelinated and the basal ganglia are mature.

CLINICAL FINDINGS

Shortly after birth, the infant with CP may exhibit some typical signs and symptoms, including:

● excessive lethargy or irritability
● high-pitched cry
● poor head control
● weak sucking reflex.

Additional physical findings that may suggest CP include:

● delayed motor development (inability to meet major developmental milestones)
● abnormal head circumference, typically smaller than normal for age (because the head grows as the brain grows)

● abnormal postures, such as straightening legs when on back, toes down; holding head higher than normal when prone due to arching of back
● abnormal reflexes (neonatal reflexes lasting longer than expected, extreme reflexes, or clonus)
● abnormal muscle tone and performance (scooting on back to crawl, toe-first walking).

Each type of CP typically produces a distinctive set of clinical features, although some children display a mixed form of the disease. (See *Assessing signs of cerebral palsy.*)

Alert *Complications depend on the type of CP and the severity of the involvement. Possible complications include contractures; skin breakdown and ulcer formation; muscle atrophy; malnutrition; seizure disorders; speech, hearing, and vision problems; language and perceptual deficits; mental retardation; dental problems; and respiratory difficulties, including aspiration from poor gag and swallowing reflexes.*

TEST RESULTS

No diagnostic tests are specific to CP. However, neurologic screening will exclude other possible conditions, such as infection, spina bifida, or muscular dystrophy. Other screenings and tests may be performed.

● Developmental screening reveals delay in achieving milestones.
● Vision and hearing screening demonstrates degree of impairment.
● EEG identifies the source of seizure activity.

Alert *Suspect CP whenever an infant exhibits an alteration in neurologic function during clinical observation. This may include difficulty in sucking or moving voluntarily. Infants particularly at risk include those with a low birth weight,*

ASSESSING SIGNS OF CEREBRAL PALSY

Each type of cerebral palsy (CP) is manifested by specific findings. This chart highlights the major signs associated with each type of CP. The manifestations reflect impaired upper motor neuron function and disruption of the normal stretch reflex.

TYPE OF CP	SIGNS
Spastic CP (due to impairment of the pyramidal tract [most common type])	◆ Hyperactive deep tendon reflexes ◆ Increased stretch reflexes ◆ Rapid alternating muscle contraction and relaxation ◆ Muscle weakness ◆ Underdevelopment of affected limbs ◆ Muscle contraction in response to manipulation ◆ Tendency toward contractures ◆ Typical walking on toes with a scissors gait, crossing one foot in front of the other

Athetoid CP (due to impairment of the extrapyramidal tract)	◆ Involuntary movements usually affecting arms more severely than legs, including:
	  – grimacing
	  – wormlike writhing
	  – dystonia
	  – sharp jerks
	◆ Difficulty with speech due to involuntary facial movements
	◆ Increasing severity of movements during stress; decreased with relaxation and disappearing entirely during sleep

Ataxic CP (due to impairment of the extrapyramidal tract)	◆ Disturbed balance ◆ Incoordination (especially of the arms) ◆ Hypoactive reflexes ◆ Nystagmus ◆ Muscle weakness ◆ Tremor ◆ Lack of leg movement during infancy ◆ Wide gait as the child begins to walk ◆ Sudden or fine movements impossible (due to ataxia)
Mixed CP	◆ Spasticity and athetoid movements ◆ Ataxic and athetoid movements (resulting in severe impairment)

low Apgar score at 5 minutes, seizures, and metabolic disturbances. However, all infants should have a screening test for CP as a regular part of their 6-month checkup.

TREATMENT

CP can't be cured, but treatment can help affected children reach their greatest potential within the limitations of the disorder. Such treatment requires a comprehensive and cooperative effort, involving physicians, nurses, teachers, psychologists, the child's family, and occupational, physical, and speech therapists. Home care is usually possible. Treatment typically includes:

● braces, casts, or splints and special appliances, such as adapted eating utensils and a low toilet seat with arms, to help the child perform activities of daily living independently

- range-of-motion exercises to minimize contractures
- an anticonvulsant to control seizures
- muscle relaxants (sometimes) to reduce spasticity
- surgery to decrease spasticity or correct contractures
- muscle transfer or tendon lengthening surgery to improve function of joints
- rehabilitation including occupational, physical, and speech therapy to maintain or improve functional abilities.

NURSING CONSIDERATIONS

A child with CP may be hospitalized for orthopedic surgery or for treatment of other complications.
- Speak slowly and distinctly. Encourage the child to ask for items he wants. Listen patiently and don't rush him.
- Plan a high-calorie diet that's adequate to meet the child's high energy needs.
- During meals, maintain a quiet, unhurried atmosphere with as few distractions as possible. The child should be encouraged to feed himself and may need special utensils and a chair with a solid footrest. Teach him to place food far back in his mouth to facilitate swallowing.
- Encourage the child to chew food thoroughly, drink through a straw, and suck on lollipops to develop the muscle control needed to minimize drooling.
- Allow the child to wash and dress independently, assisting only as needed. The child may need clothing modifications.
- Give all care in an unhurried manner; otherwise, muscle spasticity may increase.

- Encourage the child and his family to participate in the care plan so they can continue it at home.
- Care for associated hearing or vision disturbances, as necessary.
- Give frequent mouth and dental care, as necessary.
- Reduce muscle spasms that increase postoperative pain by moving and turning the child carefully after surgery; provide analgesics as needed.
- After orthopedic surgery, provide good cast care. Wash and dry the skin at the edge of the cast frequently. Reposition the child often, check for foul odor, and ventilate under the cast with a cool air blow-dryer.
- Encourage parents to set realistic individualized goals for the child; assist in planning crafts and other activities. Stress the child's need to develop peer relationships; warn the parents against being overprotective.
- Identify and deal with family stress. The parents may feel unreasonable guilt about their child's disability and may need psychological counseling.
- Suggest supportive community organizations such as the United Cerebral Palsy Association or their local chapter.

Guillain-Barré syndrome

Also known as *infectious polyneuritis, Landry-Guillain-Barré syndrome,* or *acute idiopathic polyneuritis,* Guillain-Barré syndrome is an acute, rapidly progressive, and potentially fatal form of polyneuritis that causes muscle weakness and mild distal sensory loss.

This syndrome can occur at any age but is most common between ages 30 and 50. It affects both sexes equally. Recovery is spontaneous and complete in about 95% of patients, although mild motor or reflex deficits may persist in the feet and legs. The prognosis is best when symptoms clear before 15 to 20 days after onset.

This syndrome occurs in three phases:

● Acute phase — beginning with the onset of the first definitive symptom and ends 1 to 3 weeks later; further deterioration doesn't occur after the acute phase
● Plateau phase — lasting several days to 2 weeks
● Recovery phase — believed to coincide with remyelinization and regrowth of axonal processes; extending over 4 to 6 months, but possibly lasting up to 2 to 3 years if the disease is severe.

CAUSES

The precise cause of Guillain-Barré syndrome is unknown, but it may be a cell-mediated immune response to a virus. About 50% of patients with Guillain-Barré syndrome have a recent history of minor febrile illness, usually an upper respiratory tract infection or, less commonly, gastroenteritis. When infection precedes the onset of Guillain-Barré syndrome, signs of infection subside before neurologic features appear.

Other possible precipitating factors include:
● Hodgkin's or other malignant disease
● rabies or swine influenza vaccination
● surgery
● systemic lupus erythematosus.

PATHOPHYSIOLOGY

The major pathologic manifestation is segmental demyelination of the peripheral nerves. This prevents normal transmission of electrical impulses along the sensorimotor nerve roots. Because this syndrome causes inflammation and degenerative changes in both the posterior (sensory) and the anterior (motor) nerve roots, signs of sensory and motor losses occur simultaneously. (See *Understanding sensorimotor nerve degeneration,* page 140.) Additionally, autonomic nerve transmission may be impaired.

CLINICAL FINDINGS

Symptoms are progressive and include:
● symmetrical muscle weakness (major neurologic sign) appearing in the legs first (ascending type) and then extending to the arms and facial nerves within 24 to 72 hours, from impaired anterior nerve root transmission
● muscle weakness developing in the arms first (descending type) or in the arms and legs simultaneously, from impaired anterior nerve root transmission
● muscle weakness absent or affecting only the cranial nerves (in mild forms)
● paresthesia, sometimes preceding muscle weakness but vanishing quickly, from impairment of the dorsal nerve root transmission
● diplegia, possibly with ophthalmoplegia (ocular paralysis), from impaired motor nerve root transmission and involvement of cranial nerves III, IV, and VI
● dysphagia or dysarthria and, less often, weakness of the muscles supplied by cranial nerve XI (spinal accessory nerve)

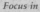
UNDERSTANDING
SENSORIMOTOR NERVE DEGENERATION

Guillain-Barré syndrome attacks the peripheral nerves so that they can't transmit messages to the brain correctly. The myelin sheath degenerates for unknown reasons. This sheath covers the nerve axons and conducts electrical impulses along the nerve pathways. Degeneration brings inflammation, swelling, and patchy demyelination. As this disorder destroys myelin, the nodes of Ranvier (at the junction of the myelin sheaths) widen. This delays and impairs impulse transmission along the dorsal and anterior nerve roots.

Because the dorsal nerve roots handle sensory function, the patient may experience tingling and numbness. Similarly, because the anterior nerve roots are responsible for motor function, impairment causes varying weakness, immobility, and paralysis.

CROSS SECTION OF THE SPINAL CORD
This cross section of the spinal cord shows the anterior and posterior segments.

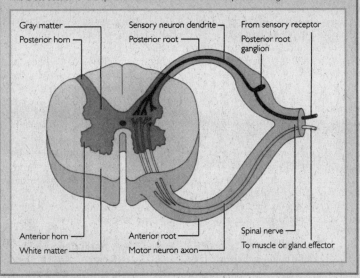

hypotonia and areflexia from interruption of the reflex arc.

  Alert Common complications of Guillain-Barré syndrome include thrombophlebitis, pressure ulcers, muscle wasting, sepsis, joint contractures aspiration, respiratory tract infections, mechanical respiratory failure, sinus tachycardia or bradycardia, hypertension and postural hypoten- *sion, and loss of bladder and bowel sphincter control.*

TEST RESULTS
Cerebrospinal fluid (CSF) analysis by lumbar puncture reveals elevated protein levels, peaking in 4 to 6 weeks, probably as a result of widespread inflammation of the nerve

roots; the CSF white blood cell count remains normal, but in severe disease, CSF pressure may rise above normal.

- Complete blood count shows leukocytosis with immature forms early in the illness, and then quickly returns to normal.
- Electromyography possibly shows repeated firing of the same motor unit, instead of widespread sectional stimulation.
- Nerve conduction velocities show slowing soon after paralysis develops.
- Serum immunoglobulin levels reveal elevated levels from inflammatory response.

TREATMENT

Primarily supportive, treatments include:

- endotracheal (ET) intubation or tracheotomy if respiratory muscle involvement causes difficulty in clearing secretions
- trial dose (7 days) of prednisone to reduce inflammatory response if the disease is relentlessly progressive; if prednisone produces no noticeable improvement, discontinue drug
- plasmapheresis useful during the initial phase but of no benefit if begun 2 weeks after onset
- continuous electrocardiogram monitoring for possible arrhythmias from autonomic dysfunction; propranolol to treat tachycardia and hypertension or atropine for bradycardia; volume replacement for severe hypotension.

NURSING CONSIDERATIONS

Monitoring the patient for escalation of symptoms is of special concern.

- Watch for ascending sensory loss, which precedes motor loss. Also, monitor vital signs and level of consciousness.
- Assess and treat respiratory dysfunction. If respiratory muscles are weak, take serial vital capacity recordings.
- Monitor pulse oximetry and end-tidal carbon dioxide measurements; obtain arterial blood gas measurements. Because neuromuscular disease results in primary hypoventilation with hypoxemia and hypercapnia, watch for partial pressure of arterial oxygen (PaO_2) below 70 mm Hg, which signals respiratory failure. Be alert for signs of rising partial pressure of arterial carbon dioxide (confusion, tachypnea).
- Auscultate breath sounds, turn and position the patient, and encourage incentive spirometry. Begin respiratory support at the first sign of dyspnea (in adults, vital capacity less than 800 ml; in children, less than 12 ml/kg body weight) or with decreasing PaO_2.
- If respiratory failure is imminent, establish an emergency airway with an ET tube.
- Give meticulous skin care to prevent skin breakdown and contractures. Establish a strict turning schedule; inspect the skin (especially sacrum, heels, and ankles) for breakdown, and reposition the patient every 2 hours. After each position change, stimulate circulation by carefully massaging pressure points. Also, use foam, gel, or alternating pressure pads at points of contact.
- Perform passive range-of-motion exercises within the patient's pain limits. When the patient's condition stabilizes, change to gentle stretching and active assistance exercises.
- To prevent aspiration, test the gag reflex, and elevate the head of the bed before giving the patient anything to eat. If the gag reflex is absent, provide alternative enteral feedings.

• As the patient regains strength and can tolerate a vertical position, be alert for postural hypotension. Monitor his blood pressure and pulse during tilting periods and, if necessary, apply toe-to-groin elastic bandages or an abdominal binder to minimize postural hypotension.

• If the patient has severe paralysis and is expected to have a long recovery period, a gastrostomy tube may be necessary to provide adequate nourishment.

• Inspect the patient's legs regularly for signs of thrombophlebitis (localized pain, tenderness, erythema, edema, and positive Homans' sign). To prevent thrombophlebitis, apply antiembolism stockings and give prophylactic anticoagulants, as ordered.

• If the patient has facial paralysis, give eye and mouth care every 4 hours. Protect the corneas with isotonic eye drops and eye shields.

• Watch for urine retention. Measure and record intake and output every 8 hours, and offer the bedpan every 3 to 4 hours. Encourage adequate fluid intake of 2 qt (2 L)/day, unless contraindicated. If urine retention develops, begin intermittent catheterization, as ordered. Because the abdominal muscles are weak, the patient may need manual pressure on the bladder (Credé's method) before he can urinate.

• To prevent and relieve constipation, offer prune juice and a high-bulk diet. If necessary, give stool softeners as ordered.

• Before discharge, prepare a home care plan. Teach the patient how to transfer from bed to wheelchair, from wheelchair to toilet or tub, and how to walk short distances with a walker or a cane. Teach the family how to help him eat, compensating for facial weakness and how to help him avoid skin breakdown. Stress the need for a regular bowel and bladder routine. Refer the patient for physical therapy, as needed.

Headache

The most common patient complaint, headache usually occurs as a symptom of an underlying disorder. Ninety percent of all headaches are vascular, muscle contraction, or a combination; 10% are due to underlying intracranial, systemic, or psychological disorders. Migraine headaches, probably the most intensely studied, are throbbing, vascular headaches that usually begin to appear in childhood or adolescence and recur throughout adulthood. Affecting up to 10% of Americans, they're more common in females and have a strong familial incidence.

CAUSES
Most chronic headaches result from tension (muscle contraction), which may be caused by:
• emotional stress or fatigue
• environmental stimuli (noise, crowds, or bright lights)
• menstruation.
    Other possible causes include:
• diseases of the scalp, teeth, extracranial arteries, external or middle ear
• glaucoma
• hypertension
• increased intracranial pressure (ICP), head trauma, tumor, intracranial bleeding, abscess, or aneurysm
• inflammation of the eyes or mucosa of the nasal or paranasal sinuses
• systemic disease
• vasodilators (nitrates, alcohol, and histamine).

PATHOPHYSIOLOGY

Headaches are believed to be associated with constriction and dilation of intracranial and extracranial arteries. During a migraine attack, certain biochemical abnormalities, including local leakage of a vasodilator polypeptide called *neurokinin* through the dilated arteries, are thought to occur as well as a decrease in the plasma level of serotonin.

Headache pain may emanate from the pain-sensitive structures of the skin, scalp, muscles, arteries, and veins; cranial nerves V, VII, IX, and X; or cervical nerves 1, 2, and 3. Intracranial mechanisms of headaches include traction or displacement of arteries, venous sinuses, or venous tributaries and inflammation or direct pressure on the cranial nerves with afferent pain fibers.

The evolution of a headache has four distinct phases:

● Normal — Cerebral and temporal arteries are innervated extracranially; parenchymal arteries are noninnervated.

● Vasoconstriction (aura) — Stress-related neurogenic local vasoconstriction of innervated cerebral arteries reduces cerebral blood flow (localized ischemia). Systematically, the prostaglandin thromboxane causes increased platelet aggregation and release of serotonin, a potent vasoconstrictor and, possibly, other vasoactive substances.

● Parenchymal artery dilation — Noninnervated parenchymal vessels dilate in response to local acidosis and anoxia (ischemia). Neurogenic or biologic factors may cause preformed arteriovenous shunts to open. Increased blood flow, increased internal pressure, and enhanced pulsations short-circuit the normal nutritive capillaries and cause pain.

● Vasodilation (headache) — Compensatory mechanisms cause marked vasodilation of the innervated arteries resulting in headache. Systemic platelet aggregation decreases, and falling serotonin levels result in vasodilation. A painful, sterile perivascular inflammation develops and persists into a postheadache phase.

CLINICAL FINDINGS

● Unilateral, pulsating pain initially, which later becomes more generalized
● Commonly preceded by a scintillating scotoma, hemianopsia, unilateral paresthesia, or speech disorders
● Irritability, anorexia, nausea, vomiting, and photophobia
● Dull, persistent ache, tender spots on the head and neck, and a feeling of tightness around the head, with a characteristic "hat-band" distribution in both muscle contraction and traction-inflammatory vascular headaches; pain often severe and unrelenting
● If caused by intracranial bleeding, headache possibly resulting in neurologic deficits, such as paresthesia and muscle weakness; opioids may fail to relieve pain in these cases
● If caused by a tumor, pain being most severe when patient awakens

Alert *Complications of headaches may include misdiagnosis, status migraines, and disruption of lifestyle.*

TEST RESULTS

Diagnosis requires a history of recurrent headaches and physical examination of the head and neck.

● Examination includes percussion, auscultation for bruits, inspection for signs of infection, and palpation for defects, crepitus, or tender spots (especially after trauma).

- Definitive diagnosis also requires a complete neurologic examination, assessment for other systemic diseases, and a psychosocial evaluation when such factors are suspected.
- Diagnostic tests include computed tomography scan or magnetic resonance imaging.
- A lumbar puncture may be performed; it isn't done if there's evidence of increased ICP or if a brain tumor is suspected because rapidly reducing pressure, by removing spinal fluid, can cause brain herniation.

TREATMENT

Depending on the type of headache, treatment includes:
- analgesics for symptomatic relief
- identification and elimination of causative factors
- stress reduction
- muscle relaxants (for chronic tension headaches)
- ergotamine alone or with caffeine (for migraine headaches) (Remember that these medications can't be taken by pregnant women because they stimulate uterine contractions. These drugs and others, such as metoclopramide (Reglan) or naproxen (Naprosyn), work best when taken early in the course of an attack. If nausea and vomiting make oral administration impossible, drugs may be given as rectal suppositories.)
- drugs in the class of sumatriptan (considered by many clinicians to be the drug of choice for acute migraine attacks or cluster headaches)
- other drugs, such as propranolol (Inderol), atenolol (Tenormen), clonidine (Catapres), and amitriptyline.

NURSING CONSIDERATIONS

Headaches seldom require hospitalization unless caused by a serious disor-

der. If that's the case, direct your care to the underlying problem.
- Obtain a complete patient history, including duration and location of the headache, time of day it usually begins, nature of the pain, concurrence with other symptoms such as blurred vision, medications taken such as oral contraceptives, prolonged fasting, and precipitating factors, such as tension, menstruation, loud noises, menopause, or alcohol. Exacerbating factors can also be assessed through ongoing observation of the patient's personality, habits, activities of daily living, family relationships, coping mechanisms, and relaxation activities.
- Using the patient's history as a guide, help him avoid exacerbating factors. Advise lying down in a dark, quiet room during an attack and to place ice packs on his forehead or a cold cloth over the eyes.
- Instruct the patient to take the prescribed medication at the onset of migraine symptoms, to prevent dehydration by drinking plenty of fluids after nausea and vomiting subside, and to use other headache relief measures.
- The patient with a migraine headache usually needs to be hospitalized only if nausea and vomiting are severe enough to induce dehydration and possible shock.
- Instruct the patient to follow up with a neurologist or pain clinic to establish an effective pain control regimen.

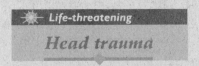

☀ Life-threatening

Head trauma

Head trauma, also known as *traumatic brain injury,* describes a traumatic insult to the brain that results in physical, intellectual, emotional, social, or vocational changes. Young children age 6 months to 2 years, persons age 15 to 24, and elderly people are at highest risk for head trauma. The risk for men is double the risk for women.

Head trauma is generally categorized as closed or open trauma. Closed trauma, or *blunt trauma* as it's sometimes called, is more common. It typically occurs when the head strikes a hard surface or a rapidly moving object strikes the head. The dura is intact, and no brain tissue is exposed to the external environment. In open trauma, as the name suggests, an opening in the scalp, skull, meninges, or brain tissue, including the dura, exposes the cranial contents to the environment, and the risk of infection is high.

Mortality from head trauma has declined with advances in preventative measures, such as seat belts and airbags, quicker emergency response and transport times, and improved treatment, including the development of regional trauma centers. Advances in technology have increased the effectiveness of rehabilitative services, even for patients with severe head injuries.

CAUSES
- Crime and assaults
- Falls
- Sports-related incidents
- Transportation or automobile crash (number one cause)

PATHOPHYSIOLOGY
The brain is shielded by the cranial vault (hair, skin, bone, meninges, and cerebrospinal fluid [CSF]), which intercepts the force of a physical blow. Below a certain level of force (the absorption capacity), the cranial vault prevents energy from affecting the brain. The degree of traumatic head injury usually is proportional to the amount of force reaching the cranial tissues. Furthermore, unless ruled out, neck injuries should be presumed present in patients with traumatic head injury.

Closed trauma is typically a sudden acceleration-deceleration injury resulting in a coup/contrecoup injury. In coup/contrecoup, the head hits a relatively stationary object, injuring cranial tissues near the point of impact (coup); then the remaining force pushes the brain against the opposite side of the skull, causing a second impact and injury (contrecoup). Contusions and lacerations may also occur during contrecoup as the brain's soft tissues slide over the rough bone of the cranial cavity. In addition, the cerebrum may endure rotational shear, damaging the upper midbrain and areas of the frontal, temporal, and occipital lobes.

Open trauma penetrates the scalp, skull, meninges, or brain. Open head injuries are associated with skull fractures, and bone fragments commonly cause hematomas and meningeal tears with consequent loss of CSF.

CLINICAL FINDINGS
Types of head trauma include concussion, contusion, epidural hematoma, subdural hematoma, intracerebral hematoma, and skull fractures. Each is associated with specific signs and symptoms. (See *Types of head trauma*, pages 146 to 149.)

Alert *Complications of head trauma may include increased intracranial pressure (ICP), infection (open trauma), respiratory depression and failure, perma-*

(Text continues on page 148.)

TYPES OF HEAD TRAUMA

This chart summarizes the signs and symptoms and diagnostic test findings for the different types of head trauma.

TYPE	DESCRIPTION
Concussion **(closed head injury)**	◆ Blow to the head hard enough to make the brain hit, or twist, within the skull but not hard enough to cause a cerebral contusion; causing temporary neural dysfunction ◆ Loss of consciousness lasting less than 6 hours ◆ Recovery usually complete within 24 to 48 hours ◆ Repeated injuries exacting a cumulative toll on the brain
Contusion **(bruising of brain** **tissue; more serious** **than concussion)**	◆ Acceleration-deceleration injuries disrupting normal nerve functions in bruised area ◆ Injury directly beneath the site of impact when the brain rebounds against the skull from the force of a blow (for example, a beating with a blunt instrument), when the force of the blow drives the brain against the opposite side of the skull, or when the head is hurled forward and stopped abruptly (as in an automobile crash when a driver's head strikes the windshield) ◆ Brain possibly striking bony prominences inside the skull (especially the sphenoidal ridges), causing intracranial hemorrhage or hematoma
Epidural hematoma	◆ Blood commonly accumulating between skull and dura; injury to middle meningeal artery in parietotemporal area most common and frequently accompanied by linear skull fractures in temporal region over middle meningeal artery ◆ Less commonly arising from dural venous sinuses

SIGNS AND SYMPTOMS	DIAGNOSTIC TEST FINDINGS
◆ Short-term loss of consciousness secondary to disruption of reticular activating system (RAS), possibly due to abrupt pressure changes in the areas responsible for consciousness, changes in polarity of the neurons, ischemia, or structural distortion of neurons ◆ Vomiting from localized injury and compression ◆ Anterograde and retrograde amnesia (patient can't recall events immediately after the injury or events that led up to the traumatic incident) correlating with severity of injury; all related to disruption of RAS ◆ Irritability or lethargy from localized injury and compression ◆ Behavior out of character due to focal injury ◆ Complaints of dizziness, nausea, or severe headache due to focal injury and compression	◆ Computed tomography (CT) scan revealing no sign of fracture, bleeding, or other nervous system lesion
◆ Severe scalp wounds from direct injury ◆ Labored respiration and loss of consciousness secondary to increased pressure from bruising ◆ Drowsiness, confusion, disorientation, agitation, or violent behavior from increased intracranial pressure (ICP) associated with trauma ◆ Hemiparesis related to interrupted blood flow to the site of injury ◆ Decorticate or decerebrate posturing from cortical damage or hemispheric dysfunction ◆ Unequal pupillary response from brain stem involvement	◆ CT scan showing changes in tissue density, possible displacement of the surrounding structures, and evidence of ischemic tissue, hematomas, and fractures
◆ Some patients possibly experiencing a brief period of unconsciousness after injury reflecting the concussive effects of head trauma, followed by a lucid interval varying from 10 to 15 minutes to hours or, rarely, days ◆ Severe headache ◆ Progressive loss of consciousness and deterioration in neurologic signs resulting from expanding lesion and extrusion of medial portion of temporal lobe through tentorial opening ◆ Compression of brain stem by temporal lobe causing clinical manifestations of intracranial hypertension ◆ Deterioration in level of consciousness resulting from compression of brain stem reticular formation as temporal lobe herniates on its upper portion ◆ Respirations, initially deep and labored, becoming shallow and irregular as brain stem becomes impacted ◆ Contralateral motor deficits reflecting compression of corticospinal tracts that pass through the brain stem ◆ Ipsilateral (same-side) pupillary dilation due to compression of third cranial nerve ◆ Seizures possible from high ICP ◆ Continued bleeding leading to progressive neurologic deterioration, evidenced by bilateral pupillary dilation, bilateral decerebrate response, increased systemic blood pressure, decreased pulse, and profound coma with irregular respiratory patterns	◆ CT scan or magnetic resonance imaging (MRI) identifying abnormal masses or structural shifts within the cranium

(continued)

TYPE	DESCRIPTION
Subdural hematoma	◆ Resulting from accumulation of blood in subdural space (between dura mater and arachnoid) ◆ May be acute, subacute, and chronic; unilateral or bilateral ◆ Usually associated with torn bridging veins that connect the cerebrum to the dura ◆ Acute hematomas being a surgical emergency
Intracerebral hematoma	◆ Shear forces from brain movement frequently causing vessel laceration and hemorrhage into the parenchyma ◆ Traumatic or spontaneous disruption of cerebral vessels in brain parenchyma causing neurologic deficits, depending on site and amount of bleeding ◆ Trauma commonly associated with intracerebral hematomas and, possibly, hypertension; frontal and temporal lobes common sites
Skull fracture	◆ Four types of skull fracture exist: linear, comminuted, depressed, and basilar ◆ Blow to the head causing one or more of the types; not problematic unless brain exposed or bone fragments driven into neural tissue ◆ Basilar skull fracture of the anterior or middle fossae associated with severe head trauma; more common than those of the posterior fossa

nent neurologic deficits, and brain herniation.

TEST RESULTS

Each type of head trauma is associated with specific diagnostic findings evident through computed tomography scan or magnetic resonance imaging and correlated with neurologic findings.

TREATMENT
Surgical

● Evacuation of the hematoma or a craniotomy to elevate or remove fragments that have been driven into the brain, and to extract foreign bodies and necrotic tissue, thereby reducing the risk of infection and further brain damage from fractures

Supportive

● Close observation to detect changes in neurologic status suggest-

SIGNS AND SYMPTOMS	DIAGNOSTIC TEST FINDINGS
◆ Similar to epidural hematoma but significantly slower in onset because bleeding is typically of venous origin ◆ Prognosis worse due to direct blood-brain contact	◆ CT scan or MRI revealing mass and altered blood flow in the area, evidence of masses and tissue shifting
◆ Unresponsive immediately or possibly experiencing a lucid period before lapsing into a coma from increasing ICP and mass effect of hemorrhage and neuronal dysruption ◆ Possible motor deficits and decorticate or decerebrate responses from compression of corticospinal tracts and brain stem	◆ CT scan identifying bleeding site
◆ Possibly asymptomatic, depending on underlying brain trauma ◆ Discontinuity and displacement of bone structure occurring with severe fracture ◆ Motor, sensory, and cranial nerve dysfunction associated with facial fractures ◆ Persons with anterior fossa basilar skull fractures possibly having periorbital ecchymosis (raccoon eyes), anosmia (loss of smell due to first cranial nerve involvement), and pupil abnormalities (second and third cranial nerve involvement) ◆ Cerebrospinal fluid (CSF) rhinorrhea (leakage through the nose), CSF otorrhea (leakage from the ear), hemotympanium (blood accumulation behind the tympanic membrane), ecchymosis over the mastoid bone (battle sign), and facial paralysis (seventh cranial nerve injury) accompanying middle fossa basilar skull fractures ◆ Signs of medullary dysfunction, such as cardiovascular and respiratory failure, accompanying posterior fossa basilar skull fracture	◆ CT scan and MRI revealing fracture type, location, and underlying brain injury

ing further damage or expanding hematoma

● Cleaning and debridement of wounds associated with skull fractures

● Osmotic diuretics, such as mannitol (Osmitrol), to reduce cerebral edema

● Analgesics, such as acetaminophen (Tylenol) and morphine (for severe headache), to relieve complaints of headache

● Anticonvulsants, such as phenytoin (Dilantin), to prevent seizures; lorazepam (Ativan) to treat seizures

● Respiratory support, including mechanical ventilation and endotracheal intubation, as indicated, for respiratory failure and airway protection

● Prophylactic antibiotics as indicated to prevent the onset of meningitis from CSF leakage associated with skull fractures

Nursing considerations

- Obtain a thorough history of the injury from the patient (if able), family members, eyewitnesses, or emergency medical services personnel. Ask whether the patient lost consciousness.
- Monitor vital signs and check for additional injuries. Palpate the skull for tenderness or hematomas.
- If the patient has an altered level of consciousness (LOC) or if a neurologic examination reveals abnormalities, observe the patient in the emergency department. Check vital signs, LOC, and pupil size every 15 minutes. The patient who's neurologic status is stable after 4 or more hours of observation can be discharged (with a head injury instruction sheet) in the care of a responsible adult.
- After the patient is stabilized, clean and dress superficial scalp wounds. (If the skin has been broken, tetanus prophylaxis may be in order.) Assist with suturing if necessary.
- If it's determined that the patient can be discharged, instruct the patient to be alert for worsening of headache, vomiting, signs of an ear bleed or CSF leak. Be sure to also include instructions for waking the patient every few hours during the night for observation of mental state and administration of medication.

For the patient with more serious head injuries, such as a cerebral contusion or skull fracture:

- Establish and maintain a patent airway; nasal airways are contraindicated in patients who may have a basilar skull fracture. Intubation is necessary for a patient with a Glasgow Coma Scale score of 8 or less. Suction the patient through the mouth, not the nose, to prevent introducing bacteria if a CSF leak is present.
- Look for CSF draining from the patient's ears, nose, or mouth. Check pillowcases and linens for CSF leaks and look for a halo sign. If the patient's nose is draining CSF, wipe it—don't let him blow it. If his ear is draining, cover it lightly with sterile gauze—don't pack it.
- If spinal injury is ruled out, position the patient with a head injury so that secretions can drain properly. Elevate the head of the bed 30 degrees if intracerebral injury is suspected.
- Institute seizure precautions as indicated. Agitated behavior may be due to hypoxia or increased ICP, so check for these symptoms. Speak in a calm, reassuring voice, and touch the patient gently.
- Use caution in giving the patient opioids or sedatives because they may depress respirations, increase carbon dioxide levels, lead to increased ICP, and mask changes in neurologic status.
- Facilitate diagnostic imaging and prepare for surgery as indicated.

Herniated intervertebral disk

Also called a *ruptured* or *slipped disk* or a *herniated nucleus pulposus,* a herniated disk occurs when all or part of the nucleus pulposus—the soft, gelatinous, central portion of an intervertebral disk—is forced through the disk's weakened or torn outer ring (anulus fibrosus). Herniated disks usually occur in adults (mostly men) under age 45. About 90% of herniated disks occur in the lumbar and lumbosacral regions, 8% occur in the cervical area, and 1% to 2% occur in the thoracic area. Patients with a congenitally small lumbar spinal canal or with osteophyte formation along the vertebrae may be more susceptible to nerve root compression and more likely to have neurologic symptoms.

CAUSES

The two major causes of herniated intervertebral disk include:

- intervertebral joint degeneration
- severe trauma or strain.

Alert *In older patients whose disks have begun to degenerate, minor trauma may cause herniation.*

PATHOPHYSIOLOGY

An intervertebral disk has two parts: the soft center called the *nucleus pulposus* and the tough, fibrous surrounding ring called the *anulus fibrosus*. The nucleus pulposus acts as a shock absorber, distributing the mechanical stress applied to the spine when the body moves. Physical stress, usually a twisting motion, can tear or rupture the anulus fibrosus so that the nucleus pulposus herniates into the spinal canal. The vertebrae move closer together and the ruptured disk material exerts pressure on the nerve roots, causing pain and, possibly, sensory and motor loss. A herniated disk also can occur with intervertebral joint degeneration. If the disk has begun to degenerate, minor trauma may cause herniation.

Herniation occurs in three steps. In protrusion, the nucleus pulposus presses against the anulus fibrosus. Next, extrusion occurs where the nucleus pulposus bulges forcibly though the anulus fibrosus, pushing against the nerve root. Finally, sequestration occurs whereby the anulus gives way as the disk's core bursts and presses against the nerve root.

CLINICAL FINDINGS

- Severe lower back pain to the buttocks, legs, and feet, usually unilaterally, from compression of nerve roots supplying these areas
- Sudden pain after trauma, subsiding in a few days, and then recurring at shorter intervals and with progressive intensity
- Sciatic pain following trauma, beginning as a dull pain in the buttocks; Valsalva's maneuver, coughing, sneezing, and bending intensify the pain, which is often accompanied by muscle spasms from pressure and irritation of the sciatic nerve root
- Sensory and motor loss in the area innervated by the compressed spinal nerve root and, in later stages, weakness and atrophy of leg muscles

Alert *Complications of a herniated disk are dependent on the severity and the specific site of herniation. Common complications include neurologic deficits and bowel and bladder problems.*

TEST RESULTS

- Straight-leg raising test is positive only if the patient has posterior leg (sciatic) pain, not back pain.
- Lasègue's test reveals resistance and pain as well as loss of ankle or knee-jerk reflex, indicating spinal root compression.
- Spinal X-rays rule out other abnormalities but may not diagnose a herniated disk because a marked disk prolapse may not be apparent on a normal X-ray.
- Computed tomography scan and magnetic resonance imaging show spinal canal compression by herniated disk material.

TREATMENT

- Heat applications to decrease muscle spasm and aid in pain relief

- Exercise program to strengthen associated muscles and prevent further deterioration
- Corticosteroids such as dexamethasone for an initial, short course or anti-inflammatory drugs, such as aspirin, and nonsteroidal anti-inflammatory drugs to reduce inflammation and edema at the site of injury; muscle relaxants, such as diazepam (Valium), methocarbamol, and cyclobenzaprine (Flexeril), to minimize muscle spasm from nerve root irritation; epidural injections at the level of the protrusion to relieve pain
- Surgery, including laminectomy to remove the extruded disk, spinal fusion to overcome segmental instability, or both to stabilize the spine

NURSING CONSIDERATIONS

A patient with a herniated disk requires supportive care, careful patient teaching, and strong emotional support to help him cope with the discomfort and frustration of chronic lower back pain.

- During conservative treatment, watch for deterioration in neurologic status (especially during the first 24 hours after admission), which may indicate an urgent need for surgery. Use sequential compression devices as prescribed, and encourage the patient to move his legs, as allowed. Encourage the patient to work closely with the physical therapy department to ensure a consistent regimen of leg- and back-strengthening exercises. Provide good skin care. Assess for bowel function.
- After laminectomy, microdiskectomy, or spinal fusion, promote bed rest, as ordered. If a blood drainage system is in use, check the tubing frequently for kinks and a secure vacuum. Empty the drainage device at the

end of each shift, and record amount and color. Report colorless moisture on dressings (possible cerebrospinal fluid leakage) or excessive drainage immediately. Observe neurovascular status of legs (color, motion, temperature, and sensation).
- Monitor vital signs and check for bowel sounds and abdominal distention. Use logrolling technique to turn the patient. Administer analgesics or provide patient controlled analgesia, as ordered, especially before initial attempts at sitting or walking. Give the patient assistance during his first attempt to walk. Provide a straight-backed chair for limited sitting.
- Teach the patient who has undergone spinal fusion how to wear a brace. Assist with straight-leg-raising and toe-pointing exercises, as ordered. Before discharge, teach proper body mechanics—bending at the knees and hips (never at the waist), standing straight, and carrying objects close to the body. Advise the patient to lie down when tired and to sleep on his side (never prone) on an extra-firm mattress or a bed board. Urge maintenance of proper weight to prevent lordosis caused by obesity.
- After chemonucleolysis, promote bed rest, as ordered. Administer analgesics and apply heat, as needed. Urge the patient to cough and deep breathe. Assist with special exercises, and tell the patient to continue these exercises after discharge.
- Inform the patient who must receive a muscle relaxant of possible adverse effects, especially drowsiness. Warn him to avoid activities that require alertness until he has built up a tolerance for the drug's sedative effects.

Hydrocephalus

An excessive accumulation of cerebrospinal fluid (CSF) within the ventricular spaces of the brain, hydrocephalus occurs most commonly in neonates. It can also occur in adults as a result of injury or disease. In infants, hydrocephalus enlarges the head and, in both infants and adults, the resulting compression can damage brain tissue. With early detection and surgical intervention, the prognosis improves. However, even after surgery, complications may persist, such as developmental delay, impaired motor function, and vision loss. Without surgery, the prognosis is poor. Mortality may result from increased intracranial pressure (ICP) in people of all ages; infants may die of infection and malnutrition.

CAUSES

Hydrocephalus may result from:
- faulty absorption of CSF (communicating hydrocephalus)
- obstruction in CSF flow (noncommunicating hydrocephalus).

Alert *Risk factors associated with the development of hydrocephalus in infants may include intrauterine infection and intracranial hemorrhage from birth trauma or prematurity. In older children and adults, risk factors may include meningitis, mastoiditis, chronic otitis media, traumatic brain injury, and brain tumors or intracranial hemorrhage.*

PATHOPHYSIOLOGY

In noncommunicating hydrocephalus, the obstruction occurs most frequently between the third and fourth ventricles, at the aqueduct of Sylvius, but it can also occur at the outlets of the fourth ventricle (foramina of Luschka and Magendie) or, rarely, at the foramen of Monro. This obstruction may result from faulty fetal development, infection (syphilis, granulomatous diseases, meningitis), a tumor, a cerebral aneurysm, or a blood clot (after intracranial hemorrhage).

In communicating hydrocephalus, faulty absorption of CSF may result from surgery to repair a myelomeningocele, adhesions between meninges at the base of the brain, or meningeal hemorrhage. Rarely, a tumor in the choroid plexus causes overproduction of CSF and consequent hydrocephalus.

In either type, both CSF pressure and volume increase. Obstruction in the ventricles causes dilation, stretching, and disruption of the lining. Underlying white matter atrophies. Compression of brain tissue and cerebral blood vessels leads to ischemia and, eventually, cell death.

CLINICAL FINDINGS
In infants
- Enlargement of the head clearly disproportionate to the infant's growth (most characteristic sign) from the increased CSF volume
- Distended scalp veins from increased CSF pressure
- Thin, shiny, fragile-looking scalp skin from the increase in CSF pressure
- Underdeveloped neck muscles from increased weight of the head
- Depressed orbital roof with downward displacement of the eyes and prominent sclerae from increased pressure
- High-pitched, shrill cry, irritability, and abnormal muscle tone in the legs from neurologic compression
- Projectile vomiting from increased ICP
- Skull widening to accommodate increased pressure

In adults and older children

- Decreased level of consciousness (LOC) from increasing ICP
- Ataxia from compression of the motor areas
- Incontinence
- Impaired intellect

Alert Complications of hydrocephalus may include mental retardation, impaired motor function, vision loss, brain herniation, death from increased ICP, infection, malnutrition, shunt infection (following surgery), septicemia (following shunt insertion); paralytic ileus, adhesions, peritonitis, and intestinal perforation (following shunt insertion).

TEST RESULTS

- Computed tomography scan and magnetic resonance imaging reveal variations in tissue density and fluid in the ventricular system.
- Lumbar puncture reveals increased fluid pressure from communicating hydrocephalus.
- Ventriculography shows ventricular dilation with excess fluid.

Alert In infants, abnormally large head size for the patient's age strongly suggests hydrocephalus. Measurement of the head circumference is the most important diagnostic technique.

TREATMENT

The only treatment for hydrocephalus is surgical correction, by insertion of:

- ventriculoperitoneal shunt, which transports excess fluid from the lateral ventricle into the peritoneal cavity
- ventriculoatrial shunt (less common), which drains fluid from the brain's lateral ventricle into the right atrium of the heart, where the fluid makes its way into the venous circulation

- temporary external ventricular or lumbar drain for head trauma or intracranial bleeding.

Supportive care is also warranted.

NURSING CONSIDERATIONS

On initial assessment, obtain a complete history from the patient or the family. Note general behavior, especially irritability, apathy, or decreased LOC. Perform a neurologic assessment. Examine the eyes; pupils should be equal and reactive to light. In adults and older children, evaluate movement and motor strength in the extremities. Watch for ataxia, confusion, and incontinence. Ask the patient if he has headaches and watch for projectile vomiting; both are signs of increased ICP. Also watch for seizures. Note changes in vital signs.

Before surgery (shunt insertion)

- Encourage maternal-infant bonding when possible.
- Check fontanels for tension or fullness, and measure and record head circumference. On the patient's chart, draw a picture showing where to measure the head so that other staff members measure it in the same place, or mark the forehead with ink.
- To prevent postfeeding aspiration and hypostatic pneumonia, place the infant on his side and reposition every 2 hours, or prop him up in an infant seat.
- To prevent skin breakdown, make sure that his earlobe is flat, and place a sheepskin or rubber foam under his head.
- When turning the infant, move his head, neck, and shoulders with his body to reduce strain on his neck.
- To lessen strain from the weight of the infant's head on your arm while

holding him during feeding, place his head, neck, and shoulders on a pillow.

After surgery
- Place the infant on the side opposite the operative site with his head level with his body unless the physician's orders specify otherwise.
- Check temperature, pulse rate, blood pressure, and LOC. Also check fontanels for fullness daily. Watch for vomiting, which may be an early sign of increased ICP and shunt malfunction.
- Watch for signs of infection, especially meningitis (fever, stiff neck, irritability, tense fontanels). Watch for redness, swelling, or other signs of local infection over the shunt tract.
- Check dressing often for drainage.
- Listen for bowel sounds after ventriculoperitoneal shunt.
- Check the infant's growth and development periodically, and help the parents set goals consistent with the child's ability and potential. Help the parents focus on their child's strengths, not his weaknesses. Discuss special education programs, and emphasize the infant's need for sensory stimulation appropriate for his age. Teach parents to watch for signs of shunt malfunction, infection, and paralytic ileus. Tell them that surgery for lengthening the shunt will be required periodically as the child grows older. Surgery may also be required to correct shunt malfunctioning or to treat infection. Emphasize that hydrocephalus is a lifelong problem and that the child will require regular, continuing evaluation.

Intracranial aneurysm

In an intracranial aneurysm, a weakness in the wall of an artery causes localized dilation. Its most common form is the berry aneurysm, a saclike outpouching in a cerebral artery. Cerebral aneurysms usually arise at an arterial junction in the Circle of Willis, the circular anastomosis forming the major cerebral arteries at the base of the brain. (See *Most common sites of intracranial aneurysm*, page 156.) Intracranial aneurysms may rupture and cause subarachnoid hemorrhage.

The incidence is slightly higher in women than in men, especially those in their late 40s or early to mid-50s, but an intracranial aneurysm may occur at any age in either sex. The prognosis is guarded. About one-half of all patients who suffer a subarachnoid hemorrhage die immediately. Of those who survive untreated, 40% die from the effects of hemorrhage and another 20% die later from recurring hemorrhage. New treatments are improving the prognosis.

CAUSES
- Combination of congenital defect and degenerative process
- Congenital defect
- Degenerative process
- Trauma

PATHOPHYSIOLOGY
Blood flow exerts pressure against a congenitally weak arterial wall, stretching it like an overblown balloon and making it likely to rupture. Such a rupture is followed by a subarachnoid hemorrhage, in which blood spills

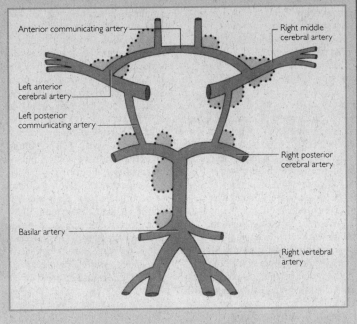

MOST COMMON SITES OF INTRACRANIAL ANEURYSM

Intracranial aneurysms usually arise at the arterial bifurcation in the Circle of Willis and its branches. This illustration shows the most common sites around this circle.

Anterior communicating artery

Right middle cerebral artery

Left anterior cerebral artery

Left posterior communicating artery

Right posterior cerebral artery

Basilar artery

Right vertebral artery

into the space normally occupied by cerebrospinal fluid. Sometimes, blood also spills into brain tissue, where a large clot can cause potentially fatal increased intracranial pressure (ICP) and brain tissue damage.

CLINICAL FINDINGS

Symptoms include:
- Headache, intermittent nausea, nuchal rigidity, stiff back and legs as premonitory symptoms resulting from oozing of blood into the subarachnoid space.

Usually, however, the rupture occurs abruptly and without warning, causing:
- sudden severe headache caused by bleeding into meningeal space
- nausea and projectile vomiting related to increased ICP
- altered level of consciousness (LOC), including deep coma, depending on the severity and location of bleeding, from increased ICP caused by increased cerebral blood volume
- meningeal irritation, resulting in nuchal rigidity, back and leg pain, fever, restlessness, irritability, occa-

sional seizures, photophobia, and blurred vision, secondary to bleeding into the subarachnoid space
• hemiparesis, hemisensory defects, dysphagia, and visual defects from bleeding into the brain tissues
• diplopia, ptosis, dilated pupil, and inability to rotate the eye caused by compression on the oculomotor nerve if the aneurysm is near the internal carotid artery.

Typically, the severity of a ruptured intracranial aneurysm is graded according to the patient's signs and symptoms. Five grades characterize a ruptured cerebral aneurysm:
• Grade I (minimal bleeding) — The patient is alert with no neurologic deficit; he may have a slight headache and nuchal rigidity.
• Grade II (mild bleeding) — The patient is alert, with a mild to severe headache and nuchal rigidity; he may have third-nerve palsy.
• Grade III (moderate bleeding) — The patient is confused or drowsy, with nuchal rigidity and, possibly, a mild focal deficit.
• Grade IV (severe bleeding) — The patient is stuporous, with nuchal rigidity and, possibly, mild to severe hemiparesis.
• Grade V (moribund; often fatal) — If the rupture is nonfatal, the patient is in a deep coma or decerebrate.

🔆 *Alert* *The major complications associated with cerebral aneurysm include death from increased ICP and brain herniation; rebleeding; and vasospasm.*

TEST RESULTS
• Cerebral angiography, computed tomography (CT) angiography, and magnetic resonance angiography reveal altered cerebral blood flow, vessel lumen dilation, and differences in arterial filling.

• Standard CT scan reveals subarachnoid or ventricular bleeding with blood in subarachnoid space and displaced midline structures.
• Standard magnetic resonance imaging shows a cerebral blood flow void.

TREATMENT
Treatment to reduce the risk of rupture if it hasn't occurred may include:
• bed rest in a quiet, darkened room with minimal stimulation
• avoidance of coffee and other stimulants to reduce the risk of blood pressure elevation
• codeine or another analgesic as needed to maintain rest and minimize risk of pressure changes
• antihypertensives if the patient is hypertensive
• phenobarbital or another sedative to prevent agitation leading to hypertension.

Other treatment may include:
• surgical repair by clipping, ligation, coiling, or wrapping (before or after rupture)
• calcium channel blockers to decrease spasm and subsequent rebleeding
• corticosteroids to manage headache and reduce edema
• phenytoin or another anticonvulsant to prevent seizures secondary to pressure and tissue irritation from bleeding.

NURSING CONSIDERATIONS
An accurate neurologic assessment, good patient care, patient and family teaching, and psychological support can speed recovery and reduce complications.
• During initial treatment after hemorrhage, establish and maintain a patent airway. Position the patient to

promote pulmonary drainage and prevent upper airway obstruction. If he's intubated, administering 100% oxygen before suctioning to remove secretions will prevent hypoxia and vasodilation from carbon dioxide accumulation. Suction no longer than 20 seconds to avoid increased ICP. Give frequent nose and mouth care.

● Until the aneurysm is repaired, implement aneurysm precautions to minimize the risk of rebleed and to avoid increased ICP. Such precautions include bed rest in a quiet, darkened room; limited visitation; avoidance of strenuous physical activity and straining with bowel movements.

● Turn the patient often. Encourage occasional deep breathing and leg movement. Assist with active range-of-motion (ROM) exercises; if the patient is paralyzed, perform regular passive ROM exercises.

● Monitor arterial blood gases, LOC, and vital signs often, and measure intake and output. Avoid taking the patient's temperature rectally because vagus nerve stimulation may cause cardiac arrest.

● Watch for danger signals, such as decreased LOC, unilateral enlarged pupil, onset or worsening of hemiparesis or motor deficit, increased blood pressure, slowed pulse, worsening of headache or sudden onset of a headache, renewed or worsened nuchal rigidity, and renewed or persistent vomiting, that may indicate an enlarging aneurysm, rebleeding, intracranial clot, vasospasm, or other complications. Intermittent signs such as restlessness, extremity weakness, and speech alterations can also indicate increasing ICP.

● Give fluids, as ordered, and monitor I.V. infusions to avoid increased ICP or vasospasm.

● If the patient has facial weakness, assess the gag reflex and assist him during meals, placing food in the unaffected side of his mouth. If he can't swallow, insert a nasogastric tube, as ordered, and give all tube feedings slowly. If the patient can eat, provide a high-fiber diet to prevent straining at stool, which can increase ICP. Get an order for a stool softener, such as docusate sodium (Colace), or a mild laxative, and administer as ordered. Implement a bowel program based on previous habits. If the patient is receiving steroids, check the stool for blood.

● With third (oculomotor) or seventh (facial) cranial nerve palsy, administer artificial tears or ointment to the patient's affected eye and tape the eye shut during sleeping hours to prevent corneal damage.

● To minimize stress, encourage relaxation techniques. If possible, avoid using restraints because they can cause agitation and raise ICP.

● Administer antihypertensives, as ordered, and carefully monitor blood pressure.

● If the patient can't speak, establish a simple means of communication or use cards or a notepad. Encourage his family to speak to him in a normal tone, even if he doesn't seem to respond.

● Provide emotional support, and include the patient's family in his care as much as possible. Encourage family members to adopt a realistic attitude, but don't discourage hope.

● Before discharge, make a referral to a visiting nurse or a rehabilitation center when necessary, and teach the patient and his family how to recognize signs of rebleeding and vasospasm.

Meningitis

In meningitis, the brain and the spinal cord meninges become inflamed, usually as a result of bacterial or viral infection. Such inflammation may involve all three meningeal membranes — the dura mater, arachnoid, and pia mater.

If the disease is recognized early and the infecting organism responds to treatment, the prognosis is good and complications are rare. However, mortality in untreated meningitis is 70% to 100%. The prognosis is poorer for infants and elderly patients.

CAUSES

- Almost always a complication of bacteremia, especially from pneumonia, empyema, osteomyelitis, and endocarditis
- Aseptic meningitis possibly resulting from chemicals, a virus, or other agent
- Other infections associated with its development include sinusitis, otitis media, encephalitis, myelitis, and brain abscess (usually caused by *Neisseria meningitidis, Haemophilus influenzae, Streptococcus pneumoniae,* and *Escherichia coli*)
- Possibly following trauma or invasive procedures, including skull fracture, penetrating head wound, lumbar puncture, craniotomy, and ventricular shunting
- Sometimes no causative organism found

PATHOPHYSIOLOGY

Meningitis commonly begins as an inflammation of the pia mater and arachnoid mater, which may progress to congestion of adjacent tissues and destroy some nerve cells. The microorganism typically enters the central nervous system by one of four routes: the blood (most common); a direct opening between the cerebrospinal fluid (CSF) and the environment as a result of trauma or surgery; along the cranial and peripheral nerves; and through the mouth or nose. Microorganisms can be transmitted to an infant via the intrauterine environment.

The invading organism triggers an inflammatory response in the meninges. In an attempt to ward off the invasion, neutrophils gather in the area and produce an exudate in the subarachnoid space, causing the CSF to thicken. The thickened CSF flows less readily around the brain and spinal cord, and it can block the arachnoid villi, obstructing absorption of CSF and causing hydrocephalus. The exudate also exacerbates the inflammatory response, increasing the pressure in the brain. It can also extend to the cranial and peripheral nerves, triggering additional inflammation. The exudates may also irritate the meninges, disrupting their cell membranes and causing edema. The consequences are elevated intracranial pressure (ICP), engorged blood vessels, disrupted cerebral blood supply, possible thrombosis or rupture and, if ICP isn't reduced, cerebral infarction. Encephalitis may also ensue as a secondary infection of the brain tissue.

In aseptic meningitis, lymphocytes infiltrate the pia-arachnoid layers, but usually not as severely as in bacterial meningitis, and no exudate is formed. Thus, this type of meningitis is self-limiting.

CLINICAL FINDINGS

Signs of meningitis typically include:
- fever, chills, and malaise resulting from infection and inflammation

- headache, vomiting and, rarely, papilledema (inflammation and edema of the optic nerve) from increased ICP.

Signs of meningeal irritation include:
- nuchal rigidity
- positive Brudzinski's and Kernig's signs
- exaggerated and symmetrical deep tendon reflexes
- opisthotonos (a spasm in which the back and extremities arch backward so that the body rests on the head and heels).

Alert Complications of meningitis may include increased ICP, hydrocephalus, cerebral infarction, cranial nerve deficits including optic neuritis and deafness, encephalitis, paresis or paralysis, endocarditis, brain abscess, syndrome of inappropriate antidiuretic hormone, seizures, shock, coma, and death.

Other features of meningitis may include:
- sinus arrhythmias from irritation of the nerves of the autonomic nervous system
- irritability from increasing ICP
- photophobia, diplopia, and other vision problems from cranial nerve irritation
- delirium, deep stupor, and coma from increased ICP and cerebral edema.

Alert An infant with meningitis may show signs of infection, but most are simply fretful and refuse to eat. In an infant, vomiting can lead to dehydration, which prevents formation of a bulging fontanel, an important sign of increased ICP. As the illness progresses, twitching, seizures (in 30% of infants), or coma may develop. Most older children have the same symptoms as adults. In subacute meningitis, onset may be insidious.

In children, complications may include mental retardation, epilepsy, unilateral or bilateral sensory hearing loss, and subdural effusions.

TEST RESULTS
- Lumbar puncture shows elevated CSF pressure (from obstructed CSF outflow at the arachnoid villi), cloudy or milky-white CSF, high protein level, positive Gram stain and culture (unless a virus is responsible), and decreased glucose concentration.
- Cultures of blood, urine, and nose and throat secretions may reveal the offending organism.
- Chest X-ray may reveal pneumonitis or lung abscess, tubercular lesions, or granulomas secondary to a fungal infection.
- Computed tomography (CT) scan may identify cranial osteomyelitis or paranasal sinusitis as the underlying infectious process, or skull fracture as the mechanism for entrance of microorganism.
- White blood cell count reveals leukocytosis.
- CT scan may reveal hydrocephalus and can rule out cerebral hematoma, hemorrhage, or tumor as the underlying cause.

TREATMENT
Treatment may include:
- appropriate I.V. antibiotics selected by culture and sensitivity testing (usual treatment)
- mannitol (Osmitrol) to decrease cerebral edema
- anticonvulsant (usually given I.V.) or a sedative to reduce restlessness and prevent or control seizure activity
- acetaminophen (Tylenol) or other analgesics to relieve headache and fever.

Supportive measures include:
- bed rest to prevent increases in ICP

- fever reduction to reduce metabolic demands that may increase ICP
- fluid therapy (given cautiously if cerebral edema and increased ICP present) to prevent dehydration
- appropriate therapy for coexisting conditions, such as endocarditis or pneumonia
- possible prophylactic antibiotics after ventricular shunting procedures, skull fracture, or penetrating head wounds, to prevent infection (use is controversial).

Staff should take droplet precautions (in addition to standard precautions) for meningitis caused by *H. influenzae* and *N. meningitidis,* until 24 hours after the start of effective therapy.

NURSING CONSIDERATIONS

Patients must be watched carefully for changes in neurologic function or other signs of worsening condition.

- Assess neurologic function often. Observe level of consciousness (LOC) and signs of increased ICP (agitation, vomiting, seizures, and a change in motor function and vital signs). Also watch for signs of cranial nerve involvement (ptosis, strabismus, and diplopia).

Alert Be especially alert for a temperature increase up to 102° F (38.9° C), deteriorating LOC, onset of seizures, and altered respirations, all of which may signal an impending crisis.

- Monitor fluid balance. Maintain adequate fluid intake to avoid dehydration, but avoid fluid overload because of the danger of cerebral edema. Measure central venous pressure and intake and output accurately.
- Position the patient carefully to prevent joint stiffness and neck pain. Turn him often, according to a planned positioning schedule. Assist with range-of-motion exercises.
- Maintain adequate nutrition and elimination. It may be necessary to provide small, frequent meals or to supplement meals with nasogastric tube or parenteral feedings. To prevent constipation and minimize the risk of increased ICP resulting from straining at stool, give the patient a mild laxative or stool softener.
- Ensure the patient's comfort. Provide mouth care regularly. Maintain a quiet environment. Darkening the room may decrease photophobia. Relieve headache with analgesics as ordered.
- Provide reassurance and support. Reorient as necessary. Reassure the family that the delirium and behavior changes caused by meningitis usually disappear. However, if a severe neurologic deficit appears permanent, refer the patient to a rehabilitation program as soon as the acute phase of this illness has passed.
- To help prevent development of meningitis, teach patients with chronic sinusitis or other chronic infections the importance of proper medical treatment. Follow strict sterile technique when treating patients with head wounds or skull fractures.

Multiple sclerosis

Multiple sclerosis (MS) causes demyelination of the white matter of the brain and spinal cord and damage to nerve fibers and their targets. Characterized by exacerbations and remissions, MS is a major cause of chronic disability in young adults. It usually becomes symptomatic between ages 20 and 40 (the average age of onset is

27). MS affects three women for every two men and five whites for every nonwhite. Incidence is generally higher among urban populations and upper socioeconomic groups. A family history of MS and living in a cold, damp climate increase the risk.

The prognosis varies. MS may progress rapidly, disabling the patient by early adulthood or causing death within months of onset. However, 70% of patients lead active, productive lives with prolonged remissions.

Several types of MS have been identified. Terms to describe MS types include:

- elapsing-remitting — clear relapses (or acute attacks or exacerbations) with full recovery or partial recovery and lasting disability (The disease doesn't worsen between the attacks.)
- primary progressive — steady progression from the onset with minor recovery or plateaus (This form is uncommon and may involve different brain and spinal cord damage than other forms.)
- secondary progressive — begins as a pattern of clear-cut relapses and recovery (This form becomes steadily progressive and worsens between acute attacks.)
- progressive relapsing — steadily progressive from the onset, but also has clear acute attacks. (This form is rare.)

CAUSES
The exact cause of MS is unknown, but current theories suggest that a slow-acting or latent viral infection triggers an autoimmune response. Other theories suggest that environmental and genetic factors may also be linked to MS.

Certain conditions appear to precede onset or exacerbation, including:

- acute respiratory infections
- emotional stress
- fatigue (physical or emotional)
- pregnancy.

PATHOPHYSIOLOGY
In MS, sporadic patches of axon demyelination and nerve fiber loss occur throughout the central nervous system (CNS), producing widely disseminated and varied neurologic dysfunction. (See *How myelin breaks down*.)

Newer evidence of nerve fiber loss may provide an explanation for the invisible neurologic deficits experienced by many patients with MS. The axons determine the presence or absence of function; loss of myelin doesn't correlate with loss of function.

CLINICAL FINDINGS
Signs and symptoms depend on the extent and site of myelin destruction, the extent of remyelination, and the adequacy of subsequent restored synaptic transmission. Flares may be transient, or they may last for hours or weeks, possibly waxing and waning with no predictable pattern, varying from day to day, and being bizarre and difficult for the patient to describe. Clinical effects may be so mild that the patient is unaware of them or so intense that they're debilitating. Typical first signs and symptoms related to conduction deficits and impaired impulse transmission along the nerve fiber include:

- vision problems
- sensory impairment, such as burning, pins and needles, and electrical sensations
- fatigue.

Other characteristic changes include:

- ocular disturbances — optic neuritis, diplopia, ophthalmoplegia, blurred

Focus in

HOW MYELIN BREAKS DOWN

Abnormal neuron

Myelin speeds electrical impulses to the brain for interpretation. This lipoprotein complex formed of glial cells or oligodendrocytes protects the neuron's axon much like the insulation on an electrical wire. Its high electrical resistance and low capacitance allow the myelin to conduct nerve impulses from one node of Ranvier to the next.

Myelin is susceptible to injury; for example, by hypoxemia, toxic chemicals, vascular insufficiencies, or autoimmune responses. The sheath becomes inflamed, and the membrane layers break down into smaller components that become well-circumscribed plaques (filled with microglial elements, macroglia, and lymphocytes). This process is called *demyelination*.

The damaged myelin sheath can't conduct normally. The partial loss or dispersion of the action potential causes neurologic dysfunction.

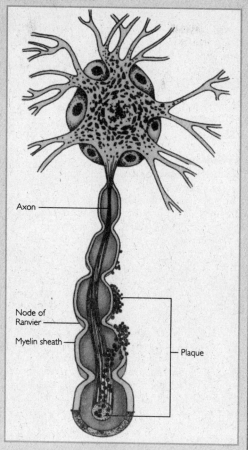

vision, and nystagmus from impaired cranial nerve dysfunction and conduction deficits to the optic nerve

● muscle dysfunction—weakness, paralysis ranging from monoplegia to quadriplegia, spasticity, hyperreflexia, intention tremor, and gait ataxia from impaired motor reflex

● urinary disturbances—incontinence, frequency, urgency, and frequent infections from impaired transmission involving sphincter innervation

- bowel disturbances — involuntary evacuation or constipation from altered impulse transmission to the internal sphincter
- fatigue — commonly the most debilitating symptom
- speech problems — poorly articulated or scanning speech and dysphagia from impaired transmission to the cranial nerves and sensory cortex.

> **Alert** *Complications of MS may include injuries from falls, urinary tract infection, constipation, joint contractures, pressure ulcers, rectal distention, pneumonia, and depression.*

TEST RESULTS

Because early symptoms may be mild, years may elapse between onset and diagnosis. Diagnosis of this disorder requires evidence of two or more neurologic attacks. Periodic testing and close observation are necessary, perhaps for years, depending on the course of the disease. Spinal cord compression, foramen magnum tumor (which may mimic the exacerbations and remissions of MS), multiple small strokes, syphilis or another infection, thyroid disease, and chronic fatigue syndrome must be ruled out.

The following tests may be useful:
- Magnetic resonance imaging reveals multifocal white matter lesions.
- EEG reveals abnormalities in brain waves in onethird of patients.
- Lumbar puncture shows normal total cerebrospinal fluid (CSF) protein but elevated immunoglobulin (Ig) G (gamma globulin); IgG reflects hyperactivity of the immune system due to chronic demyelination. An elevated CSF IgG is significant only when serum IgG is normal. CSF white blood cell count may be elevated.
- CSF electrophoresis detects bands of IgG in most patients, even when

the percentage of IgG in CSF is normal. Presence of kappa light chains provide additional support to the diagnosis.
- Evoked potential studies (visual, brain stem, auditory, and somatosensory) reveal slowed conduction of nerve impulses in most patients.

TREATMENT

The aim of treatment is threefold: Treat the acute exacerbation, treat the disease process, and treat the related signs and symptoms.
- I.V. methylprednisolone followed by oral therapy to reduce edema of the myelin sheath (speeds recovery from acute attacks); other drugs, such as azathioprine (Imuran) or methotrexate (Trexall) and cyclophosphamide (Cytoxan)
- Immune system therapy consisting of interferon and glatiramer (a combination of four amino acids) to reduce frequency and severity of relapses, and possibly slow CNS damage
- Stretching and range-of-motion exercises, coupled with correct positioning, to relieve the spasticity resulting from opposing muscle groups relaxing and contracting at the same time; helpful in relaxing muscles and maintaining function
- Baclofen (Kemstro) and tizanidine (Zanaflex) to treat spasticity; botulinum toxin injections, intrathecal injections, nerve blocks, and surgery to treat severe spasticity
- Frequent rest periods, aerobic exercise, and cooling techniques (air conditioning, breezes, water sprays) to minimize fatigue (Fatigue is characterized by an overwhelming feeling of exhaustion that can occur at any time of the day without warning. The cause is unknown and changes in en-

vironmental conditions, such as heat and humidity, can aggravate it.)
- Methylphenidate (Ritalin) or anti-depressants may be beneficial for managing fatigue
- Bladder problems (failure to store urine, failure to empty the bladder or, more commonly, both) managed by such strategies as drinking cranberry juice or insertion of an indwelling catheter and suprapubic tubes (Intermittent self-catheterization and post-void catheterization programs are helpful, as are anticholinergic medications in some patients.)
- Bowel problems (constipation and involuntary evacuation) managed by such measures as increasing fiber intake, using bulking agents, and bowel-training strategies, such as daily suppositories and rectal stimulation
- Low-dose tricyclic antidepressants, phenytoin (Dilantin), or carbamaze-pine (Tegretol) for managing sensory symptoms, such as pain, numbness, burning, and tingling sensations
- Adaptive devices and physical therapy to assist with motor dysfunction, such as problems with balance, strength, and muscle coordination
- Beta-adrenergic blockers, sedatives, or diuretics to alleviate tremors
- Speech therapy for managing dysarthria
- Antihistamines, vision therapy, or exercises to minimize vertigo
- Vision therapy or adaptive lenses for managing vision problems

NURSING CONSIDERATIONS
Management considerations focus on educating the patient and family.
- Assist with physical therapy. Increase patient comfort with massages and relaxing baths. Make sure the bath water isn't too hot because it may temporarily intensify otherwise subtle symptoms. Assist with active, resistive, and stretching exercises to maintain muscle tone and joint mobility, decrease spasticity, improve coordination, and boost morale.
- Educate the patient and his family concerning the chronic course of MS. Emphasize the need to avoid stress, infections, and fatigue and to maintain independence by developing new ways of performing daily activities. Be sure to tell the patient to avoid exposure to infections.
- Stress the importance of eating a nutritious, well-balanced diet that contains sufficient roughage and adequate fluids to prevent constipation.
- Evaluate the need for bowel and bladder training during hospitalization. Encourage adequate fluid intake and regular urination. Eventually, the patient may require urinary drainage by self-catheterization or, in men, condom drainage. Teach the correct use of suppositories to help establish a regular bowel schedule.
- Promote emotional stability. Help the patient establish a daily routine to maintain optimal functioning. Activity level is regulated by tolerance level. Encourage regular rest periods to prevent fatigue and daily physical exercise.
- Inform the patient that exacerbations are unpredictable, necessitating physical and emotional adjustments in lifestyle.
- For more information, refer the patient to the National Multiple Sclerosis Society.

Myasthenia gravis

Myasthenia gravis causes sporadic but progressive weakness and abnormal fatigability of striated (skeletal) muscles; symptoms are exacerbated by exercise and repeated movement and relieved by anticholinesterase drugs. Usually, this disorder affects muscles innervated by the cranial nerves (face, lips, tongue, neck, and throat), but it can affect any muscle group.

Myasthenia gravis follows an unpredictable course of periodic exacerbations and remissions. There's no known cure. Drug treatment has improved the prognosis and allows patients to lead relatively normal lives, except during exacerbations. When the disease involves the respiratory system, it may be life-threatening.

Myasthenia gravis affects 1 in 25,000 people at any age, but incidence peaks between ages 20 and 40. It's three times more common in women than in men in this age-group, but after age 40, the incidence is similar.

About 20% of infants born to mothers with myasthenia gravis have transient (or occasionally persistent) myasthenia. This disease may coexist with immune and thyroid disorders; 15% of patients with myasthenia gravis have thymomas. Remissions occur in about 25% of patients.

CAUSES

The exact cause of myasthenia gravis is unknown. However, it's believed to be the result of:
- autoimmune response
- inadequate muscle fiber response to acetylcholine
- ineffective acetylcholine release.

PATHOPHYSIOLOGY

Myasthenia gravis causes a failure in transmission of nerve impulses at the neuromuscular junction. The site of action is the postsynaptic membrane.

Theoretically, antireceptor antibodies block, weaken, or reduce the number of acetylcholine receptors available at each neuromuscular junction and thereby impair muscle depolarization necessary for movement. (See *Impaired transmission in myasthenia gravis*.)

CLINICAL FINDINGS

Myasthenia gravis may occur gradually or suddenly. Signs and symptoms include:
- weak eye closure, ptosis, and diplopia from impaired neuromuscular transmission to the cranial nerves supplying the eye muscles (may be the only symptom present)
- skeletal muscle weakness and fatigue, increasing through the day but decreasing with rest (In the early stages, easy fatigability of certain muscles may appear with no other findings. Later, it may be severe enough to cause paralysis.)
- progressive muscle weakness and accompanying loss of function depending on muscle group affected; becoming more intense during menses and after emotional stress, prolonged exposure to sunlight or cold, or infections
- blank and expressionless facial appearance and nasal vocal tones secondary to impaired transmission of cranial nerves innervating the facial muscles
- frequent nasal regurgitation of fluids and difficulty chewing and swallowing from cranial nerve involvement
- drooping eyelids from weakness of facial and extraocular muscles
- weakened neck muscles with head tilting back to see; neck muscles possibly becoming too weak to support the head without bobbing

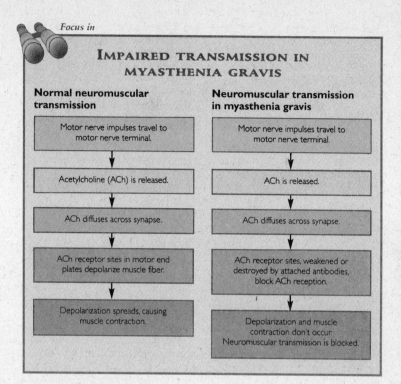

Focus in

IMPAIRED TRANSMISSION IN MYASTHENIA GRAVIS

Normal neuromuscular transmission

Motor nerve impulses travel to motor nerve terminal.

↓

Acetylcholine (ACh) is released.

↓

ACh diffuses across synapse.

↓

ACh receptor sites in motor end plates depolarize muscle fiber.

↓

Depolarization spreads, causing muscle contraction.

Neuromuscular transmission in myasthenia gravis

Motor nerve impulses travel to motor nerve terminal.

↓

ACh is released.

↓

ACh diffuses across synapse.

↓

ACh receptor sites, weakened or destroyed by attached antibodies, block ACh reception.

↓

Depolarization and muscle contraction don't occur. Neuromuscular transmission is blocked.

---

weakened respiratory muscles, decreased tidal volume and vital capacity from impaired transmission to the diaphragm making breathing difficult and predisposing the patient to pneumonia and other respiratory tract infections

● respiratory muscle weakness (myasthenic crisis) possibly severe enough to require an emergency airway and mechanical ventilation.

Alert *Complications of myasthenia gravis may include respiratory distress, pneumonia, aspiration, and myasthenic crisis.*

TEST RESULTS

● Tensilon challenge test confirms diagnosis of myasthenia gravis, revealing temporarily improved muscle function within 30 to 60 seconds after I.V. injection of edrophonium or neostigmine and lasting up to 30 minutes.

● Electromyography with repeated neural stimulation shows progressive decrease in muscle fiber contraction.

● Serum antiacetylcholine antibody titer may be elevated.

● Chest X-ray reveals thymoma (in approximately 15% of patients).

TREATMENT

● Anticholinesterase drugs, such as neostigmine (Prostigim) and pyridostigmine (Mestinon), to counteract fatigue and muscle weakness and allow about 80% of normal muscle function (drugs less effective as disease worsens)

- Immunosuppressant therapy with corticosteroids, azathioprine (Imuran), cyclosporine (Sandimmune), and cyclophosphamide (Cytoxan) used in a progressive fashion (when the previous drug response is poor, the next one is used) to decrease the immune response toward acetylcholine receptors at the neuromuscular junction
- Immunoglobulin G during acute relapses or plasmapheresis in severe exacerbations to suppress the immune system
- Thymectomy to remove thymomas and possibly induce remission in some cases of adultonset myasthenia
- Tracheotomy, positive-pressure ventilation, and vigorous suctioning to remove secretions for treatment of acute exacerbations that cause severe respiratory distress
- Discontinuation of anticholinesterase drugs in myasthenic crisis, until respiratory function improves — myasthenic crisis requires immediate hospitalization and vigorous respiratory support

NURSING CONSIDERATIONS

Careful baseline assessment, early recognition and treatment of potential crises, supportive measures, and thorough patient teaching can minimize exacerbations and complications. Continuity of care is essential.

- Establish an accurate neurologic and respiratory baseline. Thereafter, monitor tidal volume and vital capacity regularly. The patient may need a ventilator and frequent suctioning to remove accumulating secretions.
- Be alert for signs of an impending crisis (increased muscle weakness, respiratory distress, and difficulty in talking or chewing).
- To prevent relapses, adhere closely to the ordered drug administration schedule. Be prepared to give atropine for anticholinesterase overdose or toxicity.
- Plan exercise, meals, patient care, and activities to make the most of energy peaks. For example, give medication 20 to 30 minutes before meals to facilitate chewing or swallowing. Allow the patient to participate in his care.
- When swallowing is difficult, give soft, solid foods instead of liquids to lessen the risk of choking.
- Patient teaching is essential because myasthenia gravis is usually a lifelong condition. Help the patient plan daily activities to coincide with energy peaks. Stress the need for frequent rest periods throughout the day. Emphasize that periodic remissions, exacerbations, and day-to-day fluctuations are common.
- Teach the patient how to recognize the adverse effects and signs of toxicity of anticholinesterase drugs (headaches, weakness, sweating, abdominal cramps, nausea, vomiting, diarrhea, excessive salivation, and bronchospasm) and corticosteroids (euphoria, insomnia, edema, and increased appetite).
- Warn the patient to avoid strenuous exercise, stress, infection, and needless exposure to the sun or cold. All of these factors may worsen signs and symptoms. Wearing an eye patch or glasses with one frosted lens may help the patient with diplopia.
- For more information and an opportunity to meet other myasthenia gravis patients who lead full, productive lives, refer the patient to the Myasthenia Gravis Foundation.

Parkinson's disease

Named for James Parkinson, the English physician who wrote the first accurate description of the disease in 1817, Parkinson's disease (also known as *shaking palsy*) characteristically produces progressive muscle rigidity, akinesia, and involuntary tremor. Deterioration is a progressive process. Death may result from complications, such as aspiration pneumonia or some other infection.

Parkinson's disease is one of the most common crippling diseases in the United States. It strikes 1 in every 100 people over age 60 and affects men more often than women. Roughly 60,000 new cases are diagnosed annually in the United States alone, and incidence is predicted to increase as the population ages.

CAUSES

The cause of Parkinson's disease is unknown. However, study of the extrapyramidal brain nuclei (corpus striatum, globus pallidus, substantia nigra) has established that:

● Dopamine deficiency prevents affected brain cells from performing their normal inhibitory function in the central nervous system.
● Some cases are caused by exposure to toxins, such as manganese dust or carbon monoxide.

PATHOPHYSIOLOGY

Parkinson's disease is a degenerative process involving the dopaminergic neurons in the substantia nigra (the area of the basal ganglia that produces and stores the neurotransmitter dopamine). This area plays an important role in the extrapyramidal system,
which controls posture and coordination of voluntary motor movements.

Normally, stimulation of the basal ganglia results in refined motor movement because acetylcholine (excitatory) and dopamine (inhibitory) release are balanced. Degeneration of the dopaminergic neurons and loss of available dopamine leads to an excess of excitatory acetylcholine at the synapse and consequent rigidity, tremors, and bradykinesia.

Other nondopaminergic neurons may be affected, possibly contributing to depression and the other nonmotor symptoms associated with this disease. Also, the basal ganglia is interconnected to the hypothalamus, potentially affecting autonomic and endocrine function as well.

Current research on the pathogenesis of Parkinson's disease focuses on damage to the substantia nigra from oxidative stress. Oxidative stress is believed to diminish brain iron content, impair mitochondrial function, inhibit antioxidant and protective systems, reduce glutathione secretion, and damage lipids, proteins, and deoxyribonucleic acid. Brain cells are less capable of repairing oxidative damage than are other tissues.

CLINICAL FINDINGS

● Muscle rigidity, akinesia, and an insidious tremor beginning in the fingers (unilateral pill-roll tremor) that increases during stress or anxiety and decreases with purposeful movement and sleep; secondary to loss of inhibitory dopamine activity at the synapse
● Muscle rigidity with resistance to passive muscle stretching, which may be uniform (lead-pipe rigidity) or jerky (cogwheel rigidity) secondary to depletion of dopamine

- Akinesia causing difficulty walking (gait that lacks normal parallel motion and may be retropulsive or propulsive) from impaired dopamine action
- High-pitched, monotone voice from dopamine depletion
- Drooling secondary to impaired regulation of motor function
- Masklike facial expression from depletion of dopamine
- Loss of posture control (the patient walks with body bent forward) from loss of motor control due to dopamine depletion
- Difficulty speaking or swallowing, or both
- Oculogyric crises (eyes are fixed upward, with involuntary tonic movements) or blepharospasm (eyelids are completely closed)
- Excessive sweating from impaired autonomic dysfunction
- Decreased motility of GI and genitourinary smooth muscle from impaired autonomic transmission
- Orthostatic hypotension from impaired vascular smooth muscle response
- Oily skin secondary to inappropriate androgen production controlled by the hypothalamus pituitary axis

Alert *Complications of Parkinson's disease may include injury from falls, aspiration, urinary tract infections, and pressure ulcers.*

TEST RESULTS

Generally, diagnostic tests are of little value in identifying Parkinson's disease. Diagnosis is based on the patient's age and history and on the characteristic clinical picture. However, urinalysis may support the diagnosis by revealing decreased dopamine levels.

A conclusive diagnosis is possible only after ruling out other causes of tremor, involutional depression, cerebral arteriosclerosis and, in patients under age 30, intracranial tumors, Wilson's disease, or phenothiazine or other drug toxicity.

TREATMENT

The aim of treatment is to relieve symptoms and keep the patient functional as long as possible. Treatment includes:
- levodopa, a dopamine replacement most effective during early stages and given in increasing doses until symptoms are relieved or adverse effects appear (Because adverse effects can be serious, levodopa is usually given in combination with carbidopa (Lodosyn) or entacapone (Comtan) to halt peripheral dopamine synthesis. Dopamine agonists may be used early in the disease or in combination with levodopa to enhance response or decrease adverse effects.)
- non-ergot derivitaves, apomorphine (Apokyn), pramipexole (Mirapex), and ropinirole (Requip), may improve motor function by stimulating dopamine D2 receptors in the brain
- benztropine (Cogentin), an antimuscarine, or entacapone, a COMT inhibitor, may be combined with levodopa and carbidopa to maintain optimal symptom relief
- pergolide (Permax), a dopamine agonist, directly stimulates dopamine receptors in the nigrostriatal system
- alternative drug therapy, including anticholinergics such as trihexyphenidyl; antihistamines such as diphenhydramine (Benadryl); and amantadine (Symmetrel), an antiviral, or Selegiline (Eldepryl), an enzyme-inhibiting drug, for when levodopa proves ineffective to conserve dopamine and enhance the therapeutic effect of levodopa

- stereotactic neurosurgery for when drug therapy fails to prevent involuntary movement (It's most effective in young, otherwise healthy persons with unilateral tremor or muscle rigidity. Neurosurgery can only relieve symptoms, not cure the disease.)
- deep brain stimulation, an alternative for patients that fail conventional treatment, in which neurostimulator and electrodes are implanted that stimulate the globus pallidus subthalamic nucleus to decrease tremors and allow normal function
- fetal cell transplantation (controversial), in which fetal brain tissue is injected into the patient's brain, in the hope that injected cells will grow, allowing the brain to process dopamine and, thereby, halting or reducing the disease progression
- physical therapy, including active and passive range-of-motion exercises, routine daily activities, walking, and baths and massage to help relax muscles; complement drug treatment and neurosurgery attempting to maintain normal muscle tone and function.

NURSING CONSIDERATIONS

Effectively caring for the patient with Parkinson's disease requires careful monitoring of drug treatment, emphasis on teaching self-reliance, and generous psychological support.
- Monitor drug treatment and adjust dosage, if necessary, to minimize adverse effects.
- If the patient has surgery, watch for signs of hemorrhage and increased intracranial pressure by frequently checking level of consciousness and vital signs.
- Encourage independence. The patient with excessive tremor may achieve partial control of his body by sitting on a chair and using its arms to

steady himself. Advise the patient to change position slowly and dangle his legs before getting out of bed. Remember that fatigue may cause him to depend more on others.
- Help the patient overcome problems related to eating and elimination. For example, if he has difficulty eating, offer supplementary or small, frequent meals to increase caloric intake. Help establish a regular bowel routine by encouraging him to drink at least 2 qt (approximately 2 L) of liquids daily and eat high-fiber foods. He may need an elevated toilet seat to assist him from a standing to a sitting position.
- Give the patient and family emotional support. Teach them about the disease, its progressive stages, and adverse drug effects. Show the family how to prevent pressure ulcers and contractures by proper positioning. Inform them of the dietary restrictions levodopa imposes, and explain household safety measures to prevent injury. Help the patient and his family express their feelings and frustrations about the progressively debilitating effects of the disease. Establish long- and short-term treatment goals, and be aware of the patient's need for intellectual stimulation and diversion. Refer the patient and family to the National Parkinson Foundation or the United Parkinson Foundation for more information.

Reye's syndrome

Reye's syndrome is an acute illness that causes fatty infiltration of the liver with concurrent hyperammonemia, encephalopathy, and increased intracranial pressure (ICP). In addition, fatty infiltration of the kidneys, brain, and myocardium may occur. Reye's syndrome affects children from infancy to adolescence and occurs equally in boys and girls.

Prognosis depends on the severity of central nervous system depression. Until recently, mortality was as high as 90%. Today, ICP monitoring and, consequently, early treatment of increased ICP, along with other treatment measures, have reduced mortality to about 20%. Death is usually a result of cerebral edema or respiratory arrest. Comatose patients who survive may have residual brain damage.

Incidence commonly rises during influenza outbreaks and may be linked to aspirin use. For this reason, use of aspirin for children under age 15 isn't recommended.

CAUSES

Reye's syndrome typically begins within 1 to 3 days of an acute viral infection, such as an upper respiratory tract infection, type B influenza, or varicella (chickenpox).

PATHOPHYSIOLOGY

In Reye's syndrome, damaged hepatic mitochondria disrupt the urea cycle, which normally changes ammonia to urea for its excretion from the body. This results in hyperammonemia, hypoglycemia (in 15% of cases), and an increase in serum short-chain fatty acids, leading to encephalopathy. Simultaneously, fatty infiltration occurs in renal tubular cells, neuronal tissue, and muscle tissue, including the heart.

CLINICAL FINDINGS

The severity of the child's signs and symptoms varies with the degree of encephalopathy and cerebral edema. In any case, Reye's syndrome develops in five stages. After the initial viral infection, a brief recovery period follows when the child doesn't seem seriously ill. A few days later, he develops intractable vomiting; lethargy; rapidly changing mental status (mild to severe agitation, confusion, irritability, and delirium); rising blood pressure, respiratory rate, and pulse rate; and hyperactive reflexes.

Reye's syndrome commonly progresses to coma. As coma deepens, seizures develop, followed by decreased tendon reflexes and, usually, respiratory failure.

Alert *Increased ICP, a serious complication of Reye's syndrome, is now considered the result of an increased cerebral blood volume causing intracranial hypertension. Such swelling may develop as a result of acidosis, increased cerebral metabolic rate, and an impaired autoregulatory mechanism.*

Other complications may include respiratory failure and death.

TEST RESULTS

A history of a recent viral disorder with typical clinical features strongly suggests Reye's syndrome. An increased serum ammonia level, abnormal clotting studies, and hepatic dysfunction confirm it. Absence of jaundice despite increased liver aminotransferase levels rules out acute hepatic failure and hepatic encephalopathy.

Abnormal test results may include:
- liver function studies — aspartate aminotransferase and alanine aminotransferase elevated to twice normal levels
- liver biopsy — fatty droplets uniformly distributed throughout cells
- cerebrospinal fluid (CSF) analysis — white blood cell count less than

10/mm^3; with coma, increased CSF pressure
- coagulation studies — prolonged prothrombin time and partial thromboplastin time
- blood values — elevated serum ammonia levels; normal or low (in 15% of cases) serum glucose levels; increased serum fatty acid and lactate levels.

TREATMENT
For treatment guidelines, see *Stages and treatment for Reye's syndrome.*

STAGES AND TREATMENT FOR REYE'S SYNDROME

SIGNS AND SYMPTOMS	BASELINE TREATMENT	BASELINE INTERVENTIONS
Stage I Vomiting, lethargy, hepatic dysfunction	◆ To decrease intracranial pressure (ICP) and brain edema, give I.V. fluids at two-thirds maintenance. Also give an osmotic diuretic or furosemide (Lasix). ◆ To treat hypoprothrombinemia, give vitamin K; if vitamin K is unsuccessful, give fresh frozen plasma. ◆ Monitor serum ammonia and blood glucose levels and plasma osmolality every 4 to 8 hours to check progress.	◆ Monitor vital signs and check level of consciousness for increasing lethargy. Monitor vital signs more often as the patient's condition deteriorates. ◆ Monitor fluid intake and output to prevent fluid overload. Maintain urine output at 1 ml/kg/hr; plasma osmolality, 290 mOsm; and blood glucose, 150 mg/ml. Also, restrict protein.
Stage II Hyperventilation, delirium, hepatic dysfunction, hyperactive reflexes	◆ Continue baseline treatment from Stage I.	◆ Maintain seizure precautions. ◆ Immediately report signs of coma that require invasive, supportive therapy, such as intubation. ◆ Keep head of bed at 30-degree angle.
Stage III Coma, hyperventilation, decorticate rigidity, hepatic dysfunction	◆ Continue baseline treatment from Stage I and seizure treatment. ◆ Monitor ICP. ◆ Provide endotracheal intubation and mechanical ventilation to control partial pressure of arterial carbon dioxide (Paco$_2$) levels. A neuromuscular blocker may help control ventilation. ◆ Give mannitol (Osmitrol) I.V.	◆ Monitor ICP (should be < 20 mm Hg before suctioning). ◆ Keep the patient sedated. ◆ When ventilating the patient, maintain Paco$_2$ between 30 and 40 mm Hg and partial pressure of arterial oxygen between 80 and 100 mm Hg. ◆ Closely monitor cardiovascular status with a pulmonary artery catheter or central venous pressure line. ◆ Give good skin and mouth care and perform range-of-motion exercises.

(continued)

STAGES AND TREATMENT FOR REYE'S SYNDROME (continued)

SIGNS AND SYMPTOMS	BASELINE TREATMENT	BASELINE INTERVENTIONS
Stage IV Deepening coma; decerebrate rigidity; large, fixed pupils; minimal hepatic dysfunction	◆ Continue baseline treatment from Stage I and supportive care. ◆ If all previous measures fail, barbiturate coma, decompressive craniotomy, hypothermia, or exchange transfusion may be used.	◆ Check patient for loss of reflexes and signs of flaccidity. ◆ Give the family support.
Stage V Seizures, loss of deep tendon reflexes, flaccidity, respiratory arrest, ammonia level above 300 mg/dl	◆ Continue baseline treatment from Stage I and supportive care.	◆ Help the family cope with the patient's impending death.

NURSING CONSIDERATIONS

● Advise nonsalicylate analgesics and antipyretics such as acetaminophen (Tylenol) to help prevent Reye's syndrome.
● For more information, refer parents to the National Reye's Syndrome Foundation.

Seizure disorder

Seizure disorder, or epilepsy, is a condition of the brain characterized by susceptibility to recurrent seizures (paroxysmal events associated with abnormal electrical discharges of neurons in the brain). Primary seizure disorder or epilepsy is idiopathic without apparent structural changes in the brain. Secondary epilepsy, characterized by structural changes or metabolic alterations of the neuronal membranes, causes increased automaticity.

Epilepsy is believed to affect 1% to 2% of the population; approximately 2 million people have been diagnosed with the disorder. The incidence is highest in childhood and old age. The prognosis is good if the patient adheres strictly to prescribed treatment. Seizures not associated with a seizure disorder may also occur, such as child febrile seizures and postconcussive seizures.

CAUSES

About one-half of all seizure disorder cases are idiopathic; possible causes of seizures include:
● anoxia
● birth trauma (inadequate oxygen supply to the brain, blood incompatibility, or hemorrhage)
● brain tumors
● head injury or trauma
● infectious diseases (meningitis, encephalitis, or brain abscess)

- ingestion of toxins (mercury, lead, or carbon monoxide)
- inherited disorders or degenerative disease, such as phenylketonuria or tuberous sclerosis
- metabolic disorders, such as hypoglycemia, hyponatremia and hypoparathyroidism
- perinatal infection
- stroke (hemorrhage, thrombosis, or embolism).

PATHOPHYSIOLOGY

Some neurons in the brain may depolarize easily or be hyperexcitable; this epileptogenic focus fires more readily than normal when stimulated. In these neurons, the membrane potential at rest is less negative or inhibitory connections are missing, possibly as a result of decreased gamma-aminobutyric acid activity or localized shifts in electrolytes. On stimulation, the epileptogenic focus fires and spreads electrical current to surrounding cells. These cells fire in turn and the impulse cascades to one side of the brain (a partial seizure), both sides of the brain (a generalized seizure), or specific cortical, subcortical, or brain stem areas.

The brain's metabolic demand for oxygen increases dramatically during a seizure. If this demand isn't met, hypoxia and brain damage ensue. Firing of inhibitory neurons causes the excitatory neurons to slow their firing and eventually stop. If this inhibitory action doesn't occur, the result is status epilepticus: one seizure occurring right after another and another; without treatment the anoxia can be fatal.

CLINICAL FINDINGS

The hallmark of epilepsy is recurring seizures, which can be classified as partial, generalized, status epilepticus,

or unclassified (some patients may be affected by more than one type). (See *Seizure types,* page 176.)

Alert *Complications of epilepsy may include hypoxia or anoxia from airway occlusion, traumatic injury, brain damage, depression, and anxiety.*

TEST RESULTS

Clinically, the diagnosis of epilepsy is based on the occurrence of one or more seizures and underlying cause. Diagnostic tests that help support the findings include:
- Computed tomography scan or magnetic resonance imaging reveal abnormalities.
- EEG reveals paroxysmal abnormalities to confirm the diagnosis and provide evidence of the continuing tendency to have seizures. In tonic-clonic seizures, high, fast voltage spikes are present in all leads; in absence seizures, rounded spike wave complexes are diagnostic. A negative EEG doesn't rule out epilepsy because the abnormalities occur intermittently.
- Serum chemistry blood studies may reveal hypoglycemia, electrolyte imbalances, elevated liver enzymes, and elevated alcohol levels, providing clues to underlying conditions that increase the risk of seizure activity.

TREATMENT

- Drug therapy specific to the type of seizure, including phenytoin (Dilantin), carbamazepine (Tegretol), phenobarbital, gabapentin (Neurontin), and primidone for generalized tonic-clonic seizures and complex partial seizures (I.V. fosphenytoin [Cerebyx] is an alternative to phenytoin.)
- Valproic acid (Depakene), clonazepam (Klonopin), and ethosuximide (Zarontin) for absence seizures; gaba-

Seizure types

The various types of seizures—partial, generalized, status epilepticus, and unclassified— have distinct signs and symptoms.

Partial

Arising from a localized area of the brain, partial seizures cause focal symptoms. These seizures are classified by their effect on consciousness and whether they spread throughout the motor pathway, causing a generalized seizure.

◆ A *simple partial seizure* begins locally and generally doesn't cause an alteration in consciousness. It may present with sensory symptoms (lights flashing, smells, auditory hallucinations), autonomic symptoms (sweating, flushing, pupil dilation), and psychic symptoms (dream states, anger, fear). The seizure lasts for a few seconds and occurs without preceding or provoking events. This type can be motor or sensory.

◆ A *complex partial seizure* alters consciousness. Amnesia for events that occur during and immediately after the seizure is a differentiating characteristic. During the seizure, the patient may follow simple commands. This seizure generally lasts for 1 to 3 minutes.

Generalized

As the term suggests, generalized seizures cause a generalized electrical abnormality within the brain. They can be convulsive or nonconvulsive and include several types:

◆ *Absence seizures* occur most commonly in children, although they may affect adults. They usually begin with a brief change in level of consciousness, indicated by blinking or rolling of the eyes, a blank stare, and slight mouth movements. The patient retains his posture and continues preseizure activity without difficulty. Typically, each seizure lasts from 1 to 10 seconds. If not properly treated, seizures can recur as often as 100 times per day. An absence seizure is a nonconvulsive seizure, but it may progress to a generalized tonic-clonic seizure.

◆ *Myoclonic seizures* (bilateral massive epileptic myoclonus) are brief, involuntary muscular jerks of the body or extremities, which may be rhythmic. Consciousness isn't usually affected.

◆ *Generalized tonic-clonic seizures* typically begin with a loud cry, precipitated by air rushing from the lungs through the vocal cords. The patient then loses consciousness and falls to the ground. The body stiffens (tonic phase) and then alternates between episodes of muscle spasm and relaxation (clonic phase). Tongue biting, incontinence, labored breathing, apnea, and subsequent cyanosis may occur. The seizure stops in 2 to 5 minutes, when abnormal electrical conduction ceases. When the patient regains consciousness, he's confused and may have difficulty talking. If he can talk, he may complain of drowsiness, fatigue, headache, muscle soreness, and arm or leg weakness. He may fall into a deep sleep after the seizure.

◆ *Atonic seizures* are characterized by a general loss of postural tone and a temporary loss of consciousness. They occur in young children and are sometimes called *drop attacks* because they cause the child to fall.

Status epilepticus

Status epilepticus is a continuous seizure state that can occur in all seizure types. The most life-threatening example is generalized tonic-clonic status epilepticus, a continuous generalized tonic-clonic seizure. Status epilepticus is accompanied by respiratory distress leading to hypoxia or anoxia. It can result from abrupt withdrawal of anticonvulsant medications, hypoxic encephalopathy, acute head trauma, metabolic encephalopathy, or septicemia secondary to encephalitis or meningitis.

Unclassified

This category is reserved for seizures that don't fit the characteristics of partial or generalized seizures or status epilepticus. Included as unclassified are events that lack the data to make a more definitive diagnosis.

pentin and felbamate (Felbatol) as other anticonvulsant drugs
- Surgical removal of a demonstrated focal lesion, if drug therapy is ineffective; surgery to remove the underlying cause (tumor, abscess, or vascular problem)
- Vagus nerve stimulator implantation to reduce incidence of focal seizure
- I.V. diazepam (Valium), lorazepam (Ativan), or midazolam (Versed) for status epilepticus
- Administration of dextrose (when seizures are secondary to hypoglycemia) or thiamine (in chronic alcoholism or withdrawal) or toxin-specific treatment
- Supplemental oxygen

NURSING CONSIDERATIONS

A key to support is a true understanding of the nature of epilepsy and of the misconceptions that surround it.
- Encourage the patient and family to express their feelings about the patient's condition. Answer their questions, and help them cope by dispelling some of the myths about epilepsy; for example, the myth that it's contagious. Assure them that epilepsy is controllable for most patients who follow a prescribed regimen of medication and that most patients maintain a normal lifestyle.
- Stress the need for compliance with the prescribed drug schedule. Reinforce dosage instructions and stress the importance of taking medication regularly and at scheduled times. Caution the patient to monitor the quantity of medication he has so he doesn't run out of it.
- Warn against possible adverse effects — drowsiness, lethargy, hyperactivity, confusion, and visual and sleep disturbances — all of which indicate the need for dosage adjustment. Phenytoin therapy may lead to hyperplasia of the gums, which may be relieved by conscientious oral hygiene. Instruct the patient to report adverse effects immediately.
- When administering phenytoin I.V., use a large vein and monitor vital signs frequently. Avoid I.M. administration and mixing with dextrose solutions.
- Emphasize the importance of having anticonvulsant blood levels checked at regular intervals, even if the seizures are under control.
- Warn the patient against drinking alcoholic beverages.
- Know which social agencies in your community can help epileptic patients. Refer the patient to the Epilepsy Foundation of America for general information and to the state motor vehicle department for information about a driver's license.

The primary goals of the health care professional and family members caring for a patient having a seizure are protection from injury, protection from aspiration, and observation of the seizure activity. Generalized tonic-clonic seizures may necessitate first aid.

Show the patient's family members how to administer first aid correctly. Tell them to avoid restraining the patient during a seizure, help him to a lying position, loosen tight clothing, and place something flat and soft, such as a pillow under his head. The area should be cleared of hard objects. Caution them not to force anything into the patient's mouth if his teeth are clenched — a tongue blade or spoon could lacerate the mouth and lips or displace teeth, precipitating respiratory distress. However, if the patient's mouth is open, they can protect his tongue by placing a soft object (such as a folded cloth) between his teeth. His head should be turned to provide an open airway. After the seizure subsides, they should reassure the patient that he's all right, orient him to time and place, and inform him that he has had a seizure.

Spinal cord trauma

Spinal injuries include fractures, contusions, and compressions of the vertebral column, usually as the result of trauma to the head or neck. The real danger lies in spinal cord damage — cutting, pulling, twisting, or compression. Damage may involve the entire cord or be restricted to a portion of it, and can occur at any level. Fractures of the 5th, 6th, or 7th cervical, 12th thoracic, and 1st lumbar vertebrae are most common.

CAUSES
The most serious spinal cord trauma typically results from:
- accidents (automobile crashes, falls from a height, sports injuries, diving into shallow water)
- gunshot or stab wounds.
  Less serious injuries commonly occur from:
- lifting heavy objects
- minor falls.
  Spinal dysfunction may also result from:
- hyperparathyroidism
- neoplastic lesions.

PATHOPHYSIOLOGY
Like head trauma, spinal cord trauma results from acceleration, deceleration, or other deforming forces usually applied from a distance. Mechanisms involved with spinal cord trauma include:

- hyperextension from acceleration-deceleration forces and sudden reduction in the anteroposterior diameter of the spinal cord
- hyperflexion from sudden and excessive force, propelling the spine forward or causing an exaggerated movement to one side
- vertical compression from force being applied from the top of the cranium along the vertical axis through the vertebra or from the lumbar spine upward
- rotational forces from twisting, which adds shearing forces.

Injury causes microscopic hemorrhages in the gray matter and pia mater and arachnoid mater. The hemorrhages gradually increase in size until some or all of the gray matter is filled with blood, which causes necrosis. From the gray matter, the blood enters the white matter, where it impedes the circulation within the spinal cord. Ensuing edema causes compression and decreases the blood supply. Thus, the spinal cord loses perfusion and becomes ischemic. The edema and hemorrhage are greatest at and approximately two segments above and below the injury. The edema temporarily adds to the patient's dysfunction by increasing pressure and compressing the nerves. Edema at or above the 3rd to 5th cervical vertebrae may interfere with phrenic nerve impulse transmission to the diaphragm and inhibit respiratory function.

In the white matter, circulation usually returns to normal in approximately 24 hours. However, in the gray matter, an inflammatory reaction prevents restoration of circulation. Phagocytes appear at the site within 36 to 48 hours after the injury, macrophages engulf degenerating axons, and collagen replaces the normal tissue. Scar-

TYPES OF SPINAL CORD INJURY

Injury to the spinal cord can be classified as complete or incomplete. An incomplete spinal injury may be an anterior cord syndrome, central cord syndrome, or Brown-Séquard syndrome, depending on the area of the cord affected. This chart highlights the characteristic signs and symptoms of each.

TYPE	DESCRIPTION	SIGNS AND SYMPTOMS
Complete disruption	◆ All tracts of the spinal cord completely disrupted ◆ All functions involving the spinal cord below the level of disruption lost ◆ Complete and permanent loss	◆ Loss of motor function (quadriplegia) with cervical cord disruption; paraplegia with thoracic cord disruption; bowel, bladder and sexual dysfunction with lumbar or sacral disruption ◆ Muscle flaccidity ◆ Loss of all reflexes and sensory function below level of injury ◆ Bladder and bowel atony ◆ Paralytic ileus ◆ Loss of vasomotor tone below injury with low and unstable blood pressure ◆ Loss of perspiration below level of injury ◆ Dry pale skin ◆ Respiratory impairment with cervical or upper thoracic spinal injury ◆ Neurogenic shock
Incomplete transection: Central cord syndrome	◆ Center portion of the cord affected ◆ Typically from hyperextension injury	◆ Motor deficits greater in the upper than in lower extremities ◆ Variable degree of bladder dysfunction
Incomplete transection: Anterior cord syndrome	◆ Occlusion of the anterior spinal artery ◆ Occlusion occurring from pressure by bone fragments	◆ Loss of motor function below level of injury ◆ Loss of pain and temperature sensations below level of injury ◆ Intact touch, pressure, position, and vibration senses
Incomplete transection: Brown-Séquard syndrome	◆ Hemisection of the cord occurring ◆ Most commonly occurring in stabbing or gunshot wounds ◆ Damage to cord on only one side occurring	◆ Ipsilateral paralysis or paresis below level of injury ◆ Ipsilateral loss of touch, pressure, vibration, and position sense below level of injury ◆ Contralateral loss of pain and temperature sensations below level of injury

ring and meningeal thickening leaves the nerves in the area blocked or tangled.

CLINICAL FINDINGS
● Muscle spasm and back pain worsening with movement

● Mild paresthesia to quadriplegia and shock, if the injury damages the spinal cord; in milder injury, such symptoms may be delayed several days or weeks; specific signs and symptoms depending on injury type and degree (See *Types of spinal cord injury.*)

COMPLICATIONS OF SPINAL CORD INJURY

Early detection of complications, such as spinal and neurogenic shock and autonomic dysreflexia, is essential when assessing the patient with a spinal cord injury.

SPINAL SHOCK

Spinal shock is the loss of autonomic, reflex, motor, and sensory activity below the level of the cord lesion. It occurs secondary to damage to the spinal cord.

Signs of spinal shock include:
◆ flaccid paralysis
◆ loss of deep tendon and perianal reflexes
◆ loss of motor and sensory function.

Until spinal shock has resolved (usually 1 to 6 weeks after injury), the extent of actual cord damage can't be fully assessed. The earliest indicator of resolution is the return of reflex activity.

NEUROGENIC SHOCK

Neurogenic shock is an abnormal vasomotor response that occurs secondary to disruption of sympathetic impulses from the brain stem to the thoracolumbar area, and is seen in patients with major injuries above the T6 level. This temporary loss of autonomic function below the level of injury causes profound cardiovascular changes.

Signs of neurogenic shock include:
◆ orthostatic hypotension
◆ bradycardia
◆ loss of the ability to sweat below the level of the lesion

◆ poikilothermy (loss of ability to regulate body temperature; patient very sensitive to hypothermy).

Treatment is symptomatic (active warming, fluid replacement, vasopressors). Symptoms resolve when spinal cord edema resolves.

AUTONOMIC DYSREFLEXIA

Also known as *autonomic hyperreflexia*, autonomic dysreflexia is a serious medical condition that occurs after resolution of spinal shock. Emergency recognition and management is a must.

Autonomic dysreflexia should be suspected in the patient with:
◆ spinal cord trauma at or above level T6
◆ bradycardia
◆ hypertension and a severe pounding headache
◆ cold or goose-fleshed skin below the lesion.

Dysreflexia is caused by noxious stimuli, most commonly a distended bladder or skin lesion.

Treatment focuses on eliminating the stimulus; rapid identification and removal may avoid the need for pharmacologic control of the headache and hypertension.

Alert *Complications include autonomic dysreflexia, spinal shock, and neurogenic shock. (See* Complications of spinal cord injury.)

TEST RESULTS
● Spinal X-rays, the most important diagnostic measure, detect most fractures.
● Thorough neurologic evaluation locates the level of injury and detects cord damage.
● Computed tomography scan provides images of fracture; magnetic resonance imaging reveals spinal cord edema and compression and may reveal a spinal mass.

TREATMENT
● Immediate immobilization on a rigid board to stabilize the spine and prevent further cord damage (primary treatment); use of head blocks on both sides of the patient's head, a hard cervical collar, or skeletal traction with skull tongs or a halo device for cervical spine injuries
● Methylprednisolone (Solu-Medrol) to reduce inflammation with evidence of cord injury

- Bed rest on firm support (such as a bed board), analgesics, and muscle relaxants for treatment of stable fractures until surgical repair or healing
- Orthopedic devices to treat stable thoracic or lumbar fracture
- Laminectomy and spinal fusion for severe or unstable lumbar fractures
- Neurosurgery to relieve the pressure when the damage results in compression of the spinal column (If the cause of compression is a metastatic lesion, chemotherapy and radiation may be indicated.)
- Treatment of surface wounds accompanying the spinal injury; tetanus prophylaxis unless the patient has had recent immunization
- Exercises to strengthen the back muscles and a back brace or corset to provide support while walking
- Rehabilitation to maintain or improve functional level

NURSING CONSIDERATIONS

In all spinal injuries, suspect cord damage until proven otherwise.
- During the initial assessment and X-ray studies, immobilize the patient on a firm surface, with immobilization devices on both sides of his head. Tell him not to move and avoid moving him yourself because movement can damage the cord. If you must move the patient, get at least three other members of the staff to help you logroll him to avoid disturbing spinal alignment.
- Throughout assessment, offer comfort and reassurance. Remember, the fear of possible paralysis will be overwhelming. Talk to the patient quietly and calmly. Allow a family member who isn't too distraught to accompany him.
- If the injury requires surgery, administer prophylactic antibiotics as ordered. Catheterize the patient, as ordered, to avoid urine retention, and monitor bowel elimination patterns to avoid impaction.
- Explain traction methods to the patient and his family. Reassure them that skeletal traction devices don't penetrate the brain. If the patient has a halo or skull-tong traction device, clean pin sites according to facility policy, trim hair short, and provide analgesics for persistent headaches. During traction, turn the patient often to prevent pneumonia, embolism, and skin breakdown; perform passive range-of-motion exercises to maintain muscle tone. If available, use a rotating bed to facilitate turning and care as indicated.
- Turn the patient on his side during feedings to prevent aspiration. Create a relaxed atmosphere at mealtimes.
- Suggest appropriate diversionary activities to fill the patient's hours of immobility.
- Watch closely for neurologic changes. Immediately report changes in skin sensation and loss of muscle strength — either of which might indicate pressure on the spinal cord, possibly as a result of edema or shifting bone fragments.
- Help the patient walk as soon as the physician allows; he'll probably need to wear a back brace or a halo vest.
- Refer the patient to rehabilitation services.

Stroke

A stroke, also known as a *cerebrovascular accident* or *brain attack,* is a sudden impairment of the brain's circulation in one or more blood vessels. A stroke interrupts or diminishes oxygen supply and commonly causes serious damage or necrosis in the brain tissues. The sooner the circulation returns to normal after a stroke, the better the chances are for a complete recovery. However, about one-half of the patients who survive a stroke remain permanently disabled and experience a recurrence within weeks, months, or years. It's the leading cause of admission to long-term care.

Stroke is the third most common cause of death in the United States and the most common cause of neurologic disability. It strikes more than 500,000 people per year and is fatal in approximately one-half of them.

Alert *Although a stroke may occur in younger people, most patients experiencing a stroke are older than age 65. In fact, the risk of stroke doubles with each passing decade after age 55.*

Alert *The incidence of stroke is higher in Blacks than in Whites. In fact, Blacks have a 60% higher risk for stroke than Whites or Hispanics of the same age. This is believed to be the result of an increased prevalence of hypertension in Blacks. In addition, strokes in Blacks usually result from disease in the small cerebral vessels, while strokes in Whites are typically the result of disease in the large carotid arteries. Mortality for Blacks from stroke is twice the rate for Whites.*

CAUSES

Stroke typically results from one of three causes:
- embolism from a thrombus originating outside the brain, such as in the heart, aorta, or common carotid artery
- hemorrhage from an intracranial artery or vein, such as from hypertension, ruptured aneurysm, arteriovenous malformations, trauma, hemorrhagic disorder (disseminated intravascular coagulation), or septic embolism
- thrombosis of the cerebral arteries supplying the brain or of the intracranial vessels occluding blood flow. (See *Types of stroke.*)

Risk factors that have been identified as predisposing a patient to stroke include:
- cardiac disease, including arrhythmias, coronary artery disease, acute myocardial infarction, dilated cardiomyopathy, and valvular disease
- cigarette smoking
- diabetes
- familial hyperlipidemia
- family history of stroke
- head trauma
- history of transient ischemic attacks (TIAs)
- hypertension
- increased alcohol intake, stimulant use (cocaine), I.V. drug use (septic emboli)
- obesity, sedentary lifestyle
- use of hormonal contraceptives.

PATHOPHYSIOLOGY

Regardless of the cause of a stroke, the underlying event is deprivation of oxygen and nutrients to the tissues of the brain. Normally, if the arteries become blocked, autoregulatory mechanisms help maintain cerebral circulation until collateral circulation develops to deliver blood to the affected area. If the compensatory mechanisms become overworked or cerebral blood flow remains impaired for more than a few minutes, oxygen deprivation leads to infarction of brain tissue. The brain cells cease to function because they can't store glucose or glycogen for use nor engage in anaerobic metabolism.

A thrombotic or embolic stroke causes ischemia. Some of the neurons

TYPES OF STROKE

Strokes are typically classified as ischemic or hemorrhagic depending on the underlying cause. This chart describes the major types of stroke.

TYPE OF STROKE	DESCRIPTION
Ischemic: Thrombotic	◆ Most common type of stroke ◆ Frequently the result of atherosclerosis; also associated with hypertension, smoking, diabetes ◆ Thrombus in extracranial or intracranial vessel blocking blood flow to the cerebral cortex ◆ Carotid artery most commonly affected extracranial vessel ◆ Common intracranial sites including bifurcation of carotid arteries, distal intracranial portion of vertebral arteries, and proximal basilar arteries ◆ May occur during sleep or shortly after awakening, during surgery, or after a myocardial infarction
Ischemic: Embolic	◆ Second most common type of stroke ◆ Embolus from heart or extracranial arteries floating into cerebral bloodstream and commonly lodging in middle cerebral artery or branches ◆ Embolus commonly originating during atrial fibrillation ◆ Typically occurring during activity ◆ Symptoms developing rapidly
Ischemic: Lacunar	◆ Subtype of thrombotic stroke ◆ Hypertension creating tiny cavities deep in white matter of the brain, affecting the internal capsule, basal ganglia, thalamus, and pons ◆ Lipid coating lining of the small penetrating arteries thickens and weakens the wall, causing microaneurysms and dissections
Hemorrhagic	◆ Third most common type of stroke ◆ Typically caused by hypertension or rupture of aneurysm ◆ Blood supply to area supplied by the ruptured artery diminished and surrounding tissue compressed by accumulated blood

served by the occluded vessel die from lack of oxygen and nutrients. This results in infarction, in which tissue injury triggers an inflammatory response that in turn increases intracranial pressure (ICP). Injury to the surrounding cells disrupts metabolism and leads to changes in ionic transport, localized acidosis, and free radical formation. Calcium, sodium, and water accumulate in the injured cells, and excitatory neurotransmitters are released. Consequent continued cellular injury and swelling set up a vicious cycle of further damage.

When hemorrhage is the cause, not only does the impaired perfusion cause infarction, but the blood itself acts as a space-occupying mass, exerting pressure on the brain tissues. The brain's regulatory mechanisms attempt to maintain equilibrium by increasing blood pressure to maintain cerebral perfusion pressure. The increased ICP forces cerebrospinal fluid out, thus restoring the balance. If the hemorrhage is small, this may be enough to keep the patient alive with only minimal neurologic deficits. However, if the bleeding is heavy, ICP increases rapidly and perfusion stops. Even if the pressure returns to normal, many brain cells die.

Initially, the ruptured blood vessels may constrict to limit the blood loss. This vasospasm further compromises blood flow, leading to more ischemia and cellular damage. If a clot forms in the vessel, decreased blood flow also promotes ischemia. If the blood enters the subarachnoid space, meningeal irritation occurs. The blood cells that pass through the vessel wall into the surrounding tissue also may break down and block the arachnoid villi, causing communicating hydrocephalus.

CLINICAL FINDINGS

The clinical features of stroke vary according to the affected artery and the region of the brain it supplies, the severity of the damage, and the extent of collateral circulation developed. A stroke in one hemisphere causes motor weakness on the opposite side of the body; a stroke that damages cranial nerves affects structures on the same side as the infarction.

General symptoms
- Unilateral limb weakness
- Speech difficulties
- Numbness on one side
- Headache
- Vision disturbances (diplopia, hemianopsia, ptosis)
- Dizziness
- Anxiety
- Altered level of consciousness (LOC)

Additionally, symptoms are usually classified by the artery affected.

Middle cerebral artery
- Aphasia
- Dysphasia
- Visual field deficits

- Hemiparesis of affected side (more severe in the face and arm than in the leg)

Carotid artery
- Weakness
- Paralysis
- Numbness
- Sensory changes
- Vision disturbances on the affected side
- Altered LOC
- Bruits
- Headaches
- Aphasia
- Ptosis

Vertebrobasilar artery
- Weakness on the affected side
- Numbness around lips and mouth
- Visual field deficits
- Diplopia
- Poor coordination
- Dysphagia
- Slurred speech
- Dizziness
- Nystagmus
- Amnesia
- Ataxia

Anterior cerebral artery
- Confusion
- Intellectual deficits
- Weakness
- Numbness, especially in the legs on the affected side
- Incontinence
- Loss of coordination
- Impaired motor and sensory functions
- Personality changes

Posterior cerebral artery
- Visual field deficits (homonymous hemianopsia)
- Sensory impairment
- Dyslexia

- Perseveration (abnormally persistent replies to questions)
- Coma
- Cortical blindness
- Absence of paralysis (usually)

Alert *Complications of stroke vary with the severity, location, and type but may include unstable blood pressure (from loss of vasomotor control), cerebral edema, fluid imbalances, sensory impairment, infections such as pneumonia, altered LOC, aspiration, contractures, pulmonary embolism, and death.*

TEST RESULTS

- Computed tomography scan identifies an ischemic stroke within the first 72 hours of symptom onset and evidence of a hemorrhagic stroke (lesions larger than 1 cm) immediately.
- Magnetic resonance imaging assists in identifying areas of ischemia or infarction and cerebral swelling.
- Computed tomography angiography and magnetic resonance angiography detect atherosclerosis or an aneurysm.
- Cerebral angiography reveals disruption or displacement of the cerebral circulation by occlusion, such as stenosis or acute thrombus, or hemorrhage.
- Digital subtraction angiography shows evidence of occlusion of cerebral vessels, lesions, or vascular abnormalities.
- Carotid duplex scan identifies the degree of stenosis.
- Brain scan shows ischemic areas but may not be conclusive for up to 2 weeks after a stroke.
- Single-photon emission computed tomography and positron emission tomography scans identify areas of altered metabolism surrounding lesions not yet able to be detected by other diagnostic tests.

- Transesophageal echocardiogram reveals cardiac disorders, such as atrial thrombi, atrial septal defect, or patent foramen ovale, as causes of thrombotic stroke.
- Ophthalmoscopy may identify signs of hypertension and atherosclerotic changes in retinal arteries.
- EEG helps identify damaged areas of the brain.

TREATMENT

Treatment is supportive to minimize and prevent further cerebral damage. Measures include:
- stool softeners to prevent straining, which increases ICP
- anticonvulsants to treat or prevent seizures
- surgery for large cerebellar infarction to remove infarcted tissue and decompress remaining live tissue
- aneurysm repair to prevent further hemorrhage
- percutaneous transluminal angioplasty or stent insertion to open occluded vessels.

For ischemic stroke

- Thrombolytic therapy (tPA, alteplase [Activase]) within the first 3 hours after the onset of symptoms to dissolve the clot, remove occlusion, and restore blood flow, thus minimizing cerebral damage (see *Treating thrombotic stroke,* page 186)
- Anticoagulant therapy (heparin, warfarin [Coumadin]) to maintain vessel patency and prevent further clot formation in cases of high-grade carotid stenosis or in newly diagnosed cardiovascular disease

For TIAs

- Antiplatelet drugs (aspirin, ticlopidine [Ticlid], extended-release dipyridamole in combination with aspirin

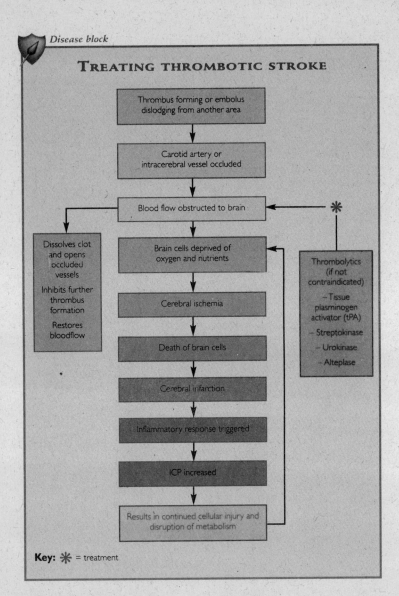

TREATING THROMBOTIC STROKE

Thrombus forming or embolus dislodging from another area

↓

Carotid artery or intracerebral vessel occluded

↓

Blood flow obstructed to brain

↓

Brain cells deprived of oxygen and nutrients

↓

Cerebral ischemia

↓

Death of brain cells

↓

Cerebral infarction

↓

Inflammatory response triggered

↓

ICP increased

↓

Results in continued cellular injury and disruption of metabolism

Dissolves clot and opens occluded vessels

Inhibits further thrombus formation

Restores bloodflow

Thrombolytics (if not contraindicated)

– Tissue plasminogen activator (tPA)

– Streptokinase

– Urokinase

– Alteplase

Key: ✳ = treatment

[Aggrenox]) to reduce the risk of platelet aggregation and subsequent clot formation

• Carotid endarterectomy to open partially (greater than 70%) occluded carotid arteries

For hemorrhagic stroke

● ICP management with monitoring, hyperventilation (to decrease partial pressure of arterial carbon dioxide [$PaCO_2$] to lower ICP), osmotic diuretics (mannitol [Osmitrol], to reduce cerebral edema), and corticosteroids (dexamethasone [Decadron], to reduce inflammation and cerebral edema)

● Analgesics to relieve headache associated with hemorrhagic stroke

NURSING CONSIDERATIONS

During the acute phase, efforts focus on survival needs and the prevention of further complications. Effective care emphasizes continuing neurologic assessment, respiratory support, continuous monitoring of vital signs, careful positioning to prevent aspiration and contractures, management of GI problems, and careful monitoring of fluid, electrolyte, and nutritional status. Patient care must also include measures to prevent such complications as infection.

● Maintain patent airway and provide supplemental oxygenation as indicated. Loosen constrictive clothing. Watch for ballooning of the cheek with respiration. The side that balloons is the side affected by the stroke. If the patient is unconscious, he could aspirate saliva so keep him in a lateral position to allow secretions to drain naturally or suction secretions, as needed. Insert an artificial airway, and start mechanical ventilation or supplemental oxygen, if necessary.

● Check vital signs and neurologic status, record observations, and report significant changes to the physician. Monitor blood pressure, LOC, pupillary changes, motor function (voluntary and involuntary movements), sensory function, speech, skin color, temperature, signs of increased ICP, and nuchal rigidity or flaccidity.

◆ *Alert* *An impending stroke may produce a sudden rise in blood pressure, rapid and bounding pulse, and the patient may complain of a headache. If the patient is unresponsive, monitor his respiratory status often and alert the physician to increased $PaCO_2$ or decreased partial pressure of arterial oxygen.*

● Maintain fluid and electrolyte balance. Administer I.V. fluids, as ordered. Offer the urinal or bedpan every 2 hours as appropriate. If the patient is incontinent, he may need an indwelling urinary catheter, but this should be avoided, if possible, because of the risk of infection.

● Ensure adequate nutrition. Check for gag reflex before offering small oral feedings of semisolid foods. Place the food tray within the patient's visual field because loss of peripheral vision is common. If oral feedings aren't possible, insert a nasogastric (NG) tube.

● Manage GI problems. Be alert for signs that the patient is straining at elimination because this increases ICP. Modify diet, administer stool softeners, as ordered, and give laxatives, if necessary. If the patient vomits (usually during the first few days), keep him positioned on his side to prevent aspiration. Consider insertion of an NG tube to suction.

● Provide careful mouth care. Clean and irrigate the patient's mouth to remove food particles. Care for his dentures, as needed.

● Provide meticulous eye care. Remove secretions with a cotton ball and sterile normal saline solution. Instill eyedrops, as ordered. Patch the patient's affected eye if he can't close the lid.

- Position the patient and align his extremities correctly. Use high-topped sneakers or other devices to prevent footdrop and contracture and a convoluted foam, flotation, or pulsating mattress or sheepskin to prevent pressure ulcers. To prevent pneumonia, turn the patient at least every 2 hours. Elevate the affected hand to control dependent edema, and place it in a functional position.
- Assist the patient with exercise. Perform range-of-motion exercises for both the affected and unaffected sides. Teach and encourage the patient to use his unaffected side to exercise his affected side.
- Establish and maintain communication with the patient. If he's aphasic, set up a simple method of communicating basic needs. Remember to phrase your questions so he'll be able to answer, using this system. Repeat yourself quietly and calmly (Remember, he doesn't have hearing difficulty.) and use gestures if necessary to help him understand. Even the unresponsive patient can hear, so don't say anything in his presence that you wouldn't want him to hear and remember.
- Provide psychological support. Set realistic short-term goals. Involve the patient's family in his care when possible, and explain his deficits and strengths.

Begin your rehabilitation of the patient with a stroke on admission. The amount of teaching you'll have to do depends on the extent of neurologic deficit.
- If necessary, teach the patient to comb his hair, dress, and wash. With the aid of a physical therapist and an occupational therapist, obtain appliances, such as walking frames, hand bars by the toilet, and ramps, as need-ed. The patient may fail to recognize that he has a paralyzed side (called *unilateral neglect*) and must be taught to inspect that side of his body for injury and to protect it from harm. If speech therapy is indicated, encourage the patient to begin as soon as possible and follow through with the speech pathologist's suggestions. To reinforce teaching, involve the patient's family in all aspects of rehabilitation. With their cooperation and support, devise a realistic discharge plan, and let them help decide when the patient can return home.
- Before discharge, warn the patient or his family to report premonitory signs of a stroke, such as severe headache, drowsiness, confusion, and dizziness. Emphasize the importance of regular follow-up visits.
- If aspirin has been prescribed to minimize the risk of thrombotic stroke, tell the patient to watch for possible GI bleeding. Make sure the patient and his family realize that acetaminophen isn't a substitute for aspirin.

To help prevent stroke:
- Stress the need to control such diseases as diabetes or hypertension.
- Teach all patients (especially those at high risk) the importance of following a low-cholesterol, low-salt diet; watching their weight; increasing activity; avoiding smoking and prolonged bed rest; and minimizing stress.
- Instruct the patient and his family to go to the emergency department immediately if symptoms develop.

4

GASTROINTESTINAL SYSTEM

The GI system has the critical task of supplying essential nutrients to fuel all the physiologic and pathophysiologic activities of the body. Its functioning profoundly affects the quality of life through its impact on overall health. The GI system has two major components: the alimentary canal, or GI tract, and the accessory organs. A malfunction anywhere in the system can produce far-reaching metabolic effects, eventually threatening life itself.

The alimentary canal is a hollow muscular tube that begins in the mouth and ends at the anus. It includes the oral cavity, pharynx, esophagus, stomach, small intestine, large intestine, rectum, and anal cavity. Peristalsis propels the ingested material along the tract; sphincters prevent its reflux. Accessory glands and organs include the salivary glands, liver, biliary duct system (gallbladder and bile ducts), and pancreas.

Together, the GI tract and accessory organs serve two major functions: digestion (breaking down food and fluids into simple chemicals that can be absorbed into the bloodstream and transported throughout the body) and elimination of waste products from the body through defecation.

Appendicitis

The most common disease requiring emergency surgery, appendicitis is inflammation and obstruction of the vermiform appendix (a blind pouch attached to the cecum). Appendicitis may occur at any age and affects both men and women equally; however, between puberty and age 25, it's more prevalent in men. Since the advent of antibiotics, the incidence and death rate of appendicitis have declined; if untreated, this disease is invariably fatal.

CAUSES
- Barium ingestion
- Fecal mass
- Mucosal ulceration
- Stricture
- Viral infection

PATHOPHYSIOLOGY
Mucosal ulceration triggers inflammation, which temporarily obstructs the appendix. The obstruction blocks mucus outflow. Pressure in the now distended appendix increases, and the appendix contracts. Bacteria multiply, and inflammation and pressure continue to increase, restricting blood

flow to the pouch and causing severe abdominal pain.

CLINICAL FINDINGS
● Abdominal pain, caused by inflammation of the appendix and bowel obstruction and distention, beginning in the epigastric region, and then shifting to the right lower quadrant
● Anorexia after the onset of pain
● Nausea or vomiting caused by the inflammation
● Low-grade fever from systemic manifestation of inflammation and leukocytosis
● Tenderness from inflammation

Alert *Complications of appendicitis may include, wound infection, intra-abdominal abscess, fecal fistula, intestinal obstruction, incisional hernia, peritonitis, and death.*

TEST RESULTS
● White blood cell count is moderately high with an increased number of immature cells.
● X-ray with radiographic contrast agent reveals failure of the appendix to fill with contrast.

TREATMENT
● Maintenance of nothing-by-mouth (NPO) status until surgery
● Fowler's position to aid in pain relief
● GI intubation for decompression
● Appendectomy
● Antibiotics to treat infection if peritonitis occurs
● Parental replacement of fluid and electrolytes to reverse possible dehydration resulting from surgery or nausea and vomiting

NURSING CONSIDERATIONS
Preparation for appendectomy
● Administer I.V. fluids to prevent dehydration. Never administer cathartics or enemas, which may rupture the appendix. Maintain NPO status, and administer analgesics judiciously because they may mask symptoms.
● To lessen pain, place the patient in Fowler's position. Never apply heat to the right lower abdomen; this may cause the appendix to rupture. An ice bag may be used for pain relief.

After appendectomy
● Monitor vital signs and intake and output. Give analgesics as ordered.
● Encourage the patient to cough, breathe deeply, and turn frequently to prevent pulmonary complications.
● Document bowel sounds, passing of flatus, and bowel movements. In a patient whose nausea and abdominal rigidity have subsided, these signs indicate readiness to resume oral fluids.
● Watch closely for possible surgical complications. Continuing pain and fever may signal an abscess. The complaint that "something gave way" may mean wound dehiscence. If an abscess or peritonitis develops, incision and drainage may be necessary. Frequently assess the dressing for wound drainage.
● In appendicitis complicated by peritonitis, a nasogastric tube may be needed to decompress the stomach and reduce nausea and vomiting. If so, record drainage and give good mouth and nose care.

Celiac disease

In Celiac disease, dietary gluten — a product of wheat, barley, rye, and oats — is toxic to the patient causing injury to the mucosal villi. The mucosa appear flat and have lost absorptive surface. Symptoms generally disappear when gluten is removed from the diet.

CAUSES

Celiac disease results from a complex interaction involving dietary, genetic, and immunologic factors.

PATHOPHYSIOLOGY

The body can't hydrolyze peptides contained in gluten. Ingestion of gluten causes injury to the villi in the upper intestine, leading to a decreased surface area and malabsorption of most nutrients. Inflammatory enteritis also results, leading to osmotic diarrhea and secretory diarrhea.

CLINICAL FINDINGS

Celiac disease may produce these symptoms due to malabsorption:
- Recurrent diarrhea, abdominal distention, stomach cramps, weakness, muscle wasting, or increased appetite without weight gain due to decreased absorption of carbohydrate, fat, protein, and other nutrients
- Normochromic, hypochromic, or macrocytic anemia due to malabsorption of vitamin B_{12}, iron, and folic acid
- Osteomalacia, osteoporosis, tetany, and bone pain in lower back, rib cage, and pelvis due to malabsorption of calcium and vitamin D
- Peripheral neuropathy, paresthesia, or seizures from malabsorption of calcium
- Dry skin, eczema, psoriasis, dermatitis, herpetiformis, and acne rosacea
- Amenorrhea, hypometabolism, and adrenocortical insufficiency
- Extreme lethargy, mood changes, and irritability

TEST RESULTS

- Stool specimen for fat reveals excretion of greater than 6 g of fat per day.
- D-xylose absorption test shows less than 20% of 25 g of D-xylose in the urine after 5 hours (reflects disorders of proximal bowel).
- Shilling test reveals deficiency of vitamin B_{12} absorption.
- GI barium studies show characteristic features of the small intestine.
- Small intestine biopsy reveals the atrophy of mucosal villi.

TREATMENT

- Identification of cause and appropriate correction of condition
- Gluten-free diet to stop progression of celiac disease and malabsorption

NURSING CONSIDERATIONS

- Explain the necessity of a gluten-free diet to the patient. Advise elimination of wheat, barley, rye, and oats and foods made from them, such as breads and baked goods; suggest substitution of corn or rice. Advise the patient to consult a dietitian for a gluten-free diet that's high in protein but low in carbohydrates and fats. Depending on individual tolerance, the diet initially consists of proteins and gradually expands to include other foods. Assess the patient's acceptance and understanding of the disease, and encourage regular reevaluation.
- Observe nutritional status and progress by daily calorie counts and weight checks. Evaluate tolerance to new foods. In the early stages, offer small frequent meals to counteract anorexia.

• Assess fluid status: Record intake, urine output, and number of stools (may exceed 10 per day). Watch for signs of dehydration, such as dry skin and mucous membranes and poor skin turgor.

• Check serum electrolyte levels. Watch for signs of hypokalemia (weakness, lethargy, rapid pulse, nausea, and diarrhea) and low calcium levels (impaired blood clotting, muscle twitching, and tetany).

• Monitor prothrombin time, hemoglobin level, and hematocrit. Protect the patient from bleeding and bruising. Administer vitamin K, iron, folic acid, and vitamin B_{12} as ordered.

• Protect patients with osteomalacia from injury by keeping the bed side rails up and assisting with ambulation, as necessary.

Cholecystitis

Cholecystitis — acute or chronic inflammation causing painful distention of the gallbladder — is usually associated with a gallstone impacted in the cystic duct.

Cholecystitis accounts for 10% to 25% of all patients requiring gallbladder surgery. The acute form is most common among middle-aged women; the chronic form, among elderly people. The prognosis is good with treatment.

CAUSES
• Abnormal metabolism of cholesterol and bile salts
• Gallstones (the most common cause)
• Poor or absent blood flow to the gallbladder

PATHOPHYSIOLOGY
In acute cholecystitis, inflammation of the gallbladder wall usually develops after a gallstone lodges in the cystic duct. (See *Understanding gallstone formation,* pages 194 and 195.) When bile flow is blocked, the gallbladder becomes inflamed and distended. Bacterial growth, usually *Escherichia coli,* may contribute to the inflammation. Edema of the gallbladder (and sometimes the cystic duct) obstructs bile flow, which chemically irritates the gallbladder. Cells in the gallbladder wall may become oxygen starved and die as the distended organ presses on vessels and impairs blood flow. The dead cells slough off, and an exudate covers ulcerated areas, causing the gallbladder to adhere to surrounding structures.

CLINICAL FINDINGS
• Acute abdominal pain in the right upper quadrant that may radiate to the back, between the shoulders, or to the front of the chest secondary to inflammation and irritation of nerve fibers
• Colic due to the passage of gallstones along the bile duct
• Nausea and vomiting triggered by the inflammatory response
• Chills related to fever
• Low-grade fever secondary to inflammation
• Jaundice from obstruction of the common bile duct by calculi

Alert *Complications of cholecystitis include perforation and abscess formation, fistula formation, gangrene, empyema, cholangitis, hepatitis, pancreatitis, gallstone ileus, and carcinoma.*

TEST RESULTS
• X-ray reveals gallstones if they contain enough calcium to be radio-

paque; also helps disclose porcelain gallbladder (hard, brittle gallbladder due to calcium deposited in wall), limy bile, and gallstone ileus.
- Ultrasonography detects gallstones as small as 2 mm and distinguishes between obstructive and nonobstructive jaundice.
- Technetium-labeled scan reveals cystic duct obstruction and acute or chronic cholecystitis if ultrasound doesn't visualize the gallbladder.
- Percutaneous transhepatic cholangiography supports the diagnosis of obstructive jaundice and reveals calculi in the ducts.
- Levels of serum alkaline phosphate, lactate dehydrogenase, aspartate aminotransferase, and total bilirubin are high; serum amylase level slightly elevated; and icteric index elevated.
- White blood cell counts are slightly elevated during cholecystitis attack.

TREATMENT
- Cholecystectomy to surgically remove the inflamed gallbladder
- Choledochostomy to surgically create an opening into the common bile duct for drainage
- Percutaneous transhepatic cholecystostomy
- Endoscopic retrograde cholangiopancreatography and transcystic choledochoscopic extraction for removal of gallstones
- Lithotripsy to break up gallstones and relieve obstruction
- Oral chenodeoxycholic acid or ursodeoxycholic acid to dissolve calculi
- Low-fat diet to prevent attacks
- Vitamin K to relieve itching, jaundice, and bleeding tendencies due to vitamin K deficiencies
- Antibiotics for use during acute attack for treatment of infection
- Nasogastric tube insertion during acute attack for abdominal decompression

NURSING CONSIDERATIONS
Care for the patient with cholecystitis focuses on supportive care and close postoperative observation.
- Before surgery, teach the patient to deep breathe, cough, expectorate, and perform leg exercises that are necessary after surgery. Also teach splinting, repositioning, and ambulation techniques. Explain the procedures that will be performed before, during, and after surgery to help ease the patient's anxiety and to help ensure his cooperation.
- After surgery, monitor vital signs for signs of bleeding, infection, or atelectasis.
- Evaluate the incision site for bleeding. Serosanguineous drainage is common during the first 24 to 48 hours if the patient has a wound drain. If, after a choledochostomy, a T-tube drain is placed in the duct and attached to a drainage bag, make sure the drainage tube has no kinks. Also check that the connecting tubing from the T tube is well secured to the patient to prevent dislodgment.
- Measure and record T-tube drainage daily (200 to 300 ml is normal).
- Teach patients who will be discharged with a T tube how to perform dressing changes and routine skin care.
- Monitor intake and output. Allow the patient nothing by mouth for 24 to 48 hours or until bowel sounds return and nausea and vomiting cease (postoperative nausea may indicate a full bladder).
- If the patient doesn't void within 8 hours (or if the amount voided is inadequate based on I.V. fluid intake), per-

UNDERSTANDING
GALLSTONE FORMATION

Abnormal metabolism of cholesterol and bile salts plays an important role in gallstone formation. The liver makes bile continuously. The gallbladder concentrates and stores it until the duodenum signals it needs it to help digest fat. Changes in the composition of bile may allow gallstones to form. Changes to the absorptive ability of the gallbladder lining may also contribute to gallstone formation.

INSIDE THE LIVER

Certain conditions, such as age, obesity, and estrogen imbalance, cause the liver to secrete bile that's abnormally high in cholesterol or lacking the proper concentration of bile salts.

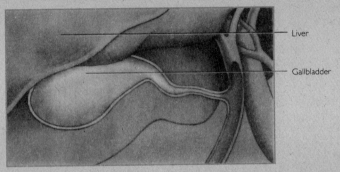

Liver

Gallbladder

INSIDE THE GALLBLADDER

When the gallbladder concentrates this bile, inflammation may occur. Excessive reabsorption of water and bile salts makes the bile less soluble. Cholesterol, calcium, and bilirubin precipitate into gallstones.

Fat entering the duodenum causes the intestinal mucosa to secrete the hormone cholecystokinin, which stimulates the gallbladder to contract and empty. If a stone lodges in the cystic duct, the gallbladder contracts but can't empty.

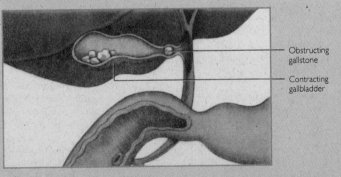

Obstructing gallstone

Contracting gallbladder

INSIDE THE COMMON BILE DUCT

If a stone lodges in the common bile duct, the bile can't flow into the duodenum. Bilirubin is absorbed into the blood and causes jaundice.

Biliary narrowing and swelling of the tissue around the stone can also cause irritation and inflammation of the common bile duct.

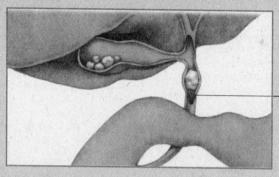

Gallstones in the common bile duct

INSIDE THE BILIARY TREE

Inflammation can progress up the biliary tree into any of the bile ducts. This causes scar tissue, fluid accumulation, cirrhosis, portal hypertension, and bleeding.

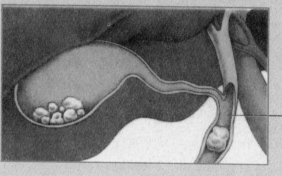

Inflammation of the common bile duct

cuss over the symphysis pubis for bladder distention (especially in patients receiving anticholinergics). Patients who have had a laparoscopic cholecystectomy may be discharged the same day or within 24 hours after surgery. These patients should have minimal pain, be able to tolerate a regular diet within 24 hours after surgery, and be able to return to normal activity within 1 week.

• Encourage deep-breathing and leg exercises every hour. The patient should ambulate after surgery. Provide elastic stockings to support leg muscles and promote venous blood flow, thus preventing stasis and clot formation.

- Evaluate the location, duration, and character of pain. Administer adequate medication to relieve pain, especially before such activities as deep breathing and ambulation, which increase pain.
- At discharge, advise the patient against heavy lifting or straining for 6 weeks. Urge him to walk daily. Tell him that food restrictions are unnecessary unless he has an intolerance to a specific food or some underlying condition (such as diabetes, atherosclerosis, or obesity) that requires such restriction.
- Instruct the patient to notify the surgeon if he has pain for more than 24 hours, anorexia, nausea or vomiting, fever, or tenderness in the abdominal area or if he notices jaundice, as these may indicate a biliary tract injury from the cholestectomy, requiring immediate attention.

Cirrhosis

Cirrhosis is a chronic disease characterized by diffuse destruction and fibrotic regeneration of hepatic cells. As necrotic tissue yields to fibrosis, this disease damages liver tissue and normal vasculature, impairs blood and lymph flow, and ultimately causes hepatic insufficiency. It's twice as common in men as in women and is especially prevalent among malnourished people over age 50 with chronic alcoholism. Mortality is high; many patients die within 5 years of onset.

CAUSES

Cirrhosis may be a result of a wide range of diseases. These clinical types of cirrhosis reflect its diverse etiology.

Hepatocellular diseases

- Autoimmune disease, such as sarcoidosis or chronic inflammatory bowel disease, possibly causing cirrhosis
- Laënnec's cirrhosis, also called *portal, nutritional,* or *alcoholic cirrhosis,* the most common type and primarily caused by hepatitis C and alcoholism; liver damage resulting from malnutrition (especially dietary protein) and chronic alcohol ingestion; fibrous tissue forming in portal areas and around central veins
- Postnecrotic cirrhosis accounting for 10% to 30% of patients and stemming from various types of hepatitis (such as Types A, B, C, D viral hepatitis) or toxic exposures

Cholestatic diseases

- Diseases of the biliary tree (biliary cirrhosis resulting from bile duct diseases suppressing bile flow)
- Sclerosing cholangitis

Metabolic diseases

- Alpha$_1$-antitrypsin
- Hemochromatosis (pigment cirrhosis)
- Wilson's disease

Other types

- Budd-Chiari syndrome (epigastric pain, liver enlargement, and ascites due to hepatic vein obstruction)
- Cardiac cirrhosis (rare; liver damage resulting from right-sided heart failure)
- Cryptogenic cirrhosis (referring to cirrhosis of unknown etiology)

PATHOPHYSIOLOGY

Cirrhosis begins with hepatic scarring or fibrosis. The scar begins as an increase in extracellular matrix components — fibril-forming collagens, proteoglycans, fibronectin, and hyaluronic acid. The site of collagen deposition varies with the cause. Hepatocyte function is eventually impaired as the matrix changes. Fat-storing cells are believed to be the source of the new matrix components. Contraction of these cells may also contribute to disruption of the lobular architecture and obstruction of the flow of blood or bile. Cellular changes producing bands of scar tissue also disrupt the lobular structure.

CLINICAL FINDINGS

Early stages

- Anorexia from distaste for certain foods
- Nausea and vomiting from inflammatory response and systemic effects of liver inflammation
- Diarrhea from malabsorption
- Dull abdominal ache from liver inflammation

Late stages

- Respiratory — pleural effusion, limited thoracic expansion due to abdominal ascites; interfering with efficient gas exchange, which causes hypoxia
- Central nervous system — progressive signs or symptoms of hepatic encephalopathy, including lethargy, mental changes, slurred speech, asterixis, peripheral neuritis, paranoia, hallucinations, extreme obtundation, and coma — secondary to the failure of ammonia metabolism into urea and consequent delivery of toxic ammonia to the brain
- Hematologic — bleeding tendencies (nosebleeds, easy bruising, bleeding gums), splenomegaly, anemia resulting from thrombocytopenia (secondary to splenomegaly and decreased vitamin K absorption), and portal hypertension
- Endocrine — testicular atrophy, menstrual irregularities, gynecomastia, and loss of chest and axillary hair from decreased hormone metabolism
- Skin — abnormal pigmentation, spider angiomas, palmar erythema, and jaundice related to impaired hepatic function; severe pruritus secondary to jaundice from bilirubinemia; extreme dryness and poor tissue turgor related to malnutrition
- Hepatic — jaundice from decreased bilirubin metabolism; hepatomegaly secondary to liver scarring and portal hypertension; ascites and edema of the legs from portal hypertension and decreased plasma proteins; hepatic encephalopathy from ammonia toxicity; and hepatorenal syndrome from advanced liver disease and subsequent renal failure
- Miscellaneous — musty breath secondary to ammonia build up; enlarged superficial abdominal veins due to portal hypertension; pain in the right upper abdominal quadrant that worsens when patient sits up or leans forward, due to inflammation and irritation of area nerve fibers; palpable liver or spleen due to organomegaly; temperature of 101° to 103° F (38.3° to 39.4° C) due to inflammatory response; hemorrhage from esophageal varices resulting from portal hypertension (see *What happens in portal hypertension*, page 198)

Alert Complications of cirrhosis may include respiratory compromise, ascites, portal hypertension, jaundice, coagulopathy, hepatic encephalopathy, bleeding esophageal varices, acute GI bleeding, liver failure, and renal failure.

WHAT HAPPENS IN PORTAL HYPERTENSION

Portal hypertension (elevated pressure in the portal vein) occurs when blood flow meets increased resistance. This common result of cirrhosis may also stem from mechanical obstruction and occlusion of the hepatic veins (Budd-Chiari syndrome).

As the pressure in the portal vein rises, blood backs up into the spleen and flows through collateral channels to the venous system, bypassing the liver. Thus, portal hypertension causes:

◆ splenomegaly with thrombocytopenia

◆ dilated collateral veins (esophageal varices, hemorrhoids, or prominent abdominal veins)

◆ ascites.

In many patients, the first sign of portal hypertension is bleeding esophageal varices (dilated tortuous veins in the submucosa of the lower esophagus).

Esophageal varices commonly cause massive hematemesis, requiring emergency care to control hemorrhage and prevent hypovolemic shock.

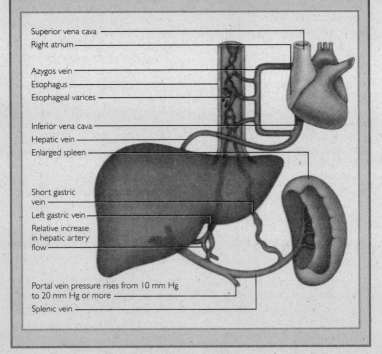

Superior vena cava
Right atrium
Azygos vein
Esophagus
Esophageal varices
Inferior vena cava
Hepatic vein
Enlarged spleen
Short gastric vein
Left gastric vein
Relative increase in hepatic artery flow
Portal vein pressure rises from 10 mm Hg to 20 mm Hg or more
Splenic vein

TEST RESULTS

● Liver biopsy reveals tissue destruction and fibrosis.

● Abdominal X-ray shows enlarged liver, cysts, or gas within the biliary tract or liver, liver calcification, and massive fluid accumulation (ascites).

- Computed tomography and liver scans show liver size, abnormal masses, and hepatic blood flow and obstruction.
- Esophagogastroduodenoscopy reveals bleeding esophageal varices, stomach irritation or ulceration, or duodenal bleeding and irritation.
- Blood studies reveal elevated levels of liver enzymes, total serum bilirubin, and indirect bilirubin; decreased levels of total serum albumin and protein; prolonged prothrombin time; decreased hemoglobin level, hematocrit, and serum electrolytes; and deficiency of vitamins A, C, and K.
- Urine studies show increased bilirubin and urobilirubinogen level.
- Fecal studies show decreased fecal urobilirubinogen level.

TREATMENT

- Vitamins and nutritional supplements to help heal damaged liver cells and improve nutritional status
- Antacids to reduce gastric distress and decrease the potential for GI bleeding
- Potassium-sparing diuretics to reduce fluid accumulation
- Vasopressin (Pitressin) to treat esophageal varices
- Esophagogastric intubation with multilumen tubes to control bleeding from esophageal varices or other hemorrhage sites by using balloons to exert pressure on the bleeding site
- Gastric lavage until the contents are clear; with antacids and histamine antagonists if the bleeding is secondary to a gastric ulcer
- Paracentesis to relieve abdominal pressure and remove ascitic fluid
- Surgical shunt placement to divert ascites into venous circulation, leading to weight loss, decreased abdominal girth, increased sodium excretion from the kidneys, and improved urine output
- Sclerosing agents injected into oozing vessels to cause clotting and sclerosis
- Surgery to create portosystemic shunt to control bleeding from esophageal varices and decrease portal hypertension (diverts a portion of the portal vein blood flow away from the liver; seldom performed)

NURSING CONSIDERATIONS

Patients with cirrhosis need close observation, intensive supportive care, and sound nutritional counseling.

- Check skin, gums, stools, and vomitus regularly for bleeding. Apply pressure to injection sites to prevent bleeding. Warn the patient against taking nonsteroidal anti-inflammatory drugs, straining at stool, and blowing his nose or sneezing too vigorously. Suggest using an electric razor and soft toothbrush.
- Observe closely for signs of behavioral or personality changes. Report increasing stupor, lethargy, hallucinations, or neuromuscular dysfunction. Awaken the patient periodically to determine level of consciousness. Watch for asterixis, a sign of developing hepatic encephalopathy.
- To assess fluid retention, weigh the patient and measure abdominal girth at least daily; inspect ankles and sacrum for dependent edema; and accurately record intake and output. Carefully evaluate the patient before, during, and after paracentesis; this drastic loss of fluid may induce shock.
- To prevent skin breakdown associated with edema and pruritus, avoid using soap when you bathe the patient; instead, use lubricating lotion or moisturizing agents. Handle the pa-

tient gently, and turn and reposition him often to keep his skin intact.

- Tell the patient that rest and good nutrition will conserve energy and decrease metabolic demands on the liver. Urge him to eat frequent small meals. Stress the need to avoid infections and abstain from alcohol. Refer the patient to Alcoholics Anonymous, if necessary.

Crohn's disease

Crohn's disease, also known as *regional enteritis* or *granulomatous colitis,* is inflammation of any part of the GI tract (usually the proximal portion of the colon and less commonly the terminal ileum), extending through all layers of the intestinal wall. It may also involve regional lymph nodes and the mesentery. Crohn's disease is most prevalent in adults ages 20 to 40.

CAUSES
The exact cause is unknown but conditions that may contribute include:
- allergies
- genetic predisposition
- immune disorders
- infection
- lymphatic obstruction.

PATHOPHYSIOLOGY
Whatever the cause of Crohn's disease, inflammation spreads slowly and progressively. Enlarged lymph nodes block lymph flow in the submucosa. Lymphatic obstruction leads to edema, mucosal ulceration and fissures, abscesses, and sometimes granulomas. Mucosal ulcerations are called *skipping lesions* because they aren't continuous, as in ulcerative colitis.

Oval, elevated patches of closely packed lymph follicles — called *Peyer's patches* — become enlarged in the lining of the small intestine. Subsequent fibrosis thickens the bowel wall and causes stenosis, or narrowing of the lumen. (See *Bowel changes in Crohn's disease.*) The serous membrane becomes inflamed (serositis), inflamed bowel loops adhere to other diseased or normal loops, and diseased bowel segments become interspersed with healthy ones. Finally, diseased parts of the bowel become thicker, narrower, and shorter.

CLINICAL FINDINGS
- Steady, colicky pain in the right lower quadrant due to acute inflammation and nerve fiber irritation
- Cramping and tenderness due to acute inflammation
- Palpable mass in the right lower quadrant
- Weight loss secondary to diarrhea and malabsorption
- Diarrhea due to bile salt malabsorption, loss of healthy intestinal surface area, and bacterial growth
- Steatorrhea secondary to fat malabsorption
- Bloody stools secondary to bleeding from inflammation and ulceration

Alert *Complications of Crohn's disease may include anal fistula, perineal abscess, fistulas to the bladder or vagina or to the skin in an old scar area, intestinal obstruction, nutrient deficiencies from poor digestion and malabsorption of bile salts and vitamin B_{12}, and fluid imbalances.*

TEST RESULTS
- Fecal occult blood test reveals minute amounts of blood in stools.
- Small bowel X-ray shows irregular mucosa, ulceration, and stiffening.

- Barium enema reveals the string sign (segments of stricture separated by normal bowel) and possibly fissures and narrowing of the bowel.
- Sigmoidoscopy and colonoscopy reveal patchy areas of inflammation (helps to rule out ulcerative colitis), with cobblestone-like mucosal surface. With colon involvement, ulcers may be seen.
- Biopsy reveals granulomas in up to one-half of all specimens.
- Blood tests reveal increased white blood cell count and erythrocyte sedimentation rate, and decreased potassium, calcium, magnesium, and hemoglobin levels.

TREATMENT
- Corticosteroids to reduce inflammation and, subsequently, diarrhea, pain, and bleeding
- Immunosuppressants to suppress the response to antigens
- Sulfasalazine (Azulfidine) to reduce inflammation
- Metronidazole (Flagyl) to treat perianal infection complications
- Antidiarrheals to combat diarrhea (not used with patients with significant bowel obstruction)
- Opioid analgesics to control pain and diarrhea
- Stress reduction and reduced physical activity to rest the bowel and allow it to heal
- Vitamin supplements to replace and compensate for the bowel's inability to absorb vitamins
- Dietary changes (elimination of fruits, vegetables, high fiber foods, dairy products, spicy and fatty foods, foods that irritate the mucosa, carbonated or caffeinated beverages, and other foods or liquids that stimulate excessive intestinal activity) to decrease

Focus in

BOWEL CHANGES IN CROHN'S DISEASE

As Crohn's disease progresses, fibrosis thickens the bowel wall and narrows the lumen. Narrowing — or stenosis — can occur in any part of the intestine and cause varying degrees of intestinal obstruction. At first, the mucosa may appear normal, but as the disease progresses it takes on a "cobblestone" appearance as shown.

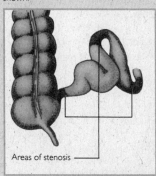

Areas of stenosis

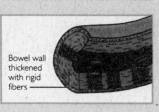

Bowel wall thickened with rigid fibers

bowel activity while still providing adequate nutrition
- Surgery, if necessary, to repair bowel perforation, drain abscesses, and correct massive hemorrhage, fistulas or acute intestinal obstruction; colectomy with ileostomy in patients with extensive disease of the large intestine and rectum

Nursing considerations

Although treatment is based largely on symptoms, you should monitor the patient's status carefully for signs of worsening.

● Record fluid intake and output (including the amount of stool), and weigh the patient daily. Watch for dehydration and maintain fluid and electrolyte balance. Be alert for signs of intestinal bleeding (bloody stools); check stools daily for occult blood.

● If the patient is receiving steroids, watch for adverse effects such as GI bleeding. Remember that steroids can mask signs of infection.

● Check hemoglobin levels and hematocrit regularly. Give iron supplements and blood transfusions, as ordered.

● Give analgesics as ordered.

● Provide good patient hygiene and meticulous mouth care if the patient is restricted to nothing by mouth. After each bowel movement, give good skin care. Always keep a clean, covered bedpan within the patient's reach. Ventilate the room to eliminate odors.

Alert *Observe the patient with Crohn's disease for fever and pain or pneumaturia, which may signal a bladder fistula. Abdominal pain and distention and fever may indicate intestinal obstruction. Watch for stools from the vagina and an enterovaginal fistula.*

● Before ileostomy, arrange for a visit by an enterostomal therapist.

● After surgery, frequently check the patient's I.V. and nasogastric tube for proper functioning. Monitor vital signs and fluid intake and output. Watch for wound infection. Provide meticulous stoma care, and teach it to the patient and family. Realize that an ileostomy changes the patient's body image, so offer reassurance and emotional support.

● Stress the need for a severely restricted diet and bed rest, which may be trying, particularly for the young patient. Encourage him to try to reduce tension. If stress is clearly an aggravating factor, refer him for counseling.

● Refer the patient to a support group such as the Crohn's and Colitis Foundation of America.

Diverticular disease

In diverticular disease, bulging pouches (diverticula) in the GI wall push the mucosal lining through the surrounding muscle. Although the most common site for diverticula is in the sigmoid colon, they may develop anywhere, from the proximal end of the pharynx to the anus. Other typical sites include the duodenum, near the pancreatic border or the ampulla of Vater, and the jejunum.

Alert *Diverticular disease is common in Western countries, suggesting that a low-fiber diet reduces stool bulk and leads to excessive colonic motility. The consequent increased intraluminal pressure causes herniation of the mucosa.*

Diverticular disease of the stomach is rare and is usually a precursor of peptic or neoplastic disease. Diverticular disease of the ileum (Meckel's diverticulum) is the most common congenital anomaly of the GI tract.

Diverticular disease has two clinical forms:

● diverticulosis, in which diverticula are present but don't cause symptoms
● diverticulitis, in which diverticula are inflamed and may cause potentially fatal obstruction, infection, or hemorrhage.

Alert *Diverticular disease is most prevalent in men older than age 40 and people who eat a low-fiber diet. More than one-half of all patients older than age 50 have colonic diverticula.*

CAUSES
- Defects in colon wall strength
- Diminished colonic motility and increased intraluminal pressure
- Low-fiber diet

PATHOPHYSIOLOGY
Diverticula probably result from high intraluminal pressure on an area of weakness in the GI wall, where blood vessels enter. Diet may be a contributing factor because insufficient fiber reduces fecal residue, narrows the bowel lumen, and leads to high intra-abdominal pressure during defecation.

In diverticulitis, retained undigested food and bacteria accumulate in the diverticular sac. This hard mass cuts off the blood supply to the thin walls of the sac, making them more susceptible to attack by colonic bacteria. Inflammation follows and may leading to perforation, abscess, peritonitis, obstruction, or hemorrhage. Occasionally, the inflamed colon segment may adhere to the bladder or other organs and cause a fistula.

CLINICAL FINDINGS
Typically the patient with diverticulosis is asymptomatic and will remain so unless diverticulitis develops.

Mild diverticulitis
- Moderate left lower abdominal pain secondary to inflammation of diverticula
- Low-grade fever from trapping of bacteria-rich stool in the diverticula

- Leukocytosis from infection secondary to trapping of bacteria-rich stool in the diverticula

Severe diverticulitis
- Abdominal rigidity from rupture of the diverticula abscesses, and peritonitis
- Left lower quadrant pain secondary to rupture of the diverticula and subsequent inflammation and infection
- High fever, chills, hypotension from sepsis, and shock from the release of fecal material from the rupture site
- Microscopic or massive hemorrhage from rupture of diverticulum near a vessel

Chronic diverticulitis
- Constipation, ribbon-like stools, intermittent diarrhea, and abdominal distention resulting from intestinal obstruction (possible when fibrosis and adhesions narrow the bowel's lumen)
- Abdominal rigidity and pain
- Diminishing or absent bowel sounds
- Nausea
- Vomiting secondary to intestinal obstruction

TEST RESULTS
- Upper GI series confirms or rules out diverticulosis of the esophagus and upper bowel.
- Barium enema reveals filling of diverticula, which confirms diagnosis.
- Biopsy reveals evidence of benign disease, ruling out cancer.
- Blood studies show an elevated erythrocyte sedimentation rate in diverticulitis.

TREATMENT
- Liquid or bland diet, stool softeners, and occasional doses of mineral

oil for symptomatic diverticulosis to relieve symptoms, minimize irritation, and lessen the risk of progression to diverticulitis

- High-residue diet for treatment of diverticulosis after pain has subsided to help decrease intra-abdominal pressure during defecation
- Exercise to increase the rate of stool passage
- Antibiotics to treat infection of the diverticula
- Analgesics, such as morphine, to control pain and to relax smooth muscle
- Antispasmodics to control muscle spasms
- Colon resection with removal of involved segment to correct cases refractory to medical treatment
- Temporary colostomy if necessary to drain abscesses and rest the colon in diverticulitis accompanied by perforation, peritonitis, obstruction, or fistula
- Blood transfusions if necessary to treat blood loss from hemorrhage and fluid replacement as needed

NURSING CONSIDERATIONS

Management of uncomplicated diverticulosis chiefly involves thorough patient education about fiber and dietary habits.

- Make sure the patient understands the importance of dietary fiber and the harmful effects of constipation and straining during defecation. Encourage increased intake of foods high in indigestible fiber, including fresh fruits and vegetables, whole grain bread, and wheat or bran cereals. Warn that a high-fiber diet may temporarily cause flatulence and discomfort. Advise the patient to relieve constipation with stool softeners or bulk-forming cathartics. However, caution against taking

bulk-forming cathartics without plenty of water; if swallowed dry, they may absorb enough moisture in the mouth and throat to swell and obstruct the esophagus or trachea.

- If the patient with diverticulosis is hospitalized, administer medications as ordered; observe his stools carefully for frequency, color, and consistency; and keep accurate pulse and temperature charts because they may signal developing inflammation or complications.

Management of diverticulitis depends on the severity of symptoms.

- In mild disease, administer medications as ordered, explain diagnostic tests and preparations for such tests, observe stools carefully, and maintain accurate records of temperature, pulse, respirations, and intake and output.
- If diverticular bleeding occurs, the patient may require blood transfusion, or angiography and catheter placement for vasopressin infusion. If so, inspect the insertion site frequently for bleeding, check pedal pulses often, and keep the patient from flexing his legs at the groin.
- Watch for vasopressin-induced fluid retention (apprehension, abdominal cramps, seizures, oliguria, or anuria) and severe hyponatremia (hypotension; rapid, thready pulse; cold, clammy skin; and cyanosis).

After surgery to resect the colon:

- Watch for signs of infection. Provide meticulous wound care because perforation may already have infected the area. Check drain sites frequently for signs of infection (purulent drainage or foul odor) or fecal drainage. Change dressings as necessary.
- Encourage coughing and deep breathing to prevent atelectasis.

- Watch for signs of postoperative bleeding (hypotension and decreased hemoglobin levels and hematocrit).
- Record intake and output accurately and keep the nasogastric tube patent.
- Teach ostomy care as needed and arrange for a visit by an enterostomal therapist.

Gastroesophageal reflux disease

Popularly known as *heartburn,* gastroesophageal reflux disease (GERD) refers to backflow of gastric or duodenal contents or both into the esophagus and past the lower esophageal sphincter (LES), without associated belching or vomiting. The reflux of gastric contents causes acute epigastric pain, usually after a meal. The pain may radiate to the chest or arms. It commonly occurs in pregnant or obese people. Lying down after a meal also contributes to reflux.

CAUSES
- Food, alcohol, or cigarettes that lower LES pressure
- Hiatal hernia
- Increased abdominal pressure, such as with obesity or pregnancy
- Medications, such as morphine, diazepam (Valium), calcium channel blockers, and anticholinergics
- Nasogastric intubation for more than 4 days
- Weakened esophageal sphincter

PATHOPHYSIOLOGY
Normally, the LES maintains enough pressure around the lower end of the esophagus to close it and prevent reflux. Typically the sphincter relaxes after each swallow to allow food into the stomach. In GERD, the sphincter doesn't remain closed (usually due to deficient LES pressure or pressure within the stomach exceeding LES pressure) and the pressure in the stomach pushes the stomach contents into the esophagus. The high acidity of the stomach contents causes pain and irritation when it enters the esophagus. (See *How heartburn occurs,* page 206.)

CLINICAL FINDINGS
- Burning pain in the epigastric area, possibly radiating to the arms and chest, from the reflux of gastric contents into the esophagus causing irritation and esophageal spasm
- Pain, usually after a meal or when lying down, secondary to increased abdominal pressure causing reflux
- Feeling of fluid accumulation in the throat without a sour or bitter taste due to hypersecretion of saliva

Alert *Complications of GERD include reflux esophagitis, esophageal stricture, esophageal ulceration, and chronic pulmonary disease from aspiration of gastric contents in the throat.*

TEST RESULTS
Diagnostic tests are aimed at determining the underlying cause of GERD:
- Esophageal acidity test evaluates the competence of the LES and provides objective measure of reflux.
- Acid perfusion test confirms esophagitis and distinguishes it from cardiac disorders.
- Esophagoscopy allows visual examination of the lining of the esophagus to reveal the extent of the disease and confirm pathologic changes in mucosa.

Focus in

HOW HEARTBURN OCCURS

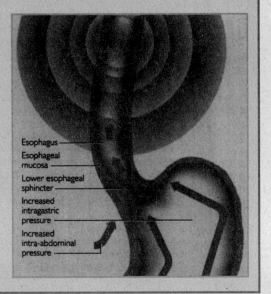

Hormonal fluctuations, mechanical stress, and the effects of certain foods and drugs can decrease lower esophageal sphincter (LES) pressure. When LES pressure falls and intra-abdominal or intragastric pressure rises, the normally contracted LES relaxes inappropriately and allows reflux of gastric acid or bile secretions into the lower esophagus. There, the reflux irritates and inflames the esophageal mucosa, causing pyrosis.

Persistent inflammation can cause LES pressure to decrease even more and may trigger a recurrent cycle of reflux and pyrosis.

Esophagus
Esophageal mucosa
Lower esophageal sphincter
Increased intragastric pressure
Increased intra-abdominal pressure

● Barium studies or upper GI series identifies hiatal hernia or shows motility problems or strictures.
● Esophageal manometry evaluates resting pressure of LES and determines sphincter competence.

TREATMENT
● Diet therapy with frequent, small meals and avoidance of eating before going to bed to reduce abdominal pressure and reduce the incidence of reflux
● Positioning—sitting up during and after meals and sleeping with head of bed elevated—to reduce abdominal pressure and prevent reflux
● Increased fluid intake to wash gastric contents out of the esophagus

● Antacids to neutralize acidic content of the stomach and minimize irritation
● Histamine-2 receptor antagonists, such as cimetidine (Tagamet), famotidine (Pepcid), and ranitidine (Zantac), to inhibit gastric acid secretion
● Proton pump inhibitors, such as esomeprazole (Nexium), lansoprazole (Prevacid), omeprazole (Prilosec), pantoprazole (Protonix), and rabeprazole (AciHex), to reduce gastric acidity
● Prokinetic drugs, such as metoclopramide (Reglan), to promote gastric emptying and increase LES pressure
● Smoking cessation to improve LES pressure (nicotine lowers LES pressure)
● Surgery if hiatal hernia is the cause or patient has refractory symptoms

- Bougie or pneumatic dilation of an esophageal stricture

NURSING CONSIDERATIONS

Teach the patient what causes GERD, how to avoid it with an antireflux regimen (medication, diet, and positional therapy), and what symptoms to watch for and report.

- Instruct the patient to avoid circumstances that increase intra-abdominal pressure (such as bending, coughing, vigorous exercise, tight clothing, constipation, and obesity) as well as substances that reduce sphincter control (cigarettes, alcohol, fatty foods, and caffeine).
- Advise the patient to sit upright, particularly after meals, and to eat small, frequent meals. Tell him to avoid highly seasoned food, acidic juices, alcoholic drinks, bedtime snacks, and foods high in fat or carbohydrates, which reduce LES pressure. He should eat meals at least 2 to 3 hours before lying down.
- Tell the patient to take antacids as ordered (usually 1 and 3 hours after meals and at bedtime).
- After surgery using a thoracic approach, carefully watch and record chest tube drainage and respiratory status. If needed, give chest physiotherapy and oxygen. Position the patient with a nasogastric tube in semi-Fowler's position to help prevent reflux. Offer reassurance and emotional support.

Hepatitis, nonviral

Nonviral hepatitis is an inflammation of the liver that usually results from exposure to certain chemicals or drugs. Most patients recover from this illness, although a few develop fulminating hepatitis or cirrhosis.

CAUSES

- Hepatotoxic chemicals
- Hepatotoxic drugs

PATHOPHYSIOLOGY

Various hepatotoxins—such as carbon tetrachloride, acetaminophen (Tylenol), trichloroethylene, poisonous mushrooms, and vinyl chloride—can cause hepatitis. After exposure to these agents, hepatic cellular necrosis, scarring, Kupffer cell hyperplasia, and infiltration by mononuclear phagocytes occur with varying severity. Alcohol, anoxia, and preexisting liver disease exacerbate the effects of some toxins.

Drug-induced (idiosyncratic) hepatitis may begin with a hypersensitivity reaction unique to the individual, unlike toxic hepatitis, which appears to affect all exposed people indiscriminately. Among possible causes are niacin (Niaspan), halothane, sulfonamides, isoniazid (Nydrazid), acetaminophen, methyldopa (Aldomet), and phenothiazines (cholestasis-induced hepatitis). Symptoms of hepatic dysfunction may appear at any time during or after exposure to these drugs, but it usually manifests after 2 to 5 weeks of therapy.

CLINICAL FINDINGS

- Anorexia, nausea, and vomiting due to systemic effects of liver inflammation
- Jaundice from decreased bilirubin metabolism, leading to hyperbilirubinemia
- Dark urine from elevated urobilinogen
- Hepatomegaly due to inflammation

- Possible abdominal pain from liver inflammation
- Clay-colored stool secondary to decreased bile in the GI tract from liver necrosis
- Pruritus secondary to jaundice and hyperbilirubinemia

Alert *Complications of nonviral hepatitis include cirrhosis and hepatic failure.*

TEST RESULTS

- Liver enzymes, such as serum aspartate aminotransferase and alanine aminotransferase levels, are elevated.
- Total and direct bilirubin levels are elevated.
- Alkaline phosphatase levels are elevated.
- White blood cell count and eosinophil count are elevated.
- Liver biopsy identifies underlying pathology, especially infiltration with white blood cells and eosinophils.

TREATMENT

- Lavage, catharsis, or hyperventilation, depending on the route of exposure, to remove the causative agent
- Acetylcysteine (Acetadole) as an antidote for acetaminophen poisoning
- Corticosteroids to relieve symptoms of drug-induced nonviral hepatitis

NURSING CONSIDERATIONS

Preventive measures should include instructing the patient about the proper use of drugs and the proper handling of cleaning agents and solvents.

Hepatitis, viral

Viral hepatitis is a common infection of the liver, resulting in hepatic cell destruction, necrosis, and autolysis. In most patients, hepatic cells eventually regenerate with little or no residual damage. However, old age and serious underlying disorders make complications more likely. The prognosis is poor if edema and hepatic encephalopathy develop.

Five major forms of hepatitis are currently recognized:
- Type A (infectious or short-incubation hepatitis) is most common among male homosexuals and in people with human immunodeficiency virus (HIV) infection. It's commonly spread via the fecal-oral route by the ingestion of fecal contaminants.
- Type B (serum or long-incubation hepatitis) also is most common among HIV-positive individuals. Routine screening of donor blood for the hepatitis B surface antigen has reduced the incidence of posttransfusion cases, but transmission by needles shared by drug abusers remains a major problem.
- Type C accounts for about 20% of all viral hepatitis cases and for most posttransfusion cases.
- Type D (delta hepatitis) is responsible for about 50% of all cases of fulminant hepatitis, which has a high mortality. Developing in 1% of patients with viral hepatitis, fulminant hepatitis causes unremitting liver failure with encephalopathy. It progresses to coma and commonly leads to death within 2 weeks. In the United States, type D occurs only in people who are frequently exposed to blood and blood products, such as I.V. drug users and hemophilia patients. Type D hepatitis is found only in patients with an acute or chronic episode of hepatitis B and requires the presence of hepatitis B surface antigen. The type D virus depends on the double-shelled type B

virus to replicate. (For this reason, type D infection can't outlast a type B infection.)

- Type E (formerly grouped with types C and D under the name *non-A, non-B hepatitis*) occurs primarily among patients who have recently returned from an endemic area (such as India, Africa, Asia, or Central America). It's more common in young adults and more severe in pregnant woman. (See *Viral hepatitis from A to E,* pages 210 and 211.)
- Other types continue to be identified with growing patient populations and sophisticated laboratory identification techniques.

CAUSES
The five major forms of viral hepatitis result from infection with the causative viruses: A, B, C, D, or E.

PATHOPHYSIOLOGY
Hepatic damage is usually similar in all types of viral hepatitis. Varying degrees of cell injury and necrosis occur. On entering the body, the virus causes hepatocyte injury and death, either by directly killing the cells or by activating inflammatory and immune reactions. The inflammatory and immune reactions will, in turn, injure or destroy hepatocytes by lysing the infected or neighboring cells. Later, direct antibody attack against the viral antigens causes further destruction of the infected cells. Edema and swelling of the interstitium lead to collapse of capillaries and decreased blood flow, tissue hypoxia, and scarring and fibrosis.

CLINICAL FINDINGS
Signs and symptoms reflect the stage of the disease.

Prodromal stage
- Easy fatigue and generalized malaise due to systemic effects of liver inflammation
- Anorexia and mild weight loss due to systemic effects of liver inflammation
- Arthralgia and myalgia due to systemic effects of liver inflammation
- Nausea and vomiting from GI effects of liver inflammation
- Changes in the senses of taste and smell related to liver inflammation
- Fever secondary to inflammatory process
- Right upper quadrant tenderness from liver inflammation and irritation of area nerve fibers
- Dark urine from urobilinogen
- Clay-colored stools from decreased bile in the GI tract

Clinical stage
- Worsening of all symptoms of prodromal stage
- Itching from increased bilirubin in the blood
- Abdominal pain or tenderness from continued liver inflammation
- Jaundice from elevated bilirubin in the blood

Recovery stage
- Symptoms subside and patient's appetite returns

Alert Complications of viral hepatitis may include chronic persistent hepatitis, which may prolong recovery up to 8 months; chronic active hepatitis; cirrhosis; primary hepatocellular carcinoma; hepatic failure and death.

TEST RESULTS
- Hepatitis profile study identifies antibodies specific to the causative virus, establishing the type of hepatitis.

VIRAL HEPATITIS FROM A TO E

This chart compares the features of each type of viral hepatitis. Other types are emerging.

FEATURE	HEPATITIS A	HEPATITIS B
Incubation	15 to 45 days	30 to 180 days
Onset	Acute	Insidious
Age-group most affected	Children, young adults	Any age
Transmission	Fecal-oral, sexual (especially oral-anal contact), nonpercutaneous (sexual, maternal-neonatal), percutaneous (rare)	Blood-borne; parenteral route, sexual, maternal-neonatal; virus shed in all body fluids
Severity	Mild	Commonly severe
Prognosis	Generally good	Worsens with age and debility
Progression to chronicity	None	Occasional

- Serum aspartate aminotransferase and serum alanine aminotransferase levels are increased in the prodromal stage.
- Serum alkaline phosphatase level is slightly increased.
- Serum bilirubin level may remain high into late disease, especially in severe cases.
- Prothrombin time is prolonged (greater than 3 seconds longer than normal indicates severe liver damage).
- White blood cell counts reveal transient neutropenia and lymphopenia followed by lymphocytosis.
- Liver biopsy confirms suspicion of chronic hepatitis.

TREATMENT
- Rest to minimize energy demands
- Avoidance of alcohol or other drugs to prevent further hepatic damage
- Diet therapy with small, high-calorie meals to combat anorexia
- Parental nutrition if patient can't eat due to persistent vomiting
- Vaccination against hepatitis A and B to provide immunity to these viruses before transmission occurs

NURSING CONSIDERATIONS
Use enteric precautions when caring for patients with type A or E hepatitis. Practice standard precautions for all patients. Inform visitors about isolation precautions.
- Provide rest periods throughout the day. Schedule treatments and tests so that the patient can rest between bouts of activity.
- Because inactivity may make the patient anxious, include diversionary activities as part of his care. Gradually add activities to his schedule as he begins to recover.

HEPATITIS C	HEPATITIS D	HEPATITIS E
15 to 160 days	14 to 64 days	14 to 60 days
Insidious	Acute and chronic	Acute
More common in adults	Any age	Ages 20 to 40
Blood-borne; parenteral route	Parenteral route; most people infected with hepatitis D are also infected with hepatitis B	Primarily fecal-oral
Moderate	Can be severe and lead to fulminant hepatitis	Highly virulent with common progression to fulminant hepatitis and hepatic failure, especially in pregnant patients
Moderate	Fair; worsens in chronic cases; can lead to chronic hepatitis D and chronic liver disease	Good unless pregnant
10% to 50% of cases	Occasional	None

- Encourage the patient to eat. Don't overload his meal tray or overmedicate him because this will diminish his appetite.
- Force fluids (at least 4 L/day). Encourage the anorectic patient to drink fruit juices. Also offer chipped ice and effervescent soft drinks to maintain hydration without inducing vomiting.
- Administer supplemental vitamins and commercial feedings, as ordered. If symptoms are severe and the patient can't tolerate oral intake, provide I.V. therapy and parenteral nutrition, as ordered by the physician.
- Record the patient's weight daily, and keep intake and output records. Observe stools for color, consistency, and amount, and record the frequency of bowel movements.
- Watch for signs of fluid shift, such as weight gain and orthostasis.

- Watch for signs of hepatic coma, dehydration, pneumonia, vascular problems, and pressure ulcers.
- In fulminant hepatitis, maintain electrolyte balance and a patent airway, prevent infections, and control bleeding. Correct hypoglycemia and other complications while awaiting liver regeneration and repair.
- Before discharge, emphasize the importance of having regular medical checkups for at least 1 year. The patient will have an increased risk of developing hepatoma. Warn the patient against using alcohol or over-the-counter drugs during this period. Teach him to recognize the signs of a recurrence.

Hyperbilirubinemia

Hyperbilirubinemia, also called *neonatal jaundice,* is the result of hemolytic processes in the neonate marked by elevated serum bilirubin levels and mild jaundice. It can be physiologic (with jaundice the only symptom) or pathologic (resulting from an underlying disease).

Physiologic jaundice generally develops 24 to 48 hours after birth and disappears by day 7 in full-term neonates and by day 9 or 10 in premature neonates. Serum unconjugated bilirubin levels don't exceed 12 mg/dl. Pathologic jaundice may appear anytime after the first day of life and persist beyond 7 days. Serum bilirubin levels are greater than 12 mg/dl in a term neonate, 15 mg/dl in a premature neonate, or increase more than 5 mg/dl in 24 hours. Physiologic jaundice is self-limiting; pathologic jaundice varies, depending on the cause.

CAUSES

- Abnormal red blood cell (RBC) morphology or deficiencies of RBC enzymes (glucose 6-phosphate dehydrogenase, hexokinase)
- Blood type incompatibility
- Breast-feeding
- Crigler-Najjar syndrome
- Enclosed hemorrhages (bruises, subdural hematoma)
- Gilbert syndrome, galactosemia, or hypothyroidism
- Heinz body anemia from drugs and toxins (vitamin K_3, sodium nitrate)
- Herpes simplex
- Infection (gram-negative bacteria)
- Intrauterine infection (rubella, cytomegalic inclusion body disease, toxoplasmosis, syphilis and, occasionally, bacteria such as *Escherichia coli, Staphylococcus, Pseudomonas, Klebsiella, Proteus,* and *Streptococcus*)
- Maternal diabetes
- Physiologic jaundice and neonatal giant cell hepatitis
- Polycythemia
- Pyloric stenosis, bile duct atresia, or choledochal cyst
- Respiratory distress syndrome (hyaline membrane disease)
- Transient neonatal hyperbilirubinemia

PATHOPHYSIOLOGY

As erythrocytes break down at the end of their neonatal life cycle, hemoglobin separates into globin (protein) and heme (iron) fragments. Heme fragments form unconjugated (indirect) bilirubin, which binds to albumin for transport to liver cells to conjugate with glucuronide, forming direct bilirubin. Because unconjugated bilirubin is fat-soluble and can't be excreted in the urine or bile, serum concentration increases causing hyperbilirubinemia and it may escape to extravascular tissue, especially fatty tissue and the brain.

Certain drugs (such as aspirin, tranquilizers, and sulfonamides) and conditions (such as hypothermia, anoxia, hypoglycemia, and hypoalbuminemia) can disrupt conjugation and usurp albumin-binding sites.

Decreased hepatic function also reduces bilirubin conjugation. Biliary obstruction or hepatitis can cause hyperbilirubinemia by blocking normal bile flow.

Increased erythrocyte production or breakdown in hemolytic disorders or in Rh or ABO incompatibility, can cause hyperbilirubinemia. Lysis releases bilirubin and stimulates cell agglutination. As a result, the liver's capacity to conjugate bilirubin becomes overloaded.

Finally, maternal enzymes in breast milk inhibit the infant's glucuronyltransferase conjugating activity.

CLINICAL FINDINGS

Signs and symptoms include jaundice from the escape of unconjugated bilirubin to extravascular tissue (primary sign of hyperbilirubinemia).

Alert Complications of hyperbilirubinemia include kernicterus, cerebral palsy, epilepsy, mental retardation, perceptual-motor disabilities, and learning disorders.

TEST RESULTS
- Elevated serum bilirubin levels

TREATMENT
- Phototherapy (treatment of choice for physiologic jaundice and pathologic jaundice due to erythroblastosis fetalis, after the initial exchange transfusion) with fluorescent lights to decompose bilirubin in the skin by oxidation (usually discontinued after bilirubin levels fall below 10 mg/dl and continue to decrease for 24 hours)
- Exchange transfusion to replace the infant's blood with fresh blood (less then 48 hours old), removing some of the unconjugated bilirubin in serum; indicated for conditions such as hydrops fetalis, polycythemia, erythroblastosis fetalis; marked reticulocytosis, drug toxicity, and jaundice that develops within the first 6 hours after birth
- Albumin administration to provide additional albumin for binding unconjugated bilirubin
- Phenobarbital administration (rare) to the mother before delivery and to the neonate several days after delivery to stimulate the hepatic glucuronide-conjugating system

NURSING CONSIDERATIONS
- Assess and record the infant's jaundice, and note the time it began. Report the jaundice and serum bilirubin levels immediately.
- Reassure parents that most infants experience some degree of jaundice. Explain hyperbilirubinemia, its causes, diagnostic tests, and treatment. In addition, explain that the infant's stool contains some bile and may be greenish.

For phototherapy
- Keep a record of how long each bilirubin light bulb is in use because these bulbs require frequent changing for optimum effectiveness.
- Undress the infant, so that his entire body surface is exposed to the light rays. Keep him 18″ to 30″ (45.5 to 76 cm) from the light source. Protect his eyes with shields that filter the light.
- Monitor and maintain the infant's body temperature; high and low temperatures predispose him to kernicterus. Remove the infant from the light source every 3 to 4 hours, and take off the eye shields. Allow his parents to visit and feed him.
- The infant usually shows a decrease in serum bilirubin level 1 to 12 hours after the start of phototherapy. When the infant's bilirubin level is less than 10 mg/dl and has been decreasing for 24 hours, discontinue phototherapy, as ordered. Resume therapy, as ordered, if serum bilirubin increases several milligrams per deciliter, as it often does because of a rebound effect.

For exchange transfusions
- Prepare the infant warmer and tray before the transfusion. Try to keep the infant quiet. Give him nothing by

mouth for 3 to 4 hours before the procedure.

- Check the type, Rh, and age of the blood to be used for the exchange. Keep emergency resuscitative and intubation equipment and oxygen available. During the procedure, monitor respiratory and heart rates every 15 minutes; check the infant's temperature every 30 minutes. Continue to monitor vital signs every 15 to 30 minutes for 2 hours.
- Measure intake and output. Observe for cord bleeding and complications, such as hemorrhage, hypocalcemia, sepsis, and shock. Report serum bilirubin and hemoglobin levels. Bilirubin levels may rise, as a result of a rebound effect, within 30 minutes after transfusion, necessitating repeat transfusions.

Preventive measures

- Maintain oral intake. Don't skip feedings because fasting stimulates the conversion of heme to bilirubin.
- Administer $Rh_O(D)$ immune globulin (human), as ordered, to an Rh-negative mother after amniocentesis, or to an Rh-negative mother during the third trimester, after the birth of an Rh-positive infant, or after spontaneous or elective abortion (to prevent hemolytic disease in subsequent infants).

Irritable bowel syndrome

Also referred to as *spastic colon* or *spastic colitis,* irritable bowel syndrome (IBS) is marked by chronic symptoms of abdominal pain, alternating constipation and diarrhea, excess flatus, a sense of incomplete evacuation, and abdominal distention. Irritable bowel syndrome is a common, stress-related disorder. However, 20% of patients never seek medical attention. IBS is a benign condition that has no anatomical abnormality or inflammatory component. It occurs in women twice as often as men.

CAUSES

- Hormonal changes (menstruation)
- Ingestion of irritants (coffee, raw fruit, or vegetables)
- Lactose intolerance
- Laxative abuse
- Psychological stress (most common)

PATHOPHYSIOLOGY

IBS appears to reflect motor disturbances of the entire colon in response to stimuli. Some muscles of the small bowel are particularly sensitive to motor abnormalities and distention; others are particularly sensitive to certain foods and drugs. The patient may be hypersensitive to the hormones gastrin and cholecystokinin. The pain of IBS seems to be caused by abnormally strong contractions of the intestinal smooth muscle as it reacts to distention, irritants, or stress. (See *What happens in irritable bowel syndrome.*)

CLINICAL FINDINGS

- Crampy lower abdominal pain secondary to muscle contraction; usually occurring during the day and relieved by defecation or passage of flatus
- Pain that intensifies 1 to 2 hours after a meal from irritation of nerve fibers by causative stimulus
- Constipation alternating with diarrhea, with one dominant; secondary to motor disturbances from causative stimulus

Focus in

WHAT HAPPENS IN
IRRITABLE BOWEL SYNDROME

Typically, the patient with irritable bowel syndrome (IBS) has a normal-appearing GI tract. However, careful examination of the colon may reveal functional irritability — an abnormality in colonic smooth-muscle function marked by excessive peristalsis and spasms, even during remission.

INTESTINAL FUNCTION

To understand what happens in IBS, consider how smooth muscle controls bowel function. Normally, segmental muscle contractions mix intestinal contents while peristalsis propels the contents through the GI tract. Motor activity is most propulsive in the proximal (stomach) and the distal (sigmoid) portions of the intestine. Activity in the rest of the intestines is slower, permitting nutrient and water absorption.

In IBS, the autonomic nervous system, which innervates the large intestine, doesn't cause the alternating contractions and relaxations that propel stools smoothly toward the rectum.

The result is constipation or diarrhea or both.

CONSTIPATION

Some patients have spasmodic intestinal contractions that set up a partial obstruction by trapping gas and stools. This causes distention, bloating, gas pain, and constipation.

DIARRHEA

Other patients have dramatically increased intestinal motility. Eating or cholinergic stimulation triggers the small intestine's contents to rush into the large intestine, dumping watery stools and irritating the mucosa. The result is diarrhea.

MIXED SYMPTOMS

If further spasms trap liquid stools, the intestinal mucosa absorbs water from the stools, leaving them dry, hard, and difficult to pass. The result: a pattern of alternating diarrhea and constipation.

• Mucus passed through the rectum from altered secretion in intestinal lumen due to motor abnormalities
• Abdominal distention and bloating caused by flatus and constipation

TEST RESULTS

• Stool samples for ova, parasites, bacteria, and blood rule out infection.
• Lactose intolerance test rules out lactose intolerance.
• Barium enema may reveal colon spasm and tubular appearance of descending colon without evidence of cancers and diverticulosis.
• Sigmoidoscopy or colonoscopy may reveal spastic contractions without evidence of colon cancer or inflammatory bowel disease.
• Rectal biopsy rules out malignancy.

TREATMENT

• Stress relief measures, including counseling or mild anti-anxiety drugs
• Investigation and avoidance of food irritants
• Application of heat to abdomen
• Bulking agents to reduce episodes of diarrhea and minimize effect of nonpropulsive colonic contractions
• Antispasmodics (propantheline or diphenoxylate with atropine sulfate [Lomotil]) for pain

- Loperamide (Imodium) possibly to reduce urgency and fecal soiling in patients with persistent diarrhea
- Tegaserod (Zelnorm) for short-term treatment of women with IBS when the primary bowel symptom is constipation to stimulate the peristaltic reflex and intestinal secretion
- Alosetron (Lotronex) for women with severe IBS who haven't responded to conventional therapy and whose primary symptom is diarrhea to reduce pain, colonic transit, and GI secretions
- Bowel training (if the cause of IBS is chronic laxative abuse) to regain muscle control

NURSING CONSIDERATIONS

Because the patient with IBS isn't hospitalized, focus your care on patient teaching.
- Tell the patient to avoid irritating foods, and encourage her to develop regular bowel habits. Help the patient deal with stress, and warn against dependence on sedatives or antispasmodics.
- Encourage regular checkups because IBS is associated with a higher-than-normal incidence of diverticulitis and colon cancer. For patients over age 40, emphasize the need for an annual sigmoidoscopy and rectal examination.

Obesity

Obesity is defined as an excess of body fat with a body mass index (BMI) greater than or equal to 30. It may result from excessive caloric intake and inadequate expenditure of energy.

CAUSES

Explanatory theories include:
- abnormal absorption of nutrients
- genetic predisposition
- hypothalamic dysfunction of hunger and satiety centers
- impaired action of GI and growth hormones and of hormonal regulators such as insulin and hypothyroidism.

An inverse relationship between socioeconomic status and the prevalence of obesity has been documented, especially in women.

PATHOPHYSIOLOGY

Excess calorie intake results in the conversion of nutrients into fat, which is stored in the body. If the individual continues to have excessive caloric intake and decreased caloric expenditure, fat continues to accumulate in the body leading to obesity. Obesity may lead to serious complications, such as respiratory difficulties, hypertension, cardiovascular disease, diabetes mellitus, renal disease, gallbladder disease, psychosocial difficulties, and premature death.

CLINICAL FINDINGS

In addition to the BMI, other indices may support diagnosis of obesity, such as anthropometric parameters and a standard detailed examination of the person.
- Degree and distribution of obesity may be estimated by standard skin thicknesses, such as subscapular, triceps, biceps, and suprailiac. Various anthropometric measurements of the waist and hip circumferences are most important.
- Chronic multisystemic disorder may be found in some individuals. In the skin examination, include a search for rashes, contact dermatoses, or oth-

er indications of problems related to obesity.

TEST RESULTS

In addition to anthropometric measurements and skin thickness estimates, supportive laboratory studies include:

- full lipid panel, which may be normal or elevated
- hepatic panel, which may be normal or abnormal if liver problems exist
- thyroid function tests may reveal hypothyroidism
- 24-hour urinary free cortisol level is elevated with Cushing syndrome or other hypercortisolemic states
- fasting glucose levels may be elevated.

TREATMENT

The patient must increase his activity level while reducing daily calorie intake through a balanced, low-calorie diet that reduces fat and sugar intake. Fat substitutes may be used, such as Olestra (Olean) and Sitostanol (Benacol). Treatment options may include hypnosis, behavior modification techniques, and psychotherapy.

- Amphetamines, amphetamine congeners, and sibutramine (Meridia) may be used temporarily to enhance compliance by suppressing appetite and creating a feeling of well-being.
- Morbid obesity (BMI greater than 40) may be treated surgically with bariatric surgery. If a patient undergoes surgery for obesity, micronutrient deficiencies can occur, especially calcium, vitamin B_{12}, folate and iron. Complications can also occur in malabsorptive operations such as uncontrolled diarrhea, potassium or magnesium deficiency, gallstone development and metabolic encephalopathy.

NURSING CONSIDERATIONS

- Obtain an accurate diet history to identify the patient's eating patterns and the importance of food to his lifestyle. Ask the patient to keep a careful record of what, where, and when he eats to help identify situations that normally provoke overeating.
- Explain the prescribed diet carefully, and encourage compliance to improve health status.
- To increase calorie expenditure, promote increased physical activity, including an exercise program. Recommend varying activity levels according to the patient's general condition and cardiovascular status.
- Watch carefully for signs of dependence or abuse if the patient is taking appetite-suppressing drugs; also watch for adverse effects, such as insomnia, excitability, dry mouth, and GI disturbances.
- Teach the grossly obese patient the importance of good skin care to prevent breakdown in moist skin folds. Recommend the regular use of powder to keep skin dry.
- To help prevent obesity in children, teach parents to avoid overfeeding their infants and to familiarize themselves with actual nutritional needs and optimum growth rates. Discourage parents from using food to reward or console their children, from emphasizing the importance of "clean plates," and from allowing eating to prevent hunger rather than to satisfy it.
- Encourage physical activity and exercise, especially in children and young adults, to establish lifelong patterns. Suggest low-calorie snacks such as raw vegetables.

Pancreatitis

Pancreatitis, inflammation of the pancreas, occurs in acute and chronic forms and may be due to edema, necrosis, or hemorrhage. This disease is commonly associated with alcoholism, trauma, peptic ulcer, and biliary tract disease. The prognosis is good in pancreatitis associated with biliary tract disease, but poor when associated with alcoholism. Mortality is as high as 60% when pancreatitis is associated with necrosis and hemorrhage.

CAUSES

- Abnormal organ structure
- Alcoholism
- Biliary tract disease
- Blunt trauma or surgical trauma
- Drugs, such as glucocorticoids, sulfonamides, thiazides, oral contraceptives, and nonsteroidal anti-inflammatory drugs
- Endoscopic examination of the bile ducts and pancreas
- Kidney failure or transplantation
- Metabolic or endocrine disorders, such as high cholesterol levels or overactive thyroid
- Pancreatic cysts or tumors
- Penetrating peptic ulcers

PATHOPHYSIOLOGY

Acute pancreatitis occurs in two forms: edematous (interstitial) and necrotizing (hemorrhagic). Edematous pancreatitis causes fluid accumulation and swelling. Necrotizing pancreatitis causes cell death and tissue damage. The inflammation that occurs with both types is caused by premature activation of enzymes, which causes tissue damage. Enzymes back up and spill out into the pancreatic tissue resulting in autodigestion of the pancreas.

Normally, the acini in the pancreas secrete enzymes in an inactive form. Two theories explain why enzymes become prematurely activated.

In one view, a toxic agent such as alcohol alters the way the pancreas secretes enzymes. Alcohol probably increases pancreatic secretion, alters the metabolism of the acinar cells, and encourages duct obstruction by causing pancreatic secretory proteins to precipitate.

Another theory is that a reflux of duodenal contents containing activated enzymes enters the pancreatic duct, activating other enzymes and setting up a cycle of more pancreatic damage.

In chronic pancreatitis, persistent inflammation produces irreversible changes in the structure and function of the pancreas. It sometimes follows an episode of acute pancreatitis. Protein precipitates block the pancreatic duct and eventually harden or calcify. Structural changes lead to fibrosis and atrophy of the glands. Growths called *pseudocysts* contain pancreatic enzymes and tissue debris. An abscess results if pseudocysts become infected.

If pancreatitis damages the islets of Langerhans, diabetes mellitus may result. Sudden severe pancreatitis causes massive hemorrhage and total destruction of the pancreas, manifested as diabetic acidosis, shock, or coma.

CLINICAL FINDINGS

- Midepigastric abdominal pain, which can radiate to the back, caused by the escape of inflammatory exudate and enzymes into the back of the

peritoneum, edema and distention of the pancreatic capsule, and obstruction of the biliary tract
- Persistent vomiting (in a severe attack) from hypomotility or paralytic ileus secondary to pancreatitis or peritonitis
- Abdominal distention (in a severe attack) from bowel hypomotility and the accumulation of fluids in the abdominal cavity
- Diminished bowel activity (in severe attack) suggesting altered motility secondary to peritonitis
- Crackles at lung bases (in a severe attack) secondary to heart failure
- Left pleural effusion (in a severe attack) from circulating pancreatic enzymes and adjacent inflammation
- Mottled skin from hemorrhagic necrosis of the pancreas
- Tachycardia secondary to dehydration and possible hypovolemia
- Low-grade fever resulting from the inflammatory response
- Cold, sweaty extremities secondary to cardiovascular collapse
- Restlessness related to pain associated with acute pancreatitis
- Extreme malaise (in chronic pancreatitis) related to malabsorption or diabetes

🔴 *Alert* *Complications of pancreatitis include massive hemorrhage and shock, pseudocysts, biliary and duodenal obstruction, portal and splenic vein thrombosis, diabetes mellitus, and respiratory failure.*

TEST RESULTS
- Elevated serum amylase and lipase confirm diagnosis.
- Blood and urine glucose tests reveal transient glucose in urine and hyperglycemia. In chronic pancreatitis, serum glucose levels may be transiently elevated.

- White blood cell count is elevated.
- Serum bilirubin levels are elevated in both acute and chronic pancreatitis.
- Blood calcium levels may be decreased.
- Stool analysis shows elevated lipid and trypsin levels in chronic pancreatitis.
- Abdominal and chest X-rays detect pleural effusions and differentiate pancreatitis from diseases that cause similar symptoms; may detect pancreatic calculi.
- Computed tomography scan and ultrasonography show enlarged pancreas with cysts and pseudocysts.
- Endoscopic retrograde cholangiopancreatography identifies ductal system abnormalities, such as calcification or strictures; helps differentiate pancreatitis from other disorders such as pancreatic cancer.

TREATMENT
- I.V. replacement of fluids, protein, and electrolytes to treat shock
- Fluid volume replacement to help correct metabolic acidosis
- Blood transfusions to replace blood loss from hemorrhage
- Withholding of food and oral fluids to rest the pancreas and reduce pancreatic enzyme secretion; administration of total parenteral nutrition
- Nasogastric (NG) tube suctioning to decrease stomach distention and suppress pancreatic secretions
- Antiemetics to alleviate nausea and vomiting
- Morphine to relieve abdominal pain
- Antacids to neutralize gastric secretions
- Histamine antagonists to decrease hydrochloric acid production
- Antibiotics to fight bacterial infections

- Anticholinergics to reduce vagal stimulation, decrease GI motility, and inhibit pancreatic enzyme secretion
- Insulin to correct hyperglycemia
- Surgical drainage to treat a pancreatic abscess or pseudocyst or to reestablish drainage of the pancreas
- Laparotomy (if biliary tract obstruction causes acute pancreatitis) to remove obstruction

NURSING CONSIDERATIONS

Acute pancreatitis is a life-threatening emergency, requiring meticulous supportive care and continuous monitoring of vital systems.

- Monitor vital signs and pulmonary artery pressure closely. If the patient has a central venous pressure line instead of a pulmonary artery catheter, monitor it closely for volume expansion (it shouldn't rise above 10 cm H_2O). Give plasma or albumin, if ordered, to maintain blood pressure. Record fluid intake and output; check urine output hourly, and monitor electrolyte levels. Assess for crackles, rhonchi, or decreased breath sounds.
- For bowel decompression, maintain constant NG suctioning, and give nothing by mouth. Perform good mouth and nose care.

Alert Watch for signs and symptoms of calcium deficiency — tetany, cramps, carpopedal spasm, and seizures. If you suspect hypocalcemia, keep airway and suction apparatus handy and pad side rails.

- Administer analgesics as needed to relieve the patient's pain and anxiety.
- Watch for complications due to total parenteral nutrition, such as sepsis, hypokalemia, overhydration, and metabolic acidosis. Watch for fever, cardiac irregularities, changes in arterial blood gas measurements, and deep respirations. Use strict aseptic technique when caring for the catheter insertion site.

Peptic ulcers

Peptic ulcers, circumscribed lesions in the mucosal membrane extending below the epithelium, can develop in the lower esophagus, stomach, pylorus, duodenum, or jejunum. Although erosions are often referred to as ulcers, erosions are breaks in the mucosal membranes that don't extend below the epithelium. Ulcers may be acute or chronic in nature. Chronic ulcers are identified by scar tissue at their base. (See *Understanding peptic ulcers.*) About 80% of all peptic ulcers are duodenal ulcers, which affect the proximal part of the small intestine and occur most commonly in men between ages 20 and 50. Duodenal ulcers usually follow a chronic course with remissions and exacerbations; 5% to 10% of patients develop complications that necessitate surgery. Gastric ulcers are most common in middle-aged and elderly men, especially in chronic users of nonsteroidal anti-inflammatory drugs (NSAIDs), alcohol, or tobacco.

CAUSES
- *Helicobacter pylori* infection
- NSAID use
- Pathologic hypersecretory disorders

PATHOPHYSIOLOGY
Although the stomach contains acidic secretions that can digest substances, intrinsic defenses protect the gastric mucosal membrane from injury. A thick, tenacious layer of gastric mucus protects the stomach from autodiges-

Focus in

UNDERSTANDING PEPTIC ULCERS

A GI lesion isn't necessarily an ulcer. Lesions that don't extend below the mucosal lining (epithelium) are called *erosions*. Lesions of both acute and chronic ulcers can extend through the epithelium and perforate the stomach wall. Chronic ulcers also have scar tissue at the base.

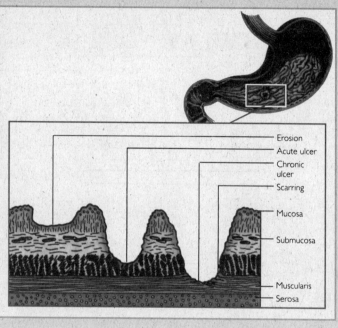

tion, mechanical trauma, and chemical trauma. Prostaglandins provide another line of defense. Gastric ulcers may be a result of destruction of the mucosal barrier.

The duodenum is protected from ulceration by the function of Brunner's glands. These glands produce a viscid, mucoid, alkaline secretion that neutralizes the acid chyme. Duodenal ulcers appear to result from excessive acid protection.

H. pylori releases a toxin that destroys the gastric and duodenal mucosa, reducing the epithelium's resistance to acid digestion and causing gastritis and ulcer disease.

Salicylates and other NSAIDs inhibit the secretion of prostaglandins (substances that block ulceration). Certain illnesses, such as pancreatitis, hepatic disease, Crohn's disease, pre-existing gastritis, and Zollinger-Ellison

(Text continues on page 224.)

TREATING PEPTIC ULCERS

This flowchart highlights the major treatments used for peptic ulcers and where they interfere with the pathophysiologic chain of events.

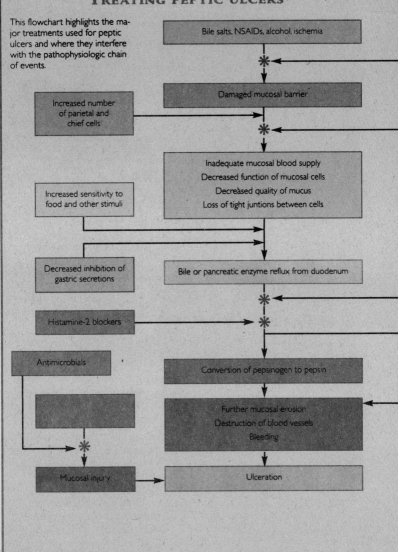

Bile salts, NSAIDs, alcohol, ischemia

Damaged mucosal barrier

Increased number of parietal and chief cells

Inadequate mucosal blood supply
Decreased function of mucosal cells
Decreased quality of mucus
Loss of tight juntions between cells

Increased sensitivity to food and other stimuli

Decreased inhibition of gastric secretions

Bile or pancreatic enzyme reflux from duodenum

Histamine-2 blockers

Antimicrobials

Conversion of pepsinogen to pepsin

Further mucosal erosion
Destruction of blood vessels
Bleeding

Mucosal injury

Ulceration

Key: ✳ = treatment

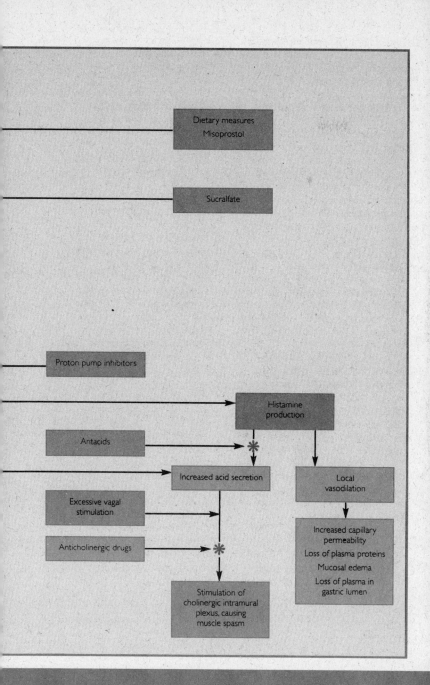

Dietary measures
Misoprostol

Sucralfate

Proton pump inhibitors

Histamine
production

Antacids

Increased acid secretion

Local
vasodilation

Excessive vagal
stimulation

Anticholinergic drugs

Stimulation of
cholinergic intramural
plexus, causing
muscle spasm

Increased capillary
permeability
Loss of plasma proteins
Mucosal edema
Loss of plasma in
gastric lumen

In addition to peptic ulcer's main causes, several predisposing factors are acknowledged. They include blood type (gastric ulcers and type A; duodenal ulcers and type O) and other genetic factors. Exposure to irritants, such as alcohol, coffee, and tobacco, may contribute by accelerating gastric acid emptying and promoting mucosal breakdown. Emotional stress also contributes to ulcer formation because of the increased stimulation of acid and pepsin secretion and decreased mucosal defense. Physical trauma and normal aging are additional predisposing conditions.

CLINICAL FINDINGS

Symptoms vary by the type of ulcer.
- Gastric ulcer — producing pain that worsens with eating due to stretching of the mucosa by food, and nausea and anorexia secondary to mucosal stretching
- Duodenal ulcer — producing epigastric pain that's gnawing, dull, aching, or "hunger-like" due to excessive acid production; and pain relieved by food or antacids, but usually recurring 2 to 4 hours later secondary to food acting as a buffer for acid

Alert Complications of peptic ulcers include hemorrhage, shock, gastric perforation, and gastric outlet obstruction.

TEST RESULTS

- Barium studies or upper GI and small bowel series may reveal the presence of the ulcer. This is the first test performed on a patient when symptoms aren't severe.
- Esophagogastroduodenoscopy confirms the presence of an ulcer and permits cytologic studies and biopsy to rule out *H. pylori* or cancer.

- Upper GI tract X-rays reveal mucosal abnormalities.
- Stool analysis may reveal occult blood.
- Serologic testing may disclose clinical signs of infection, such as elevated white blood cell count.
- Gastric secretory studies show hyperchlorhydria.
- Urea breath test results reflect activity of *H. pylori*.

TREATMENT

- Antimicrobials (tetracycline [Sumycin], bismuth subsalicylate, and metronidazole [Flagyl]) to eradicate *H. pylori* infection (see *Treating peptic ulcers*, pages 222 and 223)
- Misoprostol (Cytotec) (a prostaglandin analog) to inhibit gastric acid secretion and increase carbonate and mucus production, to protect the stomach lining
- Antacids to neutralize acid gastric contents by elevating the gastric pH, thus protecting the mucosa and relieving pain
- Avoidance of caffeine and alcohol to avoid stimulation of gastric acid secretion
- Anticholinergic drugs to inhibit the effect of the vagal nerve on acid-secreting cells
- Histamine-2 blockers to reduce acid secretion
- Sucralfate (Carafate), a mucosal protectant to form an acid-impermeable membrane that adheres to the mucous membrane and also accelerates mucus production
- Proton gastric acid pump inhibitors to decrease gastric acid secretion
- Dietary therapy with small infrequent meals and avoidance of eating before bedtime to neutralize gastric contents

- Insertion of a nasogastric (NG) tube (in instances of GI bleeding) for gastric decompression and rest and, also, to permit iced saline lavage that may contain norepinephrine
- Gastroscopy to allow visualization of the bleeding site and coagulation by laser or cautery to control bleeding
- Surgery to repair perforation or to treat unresponsiveness to conservative treatment or suspected malignancy

NURSING CONSIDERATIONS

- Advise the patient who uses antacids, has a history of cardiac disease, or follows a sodium-restricted diet to take only those antacids that contain low amounts of sodium.
- Warn the patient to avoid steroids and NSAIDs because they irritate the gastric mucosa. For the same reason, advise the patient to stop smoking and to avoid stressful situations, excessive intake of coffee, and ingestion of alcoholic beverages during exacerbations of peptic ulcer disease.

After gastric surgery

- Keep the NG tube patent. If the tube isn't functioning, don't reposition it; you might damage the suture line or anastomosis. Notify the surgeon promptly.
- Monitor intake and output, including NG tube drainage. Check for bowel sounds, and allow the patient nothing by mouth until peristalsis resumes and the NG tube is removed or clamped.
- Replace fluids and electrolytes. Assess for signs of dehydration, sodium deficiency, and metabolic alkalosis, which may occur secondary to gastric suction.

Alert *Monitor for possible complications: hemorrhage; shock; iron, folate, or vitamin B$_{12}$ deficiency anemia from* *malabsorption (pernicious anemia) due to lack of intrinsic factor; and dumping syndrome (a rapid gastric emptying, causing distention of the duodenum or jejunum produced by a bolus of food). Signs and symptoms of dumping syndrome include diaphoresis, weakness, nausea, flatulence, explosive diarrhea, distention, and palpitations within 30 minutes after a meal.*

- To avoid dumping syndrome, advise the patient to lie down after meals, to drink fluids between meals rather than with meals, to avoid eating large amounts of carbohydrates, and to eat four to six small, high-protein, low-carbohydrate meals during the day.

Ulcerative colitis

Ulcerative colitis is an inflammatory, usually chronic, disease that affects the mucosa of the colon. It invariably begins in the rectum and sigmoid colon, and commonly extends upward into the entire colon, rarely affecting the small intestine. Ulcerative colitis produces edema (leading to mucosal friability) and ulcerations. Severity ranges from a mild, localized disorder to a fulminant disease that may cause a perforated colon, progressing to potentially fatal peritonitis and toxemia. The disease cycles between exacerbation and remission.

Ulcerative colitis occurs primarily in young adults, especially women. It's more prevalent among Ashkenazic Jews and in higher socioeconomic groups; there seems to be a familial tendency. Onset of symptoms seems to peak between ages 15 and 20 and between ages 55 and 60.

Causes

Specific causes of ulcerative colitis are unknown but may be related to abnormal immune response in the GI tract, possibly associated with food or bacteria such as *Escherichia coli*.

Pathophysiology

Ulcerative colitis usually begins as inflammation in the base of the mucosal layer of the large intestine. The colon's mucosal surface becomes dark, red, and velvety. Inflammation leads to erosions that coalesce and form ulcers. The mucosa becomes diffusely ulcerated, with hemorrhage, congestion, edema, and exudative inflammation. Ulcerations are continuous. Abscesses in the mucosa drain purulent exudate, become necrotic, and ulcerate. Sloughing causes bloody, mucus-filled stools. As abscesses heal, scarring and thickening may appear in the bowel's inner muscle layer. As granulation tissue replaces the muscle layer, the colon narrows, shortens, and loses its characteristic pouches (haustral folds).

Clinical findings

- Recurrent bloody diarrhea (as many as 20 stools per day), typically containing pus and mucus (hallmark sign), from accumulated blood and mucus in the bowel
- Abdominal cramping and rectal urgency from accumulated blood and mucus
- Weight loss secondary to malabsorption
- Weakness related to possible malabsorption and subsequent anemia

Alert Complications of ulcerative colitis may include perforation, toxic megacolon, liver disease, stricture formation colon cancer, and anemia.

Test results

- Sigmoidoscopy confirms rectal involvement: specifically, mucosal friability and flattening and thick, inflammatory exudate.
- Colonoscopy reveals extent of the disease, stricture areas, and pseudopolyps (not performed when the patient has active signs and symptoms).
- Biopsy with colonoscopy confirms the diagnosis.
- Barium enema reveals the extent of the disease, detects complications, and identifies cancer (not performed when the patient has active signs and symptoms).
- Stool specimen analysis reveals blood, pus, and mucus but no disease-causing organisms.
- Serology shows decreased serum potassium, magnesium, and albumin levels; decreased white blood cell count; decreased hemoglobin level; and prolonged prothrombin time. Elevated erythrocyte sedimentation rate correlates with severity of the attack.

Treatment

- Corticotropin and adrenal corticosteroids to control inflammation
- Sulfasalazine (Azulfadine) for its anti-inflammatory and antimicrobial effects
- Antidiarrheals to relieve frequent, troublesome diarrhea in patients whose ulcerative colitis is otherwise under control
- Iron supplements to correct anemia
- Total parenteral nutrition and nothing by mouth (NPO) for patients with severe disease, to rest the intestinal tract, decrease stool volume, and restore nitrogen balance; I.V. hydration to replace fluid loss from diarrhea
- Surgery to correct massive dilation of the colon and to treat patients with symptoms that are unbearable or un-

responsive to drugs and supportive measures; proctocolectomy with ileostomy removing all the potentially malignant epithelia of the rectum and colon

NURSING CONSIDERATIONS

Patient care includes close monitoring for changes in status.
- Accurately record intake and output, particularly the frequency and volume of stools. Watch for signs of dehydration and electrolyte imbalances, especially signs and symptoms of hypokalemia (muscle weakness and paresthesia) and hypernatremia (tachycardia, flushed skin, fever, and dry tongue). Monitor the patient's hemoglobin level and hematocrit, and give blood transfusions, as ordered. Provide good mouth care for the patient who's NPO.
- After each bowel movement, thoroughly clean the skin around the rectum. Provide an air mattress or sheepskin to help prevent skin breakdown.
- Take precautionary measures if the patient is prone to bleeding. Watch closely for signs of complications, such as a perforated colon and peritonitis (fever, severe abdominal pain, abdominal rigidity and tenderness, and cool, clammy skin), and toxic megacolon (abdominal distention and decreased bowel sounds).

For patients requiring surgery:
- After surgery, provide meticulous supportive care and continue teaching correct stoma care.
- Keep the nasogastric tube patent. After removal of the tube, provide a clear-liquid diet, and gradually advance to a low-residue diet, as tolerated.
- After a proctocolectomy and ileostomy, teach good stoma care. Wash the skin around the stoma with soapy water and dry it thoroughly. Apply karaya gum around the stoma's base to avoid irritation, and make a watertight seal. Attach the pouch over the karaya ring. Cut an opening in the ring to fit over the stoma, and secure the pouch to the skin. Empty the pouch when it's one-third full.
- After a pouch ileostomy, uncork the catheter every hour to allow contents to drain. After 10 to 14 days, gradually increase the length of time the catheter is left corked until it can be opened every 3 hours. Then remove the catheter and reinsert it every 3 to 4 hours for drainage. Teach the patient how to insert the catheter and how to take care of the stoma.
- Encourage the patient to have regular physical examinations.

5

RENAL SYSTEM

The components of the renal system are the kidneys, ureters, bladder, and urethra. The kidneys, located retroperitoneally in the lumbar area, produce and excrete urine to maintain homeostasis. They regulate the volume, electrolyte concentration, and acid-base balance of body fluids; detoxify the blood and eliminate wastes; regulate blood pressure; and support red blood cell production (erythropoiesis). The ureters are tubes that extend from the kidneys to the bladder; their only function is to transport urine to the bladder. The bladder is a muscular bag that serves as reservoir for urine until it leaves the body through the urethra.

Renal disorders include acute pyelonephritis, acute and chronic renal failure, acute tubular necrosis, glomerulonephritis, nephrotic syndrome, neurogenic bladder, polycystic kidney disease, and renal calculi.

Acute pyelonephritis

Acute pyelonephritis, also known as *acute infective tubulointerstitial nephritis,* is a sudden inflammation caused by bacteria that primarily affects the interstitial area and renal pelvis or, less commonly, the renal tubules. It's one of the most common renal diseases and may affect one or both kidneys. With treatment and continued follow-up care, the prognosis is good, and extensive permanent damage is rare.

Pyelonephritis is more common in females, probably because of a shorter urethra and the proximity of the urinary meatus to the vagina and rectum — both conditions allow bacteria to reach the bladder more easily — and a lack of the antibacterial prostatic secretions produced in males. Incidence increases with age and is higher in the following groups:

- sexually active women — intercourse increases the risk of bacterial contamination
- pregnant women — about 5% develop asymptomatic bacteriuria; if untreated, about 40% develop pyelonephritis
- people with diabetes — neurogenic bladder causes incomplete emptying and urinary stasis; glycosuria may support bacterial growth in urine
- people with other renal diseases — compromised renal function aggravates susceptibility.

CAUSES

- Bacterial infection of the kidneys, including normal intestinal and fecal flora that grow readily in urine
- *Escherichia coli* most common causative organism
- Other causative organisms
  - *Enterococcus faecalis* (formerly *Streptococcus faecalis*)
  - *Klebsiella*
  - *Proteus*
  - *Pseudomonas*
  - *Staphylococcus aureus*

PATHOPHYSIOLOGY

Typically, the infection spreads from the bladder to the ureters, and then to the kidneys, such as in vesicoureteral reflux. Vesicoureteral reflux may result from congenital weakness at the junction of the ureter and bladder. Bacteria refluxed to intrarenal tissues may create colonies of infection within 24 to 48 hours. Infection may also result from instrumentation, such as catheterization, cystoscopy, or urologic surgery; from a hematogenic infection, such as in septicemia or endocarditis; or, possibly, from a lymphatic infection.

Pyelonephritis may also result from an inability to empty the bladder (for example, in patients with neurogenic bladder), urinary stasis, or urinary obstruction due to tumors, strictures, or benign prostatic hyperplasia.

Recurrent episodes of acute pyelonephritis can eventually result in chronic pyelonephritis. (See *Chronic pyelonephritis*.)

CLINICAL FINDINGS

The following symptoms characteristically develop rapidly over a few hours or a few days. Although they may disappear within days, even without treatment, residual bacterial

---

CHRONIC PYELONEPHRITIS

Chronic pyelonephritis is a persistent kidney inflammation that can scar the kidneys and may lead to chronic renal failure. Its etiology may be bacterial, metastatic, or urogenous. This disease is most common in patients who are predisposed to recurrent acute pyelonephritis such as those with urinary obstructions or vesicoureteral reflux.

Patients with chronic pyelonephritis may have a childhood history of unexplained fevers or bed-wetting. Clinical effects may include flank pain, anemia, low urine specific gravity, proteinuria, leukocytes in urine and, especially in late stages, hypertension. Uremia rarely develops from chronic pyelonephritis unless structural abnormalities exist in the excretory system. Bacteriuria may be intermittent. When no bacteria are found in the urine, diagnosis depends on excretory urography (renal pelvis may appear small and flattened) and renal biopsy.

Effective treatment of chronic pyelonephritis requires control of hypertension, elimination of the existing obstruction (when possible), and long-term antimicrobial therapy.

---

infection is likely and may cause symptoms to recur later.

- Urinary urgency and frequency, burning during urination, dysuria, nocturia, and hematuria (usually microscopic but may be gross)
- Cloudy urine that has an ammonia-like or fishy odor
- Temperature of 102° F (38.9° C) or higher, shaking chills, nausea and vomiting, flank pain, anorexia, and general fatigue.

Alert *Elderly patients may exhibit GI or pulmonary symptoms rather than the usual febrile responses to pyelonephritis. In children younger than age 2, fever, vomiting, nonspecific abdominal com-*

plaints, or failure to thrive may be the only signs of acute pyelonephritis.

TEST RESULTS

- Urine sediment reveals pyuria (pus in urine) with the presence of leukocytes singly, in clumps, and in casts and, possibly, a few red blood cells.
- Urine culture reveals significant bacteriuria — more than 100,000 organisms/mm^3 of urine.
- Low specific gravity and osmolality.
- Slightly alkaline urine pH.
- Proteinuria, glycosuria, and ketonuria are less common conditions revealed by testing.
- Computed tomography scan of the kidneys, ureters, and bladder may reveal calculi, tumors, or cysts in the kidneys and urinary tract.
- Excretory urography may show asymmetrical kidneys.

TREATMENT

Treatment centers on antibiotic therapy appropriate to the specific infecting organism after identification by urine culture and sensitivity studies. For example:

- *Enterococcus* requiring treatment with ampicillin, penicillin G, or vancomycin (Vancocin)
- *Staphylococcus* requiring penicillin G or, if resistance develops, a semisynthetic penicillin, such as nafcillin, or a cephalosporin
- *E. coli* possibly treated with sulfisoxazole, nalidixic acid (NegGram), and nitrofurantoin (Macrobid)
- *Proteus* possibly treated with ampicillin, sulfisoxazole, nalidixic acid, and a cephalosporin
- *Pseudomonas* requiring gentamicin or tobramycin
- When the infecting organism can't be identified, therapy usually consisting of a broad-spectrum antibiotic, such as ampicillin or cephalexin (Keflex)
- If the patient is pregnant or elderly, antibiotics given with caution (Symptoms may disappear after several days of antibiotic therapy. Although urine usually becomes sterile within 48 to 72 hours, the course of such therapy is 10 to 14 days.)

Other treatments

- Urinary analgesics such as phenazopyridine (Pyridium).
- Reculturing of urine 1 week after drug therapy stops, and then periodically for the next year to detect residual or recurring infection. (Most patients with uncomplicated infections respond well to therapy and don't suffer reinfection.)
- Surgery to relieve the obstruction or correct the anomaly if infection is caused by an obstruction or a vesicoureteral reflux.
- Long-term follow-up for patients at high risk for recurring urinary tract and kidney infections, such as those with prolonged use of an indwelling catheter or those taking maintenance antibiotic therapy.

NURSING CONSIDERATIONS

- Administer antipyretics for fever.
- Encourage fluids to achieve a urine output of more than 2 qt (2 L)/day. This helps to empty the bladder of contaminated urine and prevents calculi formation. Don't encourage intake of more than 3 qt (3 L) because this may decrease the effectiveness of the antibiotics.
- Provide an acid-ash diet to prevent calculus formation.
- Teach proper technique for collecting a clean-catch urine specimen. Refrigerate or culture a urine specimen

within 30 minutes of collection to prevent overgrowth of bacteria.
- Stress the need to complete prescribed antibiotic therapy even after symptoms subside. Encourage long-term follow-up care for high-risk patients.

To prevent acute pyelonephritis:
- Observe strict sterile technique during catheter insertion and care.
- Instruct females to prevent bacterial contamination by wiping the perineum from front to back after defecation.
- Advise routine checkups for patients with a history of urinary tract infections. Teach them to recognize signs of infection, such as cloudy urine, burning on urination, urgency, and frequency, especially when accompanied by flank pain and a low-grade fever.

✳ Life-threatening
Acute renal failure

Acute renal failure, the sudden interruption of renal function, can be caused by obstruction, poor circulation, or underlying kidney disease. Whether prerenal, intrarenal, or postrenal, it usually passes through three distinct phases: oliguric, diuretic, and recovery. About 5% of hospitalized patients develop acute renal failure. The condition is usually reversible with treatment, but if not treated, it may progress to end-stage renal disease, prerenal azotemia, and death.

CAUSES
Prerenal failure
- Antihypertensive drugs
- Arrhythmias that cause reduced cardiac output

- Arterial embolism
- Arterial or venous thrombosis
- Ascites
- Burns
- Cardiac tamponade
- Cardiogenic shock
- Dehydration
- Disseminated intravascular coagulation
- Diuretic overuse
- Eclampsia
- Heart failure
- Hemorrhage
- Hypovolemic shock
- Malignant hypertension
- Myocardial infarction
- Pulmonary embolism
- Sepsis
- Trauma
- Tumor
- Vasculitis

Intrarenal failure
- Acute glomerulonephritis
- Acute interstitial nephritis
- Acute pyelonephritis
- Bilateral renal vein thrombosis
- Crush injuries
- Malignant nephrosclerosis
- Myopathy
- Nephrotoxins
- Obstetric complications
- Papillary necrosis
- Polyarteritis nodosa
- Poorly treated prerenal failure
- Renal myeloma
- Sickle cell disease
- Systemic lupus erythematosus
- Transfusion reaction
- Vasculitis

Postrenal failure
- Benign prostatic hyperplasia
- Bladder obstruction
- Ureteral obstruction
- Urethral obstruction

PATHOPHYSIOLOGY

The pathophysiology of prerenal, intrarenal, and postrenal failure differs.

Prerenal failure

Prerenal failure ensues when a condition that diminishes blood flow to the kidneys leads to hypoperfusion. Examples include hypovolemia, hypotension, vasoconstriction, or inadequate cardiac output. Azotemia (excess nitrogenous waste products in the blood) develops in 40% to 80% of acute renal failure cases.

When renal blood flow is interrupted, so is oxygen delivery. The ensuing hypoxemia and ischemia can rapidly and irreversibly damage the kidneys. The tubules are most susceptible to hypoxemia's effects.

Azotemia is a consequence of renal hypoperfusion. The impaired blood flow results in decreased glomerular filtration rate (GFR) and increased tubular reabsorption of sodium and water. A decrease in the GFR causes electrolyte imbalance and metabolic acidosis. Usually, restoring renal blood flow and glomerular filtration reverses azotemia.

Intrarenal failure

Intrarenal failure, also called *intrinsic* or *parenchymal renal failure,* results from damage to the filtering structures of the kidneys. Causes of intrarenal failure are classified as nephrotoxic, inflammatory, or ischemic. When the damage is caused by nephrotoxicity or inflammation, the delicate layer under the epithelium (the basement membrane) becomes irreparably damaged, typically leading to chronic renal failure. Severe or prolonged lack of blood flow caused by ischemia may lead to renal damage (ischemic parenchymal injury) and excess nitrogen in the blood (intrinsic renal azotemia).

Acute tubular necrosis (ATN), the precursor to intrarenal failure, can result from ischemic damage to renal parenchyma during unrecognized or poorly treated prerenal failure or from obstetric complications, such as eclampsia, postpartum renal failure, septic abortion, or uterine hemorrhage.

The fluid loss causes hypotension, which leads to ischemia. The ischemic tissue generates toxic oxygen-free radicals, which cause swelling, injury, and necrosis.

Another cause of acute failure is the use of nephrotoxins, including analgesics, anesthetics, heavy metals, radiographic contrast media, organic solvents, and antimicrobials, particularly aminoglycoside antibiotics. These drugs accumulate in the renal cortex, causing renal failure that manifests well after treatment or other toxin exposure. The necrosis caused by nephrotoxins tends to be uniform and limited to the proximal tubules, whereas ischemia necrosis tends to be patchy and distributed along various parts of the nephron.

Postrenal failure

Bilateral obstruction of urine outflow leads to postrenal failure. The cause may be in the bladder, ureters, or urethra.

Bladder obstruction can result from:
- anticholinergic drugs
- autonomic nerve dysfunction
- infection
- tumors.

Ureteral obstructions, which restrict urine flow from the kidneys to the bladder, can result from:
- blood clots

- calculi
- edema or inflammation
- necrotic renal papillae
- retroperitoneal fibrosis or hemorrhage
- surgery (accidental ligation and strictures)
- tumor or uric acid crystals.

Urethral obstruction can be the result of prostatic hyperplasia, a tumor, or strictures.

The three types of acute renal failure (prerenal, intrarenal, or postrenal) usually pass through three distinct phases: oliguric, diuretic, and recovery.

Oliguric phase

Oliguria may be the result of one or several factors. Necrosis of the tubules can cause sloughing of cells, cast formation, and ischemic edema. The resulting tubular obstruction causes a retrograde increase in pressure and a decrease in the GFR. Renal failure can occur within 24 hours from this effect. Glomerular filtration may remain normal in some cases of renal failure, but tubular reabsorption of filtrate may be accelerated. In this instance, ischemia may increase tubular permeability and cause backleak. Another concept is that the intrarenal release of angiotensin II or the redistribution of blood flow from the cortex to the medulla may constrict the afferent arterioles, increasing glomerular permeability and decreasing the GFR.

Urine output may remain at less than 30 ml/hour or 400 ml/day for a few days to weeks. Before damage occurs, the kidneys respond to decreased blood flow by conserving sodium and water.

Damage impairs the kidneys' ability to conserve sodium. Fluid (water) volume excess, azotemia (elevated serum levels of urea, creatinine, and uric acid), and electrolyte imbalance occur. Ischemic or toxic injury leads to the release of mediators and intrarenal vasoconstriction. Medullary hypoxia results in the swelling of tubular and endothelial cells, adherence of neutrophils to capillaries and venules, and inappropriate platelet activation. Increasing ischemia and vasoconstriction further limit perfusion.

Injured cells lose polarity, and the ensuing disruption of tight junctions between the cells promotes backleak of filtrate. Ischemia impairs the function of energy-dependent membrane pumps, and calcium accumulates in the cells. This excess calcium further stimulates vasoconstriction and activates proteases and other enzymes. Untreated prerenal oliguria may lead to ATN.

Diuretic phase

As the kidneys become unable to conserve sodium and water, the diuretic phase, marked by increased urine secretion of more than 400 ml/24 hours, ensues. The GFR may be normal or increased, but tubular support mechanisms are abnormal. Excretion of dilute urine causes dehydration and electrolyte imbalances. High blood urea nitrogen (BUN) levels produce osmotic diuresis and consequent deficits of potassium, sodium, and water. The diuretic phase may last days or weeks.

Recovery phase

If the cause of diuresis is corrected, azotemia gradually disappears and recovery occurs. The recovery phase is a gradual return to normal or near-normal renal function over 3 to 12 months.

Alert *Even with treatment, the elderly patient is particularly susceptible to volume overload, precipitating acute pulmonary edema, hypertensive crisis, hyperkalemia, and infection.*

CLINICAL FINDINGS

Early signs include:
- oliguria
- azotemia
- anuria (rare).

As the patient becomes increasingly uremic, electrolyte imbalance and metabolic acidosis occur along with disruptions of other body systems, including:
- GI—anorexia, nausea, vomiting, diarrhea or constipation, stomatitis, bleeding, hematemesis, dry mucous membranes, uremic breath
- Central nervous system (CNS)—headache, drowsiness, irritability, confusion, peripheral neuropathy, seizures, coma
- Cutaneous—dryness, pruritus, pallor, purpura and, rarely, uremic frost
- Cardiovascular—early in the disease, hypotension; later, hypertension, arrhythmias, fluid overload, heart failure, systemic edema, anemia, altered clotting mechanisms
- Respiratory—pulmonary edema, Kussmaul's respirations.

TEST RESULTS

- Blood studies show elevated BUN, serum creatinine, and potassium levels; decreased hematocrit and hemoglobin and bicarbonate levels; and low blood pH.
- Urine studies show casts, cellular debris, and decreased specific gravity; in glomerular diseases, proteinuria and urine osmolality are close to serum osmolality; urine sodium level less than 20 mEq/L if oliguria results from de-

creased perfusion, and more than 40 mEq/L if the cause is intrarenal.
- Creatinine clearance test measures the GFR and reflects the number of remaining functioning nephrons.
- Electrocardiogram (ECG) shows tall, peaked T waves; widening QRS complex; and disappearing P waves if hyperkalemia is present.
- Ultrasonography, plain films of the abdomen, kidney-ureter-bladder radiography, excretory urography, renal scan, retrograde pyelography, computed tomography scans, and nephrotomography show the cause of renal failure.

TREATMENT

- High-calorie diet, restricted protein, low sodium, and potassium to meet metabolic needs
- Careful monitoring of electrolytes; I.V. therapy to maintain and correct fluid and electrolyte balance
- Fluid restriction to minimize edema
- Diuretic therapy to treat oliguric phase
- Fluid restoration and maintenance to treat diuretic phase
- Sodium polystyrene sulfonate (Kayexalate) by mouth or enema to reverse hyperkalemia with mild hyperkalemic symptoms (malaise, loss of appetite, muscle weakness)
- Hypertonic glucose with insulin I.V.—for more severe hyperkalemic symptoms (ECG changes, numbness and tingling)
- Sodium bicarbonate I.V. to treat metabolic acidosis
- Hemodialysis or peritoneal dialysis to correct electrolyte and fluid imbalances

Nursing considerations

- Measure and record intake and output, including all body fluids, and weigh the patient daily.
- Assess hemoglobin level and hematocrit and replace blood components, as ordered. Packed red cells deliver the necessary blood components without added volume.
- Monitor the patient's vital signs. Watch for and report signs of pericarditis (pleuritic chest pain, tachycardia, pericardial friction rub), inadequate renal perfusion (hypotension), and acidosis (Kussmaul's respirations).
- Maintain proper electrolyte balance. Strictly monitor potassium level. Watch for symptoms of hyperkalemia (malaise, anorexia, paresthesia, or muscle weakness) and ECG changes (tall, peaked T waves; widening QRS segment; and disappearing P waves), and report them immediately. Avoid administering medications containing potassium.
- Assess the patient frequently, especially during emergency treatment to lower the potassium level. If the patient receives hypertonic glucose and insulin infusions, monitor potassium and glucose levels. If you give sodium polystyrene sulfonate rectally, make sure that the patient doesn't retain it and become constipated, to prevent bowel perforation.
- Maintain the patient's nutritional status. Give the anorexic patient small, frequent meals.
- Use sterile technique because the patient with acute renal failure is highly susceptible to infection. Don't allow personnel with upper respiratory tract infections to care for the patient.
- Prevent complications of immobility by encouraging frequent coughing and deep breathing and by performing passive range-of-motion exercises.

Help the patient walk as soon as possible. Add lubricating lotion to the patient's bath water to combat skin dryness.
- Provide good mouth care frequently because mucous membranes are dry. If stomatitis occurs, an antibiotic solution may be ordered. Have the patient swish the solution around in his mouth before swallowing.
- Monitor for GI bleeding by performing a guaiac test. Administer medications carefully, especially antacids and stool softeners. Use aluminum-hydroxide–based antacids; magnesium-based antacids can cause the serum magnesium level to rise to critical levels.
- Use appropriate safety measures, such as side rails and restraints, because the patient with CNS involvement may be dizzy or confused.
- Provide emotional support to the patient and his family. Reassure them by clearly explaining procedures.
- During peritoneal dialysis, position the patient carefully. Elevate the head of the bed to reduce pressure on the diaphragm and aid respiration. Stay alert for signs of infection (cloudy drainage, elevated temperature) and, rarely, bleeding. If pain occurs, reduce the amount of dialysate. Monitor the diabetic patient's blood glucose periodically and administer insulin, as ordered. Watch for complications, such as peritonitis, atelectasis, hypokalemia, pneumonia, and shock.
- If the patient requires hemodialysis, check the blood access site (arteriovenous fistula, subclavian or femoral catheter) every 2 hours for patency and signs of clotting (palpate a thrill, auscultate a bruit). Don't use the arm with the shunt or fistula for taking blood pressure or drawing blood. Weigh the patient before beginning

dialysis. During dialysis, monitor his vital signs, clotting times, blood flow, the function of the vascular access site, and arterial and venous pressures. Watch for complications, such as septicemia, embolism, hepatitis, and rapid fluid and electrolyte loss. After dialysis, monitor the patient's vital signs and the vascular access site, weigh the patient, and watch for signs of fluid and electrolyte imbalances.

Acute tubular necrosis

Acute tubular necrosis (ATN), also known as *acute tubulointerstitial nephritis,* accounts for about 75% of acute renal failure cases and is the most common cause of acute renal failure in critically ill patients. ATN injures the nephron's tubular segment, causing renal failure and uremic syndrome. The mortality rate ranges from 40% to 70%, depending on complications from underlying diseases. Nonoliguric forms of ATN have a better prognosis.

CAUSES
- Diseased tubular epithelium that allows leakage of glomerular filtrate across the membranes and reabsorption of filtrate into the blood
- Ischemic injury to glomerular epithelial cells, resulting in cellular collapse and decreased glomerular capillary permeability
- Ischemic injury to vascular endothelium, eventually resulting in cellular swelling and tubular obstruction
- Obstruction of urine flow by the collection of damaged cells, casts, red blood cells (RBCs), and other cellular debris within the tubular walls

PATHOPHYSIOLOGY
ATN results from ischemic or nephrotoxic injury, most commonly in debilitated patients, such as the critically ill or those who have undergone extensive surgery. In ischemic injury, disruption of blood flow to the kidneys may result from circulatory collapse, severe hypotension, trauma, hemorrhage, dehydration, cardiogenic or septic shock, surgery, anesthetics, or reactions to transfusions. Nephrotoxic injury may follow ingestion of certain chemical agents, such as contrast agents administered during radiologic procedures or administration of antibiotics (aminoglycosides), or may result from a hypersensitive reaction of the kidneys. Because nephrotoxic ATN doesn't damage the basement membrane of the nephron, it's potentially reversible. However, ischemic ATN can damage the epithelial and basement membranes and can cause lesions in the renal interstitium.

CLINICAL FINDINGS
ATN is usually difficult to recognize in its early stages because effects of the critically ill patient's primary disease may mask the symptoms of ATN. However, signs and symptoms may include:
- decreased urine output, generally the first recognizable effect
- hyperkalemia
- uremic syndrome with oliguria (or, rarely, anuria) and confusion, which may progress to uremic coma
- dry mucous membranes and skin
- central nervous system symptoms, such as lethargy, twitching, and seizures.

Alert *Fever and chills may signal the onset of an infection, which is the leading cause of death in ATN.*

TEST RESULTS

Diagnosis is usually delayed until the condition has progressed to an advanced stage.

● The most significant laboratory clues are urinary sediment containing RBCs and casts, and dilute urine of low specific gravity (1.010), low osmolality (less than 400 mOsm/kg), and a high sodium level (40 to 60 mEq/L).

● Blood studies reveal elevated blood urea nitrogen and serum creatinine levels, anemia, defects in platelet adherence, metabolic acidosis, and hyperkalemia.

● An electrocardiogram may show arrhythmias (due to electrolyte imbalances) and, with hyperkalemia, widening QRS segment, disappearing P waves, and tall, peaked T waves.

TREATMENT
Acute phase

● Vigorous supportive measures until normal kidney function resumes

● Initially, possible administration of diuretics and infusion of a large volume of fluids to flush tubules of cellular casts and debris and to replace fluid loss (risk of fluid overload with this treatment)

Long-term fluid management

● Daily replacement of projected and calculated losses (including insensible loss)

Other treatments

● Transfusion of packed RBCs for anemia; epoetin alfa (Epogen) to stimulate RBC production as an alternative to blood transfusion

● Antibiotics for infection

● Emergency I.V. administration of 50% glucose, regular insulin, and sodium bicarbonate for hyperkalemia

● Sodium polystyrene sulfonate (Kayexalate, SPS) by mouth or by enema to reduce extracellular potassium levels

● Peritoneal dialysis or hemodialysis if the patient is catabolic or if hyperkalemia and fluid volume overload aren't controlled by other measures

NURSING CONSIDERATIONS

● Maintain fluid balance. Watch for fluid overload, a common complication of therapy. Accurately record intake and output, including wound drainage, nasogastric tube output, and hemodialysis and peritoneal dialysis balances. Weigh the patient daily.

● Monitor hemoglobin level and hematocrit, and administer blood products as needed. Use fresh packed cells instead of whole blood to prevent fluid overload and heart failure.

● Maintain electrolyte balance. Monitor laboratory results, and report imbalances. Enforce dietary restriction of foods containing sodium and potassium, such as bananas, orange juice, and baked potatoes. Check for potassium content in prescribed medications (for example, potassium penicillin). Provide adequate calories and essential amino acids while restricting protein intake to maintain an anabolic state. Total parenteral nutrition may be indicated in the severely debilitated or catabolic patient.

● Use sterile technique, particularly when handling catheters, because the debilitated patient is vulnerable to infection. Immediately report fever, chills, delayed wound healing, or flank pain if the patient has an indwelling catheter.

● Watch for complications. If anemia worsens (pallor, weakness, lethargy with decreased hemoglobin level), administer RBCs as ordered. For acidosis, give sodium bicarbonate or assist with dialysis in severe cases, as ordered. Watch for signs of diminishing renal perfusion (hypotension and decreased urine output). Encourage coughing and deep breathing to prevent pulmonary complications.

● Perform passive range-of-motion exercises. Provide good skin care; apply lotion or bath oil to dry skin. Help the patient walk as soon as possible, but guard against exhaustion.

● Provide reassurance and emotional support.

● To prevent ATN, make sure that patients are well hydrated before surgery or after X-rays that use a contrast medium. Administer mannitol (Osmitrol), as ordered, to high-risk patients before and during these procedures. Carefully monitor patients receiving blood transfusions to detect early signs of transfusion reaction (fever, rash, chills), and discontinue such transfusions immediately.

Chronic renal failure

Chronic renal failure (CRF) represents a destruction of renal tissue with irreversible sclerosis and loss of nephron function. It can result from chronic illness or from a rapidly progressing disease. CRF is irreversible. Few symptoms develop until less than 25% of glomerular filtration remains. The normal parenchyma deteriorates rapidly, and symptoms worsen as renal function decreases. This disease is fatal without treatment, but maintenance on dialysis or a kidney transplant can sustain life.

CAUSES

● Chronic glomerular disease (glomerulonephritis)
● Chronic infection (chronic pyelonephritis and tuberculosis)
● Collagen disease (lupus erythematosus)
● Congenital anomalies (polycystic kidney disease)
● Endocrine disease (diabetic neuropathy)
● Nephrotoxic agents (long-term aminoglycoside therapy)
● Obstruction (renal calculi)
● Vascular disease (hypertension, nephrosclerosis)

PATHOPHYSIOLOGY

CRF commonly progresses through four stages. Reduced renal reserve shows a glomerular filtration rate (GFR) of 35% to 50% of normal; renal insufficiency has a GFR of 20% to 35% of normal; renal failure has a GFR of 20% to 25% of normal; and end-stage renal disease has a GFR less than 20% of normal.

Nephron damage is progressive; damaged nephrons can't function and don't recover. The kidneys can maintain relatively normal function until about 75% of the nephrons are nonfunctional. Surviving nephrons hypertrophy and increase their rate of filtration, reabsorption, and secretion. Compensatory excretion continues as the GFR diminishes.

Urine may contain abnormal amounts of protein, red blood cells (RBCs), and white blood cells or casts. The major end products of excretion remain essentially normal, and nephron loss becomes significant. As the GFR decreases, plasma creatinine level increases proportionately without regulatory adjustment. As sodium delivery to the nephron increases, less is reabsorbed, and sodium deficits and volume depletion follow. The kidney becomes incapable of concentrating and diluting urine.

If tubular interstitial disease is the cause of CRF, primary damage to the tubules — the medullary portion of the nephron — precedes failure, as do such problems as renal tubular acidosis, salt wasting, and difficulty diluting and concentrating urine. If vascular or glomerular damage is the primary cause, proteinuria, hematuria, and nephrotic syndrome are more prominent.

Changes in acid-base balance affect phosphorus and calcium balance. Renal phosphate excretion and $1,25(OH)_2$ vitamin D_3 synthesis are diminished. Hypocalcemia results in secondary hypoparathyroidism, a diminished GFR, and progressive hyperphosphatemia, hypocalcemia, and dissolution of bone. In early renal insufficiency, acid excretion and phosphate reabsorption increase to maintain normal pH. When the GFR decreases by 30% to 40%, progressive metabolic acidosis ensues and tubular secretion of potassium increases. Total-body potassium levels may increase to life-threatening levels, requiring dialysis.

In glomerulosclerosis, distortion of filtration slits and erosion of the glomerular epithelial cells lead to increased fluid transport across the glomerular wall. Large proteins traverse the slits but become trapped in glomerular basement membranes, obstructing the glomerular capillaries. Epithelial and endothelial injury cause proteinuria. Mesangial-cell proliferation, increased production of extracellular matrix, and intraglomerular coagulation cause the sclerosis.

Tubulointerstitial injury occurs from toxic or ischemic tubular damage, as with acute tubular necrosis. Debris and calcium deposits obstruct the tubules. The resulting defective tubular transport is associated with interstitial edema, leukocyte infiltration, and tubular necrosis. Vascular injury causes diffuse or focal ischemia of renal parenchyma, associated with thickening, fibrosis, or focal lesions of renal blood vessels. Decreased blood flow then leads to tubular atrophy, interstitial fibrosis, and functional disruption of glomerular filtration, medullary gradients, and concentration.

The structural changes trigger an inflammatory response. Fibrin deposits begin to form around the interstitium. Microaneurysms result from vascular wall damage and increased pressure secondary to obstruction or hypertension. Eventual loss of the nephron triggers compensatory hyperfunction of uninjured nephrons, which initiates a positive-feedback loop of increasing vulnerability.

Eventually, the healthy glomeruli are so overburdened that they become sclerotic, stiff, and necrotic. Toxins accumulate and potentially fatal changes ensue in all major organ systems.

Extrarenal consequences

Physiologic changes affect more than one system, and the presence and severity of manifestations depend on the duration of renal failure and its response to treatment. In some fluid and electrolyte imbalances, the kidneys can't retain salt, and hyponatremia results. Dry mouth, fatigue, nausea, hypotension, loss of skin turgor, and listlessness can progress to somnolence and confusion. Later, as the number of functioning nephrons decreases, so does the capacity to excrete sodium and potassium. Sodium retention leads to fluid overload and edema; the potassium overload leads to muscle irritability and weakness and life-threatening cardiac arrhythmias.

As the cardiovascular system becomes involved, hypertension occurs, and irregular distant heart sounds may be auscultated if pericardial effusion occurs. Bibasilar crackles in the lungs and peripheral edema reflect heart failure.

Pulmonary changes include reduced macrophage activity and increasing susceptibility to infection. Decreased breath sounds in areas of consolidation reflect the presence of pneumonia. As the pleurae become more involved, the patient may experience pleuritic pain and friction rubs.

Kussmaul's respirations may be noted as a result of metabolic acidosis. The GI mucosa becomes inflamed and ulcerated, and gums may also be ulcerated and bleeding. Stomatitis, uremic fetor (an ammonia smell to the breath), hiccups, peptic ulcer, and pancreatitis in end-stage renal failure are believed to be due to retention of metabolic acids and other metabolic waste products. Malnutrition may be secondary to anorexia, malaise, and reduced dietary intake of protein. The reduced protein intake also affects capillary fragility and results in decreased immune functioning and poor wound healing.

Normochromic normocytic anemia and platelet disorders with prolonged bleeding time ensue. Diminished erythropoietin secretion leads to reduced RBC production in the bone marrow. Uremic toxins associated with CRF shorten RBC survival time. The patient experiences lethargy and dizziness.

Demineralization of the bone (renal osteodystrophy) manifested by bone pain and pathologic fractures is due to several factors:

- decreased renal activation of vitamin D, decreasing dietary calcium absorption
- phosphate retention resulting in decreased serum calcium
- increased parathyroid hormone (PTH) circulation due to decreased urinary excretion of phosphorus.

The skin acquires a grayish-yellow tint as urine pigments (urochromes) accumulate. Inflammatory mediators released by retained toxins in the skin cause pruritus. Uric acid and other substances in sweat crystallize and accumulate on the skin as uremic frost. A high plasma calcium level is also associated with pruritus.

Restless leg syndrome (abnormal sensation and spontaneous movement of the feet and lower legs), muscle weakness, and decreased deep tendon reflexes are believed to result from the effect of toxins on the nervous system.

Alert Restless leg syndrome is one of the first signs of peripheral neuropathy. This condition eventually progresses to paresthesia and motor nerve dysfunction (bilateral footdrop) unless dialysis is initiated.

CRF increases the risk of death from infection. This failure is related to suppression of cell-mediated immunity and a reduction in the number and function of lymphocytes and phagocytes.

All hormone levels are impaired in excretion and activation. Females may be anovulatory, amenorrheic, or unable to carry pregnancy to full term. Males tend to have decreased sperm counts and impotence.

CLINICAL FINDINGS

- Hypervolemia due to sodium retention
- Hyperphosphatemia and hyperkalemia due to electrolyte imbalance
- Hypocalcemia due to decreased intestinal calcium absorption and hyperphosphatemia
- Azotemia due to retention of nitrogenous wastes
- Metabolic acidosis due to loss of bicarbonate
- Bone and muscle pain and fractures caused by calcium-phosphorus imbalance and consequent PTH imbalances
- Peripheral neuropathy due to accumulation of toxins
- Dry mouth, fatigue, and nausea due to hyponatremia
- Hypotension due to sodium loss
- Altered mental state due to hyponatremia and toxin accumulation
- Irregular heart rate due to hyperkalemia
- Hypertension due to fluid overload
- Gum sores and bleeding due to coagulopathies
- Yellow-bronze skin due to altered metabolic processes
- Dry, scaly skin and severe itching due to uremic frost
- Muscle cramps and twitching, including cardiac irritability, due to hyperkalemia
- Malnutrition, fatigue, erectile dysfunction, decreased libido, and amenorrhea due to uremia
- Kussmaul's respirations due to metabolic acidosis

Alert *Growth retardation in children occurs from endocrine abnormalities induced by renal failure. Impaired bone growth and bowlegs in children are also due to rickets.*

- Infertility, decreased libido, amenorrhea, and impotence due to endocrine disturbances
- GI bleeding, hemorrhage, and bruising due to thrombocytopenia and platelet defects
- Pain, burning, and itching in legs and feet associated with peripheral neuropathy
- Infection related to decreased macrophage activity

TEST RESULTS

Blood study results that help diagnose CRF include:

- decreased arterial pH and bicarbonate, low hemoglobin level and hematocrit
- decreased RBC survival time, mild thrombocytopenia, platelet defects
- elevated blood urea nitrogen, serum creatinine, sodium, and potassium levels
- increased aldosterone secretion related to increased renin production
- hyperglycemia (a sign of impaired carbohydrate metabolism)
- hypertriglyceridemia and low levels of high-density lipoprotein.

Urinalysis results include:

- specific gravity fixed at 1.010
- proteinuria, glycosuria, RBCs, leukocytes, casts, or crystals, depending on the cause.

Other study results used to diagnose CRF include:

- reduced kidney size on kidney-ureter-bladder radiography, excretory urography, nephrotomography, renal scan, or renal arteriography
- renal biopsy to identify underlying disease
- EEG to identify metabolic encephalopathy.

TREATMENT

- Calculated restricted protein diet to limit accumulation of end products of protein metabolism that the kidneys can't excrete
- High-protein diet for patients on continuous peritoneal dialysis
- High-calorie diet to prevent ketoacidosis and tissue atrophy
- Sodium, phosphorus, and potassium restrictions to prevent elevated levels
- Fluid restriction to maintain fluid balance
- Loop diuretics, such as furosemide (Lasix), to maintain fluid balance
- Cardiac glycosides, such as digoxin (Lanoxin), to mobilize fluids causing edema
- Calcium carbonate (Caltrate) or calcium acetate (PhosLo) to treat renal osteodystrophy by binding to and excreting phosphate and supplementing calcium
- Antihypertensives to control blood pressure and edema
- Antiemetics to relieve nausea and vomiting
- Famotidine (Pepcid) or ranitidine (Zantac) to decrease gastric irritation
- Methylcellulose (Citrucel) or docusate sodium (Colace) to prevent constipation
- Iron and folate supplements or an RBC transfusion for anemia
- Synthetic erythropoietin to stimulate the bone marrow to produce RBCs; supplemental iron, conjugated estrogens, and desmopressin (DDAVP) to combat hematologic effects
- Antipruritics, such as diphenhydramine (Benadryl), to relieve itching
- Aluminum hydroxide gel to reduce serum phosphate levels
- Supplementary vitamins, particularly B and D, and essential amino acids
- Dialysis for hyperkalemia and fluid imbalances
- Oral or rectal administration of cation exchange resins, such as sodium polystyrene sulfonate (Kayexalate), and I.V. administration of 50% dextrose, and regular insulin, to reverse hyperkalemia
- Calcium gluconate to protect the heart from hyperkalemia
- Sodium bicarbonate to treat metabolic acidosis
- Emergency pericardiocentesis or surgery for cardiac tamponade
- Intensive dialysis and thoracentesis to relieve pulmonary edema and pleural effusion
- Peritoneal dialysis or hemodialysis to help control end-stage renal disease
- Kidney transplantation (usually the treatment of choice if a donor is available)

NURSING CONSIDERATIONS

- Bathe the patient daily using superfatted soaps, oatmeal baths, and skin lotion without alcohol to ease pruritus. Don't use glycerin-containing soaps because they'll cause skin drying. Give good perineal care using mild soap and water. Pad the side rails to guard against ecchymoses. Turn the patient often, and use a convoluted foam mattress to prevent skin breakdown.
- Brush the patient's teeth often with a soft brush or sponge tip to reduce breath odor. Sugarless hard candy and mouthwash minimize metallic taste in the mouth and alleviate thirst.
- Offer small, palatable meals. Encourage intake of high-calorie foods. Instruct the outpatient to avoid high-sodium and high-potassium foods.

Encourage adherence to fluid and protein restrictions. To prevent constipation, stress the need for exercise and sufficient dietary bulk.

- Watch for hyperkalemia, cramping of the legs and abdomen, diarrhea, muscle irritability, and a weak pulse rate. Monitor the electrocardiogram for tall, peaked T waves; widening QRS segment; prolonged PR interval; and disappearance of P waves, indicating hyperkalemia.

- Assess the patient's hydration status carefully. Check for jugular vein distention, and auscultate the lungs for crackles. Measure daily intake and output carefully, including all body fluids. Record daily weight, presence or absence of thirst, axillary sweat, dryness of tongue, hypertension, and peripheral edema.

- Monitor the patient for bone or joint complications. Prevent pathologic fractures by turning him carefully and ensuring his safety. Provide passive range-of-motion exercises for the bedridden patient.

- Encourage deep breathing and coughing to prevent pulmonary congestion. Listen often for crackles, rhonchi, and decreased breath sounds. Stay alert for clinical effects of pulmonary edema (dyspnea, restlessness, crackles). Administer diuretics and other medications as ordered.

- Maintain strict sterile technique. Use a micropore filter during I.V. therapy. Watch for signs of infection (listlessness, high fever, leukocytosis). Urge the outpatient to avoid contact with infected people during the cold and flu season.

- Carefully observe and document seizure activity. Infuse sodium bicarbonate for acidosis, and sedatives or anticonvulsants for seizures, as ordered. Pad the side rails and keep an oral airway and suction setup at the bedside. Assess the patient's neurologic status periodically, and check for Chvostek's and Trousseau's signs, indicators of a low serum calcium level.

- Observe for signs of bleeding. Watch for prolonged bleeding at puncture sites and at the vascular access site used for hemodialysis. Monitor hemoglobin level and hematocrit, and check stool, urine, and vomitus for blood.

- Report signs of pericarditis, such as a pericardial friction rub and chest pain.

Alert Watch for the disappearance of friction rub, with a drop of 15 to 20 mm Hg in blood pressure during inspiration (paradoxical pulse) — an early sign of pericardial tamponade.

- Schedule medications carefully. Give iron before meals, aluminum hydroxide gels after meals, and antiemetics, as necessary, ½ hour before meals. Administer antihypertensives at appropriate intervals. If the patient requires a rectal infusion of sodium polystyrene sulfonate for a dangerously high potassium level, apply an emollient to soothe the perianal area. Make sure that the sodium polystyrene sulfonate enema is expelled; otherwise, it will cause constipation and won't lower the potassium level. Recommend antacid cookies as an alternative to aluminum hydroxide gels needed to bind GI phosphate.

For dialysis

- Prepare the patient by fully explaining the procedure. Make sure that he understands how to protect and care for the arteriovenous shunt, fistula, or other vascular access. Check the vascular access site every 2 hours for patency and the extremity for adequate blood supply and intact nervous function (temperature, pulse rate, capillary refill, and sensation). If a fistula is present, feel for a thrill and listen for a bruit. Use a gentle touch to avoid occluding the fistula. Report signs of possible clotting. Don't use the arm with the vascular access site to take blood pressure readings, draw blood, or give injections because these procedures may rupture the fistula or occlude blood flow.

● Withhold the 6 a.m. (or morning) dose of antihypertensive on the morning of dialysis, and instruct the outpatient to do the same.

● Use standard precautions when handling body fluids and needles.

● Monitor hemoglobin level and hematocrit. Assess the patient's tolerance of his levels. Some individuals are more sensitive to lower levels than others. Instruct the anemic patient to conserve energy and to rest frequently.

● After dialysis, check for disequilibrium syndrome, a result of sudden correction of blood chemistry abnormalities. Symptoms range from a headache to seizures. Also, check for excessive bleeding from the dialysis site. Apply a pressure dressing or an absorbable gelatin sponge, as indicated. Monitor blood pressure carefully after dialysis.

● A patient undergoing dialysis is under a great deal of stress, as is his family. Refer him to appropriate counseling agencies for assistance in coping with CRF.

Glomerulonephritis

Glomerulonephritis is a bilateral inflammation of the glomeruli, typically following a streptococcal infection.

Acute glomerulonephritis is also called *acute poststreptococcal glomerulonephritis.*

Acute glomerulonephritis is most common in boys ages 3 to 7, but it can occur at any age. Up to 95% of children and 70% of adults recover fully; the rest, especially elderly patients, may progress to chronic renal failure (CRF) within months.

Rapidly progressive glomerulonephritis (RPGN) — also called *subacute, crescentic,* or *extracapillary glomerulonephritis* — most commonly occurs in patients ages 50 to 60. It may be idiopathic or associated with a proliferative glomerular disease such as poststreptococcal glomerulonephritis.

Alert *Goodpasture's syndrome, a type of RPGN, is rare, but occurs most commonly in men ages 20 to 30. (See* chapter 8, Immune system.)

Chronic glomerulonephritis is a slowly progressive disease characterized by inflammation, sclerosis, scarring and, eventually, renal failure. It usually remains undetected until the progressive phase, which is usually irreversible.

CAUSES
Acute and RPGN
● Immunoglobulin (Ig) A nephropathy (Berger's disease)
● Impetigo
● Lipid nephrosis
● Streptococcal infection of the respiratory tract

Chronic glomerulonephritis
● Focal glomerulosclerosis
● Goodpasture's syndrome
● Hemolytic uremic syndrome
● Membranoproliferative glomerulonephritis
● Membranous glomerulopathy
● Poststreptococcal glomerulonephritis

- RPGN
- Systemic lupus erythematosus (SLE)

PATHOPHYSIOLOGY

In nearly all types of glomerulonephritis, the epithelial or podocyte layer of the glomerular membrane is disturbed. This results in a loss of negative charge. (See *Characteristics of glomerular lesions*.)

Acute poststreptococcal glomerulonephritis results from the entrapment and collection of antigen-antibody complexes in the glomerular capillary membranes, after infection with a group A beta-hemolytic streptococcus. The antigens, which are endogenous or exogenous, stimulate antibody formation. Circulating antigen-antibody complexes become lodged in the glomerular capillaries. Glomerular injury occurs when the complexes initiate complement activation and the release of immunologic substances that lyse cells and increase membrane permeability. Antibody damage to basement membranes causes crescent formation. The severity of glomerular damage and renal insufficiency is related to the size, number, location (focal or diffuse), duration of exposure, and type of antigen-antibody complexes.

Antibody or antigen-antibody complexes in the glomerular capillary wall activate biochemical mediators of inflammation — complement, leukocytes, and fibrin. Activated complement attracts neutrophils and monocytes, which release lysosomal enzymes that damage the glomerular cell walls and cause a proliferation of the extracellular matrix, affecting glomerular blood flow. Those events increase membrane permeability, which causes a loss of negative charge across the

---

CHARACTERISTICS OF GLOMERULAR LESIONS

The types of glomerular lesions and their characteristics include:
- diffuse lesions — relatively uniform, involve most or all glomeruli (for example, glomerulonephritis)
- focal lesions — involve only some glomeruli; others normal
- segmental-local — involve only one part of the glomerulus
- mesangial — deposits of immunoglobulins in mesangial matrix
- membranous — thickening of glomerular capillary wall
- proliferative lesions — increased number of glomerular cells
- sclerotic lesions — glomerular scarring from previous glomerular injury
- crescent lesions — accumulation of proliferating cells in Bowman's space.

---

glomerular membrane as well as enhanced protein filtration.

Membrane damage leads to platelet aggregation, and platelet degranulation releases substances that increase glomerular permeability. Protein molecules and red blood cells (RBCs) can now pass into urine, resulting in proteinuria or hematuria. Activation of the coagulation system leads to fibrin deposits in Bowman's space. The result is crescent formation and diminished renal blood flow and glomerular filtration rate (GFR). Glomerular bleeding causes acidic urine, which transforms hemoglobin to methemoglobin and results in brown urine without clots.

The inflammatory response decreases the GFR, which causes fluid retention and decreased urine output, extracellular fluid volume expansion, and hypertension. Gross proteinuria is associated with nephrotic syndrome.

After 10 to 20 years, renal insufficiency develops, followed by nephrotic syndrome and end-stage renal failure.

Goodpasture's syndrome is an RPGN in which antibodies are produced against the pulmonary capillaries and glomerular basement membrane. Diffuse intracellular antibody proliferation in Bowman's space leads to a crescent-shaped structure that obliterates the space. The crescent is composed of fibrin and endothelial, mesangial, and phagocytic cells, which compress the glomerular capillaries, diminish blood flow, and cause extensive scarring of the glomeruli. The GFR is reduced, and renal failure occurs within weeks or months.

IgA nephropathy, or Berger's disease, is usually idiopathic. The plasma IgA level is elevated, and IgA and inflammatory cells are deposited into Bowman's space. The result is sclerosis and fibrosis of the glomerulus and a reduced GFR.

Lipid nephrosis causes disruption of the capillary filtration membrane and loss of its negative charge. This increased permeability with resultant loss of protein leads to nephrotic syndrome.

Systemic diseases, such as hepatitis B virus, SLE, or solid malignant tumors, cause a membranous nephropathy. An inflammatory process causes thickening of the glomerular capillary wall. Increased permeability and proteinuria lead to nephrotic syndrome.

Sometimes the immune complement further damages the glomerular membrane. The damaged and inflamed glomeruli lose the ability to be selectively permeable so that RBCs and proteins filter through as the GFR decreases. Uremic poisoning may result. Renal function may deteriorate, especially in adults with sporadic acute poststreptococcal glomerulonephritis, commonly in the form of glomerulosclerosis accompanied by hypertension. The more severe the disorder, the more likely the occurrence of complications. Hypervolemia leads to hypertension, resulting from either sodium and water retention (caused by the decreased GFR) or inappropriate renin release. The patient develops pulmonary edema and heart failure.

CLINICAL FINDINGS

- Decreased urination or oliguria due to a decreased GFR
- Smoky or coffee-colored urine due to hematuria
- Dyspnea and orthopnea due to pulmonary edema secondary to hypervolemia
- Periorbital edema due to hypervolemia
- Mild to severe hypertension due to a decreased GFR, sodium or water retention, and the inappropriate release of renin
- Bibasilar crackles due to heart failure

Alert *The presenting features of glomerulonephritis in a child may be encephalopathy with seizures and local neurologic deficits. An elderly patient with glomerulonephritis may report vague, nonspecific symptoms, such as nausea, malaise, and arthralgia.*

TEST RESULTS

Blood study results that aid in diagnosis include:
- elevated electrolyte, blood urea nitrogen (BUN), and creatinine levels
- decreased serum protein level
- decreased hemoglobin level in chronic glomerulonephritis
- elevated antistreptolysin-O titers in 80% of patients, elevated streptozyme

(a hemagglutination test that detects antibodies to several streptococcal antigens) and anti-DNase B (a test to determine a previous infection of group A beta-hemolytic streptococcus) titers, and low serum complement levels indicating recent streptococcal infection.

Urinalysis results that help diagnose glomerulonephritis include:
- RBCs, white blood cells, mixed cell casts, and protein indicating renal failure
- fibrin-degradation products and C3 protein.

Alert *Significant proteinuria isn't a common finding in an elderly patient.*

Other test results that help diagnose glomerulonephritis are:
- throat culture showing group A beta-hemolytic streptococcus
- bilateral kidney enlargement on kidney-ureter-bladder X-ray (acute glomerulonephritis)
- symmetrical contraction with normal pelves and calyces (chronic glomerulonephritis) as seen on X-ray
- renal biopsy confirming the diagnosis or assessing renal tissue status.

TREATMENT
- Primary disease treatment to alter immunologic cascade (see *Averting renal failure in glomerulonephritis,* page 248)
- Antibiotics for 7 to 10 days to treat infections contributing to ongoing antigen-antibody response
- Anticoagulants to control fibrin crescent formation in RPGN
- Bed rest to reduce metabolic demands
- Fluid restrictions to decrease edema
- Dietary sodium restriction to prevent fluid retention
- Correction of electrolyte imbalances
- Loop diuretics, such as metolazone (Zaroxolyn) or furosemide (Lasix), to reduce extracellular fluid overload
- Vasodilators, such as hydralazine (Apresoline), to decrease hypertension
- Dialysis or kidney transplantation for chronic glomerulonephritis progressing to CRF
- Corticosteroids to decrease antibody synthesis and suppress inflammatory response
- Plasmapheresis in RPGN to suppress rebound antibody production, possibly combined with corticosteroids and cyclophosphamide (Cytotan)

NURSING CONSIDERATIONS
- Check the patient's vital signs and electrolyte values. Monitor intake and output and daily weight. Assess renal function daily through serum creatinine, BUN, and urine creatinine clearance levels. Watch for and immediately report signs of acute renal failure (oliguria, azotemia, and acidosis). Monitor for ascites and edema.
- Consult the dietitian to provide a diet high in calories and low in protein, sodium, potassium, and fluids.
- Administer medications as ordered, and provide good skin care (because of pruritus and edema) and oral hygiene. Instruct the patient to continue taking prescribed antihypertensives as scheduled, even if he's feeling better, and to report adverse effects. Advise him to take diuretics in the morning so he won't have to disrupt his sleep to void. Teach him how to assess ankle edema.
- Protect the debilitated patient against secondary infection by providing good nutrition, using good hy-

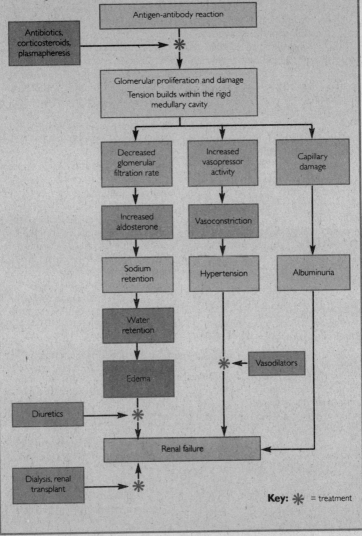

AVERTING RENAL FAILURE IN GLOMERULONEPHRITIS

This flowchart shows pathophysiologic occurrences and the treatments that can alter the course of glomerulonephritis.

Antigen-antibody reaction

Antibiotics, corticosteroids, plasmapheresis ✳

Glomerular proliferation and damage
Tension builds within the rigid medullary cavity

Decreased glomerular filtration rate

Increased vasopressor activity

Capillary damage

Increased aldosterone

Vasoconstriction

Sodium retention

Hypertension

Albuminuria

Water retention

Edema

Vasodilators ✳

Diuretics ✳

Renal failure

Dialysis, renal transplant ✳

Key: ✳ = treatment

gienic technique, and preventing contact with infected people.

- Bed rest is necessary during the acute phase. Allow the patient to gradually resume normal activities as symptoms subside.
- Advise the patient with a history of chronic upper respiratory tract infections to immediately report signs of infection (fever, sore throat).
- Tell the patient that follow-up examinations are necessary to detect CRF. Stress the need for regular blood pressure, urinary protein, and renal function assessments during the convalescent months to detect recurrence. After acute glomerulonephritis, gross hematuria may recur during nonspecific viral infections; abnormal urinary findings may persist for years.
- Encourage pregnant women with a history of glomerulonephritis to have frequent medical evaluations because pregnancy further stresses the kidneys and increases the risk of CRF.
- Help the patient adjust to this illness by encouraging him to express his feelings. Explain all necessary procedures beforehand, and answer the patient's questions about them.

Nephrotic syndrome

Marked proteinuria, hypoalbuminemia, hyperlipidemia, and edema characterize nephrotic syndrome. It results from a defect in the permeability of glomerular vessels. About 75% of all cases result from primary (idiopathic) glomerulonephritis. The prognosis is highly variable, depending on the underlying cause.

Alert *Age has no part in the progression or prognosis of nephrotic syndrome. Primary nephrotic syndrome is found predominantly in the preschool child. Incidence peaks from ages 2 to 3, and is rare after age 8.*

Primary nephrotic syndrome is more common in boys than in girls; incidence is 3 per 100,000 children per year. Some forms of nephrotic syndrome may eventually progress to end-stage renal failure.

CAUSES
- Allergic reactions
- Circulatory diseases, such as heart failure, sickle cell anemia, and renal vein thrombosis
- Collagen-vascular disorders, such as systemic lupus erythematosus and periarteritis nodosa
- Focal glomerulosclerosis
- Hereditary nephritis
- Infections, such as tuberculosis and enteritis
- Lipid nephrosis (nil lesions)

Alert *Lipid nephrosis is the main cause of nephrotic syndrome in children younger than age 8.*

- Membranoproliferative glomerulonephritis
- Membranous glomerulonephritis

Alert *Membranous glomerulonephritis is the most common lesion in adult idiopathic nephrotic syndrome.*

- Metabolic diseases such as diabetes mellitus
- Neoplastic diseases such as multiple myeloma
- Nephrotoxins, such as mercury, gold, and bismuth
- Pregnancy

PATHOPHYSIOLOGY
In lipid nephrosis, the glomeruli appear normal by light microscopy, and some tubules may contain increased lipid deposits. Membranous glomerulonephritis is characterized by the appearance of immune complexes, seen

as dense deposits in the glomerular basement membrane, and by the uniform thickening of the basement membrane. It eventually progresses to renal failure.

Focal glomerulosclerosis can develop spontaneously at any age, can occur after kidney transplantation, or may result from heroin injection. Ten percent of children and up to 20% of adults with nephrotic syndrome develop this condition. Lesions initially affect some of the deeper glomeruli, causing hyaline sclerosis. Involvement of the superficial glomeruli occurs later. These lesions usually cause slowly progressive deterioration in renal function, although remission may occur in children.

Membranoproliferative glomerulonephritis causes slowly progressive lesions in the subendothelial region of the basement membrane. This disorder may follow infection, particularly streptococcal infection, and occurs primarily in children and young adults.

Regardless of the cause, the injured glomerular filtration membrane allows the loss of plasma proteins, especially albumin and immunoglobulin. In addition, metabolic, biochemical, or physiochemical disturbances in the glomerular basement membrane result in the loss of negative charge as well as increased permeability to protein. Hypoalbuminemia results not only from urinary loss, but also from decreased hepatic synthesis of replacement albumin. Increased plasma concentration and low molecular weight accentuate albumin loss. Hypoalbuminemia stimulates the liver to synthesize lipoprotein, with consequent hyperlipidemia, and clotting factors. Decreased dietary intake, as with anorexia, malnutrition, or concomitant disease, further contributes to decreased plasma albumin levels. Loss of immunoglobulin also increases susceptibility to infections.

Extensive proteinuria (more than 3.5 g/day) and a low serum albumin level, secondary to renal loss, lead to low serum colloid osmotic pressure and edema. The low serum albumin level also leads to hypovolemia and compensatory salt and water retention. Consequent hypertension may precipitate heart failure in compromised patients.

CLINICAL FINDINGS

- Periorbital edema due to fluid overload (generally occurs in the morning)
- Mild to severe dependent edema of the ankles or sacrum
- Orthostatic hypotension due to fluid imbalance
- Ascites due to fluid imbalance
- Swollen external genitalia due to edema in dependent areas
- Respiratory difficulty due to pleural effusion
- Anorexia due to edema of intestinal mucosa
- Pallor and shiny skin with prominent veins
- Diarrhea due to edema of intestinal mucosa
- Frothy urine (in children)
- Change in quality of hair related to protein deficiency
- Pneumonia due to susceptibility to infections

TEST RESULTS

- Consistent heavy proteinuria (24-hour protein more than 3.5 mg/dl)
- Urinalysis showing hyaline, granular, and waxy fatty casts and oval fat bodies
- Increased serum cholesterol, phospholipid (especially low-density and

very-low-density lipoproteins), and triglyceride levels and a decreased albumin level
● Renal biopsy provides histologic identification of the lesion

TREATMENT
● The underlying cause is corrected, if possible.
● A nutritious diet is recommended, including 0.6 g of protein/kg of body weight.
● Restricted sodium intake reduces edema.
● Diuretics help to diminish edema.
● Antibiotics aid in treating infection.
● An 8-week course of a corticosteroid, such as prednisone, followed by maintenance therapy or a combination of prednisone and azathioprine (Imuran) or cyclophosphamide (Cytoxan) is recommended.
● Treatment for hyperlipidemia may be unsuccessful.
● Paracentesis is used to treat ascites.
● Thoracentesis is used to treat pleural effusion.

NURSING CONSIDERATIONS
● Frequently check urine protein. (Urine containing protein appears frothy.)
● Measure blood pressure while the patient is supine and while he's standing; immediately report a drop in blood pressure that exceeds 20 mm Hg.
● Monitor and document the location and degree of edema.
● After kidney biopsy, watch for bleeding and shock.
● Monitor intake and output and check weight at the same time each morning — after the patient voids and before he eats — and while he's wearing the same kind of clothing. Ask the dietitian to plan a moderate-protein, low-sodium diet.
● Provide good skin care because the patient with nephrotic syndrome usually has edema.
● To avoid thrombophlebitis, encourage activity and exercise, and provide antiembolism stockings as ordered.
● Watch for and teach the patient and his family how to recognize adverse drug effects, such as bone marrow toxicity from cytotoxic immunosuppressants and cushingoid symptoms (muscle weakness, mental changes, acne, moon face, hirsutism, girdle obesity, purple striae, amenorrhea) from long-term steroid therapy. Other steroid complications include masked infections, increased susceptibility to infections, ulcers, GI bleeding, and steroid-induced diabetes; a steroid crisis may occur if the drug is discontinued abruptly. To prevent GI complications, administer steroids with an antacid or with cimetidine (Tagamet) or ranitidine (Zantac). Explain that steroid adverse effects will subside when therapy stops.
● Offer the patient and his family reassurance and support, especially during the acute phase, when edema is severe and the patient's body image changes.

Neurogenic bladder

All types of bladder dysfunction caused by an interruption of normal bladder innervation by the nervous system are referred to as neurogenic bladder. Other names for this disorder include *neuromuscular dysfunction of the lower urinary tract, neurologic bladder dysfunction,* and *neuropathic bladder.* Neurogenic bladder can be hyperreflexic (hypertonic, spastic, or automatic) or flaccid (hypotonic, atonic, or autonomous).

CAUSES

Many factors can interrupt bladder innervation. Cerebral disorders causing neurogenic bladder include:

- brain tumor (meningioma and glioma)
- dementia
- incontinence associated with aging
- multiple sclerosis
- Parkinson's disease
- stroke.

Spinal cord disease or trauma can also cause neurogenic bladder, including:

- arachnoiditis (inflammation of the membrane between the dura and pia mater) causing adhesions between membranes covering the cord
- cervical spondylosis
- disorders of peripheral innervation, including autonomic neuropathies, due to endocrine disturbances such as diabetes mellitus (most common)
- myelopathies from hereditary or nutritional deficiencies
- poliomyelitis
- spina bifida
- spinal stenosis causing cord compression
- tabes dorsalis (degeneration of the dorsal columns of the spinal cord).

Other causes of neurogenic bladder include:

- acute infectious diseases, such as Guillain-Barré syndrome or transverse myelitis (pathologic changes extending across the spinal cord)
- chronic alcoholism
- collagen diseases such as systemic lupus erythematosus

- distant effects of certain cancers such as primary oat cell carcinoma of the lung
- heavy metal toxicity
- herpes zoster
- metabolic disturbances, such as hypothyroidism or uremia
- sacral agenesis (absence of a completely formed sacrum)
- vascular diseases such as atherosclerosis.

PATHOPHYSIOLOGY

An upper motor neuron lesion (at or above T12) causes spastic neurogenic bladder, with spontaneous contractions of detrusor muscles, increased intravesical voiding pressure, bladder wall hypertrophy with trabeculation, and urinary sphincter spasms. The patient may experience small urine volume, incomplete emptying, and loss of voluntary voiding control. Urinary retention also sets the stage for infection.

A lower motor neuron lesion (at or below S2 to S4) affects the spinal reflex that controls micturition. The result is a flaccid neurogenic bladder with decreased intravesical pressure, and increased bladder capacity, residual urine retention, and poor detrusor contraction. The bladder may not empty spontaneously. The patient experiences the loss of voluntary and involuntary control of urination. Lower motor neuron lesions lead to overflow incontinence. When sensory neurons are interrupted, the patient can't perceive the need to void.

Interruption of the efferent nerves at the cortical, or upper motor neuron, level results in loss of voluntary control. Higher centers also control micturition, and voiding may be incomplete. Sensory neuron interruption leads to dribbling and overflow incon-

TYPES OF NEUROGENIC BLADDER

NEURAL LESION	TYPE	CAUSE
Upper motor	Uninhibited	◆ Lack of voluntary control in infancy ◆ Multiple sclerosis
	Reflex or automatic	◆ Spinal cord transection ◆ Cord tumors ◆ Multiple sclerosis
Lower motor	Autonomous	◆ Sacral cord trauma ◆ Tumors ◆ Herniated disk ◆ Abdominal surgery with transection of pelvic parasympathetic nerves
	Motor paralysis	◆ Lesions at levels S2, S3, S4 ◆ Poliomyelitis ◆ Trauma ◆ Tumors
	Sensory paralysis	◆ Posterior lumbar nerve roots ◆ Diabetes mellitus ◆ Tabes dorsalis

tinence. Altered bladder sensation commonly makes symptoms difficult to discern.

Urine retention contributes to renal calculi as well as infection. Neurogenic bladder can lead to the deterioration of renal function if not promptly diagnosed and treated.

CLINICAL FINDINGS

● Some degree of incontinence, changes in initiation or interruption of micturition, inability to completely empty the bladder
● Frequent urinary tract infections due to urine retention
● Hyperactive autonomic reflexes (autonomic dysreflexia) when the bladder is distended and the lesion is at upper thoracic or cervical level
● Severe hypertension, bradycardia, and vasodilation (blotchy skin) above the level of the lesion
● Piloerection and profuse sweating above the level of the lesion
● Involuntary or frequent, scant urination without a feeling of bladder fullness, due to hyperreflexic neurogenic bladder
● Spontaneous spasms (caused by voiding) of the arms and legs, due to hyperreflexic neurogenic bladder
● Increased anal sphincter tone due to hyperreflexic neurogenic bladder
● Voiding and spontaneous contractions of the arms and legs due to tactile stimulation of the abdomen, thighs, or genitalia
● Overflow incontinence and diminished anal sphincter tone due to flaccid neurogenic bladder
● Greatly distended bladder without feeling of bladder fullness due to sensory impairment (see *Types of neurogenic bladder*)

TEST RESULTS

● Voiding cystourethrography evaluates bladder neck function, vesicoureteral reflux, and continence.

● Urodynamic studies evaluate how urine is stored in the bladder, how well the bladder empties urine, and the rate of movement of urine out of the bladder during voiding.

● Urine flow study (uroflow) shows diminished or impaired urine flow.

● Cystometry evaluates bladder nerve supply, detrusor muscle tone, and intravesical pressures during bladder filling and contraction.

● Urethral pressure profile determines urethral function with respect to the urethra's length and outlet pressure resistance.

● Sphincter electromyelography correlates neuromuscular function of the external sphincter with bladder muscle function during bladder filling and contraction and how well the bladder and urinary sphincter muscles work together.

● Videourodynamic studies correlate visual documentation of bladder function with pressure studies.

● Retrograde urethrography shows strictures and diverticula.

TREATMENT

● Intermittent self-catheterization to empty the bladder

● Anticholinergics and alpha-adrenergic stimulators for the patient with hyperreflexic neurogenic bladder until intermittent self-catheterization is performed

● Terazosin (Hytrin) and doxazosin (Cardura) to facilitate bladder emptying in neurogenic bladder

● Propantheline (Pro-Banthine), flavoxate (Urispas), dicyclomine (Bentyl), imipramine (Tofranil), and pseudoephedrine (Sudafed) to facilitate urine storage

● Surgery to correct structural impairment through transurethral resection of the bladder neck, urethral dilatation, external sphincterotomy, or urinary diversion procedures

● Implantation of an artificial urinary sphincter, if permanent incontinence follows surgery

NURSING CONSIDERATIONS

● Explain diagnostic tests clearly so the patient understands the procedure, the time involved, and the possible results. Assure the patient that the lengthy diagnostic process is necessary to identify the most effective treatment plan. After the treatment plan is chosen, explain it to the patient in detail.

● Use strict sterile technique during insertion of an indwelling catheter (a temporary measure to drain the incontinent patient's bladder). Don't interrupt the closed drainage system for any reason. Obtain urine specimens with a syringe and small-bore needle inserted through the aspirating port of the catheter itself (below the junction of the balloon instillation site). Irrigate in the same manner if ordered.

● Clean the catheter insertion site with soap and water at least twice per day. Don't allow the catheter to become encrusted. Use a sterile applicator to apply antibiotic ointment around the meatus after catheter care. Keep the drainage bag below the tubing, and don't raise the bag above the level of the bladder. Clamp the tubing or empty the bag before transferring the patient to a wheelchair or stretcher to prevent accidental urine reflux. If urine output is considerable, empty the bag more frequently than once every 8 hours because bacteria can multiply in standing urine and migrate up the catheter and into the bladder.

● Watch for signs of infection (fever, cloudy or foul-smelling urine). Encourage fluids to prevent calculus formation and infection from urinary stasis. Try to keep the patient as mobile as possible. Perform passive range-of-motion exercises if necessary.

● If a urinary diversion procedure is to be performed, arrange for consultation with an enterostomal therapist, and coordinate the care plans.

● Before discharge, teach the patient and his family evacuation techniques, as necessary (Credé's method, intermittent catheterization). Counsel him regarding sexual activities. The incontinent patient feels distressed. Provide emotional support.

Polycystic kidney disease

Polycystic kidney disease is an inherited disorder characterized by multiple, bilateral, grapelike clusters of fluid-filled cysts that enlarge the kidneys, compressing and eventually replacing functioning renal tissue. (See *Polycystic kidney*.) The disease affects males and females equally and appears in two distinct forms. Autosomal dominant polycystic kidney disease (ADPKD) occurs in 1 in 1,000 to 1 in 3,000 people and accounts for about 10% of end-stage renal disease in the United States. The rare infantile form causes stillbirth or early neonatal death. The adult form has an insidious onset but usually becomes obvious between ages 30 to 50; rarely, it remains asymptomatic until the patient is in his 70s.

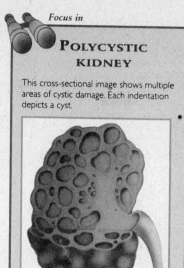

Focus in

POLYCYSTIC KIDNEY

This cross-sectional image shows multiple areas of cystic damage. Each indentation depicts a cyst.

Alert *Renal deterioration is more gradual in adults than in infants, but in both age-groups, the disease progresses relentlessly to fatal uremia.*

Prognosis in adults is very variable. Progression may be slow, even after symptoms of renal insufficiency appear. After uremia symptoms develop, polycystic disease is usually fatal within 4 years unless the patient receives dialysis. Three genetic variants of the autosomal dominant form have been identified. (See "Pathophysiology.")

CAUSES
Inherited from:
● autosomal dominant trait (adult type)
● autosomal recessive trait (infantile type).

PATHOPHYSIOLOGY

ADPKD occurs as ADPKD-1, mapped to the short arm of chromosome 16 and encoded for a 4,300–amino-acid protein; ADPKD-2, mapped to the short arm of chromosome 4 with later onset of symptoms; and a third variety not yet mapped. Autosomal recessive polycystic kidney disease occurs in 1 in 10,000 to 1 in 40,000 live births, and has been localized to chromosome 6.

Grossly enlarged kidneys are caused by multiple spherical cysts, a few millimeters to centimeters in diameter, that contain straw-colored or hemorrhagic fluid. The cysts are distributed evenly throughout the cortex and medulla. Hyperplastic polyps and renal adenomas are common. Renal parenchyma may have varying degrees of tubular atrophy, interstitial fibrosis, and nephrosclerosis. The cysts cause elongation of the pelvis, flattening of the calyces, and indentations in the kidney.

Characteristically, an affected infant shows signs of respiratory distress, heart failure and, eventually, uremia and renal failure. Accompanying hepatic fibrosis and intrahepatic bile duct abnormalities may cause portal hypertension and bleeding varices.

In most cases, about 10 years after symptoms appear, progressive compression of kidney structures by the enlarging mass causes renal failure.

Cysts also form elsewhere — such as on the liver, spleen, pancreas, and ovaries. Intracranial aneurysms, colonic diverticula, and mitral valve prolapse also occur.

In the autosomal recessive form, death in the neonatal period is most commonly due to pulmonary hypoplasia.

Alert *A few infants with this disease survive for 2 years, and then die of hepatic complications or renal, heart, or respiratory failure.*

CLINICAL FINDINGS

In neonates

- Pronounced epicanthic folds (vertical fold of skin on either side of the nose); a pointed nose; small chin; and floppy, low-set ears (Potter facies), due to genetic abnormalities
- Huge, bilateral, symmetrical masses on the flanks that are tense and can't be transilluminated, due to kidney enlargement
- Respiratory distress
- Uremia, due to renal failure

In adults

- Hypertension, due to activation of the renin-angiotensin system
- Lumbar pain, due to an enlarging kidney mass
- Widening abdominal girth, due to enlarged kidneys
- Swollen or tender abdomen caused by the enlarging kidney mass, worsened by exertion and relieved by lying down
- Grossly enlarged kidneys on palpation

TEST RESULTS

- Excretory or retrograde urography shows enlarged kidneys, with elongation of the pelvis, flattening of the calyces, and indentations in the kidney caused by cysts.
- Excretory urography of the neonate shows poor excretion of contrast medium.
- Ultrasonography, tomography, and radioisotope scans shows kidney enlargement and cysts; tomography, computed tomography, and magnetic

resonance imaging shows multiple areas of cystic damage.
- Urinalysis and creatinine clearance tests show nonspecific results indicating abnormalities.

TREATMENT
- Antibiotics for infections
- Adequate hydration to maintain fluid balance
- Surgical drainage of cystic abscess or retroperitoneal bleeding
- Surgery for intractable pain (uncommon symptom) or analgesics for abdominal pain
- Dialysis or kidney transplantation for progressive renal failure
- Nephrectomy not recommended (Polycystic kidney disease occurs bilaterally, and the infection could recur in the remaining kidney.)

NURSING CONSIDERATIONS
- Because polycystic kidney disease is usually relentlessly progressive, comprehensive patient teaching and emotional support are essential.
- Refer the young adult patient or the parents of infants with polycystic kidney disease for genetic counseling. Parents will probably have many questions about the risk to other offspring.
- Provide supportive care to minimize associated symptoms. Carefully assess the patient's lifestyle and his physical and mental status; determine how rapidly the disease is progressing. Use this information to plan individualized patient care.
- Acquaint yourself with all aspects of end-stage renal disease, including dialysis and transplantation, so you can provide appropriate care and patient teaching as the disease progresses.

- Explain all diagnostic procedures to the patient or to his family if the patient is an infant. Before beginning excretory urography or other procedures that use an iodine-based contrast medium, determine whether the patient has ever had an allergic reaction to iodine or shellfish. Even if the patient has no history of allergy, watch him for an allergic reaction during and after undergoing the procedures.
- Administer antibiotics, as ordered, for urinary tract infection. Stress to the patient the need to take the medication exactly as prescribed, even if symptoms are minimal or absent.

Renal calculi

Renal calculi, or stones (nephrolithiasis), can form anywhere in the urinary tract, although they most commonly develop on the renal pelves or calyces. They may vary in size and may be solitary or multiple. (See *Renal calculi,* page 258.)

Renal calculi are more common in men than in women and rarely occur in children. Calcium calculi generally occur in middle-age men with a family history of calculus formation.

Renal calculi rarely occur in blacks. They're prevalent in certain geographic areas, such as the southeastern United States (called the "stone belt"), possibly because a hot climate promotes dehydration and concentrates calculus-forming substances, or because of regional dietary habits.

CAUSES
Although the exact cause is unknown, predisposing factors of renal calculi include:

RENAL CALCULI

Renal calculi vary in size and type. Small calculi may remain in the renal pelvis or pass down the ureter. A staghorn calculus (a cast of the calyceal and pelvic collecting system) may develop from a calculus that stays in the kidney.

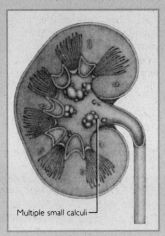

Multiple small calculi

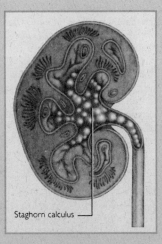

Staghorn calculus

- changes in urine pH (calcium carbonate calculi, high pH; uric acid calculi, lower pH)
- dehydration
- dietary factors
- gout (a disease of increased uric acid production or decreased excretion)
- immobilization causing calcium to be released into the blood, which is filtered by the kidneys
- infection
- metabolic factors
- obstruction to urine flow leading to stasis in the urinary tract
- renal disease.

PATHOPHYSIOLOGY

The major types of renal calculi are calcium oxalate and calcium phosphate, accounting for 75% to 80% of calculi; struvite (magnesium, ammonium, and phosphate), 15%; and uric acid, 7%. Cystine calculi are relatively rare, making up 1% of all renal calculi.

Calculi form when substances that are normally dissolved in urine, such as calcium oxalate and calcium phosphate, precipitate. Dehydration may lead to renal calculi as calculus-forming substances concentrate in urine.

Calculi form around a nucleus or nidus in the appropriate environment. A crystal evolves in the presence of calculus-forming substances (calcium oxalate, calcium carbonate, magnesium, ammonium, phosphate, or uric acid) and becomes trapped in the urinary tract, where it attracts other crystals to form a calculus. A high urine saturation of these substances encourages crystal formation and results in calculus growth.

Calculi may be composed of different substances, and urine pH affects the solubility of many calculus-forming substances. Formation of calcium oxalate and cystine calculi is independent of urine pH.

Calculi may occur on the papillae, renal tubules, calyces, renal pelves, ureter, or bladder. Many calculi are less than 5 mm in diameter and are usually passed in urine. Staghorn calculi can continue to grow in the pelvis, extending to the calyces, forming a branching calculus, and ultimately resulting in renal failure if not surgically removed.

Calcium calculi are the smallest. Most are calcium oxalate or a combination of oxalate and phosphate. Although 80% are idiopathic, they commonly occur with hyperuricosuria (a high level of uric acid in urine). Prolonged immobilization can lead to bone demineralization, hypercalciuria, and calculus formation. In addition, hyperparathyroidism, renal tubular acidosis, and excessive intake of vitamin D or dietary calcium may predispose the patient to renal calculi.

Struvite calculi are typically precipitated by an infection, particularly with *Pseudomonas* or *Proteus* species. These urea-splitting organisms are more common in women. Struvite calculi can destroy renal parenchyma.

Gout results in high uric acid production, hyperuricosuria, and uric acid calculi. Diets high in purine (such as meat, fish, and poultry) elevate the uric acid level in the body. Regional enteritis and ulcerative colitis can precipitate uric acid calculi formation. These diseases commonly result in the loss of fluid and bicarbonate, leading to metabolic acidosis. Acidic urine enhances the formation of uric acid calculi.

Cystinuria is a rare hereditary disorder in which a metabolic error causes decreased tubular reabsorption of cystine. This causes an increased amount of cystine in urine. Because cystine is a relatively insoluble substance, its presence contributes to calculus formation.

Infected, scarred tissue may be an ideal site for calculus development. In addition, infected calculi (usually magnesium ammonium phosphate or staghorn calculi) may develop if bacteria serve as the nucleus in calculus formation.

Urinary stasis allows calculus constituents to collect and adhere and encourages infection, which compounds the obstruction.

Calculi may either enter the ureter or remain in the renal pelvis, where they damage or destroy renal parenchyma and may cause pressure necrosis.

In ureters, calculi cause obstruction with resulting hydronephrosis and tend to recur. Intractable pain and serious bleeding also can result from calculi and the damage they cause. Large, rough calculi occlude the opening to the ureteropelvic junction and increase the frequency and force of peristaltic contractions, causing hematuria from trauma. The patient usually reports pain traveling from the costovertebral angle to the flank and then to the suprapubic region and external genitalia (classic renal colic pain). Pain intensity fluctuates and may be excruciating at its peak. The patient with calculi in the renal pelvis and calyces may report a constant dull pain. He may also report back pain if calculi are causing obstruction within a kidney and severe abdominal pain from calculi traveling down a ureter. Infection can develop in static urine or after trauma as the calculus abrades surfaces. If the calculus lodges and blocks urine, hydronephrosis can occur.

CLINICAL FINDINGS

- Mild to severe flank pain resulting from obstruction
- Nausea with or without vomiting
- Fever and chills from infection
- Hematuria when calculi abrade a ureter
- Abdominal distention
- Urinary frequency, hesitancy and dysuria
- Anuria from bilateral obstruction or obstruction of a patient's only kidney

TEST RESULTS

- Kidney-ureter-bladder (KUB) radiography shows most renal calculi.
- Excretory urography helps confirm the diagnosis and determine the size and location of calculi.
- Computed tomography scan of the kidney diagnoses ureterolithiasis.
- Kidney ultrasonography detects obstructive changes, such as unilateral or bilateral hydronephrosis and radiolucent calculi, not seen on KUB radiography.
- Urine culture shows pyuria, a sign of urinary tract infection, and detects the causative agent.
- Twenty-four–hour urine collection reveals calcium oxalate, phosphorus, and uric acid excretion levels.
- Calculus analysis shows mineral content.
- Serial blood calcium and phosphorus levels show hyperparathyroidism and increased calcium, relative to normal serum protein.
- Blood protein level determines the level of free calcium unbound to protein.

TREATMENT

- Increased fluid intake to more than 3 qt (3 L)/day to promote hydration

- Antimicrobial agents to treat infection, varying with the cultured organism
- Analgesics, such as morphine, for pain
- Diuretics to prevent urinary stasis and further calculus formation; thiazides to decrease calcium excretion into urine
- Methenamine (Urex) to suppress calculus formation when infection is present
- A low-calcium diet to prevent recurrence
- Oxalate-binding cholestyramine (Questran) for absorptive hypercalciuria
- Parathyroidectomy for hyperparathyroidism
- Allopurinol (Zyloprim) for uric acid calculi
- Daily small doses of ascorbic acid to acidify urine
- Cystoscope with manipulation of the calculus to remove renal calculi too large for natural passage
- Percutaneous ultrasonic lithotripsy and extracorporeal shock wave lithotripsy or laser therapy to shatter the calculus into fragments for removal by suction or natural passage
- Surgical removal of cystine calculi or large calculi or placement of urinary diversion around the calculus to relieve obstruction

NURSING CONSIDERATIONS

- To aid diagnosis, maintain a 24- to 48-hour record of urine pH, with nitrazine pH paper; strain all urine through gauze or a tea strainer, and save all solid material recqvered for analysis.
- To facilitate spontaneous passage of calculi, encourage the patient to walk and promote intake of fluids to maintain a urine output of 2 to 4 qt

(2 to 4 L)/day (urine should be very dilute and colorless). To help acidify urine, offer fruit juices, particularly cranberry juice. If the patient can't drink the required amount of fluid, give I.V. fluids. Record intake, output, and daily weight to assess fluid status and renal function.

● Stress the importance of proper diet and compliance with drug therapy. For example, if the patient's calculus is caused by a hyperuricemic condition, advise the patient or whoever prepares his meals which foods are high in purine.

● If surgery is necessary, give reassurance by supplementing and reinforcing what the surgeon has told the patient about the procedure. Emphasize the fact that the body can adapt well to one kidney if kidney removal is necessary.

● After surgery, the patient will probably have an indwelling catheter or a nephrostomy tube. Unless one of his kidneys was removed, expect bloody drainage from the catheter. Never irrigate the catheter without a physician's order. Check dressings regularly for bloody drainage, and report suspected hemorrhage (excessive drainage, rising pulse rate). Use sterile technique when changing dressings or providing catheter care.

● Watch for signs of infection (rising fever, chills), and give antibiotics as ordered. To prevent pneumonia, encourage frequent position changes, and have the patient walk as soon as possible. Teach the patient to splint the incision and thereby facilitate deep-breathing and coughing exercises.

● Before discharge, teach the patient and his family the importance of following the prescribed dietary and medication regimens to prevent recurrence of calculi. Encourage increased fluid intake. If appropriate, show the patient how to check his urine pH, and instruct him to keep a daily record. Tell him to immediately report symptoms of acute obstruction (pain, inability to void).

6

ENDOCRINE SYSTEM

The endocrine system consists of glands, specialized cell clusters, hormones, and target tissues. The glands and cell clusters secrete hormones and chemical transmitters in response to stimulation from the nervous system and other sites. Together with the nervous system, the endocrine system regulates and integrates the body's metabolic activities and maintains internal homeostasis. Each target tissue has receptors for specific hormones. Hormones connect with the receptors, and the resulting hormone-receptor complex triggers the target cell's response.

Common dysfunctions of the endocrine system are classified as hypofunction and hyperfunction, inflammation, and tumor.

Addison's disease (adrenal hypofunction)

Adrenal hypofunction is classified as primary or secondary. Primary adrenal hypofunction or insufficiency (Addison's disease) originates within the adrenal gland and is characterized by the decreased secretion of mineralocorticoids, glucocorticoids, and androgens. Secondary adrenal hypofunction is due to a disorder outside the gland such as impaired pituitary secretion of corticotropin. It's characterized by decreased glucocorticoid secretion. The secretion of aldosterone, the major mineralocorticoid, is commonly unaffected.

Addison's disease is relatively uncommon and can occur at any age and in both sexes. Secondary adrenal hypofunction occurs when a patient abruptly stops long-term exogenous steroid therapy or when the pituitary gland is injured by a tumor or by infiltrative or autoimmune processes — these occur when circulating antibodies react specifically against adrenal tissue, causing inflammation and infiltration of the cells by lymphocytes. With early diagnosis and adequate replacement therapy, the prognosis for primary and secondary adrenal hypofunction is good.

Adrenal crisis (addisonian crisis), a critical deficiency of mineralocorticoids and glucocorticoids, generally follows acute stress, sepsis, trauma, surgery, or the omission of steroid therapy in patients who have chronic adrenal insufficiency. Adrenal crisis is a medical emergency that needs immediate, vigorous treatment.

Autoimmune Addison's disease is most common in white females, and a genetic predisposition is likely. It's more common in patients with a familial predisposition to autoimmune endocrine diseases. Most people with Addison's disease are diagnosed in their third to fifth decades.

CAUSES
Primary hypofunction
- Addison's disease (most common), causing destruction of more than 90% of both adrenal glands (usually due to an autoimmune process in which circulating antibodies react specifically against the adrenal tissue)
- Bilateral adrenalectomy
- Family history of autoimmune disease (may predispose the patient to Addison's disease and other endocrinopathies)
- Hemorrhage into the adrenal gland
- Infections (histoplasmosis, cytomegalovirus [CMV])
- Neoplasms
- Tuberculosis (once the chief cause, now responsible for less than 20% of adult cases)

Secondary hypofunction (glucocorticoid deficiency)
- Hypopituitarism (causing decreased corticotropin secretion)
- Abrupt withdrawal of long-term corticosteroid therapy (Long-term exogenous corticosteroid stimulation suppresses pituitary corticotropin secretion, resulting in adrenal gland atrophy.)
- Removal of a corticotropin-secreting tumor

Adrenal crisis
- Exhausted body stores of glucocorticoids in a person with adrenal hypofunction after trauma, surgery, or other physiologic stress

PATHOPHYSIOLOGY
Addison's disease is a chronic condition that results from the partial or complete destruction of the adrenal cortex. It manifests as a clinical syndrome in which the symptoms are associated with deficient production of adrenocortical hormones, cortisol, aldosterone, and androgens. High levels of corticotropin and corticotropin-releasing hormone (CRH) accompany a low glucocorticoid level.

Corticotropin acts primarily to regulate the adrenal release of glucocorticoids (primarily cortisol); mineralocorticoids, including aldosterone; and sex steroids that supplement those produced by the gonads. Corticotropin secretion is controlled by CRH from the hypothalamus and by negative feedback control by the glucocorticoids.

Addison's disease involves all zones of the cortex, causing deficiencies of adrenocortical secretions, glucocorticoids, androgens, and mineralocorticoids.

Manifestations of adrenocortical hormone deficiency become apparent when 90% of the functional cells in both glands are lost. Usually, cellular atrophy is limited to the cortex, although medullary involvement may occur, resulting in catecholamine deficiency. Cortisol deficiency causes decreased liver gluconeogenesis (formation of glucose from molecules that aren't carbohydrates). The resulting low blood glucose levels can become dangerously low in patients who take insulin routinely.

Aldosterone deficiency causes increased renal sodium loss and enhances potassium reabsorption. Sodium excretion causes a reduction in water volume that leads to hypotension. Patients with Addison's disease may have normal blood pressure when supine, but show marked hypotension and tachycardia after standing for several minutes. Low plasma volume and arteriolar pressure stimulate renin release and a resulting increased production of angiotensin II.

Androgen deficiency may decrease hair growth in axillary and pubic areas as well as on the extremities of women. The metabolic effects of testicular androgens make such hair growth less noticeable in men.

Addison's disease is a decrease in the biosynthesis, storage, or release of adrenocortical hormones. In about 80% of patients, an autoimmune process causes partial or complete destruction of both adrenal glands. Autoimmune antibodies can block the corticotropin receptor or bind with corticotropin, preventing it from stimulating adrenal cells. Infection is the second most common cause of Addison's disease, specifically tuberculosis, which causes about 20% of cases.

Other diseases that can cause Addison's disease include acquired immunodeficiency syndrome, systemic fungal infections, CMV, adrenal tumor, and metastatic cancers. Infection can impair cellular function and affect corticotropin at any stage of regulation.

CLINICAL FINDINGS
Primary hypofunction
- Weakness
- Fatigue
- Weight loss
- Nausea, vomiting, and anorexia

- Conspicuous bronze color of the skin, especially in the creases of the hands and over the metacarpophalangeal joints (hand and finger), elbows, and knees
- Darkening of scars, areas of vitiligo (absence of pigmentation), and increased pigmentation of the mucous membranes, especially the buccal mucosa, due to decreased secretion of cortisol, causing simultaneous secretion of excessive amounts of corticotropin and melanocyte-stimulating hormone by the pituitary gland
- Associated cardiovascular abnormalities, including orthostatic hypotension, decreased cardiac size and output, and a weak, irregular pulse
- Decreased tolerance for even minor stress
- Fasting hypoglycemia due to decreased gluconeogenesis
- Craving for salty food due to decreased mineralocorticoid secretion (which normally causes salt retention)

Secondary hypofunction
- Similar to primary hypofunction, but without hyperpigmentation due to low corticotropin and melanocyte-stimulating hormone levels
- Possibly no hypotension and electrolyte abnormalities due to fairly normal aldosterone secretion
- Usually normal androgen secretion

Addisonian crisis
- Profound weakness and fatigue
- Nausea, vomiting, and dehydration
- Hypotension
- High fever followed by hypothermia (occasionally)

TEST RESULTS
The following tests help diagnose adrenal hypofunction:

- Plasma cortisol levels confirm adrenal insufficiency (corticotropin stimulation test to differentiate between primary and secondary adrenal hypofunction).
- Metyrapone test confirms suspicion of secondary adrenal hypofunction. (Oral or I.V. metyrapone blocks cortisol production and should stimulate the release of corticotropin from the hypothalamic-pituitary system; in Addison's disease, the hypothalamic-pituitary system responds normally and plasma corticotropin levels are high, but because the adrenal glands are destroyed, plasma concentrations of the cortisol precursor 11-deoxycortisol increase, as do urinary 17-hydroxycorticosteroids.)
- Rapid corticotropin stimulation test by I.V. or I.M. administration of cosyntropin (Cortrosyn), a synthetic form of corticotropin, after baseline sampling for cortisol and corticotropin (samples drawn for cortisol 30 and 60 minutes after injection), differentiates between primary and secondary adrenal hypofunction. A low corticotropin level indicates a secondary disorder. An elevated level suggests a primary disorder.

In a patient with typical Addisonian symptoms, the following laboratory findings strongly suggest acute adrenal insufficiency:
- decreased plasma cortisol level (less than 10 mcg/dl in the morning; less in the evening)
- decreased serum sodium and fasting blood glucose levels
- increased serum potassium, calcium, and blood urea nitrogen levels
- elevated hematocrit; increased lymphocyte and eosinophil counts
- X-rays showing adrenal calcification if the cause is infectious.

TREATMENT

- Lifelong corticosteroid replacement, usually with cortisone acetate or hydrocortisone (Cortef), both of which have a mineralocorticoid effect (primary or secondary adrenal hypofunction)
- Oral fludrocortisone (Florinef), a synthetic mineralocorticoid, to prevent dangerous dehydration, hypotension, hyponatremia, and hyperkalemia (Addison's disease)
- I.V. bolus of hydrocortisone, 100 mg every 6 hours for 24 hours; then, 50 to 100 mg I.M. or diluted with dextrose in saline solution and given I.V. until the patient's condition stabilizes; up to 300 mg/day of hydrocortisone and 3 to 5 qt (3 to 5 L) of I.V. saline and glucose solutions may be needed (adrenal crisis)
- With proper treatment, adrenal crisis usually subsiding quickly; blood pressure stabilizing, and water and sodium levels returning to normal; after the crisis, maintenance doses of hydrocortisone preserving physiologic stability

NURSING CONSIDERATIONS
For adrenal crisis
- Monitor the patient's vital signs carefully, especially for hypotension, volume depletion, and other signs of shock (decreased level of consciousness and urine output). Watch for hyperkalemia before treatment and for hypokalemia after treatment (from excessive mineralocorticoid effect). Watch for cardiac arrhythmias (may be caused by a serum potassium disturbance).
- If the patient also has diabetes, check blood glucose levels periodically because steroid replacement may require an adjustment of the insulin dosage.

- Record weight and intake and output carefully because the patient may have volume depletion. Until the onset of the mineralocorticoid effect, encourage fluids to replace excessive fluid loss.

For maintenance steroid therapy

- Arrange for a diet that maintains sodium and potassium balances.
- If the patient is anorexic, suggest six small meals per day to increase calorie intake. Ask the dietitian to provide a diet high in protein and carbohydrates. Keep a late-morning snack available in case the patient becomes hypoglycemic.
- Observe the patient receiving steroids for cushingoid signs such as fluid retention around the eyes and face. Watch for fluid and electrolyte imbalance, especially if the patient is receiving mineralocorticoids. Monitor weight and check blood pressure to assess body fluid status. Remember, steroids administered in the late afternoon or evening may cause stimulation of the central nervous system and insomnia. Check for petechiae because the patient can bruise easily.
- If the patient receives glucocorticoids alone, observe for orthostatic hypotension or electrolyte abnormalities, which may indicate a need for mineralocorticoid therapy.
- Explain that lifelong steroid therapy is necessary.
- Teach the patient the symptoms of steroid overdose (swelling, weight gain) and underdose (lethargy, weakness).
- Tell the patient that the dosage may need to be increased during times of stress (when he has a cold, for example).

- Warn that infection, injury, or profuse sweating in hot weather may precipitate adrenal crisis.
- Instruct the patient to always carry a medical identification card stating that he takes a steroid and giving the name of the drug and the dosage.
- Teach the patient and his family how to give a hydrocortisone injection.
- Tell the patient to keep an emergency kit available containing hydrocortisone in a prepared syringe for use in times of stress.
- Explain to the patient the importance of taking antacids while on steroids. Antacids will help to decrease gastric irritation caused by steroids.
- Warn the patient that stress may necessitate additional cortisone to prevent adrenal crisis. Review stress management techniques. Encourage adequate rest and nutrition.

Cushing's syndrome

Cushing's syndrome is a cluster of clinical abnormalities caused by excessive adrenocortical hormones (particularly cortisol) or related corticosteroids and, to a lesser extent, androgens and aldosterone. Cushing's disease (pituitary corticotropin excess) accounts for about 80% of endogenous cases of Cushing's syndrome. Cushing's disease occurs most commonly from ages 20 to 40 and is three to eight times more common in females.

Alert Cushing's syndrome caused by ectopic corticotropin secretion is more common in adult men, with the peak incidence between ages 40 to 60. In 20% of patients, Cushing's syndrome results from a cortisol-secreting tumor. Adrenal tumors, *rather than pituitary tumors, are more common in children, especially girls.*

The annual incidence of endogenous cortisol excess in the United States is 2 to 4 cases per 1 million people per year. The incidence of Cushing's syndrome resulting from exogenous administration of cortisol is uncertain, but it's known to be much greater than that of endogenous types. The prognosis for endogenous Cushing's syndrome is guardedly favorable with surgery, but morbidity and mortality are high without treatment. About 50% of individuals with untreated Cushing's syndrome die within 5 years of its onset as a result of overwhelming infection, suicide, complications from generalized arteriosclerosis (coronary artery disease), and severe hypertensive disease.

CAUSES

- Anterior pituitary hormone (corticotropin) excess
- Autonomous, ectopic corticotropin secretion by a tumor outside the pituitary gland (usually malignant, frequently oat cell carcinoma of the lung)
- Excessive glucocorticoid administration, including prolonged use

PATHOPHYSIOLOGY

Cushing's syndrome is caused by prolonged exposure to excess glucocorticoids. Cushing's syndrome can be exogenous, resulting from chronic glucocorticoid or corticotropin administration, or endogenous, resulting from increased cortisol or corticotropin secretion. Cortisol excess results in anti-inflammatory effects and excessive catabolism of protein and peripheral fat to support hepatic glucose production. The mechanism may be corticotropin dependent (elevated plasma corticotropin levels stimulate the adrenal cortex to produce excess cortisol), or corticotropin independent (excess cortisol is produced by the adrenal cortex or exogenously administered). Excess cortisol suppresses the hypothalamic-pituitary-adrenal axis, also present in ectopic corticotropin-secreting tumors.

CLINICAL FINDINGS

Cushing's syndrome induces changes in many body systems. Signs and symptoms depend on the degree and duration of hypercortisolism, the presence or absence of androgen excess, and additional tumor-related effects (adrenal carcinoma or ectopic corticotropin syndrome). Specific clinical effects vary with the system affected and include:

- diabetes mellitus, with decreased glucose tolerance, fasting hyperglycemia, and glycosuria due to cortisol-induced insulin resistance and increased gluconeogenesis in the liver (endocrine and metabolic systems)
- muscle weakness due to hypokalemia or loss of muscle mass from increased catabolism, pathologic fractures due to decreased bone mineral ionization, osteopenia, osteoporosis, and skeletal growth retardation in children (musculoskeletal system)
- purple striae; facial plethora (edema and blood vessel distention); acne; fat pads above the clavicles, over the upper back (buffalo hump), on the face (moon face), and throughout the trunk (truncal obesity) with slender arms and legs; little or no scar formation; poor wound healing due to decreased collagen and weakened tissues; spontaneous ecchymosis; hyperpigmentation; fungal skin infections (skin)
- peptic ulcer due to increased gastric secretions and pepsin production

and decreased gastric mucus, abdominal pain, increased appetite, weight gain (GI system)
- irritability and emotional lability, ranging from euphoric behavior to depression or psychosis; insomnia due to the cortisol's role in neurotransmission; headache (central nervous system [CNS])
- hypertension due to sodium and secondary fluid retention; heart failure; left ventricular hypertrophy; capillary weakness from protein loss, which leads to bleeding and ecchymosis; dyslipidemia; ankle edema (cardiovascular system)
- increased susceptibility to infection due to decreased lymphocyte production and suppressed antibody formation, decreased resistance to stress, suppressed inflammatory response masking even severe infection (immunologic system)
- fluid retention, increased potassium excretion, ureteral calculi from increased bone demineralization with hypercalciuria (renal and urologic systems)
- increased androgen production with clitoral hypertrophy, mild virilism, hirsutism, and amenorrhea or oligomenorrhea in women; sexual dysfunction; decreased libido; impotence (reproductive system).

TEST RESULTS
- Laboratory tests show hyperglycemia, hypernatremia, glycosuria, hypokalemia, and metabolic alkalosis.
- Urinary free cortisol levels are more than 150 mcg/24 hours.
- Dexamethasone suppression test confirms the diagnosis and determines the cause, possibly an adrenal tumor or a nonendocrine, corticotropin-secreting tumor.

- Blood levels of corticotropin-releasing hormone, corticotropin, and different glucocorticoids diagnose and localize the cause to the pituitary or adrenal gland.

TREATMENT
Differentiation among pituitary, adrenal, and ectopic causes of hypercortisolism is essential for effective treatment, which is specific for the cause of cortisol excess and includes medication, radiation, and surgery. Possible treatments include:
- surgery for tumors of the adrenal and pituitary glands or other tissue such as the lung
- radiation therapy (tumor)
- drug therapy, which may include metyrapone (Metopirone) and aminoglutethimide (Cytadren) to inhibit cortisol synthesis; mitotane (Lysodren) to destroy the adrenocortical cells that secrete cortisol; and bromocriptine (Parlodel) and cyproheptadine to inhibit corticotropin secretion.

NURSING CONSIDERATIONS
- Frequently monitor the patient's vital signs, especially blood pressure. Carefully observe the hypertensive patient who also has cardiac disease.
- Check laboratory reports for hypernatremia, hypokalemia, hyperglycemia, and glycosuria.
- Because the cushingoid patient is likely to retain sodium and water, check for edema and monitor daily weight and intake and output carefully. To minimize weight gain, edema, and hypertension, ask the dietary department to provide a diet that's high in protein and potassium but low in calories, carbohydrates, and sodium.
- Watch for infection, which is a particular problem in Cushing's syndrome.

- If the patient has osteoporosis and is bedridden, perform passive range-of-motion exercises carefully because of the severe risk of pathologic fractures.
- Remember, Cushing's syndrome produces emotional lability. Record incidents that upset the patient, and try to prevent such situations from occurring, if possible. Help him get the physical and mental rest he needs — by sedation, if necessary. Offer support to the emotionally labile patient throughout the difficult testing period.

After bilateral adrenalectomy and pituitary surgery:
- Report wound drainage or temperature elevation to the patient's physician immediately. Use strict sterile technique in changing the patient's dressings.
- Administer analgesics and replacement steroids as ordered.
- Monitor urine output and check the patient's vital signs carefully, watching for signs of shock (decreased blood pressure, increased pulse rate, pallor, and cold, clammy skin). To counteract shock, give vasopressors and increase the rate of I.V. fluids, as ordered. Because mitotane, aminoglutethimide, and metyrapone decrease mental alertness and produce physical weakness, assess the patient's neurologic and behavioral status, and warn him about adverse CNS effects. Also watch for severe nausea, vomiting, and diarrhea.
- Check laboratory reports for hypoglycemia due to the removal of the source of cortisol, a hormone that maintains blood glucose levels.
- Check for abdominal distention and return of bowel sounds after adrenalectomy.
- Check regularly for signs of adrenal hypofunction (orthostatic hypotension, apathy, weakness, fatigue), which indicate that steroid replacement is inadequate.
- In the patient undergoing pituitary surgery, check for and immediately report signs of increased intracranial pressure (confusion, agitation, changes in level of consciousness, nausea, and vomiting). Watch for hypopituitarism.

Provide comprehensive teaching to help the patient cope with lifelong treatment:
- Advise the patient to take replacement steroids with antacids or meals, to minimize gastric irritation. (Usually, it's helpful to take two-thirds of the dosage in the morning and the remaining one-third in the early afternoon to mimic diurnal adrenal secretion.)
- Tell the patient to carry a medical identification card and to immediately report physiologically stressful situations, such as infections, which necessitate an increased dosage.
- Instruct the patient to watch closely for signs of inadequate steroid dosage (fatigue, weakness, dizziness) and of overdosage (severe edema, weight gain). Emphatically warn against abrupt discontinuation of steroid dosage because this may produce a fatal adrenal crisis.

Diabetes insipidus

A disorder of water metabolism, diabetes insipidus results from a deficiency of circulating vasopressin (also called *antidiuretic hormone* [ADH]) or from renal resistance to this hormone. Pituitary diabetes insipidus is caused by a deficiency of vasopressin, and nephrogenic diabetes insipidus is caused by the resistance of renal tubules to vasopressin. Diabetes insipidus is characterized by excessive fluid intake and hypotonic polyuria. A decrease in ADH levels leads to altered intracellular and extracellular fluid control, causing renal excretion of a large amount of urine.

The disorder may start at any age and is slightly more common in men than in women. The incidence is slightly greater today than in the past.

In uncomplicated diabetes insipidus, the prognosis is good with adequate water replacement, and patients usually lead normal lives.

CAUSES

● Acquired, familial, idiopathic, neurogenic, or nephrogenic
● Associated with stroke, hypothalamic or pituitary tumors, and cranial trauma or surgery (neurogenic diabetes insipidus)
● Certain drugs, such as lithium (Eskalith), phenytoin (Dilantin), or alcohol (transient diabetes insipidus)
● X-linked recessive trait or end-stage renal failure (nephrogenic diabetes insipidus, less common)

PATHOPHYSIOLOGY

Diabetes insipidus is related to an insufficiency of ADH, leading to polyuria and polydipsia. The three forms of diabetes insipidus are neurogenic, nephrogenic, and psychogenic.

Neurogenic, or central, diabetes insipidus is an inadequate response of ADH to plasma osmolarity, which occurs when an organic lesion of the hypothalamus, infundibular stem, or posterior pituitary gland partially or completely blocks ADH synthesis, transport, or release. The many organic lesions that can cause diabetes insipidus include brain tumors, hypo-

physectomy, aneurysms, thrombosis, skull fractures, infections, and immunologic disorders. Neurogenic diabetes insipidus has an acute onset. A three-phase syndrome can occur, which involves:
● progressive loss of nerve tissue and increased diuresis
● normal diuresis
● polyuria and polydipsia, the manifestation of permanent loss of the ability to secrete adequate ADH.

Nephrogenic diabetes insipidus is caused by an inadequate renal response to ADH. The collecting duct permeability to water doesn't increase in response to ADH. Nephrogenic diabetes insipidus is generally related to disorders and drugs that damage the renal tubules or inhibit the generation of cyclic adenosine monophosphate in the tubules, preventing activation of the second messenger. Causative disorders include pyelonephritis, amyloidosis, destructive uropathies, polycystic disease, and intrinsic renal disease. Drugs include lithium; general anesthetics, such as methoxyflurane; and demeclocycline (Declomycin). In addition, hypokalemia or hypercalcemia impairs the renal response to ADH. A rare genetic form of nephrogenic diabetes insipidus is an X-linked recessive trait.

Psychogenic diabetes insipidus is caused by an extremely large fluid intake, which may be idiopathic or related to psychosis or sarcoidosis. The polydipsia and resultant polyuria wash out ADH more quickly than it can be replaced. Chronic polyuria may overwhelm the renal medullary concentration gradient, rendering patients partially or totally unable to concentrate urine.

Regardless of the cause, insufficient ADH causes the immediate excretion of large volumes of dilute urine and consequent plasma hyperosmolality. In conscious individuals, the thirst mechanism is stimulated, usually for cold liquids. With severe ADH deficiency, urine output may be greater than 12 L/day, with a low specific gravity. Dehydration develops rapidly if fluids aren't replaced.

CLINICAL FINDINGS
- Polydipsia (cardinal symptom) with fluid intake of 5 to 20 L/day
- Polyuria (cardinal symptom) with urine output of 2 to 20 L/24-hour period of dilute urine
- Nocturia, leading to sleep disturbance and fatigue
- Low urine specific gravity less than 1.006
- Fever
- Changes in level of consciousness
- Hypotension
- Tachycardia
- Headache and visual disturbance due to electrolyte disturbance and dehydration
- Abdominal fullness, anorexia, and weight loss due to almost continuous fluid consumption

TEST RESULTS
- Urinalysis shows almost colorless urine of low osmolality (50 to 200 mOsm/kg, less than that of plasma) and low specific gravity (less than 1.005).
- Water deprivation test identifies vasopressin deficiency, resulting in renal inability to concentrate urine.

TREATMENT
Until the cause of diabetes insipidus can be identified and eliminated, the administration of vasopressin (Pitressin) can control fluid balance and prevent dehydration.

Other medications include:
- hydrochlorothiazide (HCTZ) with a potassium supplement for central and nephrogenic diabetes insipidus
- vasopressin aqueous preparation subcutaneously (subQ) several times daily, effective for only 2 to 6 hours (used as a diagnostic agent and, rarely, in acute disease)
- desmopressin acetate (DDAVP) orally, by nasal spray absorbed through the mucous membranes, or subQ or I.V. injection, effective for 8 to 20 hours depending on the dosage
- chlorpropamide (Diabinese) to decrease thirst sensation in patients with continued hypernatremia.

NURSING CONSIDERATIONS
- Record the patient's fluid intake and output carefully. Maintain adequate fluid intake to prevent severe dehydration. Watch for signs of hypovolemic shock, and monitor blood pressure and heart and respiratory rates regularly, especially during the water deprivation test. Check the patient's weight daily.
- If the patient is dizzy or has muscle weakness, keep the bed side rails up and assist him with walking.
- Monitor urine specific gravity between doses. Watch for a decrease in specific gravity accompanied by increased urine output, indicating the recurrence of polyuria and necessitating administration of the next dose of medication or a dosage increase.
- Monitor serum electrolytes closely. Report abnormal values and treat them as ordered.
- If constipation develops, add more high-fiber foods and fruit juices to the patient's diet. If necessary, obtain an order for a mild laxative such as milk of magnesia.

- Provide meticulous skin and mouth care; apply petroleum jelly as needed to cracked or sore lips.
- Urge the patient to verbalize his feelings. Offer encouragement and a realistic assessment of his situation.
- Help the patient identify strengths that he can use in developing coping strategies.
- Refer the patient and his family to a mental health professional for additional counseling, if necessary.
- Before discharge, teach the patient how to monitor intake and output.
- Instruct the patient to administer desmopressin by nasal spray only after the onset of polyuria — not before — to prevent excess fluid retention and water intoxication.
- Tell the patient to report weight gain, which may indicate that his medication dose is too high. Recurrence of polyuria, as reflected on the intake and output sheet, indicates that the dosage is too low.
- Teach the parents of a child with diabetes insipidus about normal growth and development. Discuss how their child may differ from others at his developmental stage.
- Encourage the parents to help identify the child's strengths and to use them in developing coping strategies.
- Advise the patient with diabetes insipidus to wear a medical identification bracelet and to carry his medication with him at all times.

Diabetes mellitus

Diabetes mellitus is a metabolic disorder characterized by hyperglycemia (elevated serum glucose level) resulting from lack of insulin, lack of insulin effect, or both. Three general classifications are recognized:
- type 1, absolute insulin insufficiency
- type 2, insulin resistance with varying degrees of insulin secretory defects
- gestational diabetes, which emerges during pregnancy.

The onset of type 1 (insulin-dependent) usually occurs before age 30 (although it may occur at any age); the patient is usually thin and requires exogenous insulin and dietary management to achieve control. Conversely, type 2 (non–insulin-dependent) usually occurs in obese adults after age 40 and is treated with diet and exercise in combination with various oral antidiabetic drugs, although treatment may include insulin therapy.

Medical advances permit increased longevity and improved quality of life if the patient carefully monitors blood glucose levels, uses the data to make pharmacologic and lifestyle changes, and uses insulin delivery systems such as subcutaneous insulin pumps. In addition, medications now available enhance the body's own glucose metabolism and insulin sensitivity to optimize glycemic control and prevent progression to long-term complications.

CAUSES
- Environment (infection, diet, toxins, stress)
- Heredity
- Lifestyle changes in genetically susceptible persons
- Pregnancy

PATHOPHYSIOLOGY
In persons genetically susceptible to type 1 diabetes, a triggering event, possibly a viral infection, causes the production of autoantibodies against

the beta cells of the pancreas. The resultant destruction of the beta cells leads to a decline in and ultimate lack of insulin secretion. Insulin deficiency leads to hyperglycemia, enhanced lipolysis (decomposition of fat), and protein catabolism. These characteristics occur when more than 90% of the beta cells have been destroyed.

Type 2 diabetes mellitus is a chronic disease caused by one or more of the following factors: impaired insulin secretion, inappropriate hepatic glucose production, or peripheral insulin receptor insensitivity. Genetic factors are significant, and the onset is accelerated by obesity and a sedentary lifestyle. Again, added stress can be a pivotal factor.

Gestational diabetes mellitus occurs when a woman not previously diagnosed with diabetes shows glucose intolerance during pregnancy. This may occur if placental hormones counteract insulin, causing insulin resistance. Gestational diabetes mellitus is a significant risk factor for the future occurrence of type 2 diabetes mellitus.

Diabetes mellitus can lead to many complications, including microvascular disease (retinopathy, nephropathy, and neuropathy), dyslipidemia, macrovascular disease (coronary, peripheral, and cerebral artery disease), diabetic ketoacidosis, hyperosmolar hyperglycemic nonketotic syndrome, excessive weight gain, skin ulcerations, and chronic renal failure.

CLINICAL FINDINGS

Alert Type 1 diabetes usually presents rapidly, typically with polydipsia, polyuria, polyphagia, weakness, weight loss, dry skin, and ketoacidosis. Type 2 diabetes is typically slow and insidious in onset and usually unaccompanied by symptoms.

● Polyuria and polydipsia due to high serum osmolality caused by high serum glucose levels
● Anorexia (common) or polyphagia (occasional)
● Weight loss (usually 10% to 30%; persons with type 1 diabetes typically have almost no body fat at the time of diagnosis) due to prevention of normal metabolism of carbohydrates, fats, and proteins caused by impaired or absent insulin function
● Headaches, fatigue, lethargy, reduced energy levels, and impaired school and work performance due to low intracellular glucose levels
● Muscle cramps, irritability, and emotional lability due to electrolyte imbalance
● Vision changes, such as blurring, due to glucose-induced swelling
● Numbness and tingling due to neural tissue damage
● Abdominal discomfort and pain due to autonomic neuropathy, causing gastroparesis and constipation
● Nausea, diarrhea, or constipation due to dehydration and electrolyte imbalances or autonomic neuropathy
● Slowly healing skin infections or wounds; itching of skin
● Recurrent candida infections of the vagina or anus

TEST RESULTS

In adult men and nonpregnant women, diabetes mellitus is diagnosed by two of the following criteria obtained more than 24 hours apart, using the same test twice or any combination:
● fasting plasma glucose level of 126 mg/dl or more on at least two occasions
● typical symptoms of uncontrolled diabetes and random blood glucose level of 200 mg/dl or more

● blood glucose level of 200 mg/dl or more 2 hours after ingesting 75 g of oral dextrose.

In pregnant women, gestational diabetes may be diagnosed by:
● elevated blood glucose levels at least twice during an oral glucose tolerance test.

TREATMENT

Effective treatment of all types of diabetes mellitus optimizes blood glucose control and decreases complications.

Type I diabetes

● Insulin replacement, meal planning, and exercise (insulin replacement therapies include mixed-dose, split mixed-dose, and multiple daily injection regimens and continuous subcutaneous insulin infusions)
● Pancreas transplantation (currently requires chronic immunosuppression) (see *Treatment of type 1 diabetes mellitus*)

Type 2 diabetes

● Oral antidiabetic drugs to stimulate endogenous insulin production, increase insulin sensitivity at the cellular level, suppress hepatic gluconeogenesis, and delay GI absorption of carbohydrates (drug combinations may be used)

Both types

● Careful monitoring of blood glucose levels
● Individualized meal plan designed to meet nutritional needs, control blood glucose and lipid levels, and reach and maintain appropriate body weight (plan to be followed consistently with meals eaten at regular times)
● Weight reduction (obese patient with type 2 diabetes mellitus) or high calorie allotment, depending on growth stage and activity level (type 1 diabetes mellitus)

Gestational diabetes

● Medical nutrition therapy
● Injectable insulin if glucose isn't achieved with diet alone (because oral antidiabetic agents are teratogenic and, therefore, are contraindicated during pregnancy)
● Postpartum counseling to address the high risk of gestational diabetes in subsequent pregnancies and type 2 diabetes later in life
● Regular exercise and prevention of weight gain to help prevent type 2 diabetes

NURSING CONSIDERATIONS

● Stress the importance of complying with the prescribed treatment program.
● Tailor your teaching to the patient's needs, abilities, and developmental stage. Include diet; purpose, administration, and possible adverse effects of medications; exercise; monitoring; hygiene; and the prevention, recognition, and treatment of hypoglycemia and hyperglycemia.
● Stress the effect of blood glucose control on long-term health.
● Watch for acute complications of diabetic therapy, especially hypoglycemia (vagueness, slow cerebration, dizziness, weakness, pallor, tachycardia, diaphoresis, seizures, and coma); immediately give carbohydrates, ideally in the form of fruit juice, hard candy, honey or, if the patient is unconscious, glucagon or dextrose I.V. Also stay alert for signs of ketoacidosis (acetone breath, dehydration, weak and rapid pulse, Kussmaul's respirations) and hyperosmolar coma (polyuria, thirst, neurologic abnormal-

TREATMENT OF
TYPE 1 DIABETES MELLITUS

This flowchart shows the pathophysiologic process of diabetes and points for treatment intervention.

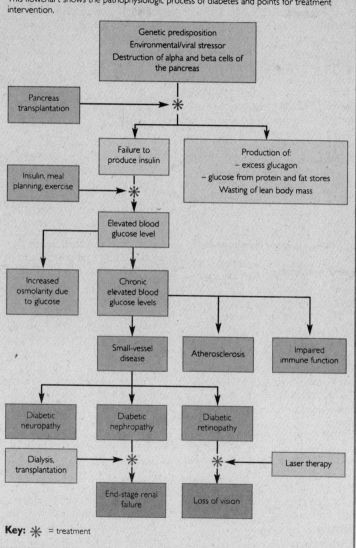

Key: ✳ = treatment

ities, stupor). These hyperglycemic crises require I.V. fluids and regular insulin.

- Monitor diabetes control by obtaining blood glucose, glycosylated hemoglobin, lipid levels, and blood pressure measurements regularly.
- Watch for diabetic effects on the cardiovascular system, such as cerebrovascular, coronary artery, and peripheral vascular impairment, and the peripheral and autonomic nervous systems. Treat all injuries, cuts, and blisters (particularly on the legs or feet) meticulously. Monitor for signs and symptoms of cellulitis. Stay alert for signs of urinary tract infection and renal disease.
- Urge regular ophthalmologic examinations to detect diabetic retinopathy.
- Assess for signs of diabetic neuropathy (numbness or pain in hands and feet, footdrop, neurogenic bladder). Stress the need for personal safety precautions because decreased sensation can mask injuries. Minimize complications by maintaining strict blood glucose control.
- Teach the patient to care for his feet by washing them daily, drying carefully between toes, and inspecting for corns, calluses, redness, swelling, bruises, and breaks in the skin. Urge him to report changes to the physician. Advise him to wear nonconstricting shoes and to avoid walking barefoot. Instruct him to use over-the-counter athlete's foot remedies and seek professional care should athlete's foot not improve. Encourage periodic visits to a podiatrist.
- Teach the patient how to manage his diabetes when he has a minor illness, such as a cold, flu, or upset stomach.

- To delay the clinical onset of diabetes, teach people at high risk to avoid risk factors. Advise genetic counseling for young adult patients with diabetes who are planning families.
- Further information may be obtained from the Juvenile Diabetes Foundation, the American Diabetes Association, and the American Association of Diabetes Educators.

Hyperthyroidism

Hyperthyroidism, or thyrotoxicosis, is a metabolic imbalance that results from the overproduction of thyroid hormone. The most common form is Graves' disease, which increases thyroxine (T_4) production, enlarges the thyroid gland (goiter), and causes multiple system changes. (See *Other forms of hyperthyroidism.*)

Alert   The incidence of Graves' disease is greatest in women ages 30 to 60, especially those with a family history of thyroid abnormalities; only 5% of patients are younger than age 15.

With treatment, most patients can lead normal lives. However, thyroid storm — an acute, severe exacerbation of thyrotoxicosis — is a medical emergency that may have life-threatening cardiac, hepatic, or renal consequences.

CAUSES
- Clinical thyrotoxicosis precipitated by excessive dietary intake of iodine or possibly stress (patients with latent disease)
- Defect in suppressor T-lymphocyte function permitting production of autoantibodies (thyroid-stimulating immunoglobulin and thyroid-stimulating

hormone [TSH]–binding inhibitory immunoglobulin)

- Increased incidence in monozygotic twins, pointing to an inherited factor, probably an autosomal recessive gene
- Medications, such as lithium (Eskalith) and amiodarone (Cordarone)
- Occasional coexistence with other endocrine abnormalities, such as type 1 diabetes mellitus, thyroiditis, and hyperparathyroidism
- Stress, such as surgery, infection, toxemia of pregnancy, or diabetic ketoacidosis, which can precipitate thyroid storm (inadequately treated thyrotoxicosis)
- Toxic nodules or tumors

PATHOPHYSIOLOGY

The thyroid gland secretes the thyroid precursor, T_4, thyroid hormone or triiodothyronine (T_3), and calcitonin. T_4 and T_3 stimulate protein, lipid, and carbohydrate metabolism primarily through catabolic pathways. Calcitonin removes calcium from the blood and incorporates it into bone.

Biosynthesis, storage, and release of thyroid hormones are controlled by the hypothalamic-pituitary axis through a negative-feedback loop. Thyrotropin-releasing hormone (TRH) from the hypothalamus stimulates the release of TSH by the pituitary gland. Circulating T_3 levels provide negative feedback through the hypothalamus to decrease TRH levels, and through the pituitary to decrease TSH levels.

Although the exact mechanism isn't understood, hyperthyroidism has a hereditary component, and it's usually associated with other autoimmune endocrinopathies.

Graves' disease is an autoimmune disorder characterized by the production of autoantibodies that attach to

---

OTHER FORMS OF HYPERTHYROIDISM

◆ Toxic adenoma — a small, benign nodule in the thyroid gland that secretes thyroid hormone (second most common cause of hyperthyroidism); cause unknown; incidence is highest in elderly patients (Clinical effects are essentially similar to those of Graves' disease, except that toxic adenoma doesn't induce ophthalmopathy, pretibial myxedema, or acropachy. Presence of adenoma is confirmed by radioactive iodine [131I] uptake and thyroid scan, which show a single hyperfunctioning nodule suppressing the rest of the gland. Treatment includes 131I therapy or surgery to remove adenoma after antithyroid drugs achieve a euthyroid state.)

◆ Thyrotoxicosis factitia — results from chronic ingestion of thyroid hormone for thyrotropin suppression in patients with thyroid carcinoma, or from thyroid hormone abuse by people who are trying to lose weight

◆ Functioning metastatic thyroid carcinoma — a rare disease that causes excess production of thyroid hormone

◆ Thyroid-stimulating hormone-secreting pituitary tumor — causes overproduction of thyroid hormone

◆ Subacute thyroiditis — a virus-induced granulomatous inflammation of the thyroid, producing transient hyperthyroidism associated with fever, pain, pharyngitis, and tenderness in the thyroid gland

◆ Silent thyroiditis — a self-limiting, transient form of hyperthyroidism, with histologic thyroiditis but no inflammatory symptoms

---

and then stimulate TSH receptors on the thyroid gland. A goiter is an enlarged thyroid gland, either the result of increased stimulation or a response to increased metabolic demand. The latter occurs in iodine-deficient areas of the world, where the incidence of goiter increases during puberty (a time of increased metabolic demand).

These goiters commonly regress to normal size after puberty in males, but not in females. Sporadic goiter in non-iodine-deficient areas is of unknown origin. Endemic and sporadic goiters are nontoxic and may be diffuse or nodular. Toxic goiters may be uninodular or multinodular and may secrete excess thyroid hormone.

Pituitary tumors with TSH-producing cells are rare, as is hypothalamic disease causing TRH excess.

Possible complications of hyperthyroidism include muscle wasting, atrophy, paralysis, vision loss or diplopia, heart failure, arrhythmias, hypoparathyroidism after surgical removal of the thyroid, and hypothyroidism after radioiodine treatment.

CLINICAL FINDINGS

- Enlarged thyroid (goiter)
- Nervousness
- Heat intolerance and sweating
- Weight loss despite increased appetite
- Frequent bowel movements
- Exophthalmos (characteristic, but absent in many patients with thyrotoxicosis)

Specific clinical effects vary with the system affected and include:

- difficulty concentrating due to accelerated cerebral function; excitability or nervousness caused by increased basal metabolic rate from T_4; fine tremor, shaky handwriting, and clumsiness from increased activity in the spinal cord area that controls muscle tone; and emotional instability and mood swings ranging from occasional outbursts to overt psychosis (central nervous system)
- moist, smooth, warm, flushed skin (patient sleeps with minimal covers and little clothing); fine, soft hair; premature patchy graying and increased hair loss in both sexes; friable nails and onycholysis (distal nail separated from the bed); pretibial myxedema (nonpitting edema of the anterior surface of the legs, dermopathy), producing thickened skin; accentuated hair follicles; sometimes itchy or painful raised red patches of skin with occasional nodule formation; and microscopic examination showing increased mucin deposits (skin, hair, and nails)
- systolic hypertension, tachycardia, full bounding pulse, wide pulse pressure, cardiomegaly, increased cardiac output and blood volume, visible point of maximal impulse, paroxysmal supraventricular tachycardia and atrial fibrillation (especially in elderly people), and occasional systolic murmur at the left sternal border (cardiovascular system)
- increased respiratory rate, and dyspnea on exertion and at rest, possibly due to cardiac decompensation and increased cellular oxygen use (respiratory system)
- excessive oral intake with weight loss; nausea and vomiting due to increased GI motility and peristalsis; increased defecation; soft stools or, in severe disease, diarrhea; and liver enlargement (GI system)
- weakness, fatigue, and muscle atrophy; rare coexistence with myasthenia gravis; possibly generalized or localized paralysis associated with hypokalemia; and, rarely, acropachy (soft-tissue swelling accompanied by underlying bone changes where new bone formation occurs) (musculoskeletal system)
- oligomenorrhea or amenorrhea, decreased fertility, increased incidence of spontaneous abortion, gynecomastia due to increased estrogen levels (males), and diminished libido (both sexes) (reproductive system)

exophthalmos due to combined effects of accumulated mucopolysaccharides and fluids in the retro-orbital tissues, forcing the eyeball outward and lid retraction, thereby producing characteristic staring gaze; occasional inflammation of conjunctivae, corneas, or eye muscles; diplopia; and increased tearing (eyes).

When thyrotoxicosis escalates to thyroid storm, these symptoms may occur:
- high fever (up to 106° F [41.1° C])
- tachycardia, pulmonary edema, hypertension, and shock
- tremors, emotional lability, extreme irritability, confusion, delirium, psychosis, apathy, stupor, and coma
- diarrhea, abdominal pain, nausea and vomiting, jaundice, and hyperglycemia.

Alert *Consider apathetic thyrotoxicosis, a morbid condition resulting from an overactive thyroid, in elderly patients with atrial fibrillation or depression.*

TEST RESULTS
- Radioimmunoassay shows increased serum T_4 and T_3 levels.
- Immunoradiometric assay shows low TSH level.
- Thyroid scan shows increased uptake of iodine 131 (^{131}I) in Graves' disease and, usually, in toxic multinodular goiter and toxic adenoma, and low radioactive uptake in thyroiditis and thyrotoxic factitia (test contraindicated in pregnancy).
- Ultrasonography confirms subclinical ophthalmopathy.

TREATMENT
Appropriate treatment depends on the severity of thyrotoxicosis, causes, the patient's age and parity, and how long surgery will be delayed if the patient is an appropriate candidate for surgery.

The primary forms of therapy include antithyroid drugs, a single oral dose of ^{131}I, and surgery.

Antithyroid therapy
- Antithyroid drugs for children, young adults, pregnant women, and patients who refuse surgery or ^{131}I treatment
- Antithyroid drugs preferred for patients with new-onset Graves' disease because of spontaneous remission in many of these patients
- Antithyroid drugs to correct the thyrotoxic state in preparation for ^{131}I treatment or surgery
- Thyroid hormone antagonists, including propylthiouracil (PTU) and methimazole (Tapazole), to block thyroid hormone synthesis (Hypermetabolic symptoms subside within 4 to 8 weeks after therapy begins, but remission of Graves' disease requires continued therapy for 6 months to 2 years.)
- Propranolol (Inderal) until antithyroid drugs reach their full effect to manage tachycardia and other peripheral effects of excessive hypersympathetic activity resulting from blocking the conversion of T_4 to the active T_3 hormone
- Minimum dosage given to keep maternal thyroid function within the high-normal range until delivery and to minimize the risk of fetal hypothyroidism; PTU preferred agent (during pregnancy)
- Possibly antithyroid medications and propranolol given to neonates for 2 to 3 months because most infants of hyperthyroid mothers are born with mild and transient thyrotoxicosis caused by placental transfer of thyroid-stimulating immunoglobulins (neonatal thyrotoxicosis)

- Continuous monitoring of maternal thyroid function for thyrotoxicosis (sometimes exacerbated in the puerperal period); antithyroid drugs gradually tapered and thyroid function reassessed 3 to 6 months postpartum
- Periodic checks of infant's thyroid function for a breast-feeding mother on low-dose antithyroid treatment due to possible presence of small amounts of the drug in breast milk, which can rapidly lead to thyrotoxicity in the neonate

Single oral dose of ^{131}I
- Treatment of choice for patients not planning to have children; patients of reproductive age must give informed consent because ^{131}I concentrates in the gonads
- During treatment, decreasing thyroid hormone production and normalizing thyroid size and function, due to the thyroid gland picking up the radioactive element (as it would regular iodine) and destroying some of the cells that normally concentrate iodine and produce T_4
- In most patients, hypermetabolic symptoms diminishing 6 to 8 weeks after such treatment; however, some patients possibly requiring a second dose (Almost all patients eventually become hypothyroid.)

Surgery
- Subtotal thyroidectomy to decrease the thyroid gland's capacity for hormone production (Patients who refuse or aren't candidates for ^{131}I treatment.)
- Iodide (Lugol's solution or saturated solution of potassium iodide), antithyroid drugs, and propranolol to relieve hyperthyroidism preoperatively (If the patient doesn't become euthyroid, surgery should be delayed and antithyroid drugs and propranolol given to decrease the systemic effects [cardiac arrhythmias] of thyrotoxicosis.)
- Lifelong regular medical supervision necessary because most patients become hypothyroid, sometimes as long as several years after surgery

For ophthalmopathy
- Local application of topical medications, such as prednisone acetate suspension, but may require high doses of corticosteroids
- Calcium channel blockers, such as diltiazem (Cardizem) and verapamil (Calan), to block the peripheral effects of thyroid hormones
- External-beam radiation therapy or surgical decompression (severe exophthalmos causing pressure on optic nerve and orbital contents)

For thyroid storm
- Antithyroid drug to stop conversion of T_4 to T_3 and to block sympathetic effect; corticosteroids to inhibit the conversion of T_4 to T_3; and iodide to block thyroid hormone release
- Supportive measures, including the administration of nutrients, vitamins, fluids, oxygen, hypothermia blankets, and sedatives

NURSING CONSIDERATIONS
- Record the patient's vital signs and weight.
- Monitor serum electrolyte level, and check periodically for hyperglycemia and glycosuria.
- Carefully monitor cardiac function if the patient is elderly or has coronary artery disease. If the heart rate is more than 100 beats/minute, check blood pressure and pulse rate often. Monitor the patient's electrocardiogram for ar-

rhythmias and changes in the ST segment.
- Check the patient's level of consciousness and urine output.
- If the patient is pregnant, tell her to watch closely during the first trimester for signs of spontaneous abortion and to report such signs immediately.
- Encourage bed rest, and keep the patient's room cool, quiet, and dark. The patient with dyspnea is most comfortable sitting upright or in high Fowler's position.
- Remember, extreme nervousness may produce bizarre behavior. Reassure the patient and his family that such behavior will probably subside with treatment. Provide sedatives as necessary.
- To promote weight gain, provide a balanced diet with six meals per day. If the patient has edema, suggest a low-sodium diet.
- If iodide is part of the treatment, mix it with milk, juice, or water to prevent GI distress, and administer it through a straw to prevent tooth discoloration.
- Watch for signs of thyroid storm (tachycardia, hyperkinesis, fever, vomiting, hypertension).
- Check intake and output carefully to ensure adequate hydration and fluid balance.
- Closely monitor blood pressure, heart rate and rhythm, and temperature. If the patient has a high fever, reduce it with appropriate hypothermic measures. Maintain an I.V. line and give drugs as ordered.
- If the patient has exophthalmos or other ophthalmopathy, suggest sunglasses or eye patches to protect his eyes from light. Moisten the conjunctivae often with isotonic eyedrops. Warn the patient with severe lid retraction to avoid sudden physical movements that might cause the lid to slip behind the eyeball.
- Avoid excessive palpation of the thyroid to avoid precipitating thyroid storm.

Thyroidectomy necessitates meticulous postoperative care to prevent complications:
- Check the patient often for respiratory distress, and keep a tracheotomy tray at the bedside.
- Watch for evidence of hemorrhage into the neck such as a tight dressing with no blood on it. Change dressings and perform wound care as ordered; check the back of the dressing for drainage. Keep the patient in semi-Fowler's position, and support his head and neck with sandbags to ease tension on the incision.
- Check for dysphagia or hoarseness from possible laryngeal nerve injury.
- Watch for signs of hypocalcemia (tetany, numbness), a complication that results from accidental removal of the parathyroid glands during surgery.
- Stress the importance of regular medical follow-up after discharge because hypothyroidism may develop 2 to 4 weeks postoperatively.

After drug therapy and ^{131}I therapy:
- After ^{131}I therapy, tell the patient not to expectorate or cough freely because his saliva will be radioactive for 24 hours. Stress the need for repeated measurement of serum T_4 level. The patient shouldn't resume antithyroid therapy.
- If the patient is taking PTU and methimazole, monitor complete blood count periodically to detect leukopenia, thrombocytopenia, and agranulocytosis. Instruct him to take these medications with meals to minimize GI distress and to avoid over-

the-counter cough preparations because many contain iodine.

- Tell him to report fever, enlarged cervical lymph nodes, sore throat, mouth sores, and other signs of blood dyscrasias and any rash or skin eruptions — signs of hypersensitivity.
- Watch the patient taking propranolol for signs of hypotension (dizziness, decreased urine output). Tell him to rise slowly after sitting or lying down to prevent orthostatic syncope.
- Instruct the patient to report symptoms of hypothyroidism.

Hypothyroidism

Hypothyroidism results from hypothalamic, pituitary, or thyroid insufficiency or resistance to thyroid hormone. The disorder can progress to life-threatening myxedema coma. Hypothyroidism is more prevalent in women in than men; in the United States, the incidence is increasing significantly in people ages 40 to 50.

Alert *Hypothyroidism occurs primarily after age 40. After age 65, the prevalence increases to as much as 10% in females and 3% in males.*

CAUSES

- Inadequate thyroid hormone production, usually after thyroidectomy or radiation therapy (particularly with iodine 131 [^{131}I]), or due to inflammation, chronic autoimmune thyroiditis (Hashimoto's disease), or such conditions as amyloidosis and sarcoidosis (rare)
- Pituitary failure to produce thyroid-stimulating hormone (TSH), hypothalamic failure to produce thyrotropin-releasing hormone (TRH), inborn errors of thyroid hormone synthesis,

iodine deficiency (usually dietary), or use of such antithyroid medications as propylthiouracil

PATHOPHYSIOLOGY

Hypothyroidism may reflect a malfunction of the hypothalamus, pituitary, or thyroid gland, all of which are part of the same negative-feedback mechanism. However, disorders of the hypothalamus and pituitary rarely cause hypothyroidism. Primary hypothyroidism, a disorder of the gland itself, is most common.

Chronic autoimmune thyroiditis, also called *chronic lymphocytic thyroiditis,* occurs when autoantibodies destroy thyroid gland tissue. Chronic autoimmune thyroiditis associated with goiter is called Hashimoto's thyroiditis. The cause of this autoimmune process is unknown, although heredity has a role, and specific human leukocyte antigen subtypes are associated with greater risk.

Outside the thyroid, antibodies can reduce the effect of thyroid hormone in two ways. First, antibodies can block the TSH receptor and prevent TSH production. Second, cytotoxic antithyroid antibodies may attack thyroid cells.

Subacute thyroiditis, painless thyroiditis, and postpartum thyroiditis are self-limited conditions that usually follow an episode of hyperthyroidism. Untreated subclinical hypothyroidism in adults is likely to become overt at a rate of 5% to 20% per year.

Complications of hypothyroidism include heart failure, myxedema coma, infection, megacolon, organic psychosis, and infertility.

CLINICAL FINDINGS

- Weakness, fatigue, forgetfulness, sensitivity to cold, unexplained weight gain, and constipation (typical, vague, early clinical features) (see *Clinical findings in acquired hypothyroidism*)

• Characteristic myxedematous signs and symptoms of decreasing mental stability; coarse, dry, flaky, inelastic skin; puffy face, hands, and feet; hoarseness; periorbital edema; upper eyelid droop; dry, sparse hair; and thick, brittle nails (as disorder progresses)

• Cardiovascular involvement, including decreased cardiac output, slow pulse rate, signs of poor peripheral circulation and, occasionally, an enlarged heart

• Anorexia, abdominal distention, menorrhagia, decreased libido, infertility, ataxia, and nystagmus; reflexes with delayed relaxation time (especially in the Achilles tendon)

• Progression to myxedema coma, usually gradual but may develop abruptly, with stress aggravating severe or prolonged hypothyroidism, including progressive stupor, hypoventilation, hypoglycemia, hyponatremia, hypotension, and hypothermia

TEST RESULTS

• Radioimmunoassay shows low triiodothyronine (T_3) and thyroxine (T_4) levels.

• TSH level is increased with cause of thyroid disorder, and decreased with hypothalamic or pituitary disorder cause.

• Thyroid panel differentiates primary hypothyroidism (thyroid gland hypofunction), secondary hypothyroidism (pituitary hyposecretion of TSH), tertiary hypothyroidism (hypothalamic hyposecretion of TRH), and euthyroid sick syndrome (impaired peripheral conversion of thyroid hormone due to a suprathyroidal illness

---

CLINICAL FINDINGS IN ACQUIRED HYPOTHYROIDISM

Typical findings in acquired hypothyroidism are listed here.

HISTORY
◆ Arthritis
◆ Cold intolerance
◆ Constipation
◆ Decreased sociability
◆ Drowsiness
◆ Dry skin
◆ Fatigue
◆ Lethargy
◆ Memory impairment
◆ Menstrual disorders
◆ Muscle cramps
◆ Psychosis
◆ Somnolence
◆ Weakness

PHYSICAL EXAMINATION
◆ Anemia
◆ Bradycardia
◆ Brittle hair
◆ Cool skin
◆ Delayed relaxation of reflexes
◆ Dementia
◆ Dry skin
◆ Gravelly voice
◆ Hypothermia
◆ Large tongue
◆ Loss of lateral third of eyebrow
◆ Puffy face and hands
◆ Slow speech
◆ Weight changes

---

such as severe infection). (See *Thyroid test results in hypothyroidism*, page 284.)

• Blood studies reveal:
– elevated serum cholesterol, alkaline phosphatase, and triglyceride levels
– normocytic, normochromic anemia
– low serum sodium level, decreased pH, and increased partial pressure of carbon dioxide, which indicates respiratory acidosis (myxedema coma).

THYROID TEST RESULTS IN HYPOTHYROIDISM

DYSFUNCTION INVOLVES	THYROTROPIN-RELEASING HORMONE	THYROID-STIMULATING HORMONE	TH (TRIIODO-THYRONINE [T_3] AND THYROXINE [T_4])
Hypothalamus	Low	Low	Low
Pituitary gland	High	Low	Low
Thyroid gland	High	High	Low
Peripheral conversion of thyroid hormone (TH)	High	Low or normal	T_3 and T_4 low, but reverse T_3 elevated

TREATMENT

- Gradual thyroid hormone replacement with synthetic T_4 and, occasionally, T_3
- Surgical excision, chemotherapy, or radiation for tumors

Alert Elderly patients should be started on a very low dose of T_4 to avoid cardiac problems; TSH levels guide gradual increases in dosage.

NURSING CONSIDERATIONS

- Provide a high-bulk, low-calorie diet and encourage activity to combat constipation and promote weight loss. Administer cathartics and stool softeners as needed.
- After thyroid replacement begins, watch for symptoms of hyperthyroidism, such as restlessness, sweating, and excessive weight loss.
- Tell the patient to report signs of aggravated cardiovascular disease, such as chest pain and tachycardia.
- To prevent myxedema coma, tell the patient to continue his course of thyroid medication even if his symptoms subside.
- Warn the patient to report infection immediately and to make sure that any physician who prescribes drugs for him knows about the underlying hypothyroidism.

Treatment of myxedema coma requires supportive care:

- Check frequently for signs of decreasing cardiac output such as decreased urine output.
- Monitor the patient's temperature until he's stable. Provide extra blankets and clothing and a warm room to compensate for hypothermia. Rapid rewarming may cause vasodilation and vascular collapse.
- Record intake and output and daily weight. As treatment begins, urine output should increase and body weight decrease; if not, report this immediately.
- Turn the edematous bedridden patient every 2 hours, and provide skin care, particularly around bony prominences, at least once per shift.

- Avoid sedation when possible or reduce dosage because hypothyroidism delays the metabolism of many drugs.
- Maintain a patent I.V. line. Monitor serum electrolyte level carefully when administering I.V. fluids.
- Monitor the patient's vital signs carefully when administering levothyroxine because rapid correction of hypothyroidism can cause adverse cardiac effects. Report chest pain or tachycardia immediately. Watch for hypertension and heart failure in the elderly patient.
- Check arterial blood gas values for hypercapnia, metabolic acidosis, and hypoxia to determine whether the patient who's severely myxedematous requires ventilatory assistance.
- Administer corticosteroids as ordered.
- Because myxedema coma may have been precipitated by an infection, check possible sources of the infection, such as blood and urine, and obtain sputum cultures.

Simple goiter

Simple, or nontoxic, goiter is a thyroid gland enlargement that isn't caused by inflammation or a neoplasm and is commonly classified as endemic or sporadic. Inherited defects may be responsible for insufficient thyroxine (T_4) synthesis or impaired iodine metabolism. Because families tend to congregate in a single geographic area, this familial factor may contribute to the incidence of endemic and sporadic goiters.

Simple goiter affects more females than males, especially during adolescence, pregnancy, and menopause, when the body's demand for thyroid hormone increases. Sporadic goiter affects no particular population segment. With appropriate treatment, the prognosis is good for either type of goiter.

CAUSES
Endemic goiter
- Inadequate dietary iodine

Sporadic goiter
- Ingestion by a pregnant woman of certain drugs, such as propylthiouracil (PTU), iodides, cobalt, and lithium (Eskalith), which may cross the placenta and affect the fetus
- Ingestion of large amounts of foods containing agents that inhibit T_4 production, such as rutabagas, cabbage, soybeans, peanuts, peaches, peas, strawberries, spinach, and radishes

PATHOPHYSIOLOGY
Goiters can occur in the presence of hypothyroidism, hyperthyroidism, or normal levels of thyroid hormone. In the presence of a severe underlying disorder, compensatory responses may cause thyroid enlargement (goiter) and hypothyroidism. Simple goiter occurs when the thyroid gland can't secrete enough thyroid hormone to meet metabolic requirements. As a result, the thyroid gland enlarges to compensate for inadequate hormone synthesis, a compensation that usually overcomes mild to moderate hormonal impairment.

Endemic goiter usually results from inadequate secretion of thyroid hormone caused by inadequate dietary intake of iodine associated with such factors as iodine-depleted soil or malnutrition. Since the introduction of iodized salt in the United States, cases

MASSIVE GOITER

Massive multinodular goiter causes gross distention and swelling of the neck, as shown here.

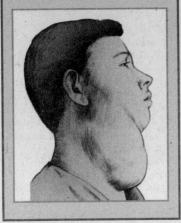

multinodular goiter. (See *Massive goiter*.)

TEST RESULTS
- Blood studies reveal normal serum thyroid levels and serum T_4 concentrations that are low-normal or normal.
- Thyroid-stimulating hormone (TSH) is at high or normal level.
- Iodine 131 uptake is normal or increased at 50% of the dose at 24 hours.

TREATMENT
- Exogenous thyroid hormone replacement with levothyroxine (treatment of choice) inhibiting TSH secretion and allowing the gland to rest
- Small doses of iodide (Lugol's iodine or potassium iodide solution) to relieve goiter due to iodine deficiency
- Avoidance of known goitrogenic drugs and foods
- For large goiter (unresponsive to treatment), subtotal thyroidectomy possibly necessary

NURSING CONSIDERATIONS
- Measure the patient's neck circumference daily to check for progressive thyroid gland enlargement, and check for the development of hard nodules in the gland, which may indicate carcinoma.
- To maintain constant hormone levels, instruct the patient to take prescribed thyroid hormone preparations at the same time each day. Advise him to avoid taking the medicine at the same time as iron-containing supplements (including prenatal vitamins), with psyllium hydrophilic mucilloid (Metamucil), or grapefruit juice. Teach the patient and his family to identify and immediately report signs of thyrotoxicosis, including increased pulse

of endemic goiter have virtually disappeared.

Sporadic goiter is triggered by certain drugs or foods that inhibit or block thyroid hormone production.

Because simple goiter doesn't alter the patient's metabolic state, complications arise solely from enlargement of the thyroid gland compressing adjacent tissues. Complications can include respiratory distress, dysphagia, venous engorgement, and development of collateral venous circulation in the chest. Also congestion of the face, some cyanosis, and distress (Pemberton sign) when the patient raises her arms until they touch the side of her head can occur.

CLINICAL FINDINGS
Thyroid enlargement may range from a mildly enlarged gland to a massive,

rate, palpitations, diarrhea, sweating, tremors, agitation, and shortness of breath.
● Instruct the patient with endemic goiter to use iodized salt to supply the daily 150 to 300 mcg of iodine necessary to prevent goiter.
● Monitor the patient taking goitrogenic drugs for signs of sporadic goiter.

Syndrome of inappropriate antidiuretic hormone

Syndrome of inappropriate antidiuretic hormone (SIADH) results when excessive antidiuretic hormone (ADH) secretion is triggered by stimuli other than increased extracellular fluid osmolarity and decreased extracellular fluid volume, reflected by hypotension. SIADH is a relatively common complication of surgery or critical illness. The prognosis varies with the degree of disease and the speed at which it develops. SIADH usually resolves within 3 days of effective treatment.

CAUSES
Common
● Oat cell carcinoma of the lung (most common), which secretes excessive levels of ADH or vasopressin-like substances
● Other neoplastic diseases — such as pancreatic and prostate cancer, Hodgkin's disease, thymoma (tumor on the thymus), and renal carcinoma

Others
● Central nervous system disorders, including brain tumor or abscess, stroke, head injury, and Guillain-Barré syndrome
● Drugs that either increase ADH production or potentiate ADH action, such as antidepressants, nonsteroidal anti-inflammatory drugs, chlorpropamide (Diabinese), vincristine, cyclophosphamide (Cytoxan), carbamazepine (Tegretol), clofibrate, metoclopramide (Reglan), and morphine
● Miscellaneous conditions, including psychosis, myxedema, acquired immunodeficiency syndrome, physiologic stress, and pain
● Pulmonary disorders, including pneumonia, tuberculosis, lung abscess, aspergillosis, bronchiectasis, and positive-pressure ventilation

PATHOPHYSIOLOGY
In the presence of excessive ADH, excessive water reabsorption from the distal convoluted tubule and collecting ducts causes hyponatremia and normal to slightly increased extracellular fluid volume. This may lead to complications, such as cerebral edema, brain herniation, and central pontine myelinosis.

CLINICAL FINDINGS
● Thirst, anorexia, fatigue, and lethargy (first signs), followed by vomiting and intestinal cramping due to hyponatremia and electrolyte imbalance manifestations
● Weight gain, edema, water retention, and decreased urine output due to hyponatremia
● Additional neurologic symptoms, such as restlessness, confusion, anorexia, headache, irritability, decreasing reflexes, seizures, and coma due to

electrolyte imbalances, worsening with the degree of water intoxication
• Decreased deep tendon reflexes

TEST RESULTS
• Blood studies reveal:
– serum osmolality less than 280 mOsm/kg of water
– hyponatremia with serum sodium level less than 135 mEq/L; lower values indicating worse condition
– elevated serum ADH level
– normal blood urea nitrogen level.
• Urine studies show elevated urinary sodium level (more than 20 mEq/L) and increased osmolality (greater than 150 mOsm/kg).

TREATMENT
• Restricted water intake (500 to 1,000 ml/day) (symptomatic treatment)
• Administration of 200 to 300 ml of 3% saline solution to slowly and steadily increase serum sodium level (severe water intoxication); if too rapid a rise, cerebral edema may result
• Correction of underlying cause of SIADH when possible
• Surgical resection, irradiation, or chemotherapy to alleviate water retention for SIADH resulting from cancer
• Demeclocycline (Declomycin) to block the renal response to ADH (if fluid restriction is ineffective)
• Furosemide (Lasix) with normal or hypertonic saline to maintain urine output and block ADH secretion

NURSING CONSIDERATIONS
• Closely monitor and record the patient's intake and output, vital signs, and daily weight. Watch for hyponatremia.
• Observe the patient for restlessness, irritability, seizures, heart failure, and unresponsiveness due to hyponatremia and water intoxication.
• To prevent water intoxication, explain to the patient and his family why he must restrict his intake.

7

HEMATOLOGIC SYSTEM

Blood, although a fluid, is one of the body's major tissues. It continuously circulates through the heart and blood vessels, carrying vital elements to every part of the body.

Blood performs several vital functions through its special components: the liquid protein (plasma) and the formed constituents (erythrocytes, leukocytes, and thrombocytes) suspended in it. Erythrocytes (red blood cells) carry oxygen to the tissues and remove carbon dioxide. Leukocytes (white blood cells) act in inflammatory and immune responses. Plasma (a clear, straw-colored fluid) carries antibodies and nutrients to tissues and carries waste away. Plasma coagulation factors and thrombocytes (platelets) control clotting.

Hematopoiesis, the process of blood formation, occurs primarily in the marrow. Primitive blood cells (stem cells) differentiate into the precursors of erythrocytes (normoblasts), leukocytes, and thrombocytes.

Specific causes of hematologic disorders include trauma, chronic disease, surgery, malnutrition, drugs, exposure to toxins or radiation, and genetic or congenital defects that disrupt the production or function of blood cells.

☀ Life-threatening
Aplastic anemias

Aplastic, or hypoplastic, anemias result from injury to or destruction of stem cells in bone marrow or the bone marrow matrix, causing pancytopenia (anemia, leukopenia, and thrombocytopenia) and bone marrow hypoplasia. Although commonly used interchangeably with other terms for bone marrow failure, aplastic anemia properly refers to pancytopenia resulting from the decreased functional capacity of a hypoplastic, fatty bone marrow.

These disorders generally produce fatal bleeding or infection, especially when they're idiopathic or caused by chloramphenicol (Chloromycetin) use or infectious hepatitis. The mortality rate for severe aplastic anemia is 80% to 90%.

CAUSES
- Autoimmune reactions (unconfirmed), severe disease (especially hepatitis), or preleukemic and neoplastic infiltration of bone marrow
- Congenital (idiopathic anemias); two identified forms of aplastic anemia including: hypoplastic or Blackfan-Diamond anemia (develops from

ages 2 to 3 months) and Fanconi's syndrome (develops from birth to age 10)
• Drugs (antibiotics, anticonvulsants) or toxic agents (such as benzene or chloramphenicol)
• Radiation (about half of such anemias)

PATHOPHYSIOLOGY
Aplastic anemias usually develop when damaged or destroyed stem cells inhibit blood cell production. Less commonly, they develop when damaged bone marrow microvasculature creates an unfavorable environment for cell growth and maturation.

CLINICAL FINDINGS
Signs and symptoms of aplastic anemias vary with the severity of pancytopenia but develop insidiously in many cases. They may include:
• progressive weakness and fatigue, shortness of breath, headache, pallor, and ultimately tachycardia and heart failure due to hypoxia and increased venous return
• ecchymosis, petechiae, and hemorrhage, especially from the mucous membranes (nose, gums, rectum, vagina) or into the retina or central nervous system due to thrombocytopenia
• infection (fever, oral and rectal ulcers, sore throat) without characteristic inflammation due to neutropenia (neutrophil deficiency).

TEST RESULTS
• Blood studies reveal 1 million/mm^3 or fewer red blood cells (RBCs) of normal color and size (normochromic and normocytic).
• RBCs may be macrocytic (larger than normal) and anisocytotic (excessive variation in size), with a very low absolute reticulocyte count.
• Elevated serum iron level (unless bleeding occurs), normal or slightly reduced total iron-binding capacity, presence of hemosiderin (a derivative of hemoglobin), and microscopically visible tissue iron storage.
• Decreased platelet, neutrophil, and lymphocyte counts.
• Abnormal coagulation test results (bleeding time) reflecting decreased platelet count.
• "Dry tap" (no cells) from bone marrow aspiration at several sites.
• Biopsy showing severely hypocellular or aplastic marrow, with varied amounts of fat, fibrous tissue, or gelatinous replacement; absence of tagged iron (because iron is deposited in the liver rather than bone marrow) and megakaryocytes (platelet precursors); and depression of RBCs and precursors (erythroid elements).
Differential diagnosis must rule out paroxysmal nocturnal hemoglobinuria and other diseases in which pancytopenia is common.

TREATMENT
Effective treatment must eliminate an identifiable cause and provide vigorous supportive measures, including:
• packed RBC or platelet transfusion; experimental histocompatibility locus antigen-matched leukocyte transfusions
• bone marrow transplantation (treatment of choice for anemia due to severe aplasia and for patients who need constant RBC transfusions)
• for patients with leukopenia, special measures to prevent infection (avoidance of exposure to communicable diseases, diligent hand washing, and so forth)

- specific antibiotics for infection (not given prophylactically because they encourage resistant strains of organisms)
- respiratory support with oxygen in addition to blood transfusions (for patients with low hemoglobin level)
- corticosteroids to stimulate erythropoiesis; marrow-stimulating agents such as androgens (controversial); antilymphocyte globulin (experimental); immunosuppressive agents (if the patient doesn't respond to other therapy); and colony-stimulating factors to encourage growth of specific cellular components.

NURSING CONSIDERATIONS

- If the platelet count is low (less than 20,000/mm^3), prevent bleeding by avoiding I.M. injections, suggesting the use of an electric razor and a soft toothbrush, humidifying oxygen to prevent drying of mucous membranes, avoiding enemas and taking rectal temperature measurements, and promoting regular bowel movements through the use of a stool softener and a proper diet to prevent constipation. Also, apply pressure to venipuncture sites until bleeding stops. Detect bleeding early by checking for blood in urine and stool and assessing skin for petechiae.
- Take safety precautions to prevent falls that could lead to prolonged bleeding or hemorrhage.
- Help prevent infection by washing your hands thoroughly before entering the patient's room, by making sure that the patient is receiving a nutritious diet (high in vitamins and proteins) to improve his resistance, and by encouraging meticulous mouth and perianal care.
- Watch for life-threatening hemorrhage, infection, adverse effects of

drug therapy, or a blood transfusion reaction. Make sure that routine throat, urine, nose, rectal, and blood cultures are done regularly and correctly to check for infection. Teach the patient to recognize signs of infection, and tell him to report them immediately.
- If the patient has a low hemoglobin level, which causes fatigue, schedule frequent rest periods. Administer oxygen therapy as needed. If blood transfusions are necessary, assess for a transfusion reaction by checking the patient's temperature and watching for the development of other signs and symptoms, such as rash, hives, itching, back pain, restlessness, and shaking chills.
- Reassure and support the patient and his family by explaining the disease and its treatment, particularly if the patient has recurring acute episodes. Explain the purpose of all prescribed drugs and discuss possible adverse effects, including which ones he should report promptly. Encourage the patient who doesn't require hospitalization to continue his normal lifestyle, with appropriate restrictions such as regular rest periods, until remission occurs.
- To prevent aplastic anemia, monitor blood studies carefully in the patient receiving anemia-inducing drugs.
- Support efforts to educate the public about the hazards of toxic agents. Tell parents to keep toxic agents out of the reach of children. Encourage people who work with radiation to wear protective clothing and a radiation-detecting badge and to observe plant safety precautions. Those who work with benzene (solvent) should know that 10 parts per million is the highest safe environmental level and

that a delayed reaction to benzene may develop.

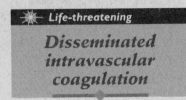

Disseminated intravascular coagulation

Disseminated intravascular coagulation (DIC) occurs as a complication of diseases and conditions that accelerate clotting, causing small blood vessel occlusion, organ necrosis, depletion of circulating clotting factors and platelets, activation of the fibrinolytic system, and consequent severe hemorrhage. Clotting in the microcirculation usually affects the kidneys and extremities, but may occur in the brain, lungs, pituitary and adrenal glands, and GI mucosa.

DIC, also called *consumption coagulopathy* or *defibrination syndrome,* is generally an acute condition but may be chronic in patients with cancer. Prognosis depends on early detection and treatment, the severity of the hemorrhage, and treatment of the underlying disease.

CAUSES

- Disorders that produce necrosis, including extensive burns and trauma, brain tissue destruction, transplant rejection, and hepatic necrosis
- Infection, including gram-negative or gram-positive septicemia and viral, fungal, rickettsial, or protozoal infection
- Neoplastic disease, including acute leukemia, metastatic carcinoma, and aplastic anemia
- Obstetric complications, including abruptio placentae, amniotic fluid em-

bolism, retained dead fetus, septic abortion, and eclampsia
- Other conditions, including heat-stroke, shock, poisonous snakebite, cirrhosis, fat embolism, incompatible blood transfusion, cardiac arrest, surgery requiring cardiopulmonary bypass, giant hemangioma, severe venous thrombosis, and purpura fulminans

PATHOPHYSIOLOGY

It isn't clear why certain disorders lead to DIC or whether they use a common mechanism. In many patients, the triggering mechanisms may be the entrance of foreign protein into the circulation and vascular endothelial injury.

Regardless of how DIC begins, the typical accelerated clotting results in generalized activation of prothrombin and a consequent excess of thrombin. The thrombin converts fibrinogen to fibrin, producing fibrin clots in the microcirculation. This process uses huge amounts of coagulation factors (especially fibrinogen, prothrombin, platelets, and factors V and VIII), causing hypofibrinogenemia, hypoprothrombinemia, thrombocytopenia, and deficiencies in factors V and VIII. Circulating thrombin also activates the fibrinolytic system, which dissolves fibrin clots into fibrin degradation products. Hemorrhage may be mostly the result of the anticoagulant activity of fibrin degradation products as well as depletion of plasma coagulation factors. DIC can lead to acute tubular necrosis, shock, and multiple organ failure. (See *Understanding DIC and its treatment.*)

CLINICAL FINDINGS

Signs and symptoms of DIC caused by the anticoagulant activity of fibrin

UNDERSTANDING DIC
AND ITS TREATMENT

This flowchart shows the pathophysiologic process of disseminated intravascular coagulation (DIC) and points for treatment intervention.

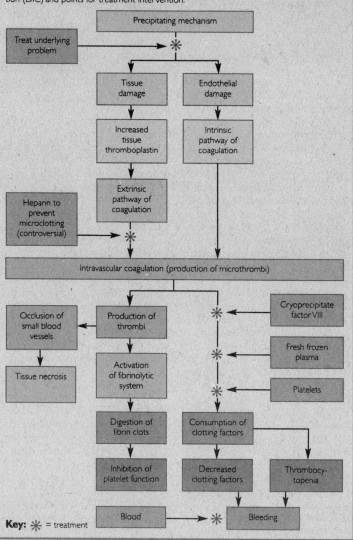

Precipitating mechanism

Treat underlying problem ──→ ✳

Tissue damage

Endothelial damage

Increased tissue thromboplastin

Intrinsic pathway of coagulation

Extrinsic pathway of coagulation

Heparin to prevent microclotting (controversial) ──→ ✳

Intravascular coagulation (production of microthrombi)

Occlusion of small blood vessels

Production of thrombi

✳ ←── Cryoprecipitate factor VIII

Tissue necrosis

Activation of fibrinolytic system

✳ ←── Fresh frozen plasma

✳ ←── Platelets

Digestion of fibrin clots

Consumption of clotting factors

Inhibition of platelet function

Decreased clotting factors

Thrombocytopenia

Key: ✳ = treatment

Blood ──→ ✳

Bleeding

degradation products and depletion of plasma coagulation factors may include:

- abnormal bleeding
- cutaneous oozing of serum
- petechiae or blood blisters
- bleeding from surgical or I.V. sites
- bleeding from the GI tract
- epistaxis
- hemoptysis.

Other signs and symptoms may include:

- cyanotic, cold, mottled fingers and toes due to fibrin clots in the microcirculation resulting in tissue ischemia
- severe muscle, back, abdominal, and chest pain from tissue hypoxia
- nausea and vomiting (may be a manifestation of GI bleeding)
- shock due to hemorrhage
- confusion, possibly due to cerebral thrombus and decreased cerebral perfusion
- dyspnea due to poor tissue perfusion and oxygenation
- oliguria due to decreased renal perfusion.

TEST RESULTS

- Platelet count is usually less than 100,000/mm^3 because platelets are consumed during thrombosis.
- Fibrinogen level is less than 150 mg/dl because fibrinogen is consumed in clot formation (level may be normal if elevated by hepatitis or pregnancy).
- Prothrombin time is greater than 15 seconds.
- Partial thromboplastin time is greater than 60 seconds.
- Increased fibrin degradation products are typically greater than 45 mcg/ml due to excess fibrinolysis by plasmin.
- D-dimer test, which shows the presence of an asymmetrical carbon

compound fragment formed in the presence of fibrin split products, is positive at less than 1:8 dilution.

- Positive fibrin monomers reveal diminished levels of factors V and VIII, red blood cell (RBC) fragmentation, and hemoglobin level less than 10 g/dl.
- Laboratory tests reveal reduced urine output (less than 30 ml/hour) and elevated blood urea nitrogen (greater than 25 mg/dl) and serum creatinine (greater than 1.3 mg/dl) levels.

TREATMENT

- Prompt recognition and treatment of underlying disorder
- Blood, fresh frozen plasma, platelet, or packed RBC transfusions to support hemostasis in active bleeding
- Heparin in early stages to prevent microclotting and as a last resort in hemorrhage (controversial in acute DIC after sepsis).

NURSING CONSIDERATIONS

- To avoid dislodging clots and causing fresh bleeding, don't scrub bleeding areas. Use pressure, cold compresses, and topical hemostatic agents to control bleeding.
- To prevent injury, enforce complete bed rest during bleeding episodes. If the patient is agitated, pad the side rails.
- Check all I.V. and venipuncture sites frequently for bleeding. Apply pressure to injection sites for at least 20 minutes. Alert other personnel to the patient's tendency to hemorrhage.
- Monitor the patient's intake and output hourly in acute DIC, especially when administering blood products. Watch for transfusion reactions and signs of fluid overload. To measure the amount of blood lost, weigh dressings and linen and record

drainage. Weigh the patient daily, particularly if there's renal involvement.
- Watch for bleeding from the GI and genitourinary tracts. If you suspect intra-abdominal bleeding, measure the patient's abdominal girth at least every 4 hours, and monitor closely for signs of shock.
- Monitor the results of serial blood studies (particularly hematocrit, hemoglobin level, and coagulation times).
- Explain all diagnostic tests and procedures. Allow time for questions.
- Inform the family of the patient's progress. Prepare them for his appearance (I.V. lines, nasogastric tubes, bruises, and dried blood). Provide emotional support for the patient and his family. As needed, enlist the aid of a social worker, chaplain, and other members of the health care team in providing such support.

FOODS HIGH IN FOLIC ACID

Here's a list of foods high in folic acid.

FOOD	MCG/100 G
Asparagus spears	109
Beef liver	294
Broccoli spears	54
Collards (cooked)	102
Mushrooms	24
Oatmeal	33
Peanut butter	57
Red beans	180
Wheat germ	305

Folic acid deficiency anemia

Folic acid deficiency anemia is a common, slowly progressive, megaloblastic anemia. It usually occurs in infants, adolescents, pregnant and lactating females, alcoholics, elderly people, and people with malignant or intestinal diseases.

CAUSES
- Alcohol abuse (alcohol may suppress metabolic effects of folate)
- Bacteria competing for available folic acid
- Excessive cooking, which can destroy a high percentage of folic acids in foods (see *Foods high in folic acid*)
- Impaired absorption (due to intestinal dysfunction from bowel resection and such disorders as celiac disease, tropical sprue, and regional jejunitis)
- Increased folic acid requirements during pregnancy, during rapid growth in infancy (common because of recent increase in survival of premature infants), during childhood and adolescence (because of general use of folate-poor cow's milk), and in patients with neoplastic diseases and some skin diseases (chronic exfoliative dermatitis)
- Limited capacity to store folic acid (in infants)
- Poor diet (common in alcoholics, elderly people living alone, and infants, especially those with infections or diarrhea)
- Prolonged drug therapy (anticonvulsants and estrogens, including hormonal contraceptives)

PATHOPHYSIOLOGY

Folic acid (pteroylglutamic acid, folacin) is found in most body tissues, where it acts as a coenzyme in metabolic processes involving one carbon transfer. It's essential for formation and maturation of red blood cells (RBCs) and for synthesis of deoxyribonucleic acid. Although its body stores are relatively small (about 70 mg), this vitamin is plentiful in most well-balanced diets.

Even so, because folic acid is water-soluble and heat-labile, it's easily destroyed by cooking. Also, approximately 20% of folic acid intake is excreted unabsorbed. Insufficient daily folic acid intake (less than 50 mcg/day) usually induces folic acid deficiency within 4 months, as the body stores in the liver are depleted. This deficiency inhibits cell growth, particularly of RBCs, leading to production of few, deformed RBCs. These enlarged red cells characteristic of the megaloblastic anemias have a shortened life span of weeks rather than months.

CLINICAL FINDINGS

Clinical features are characteristic of other megaloblastic anemias, without the neurologic manifestations.
- Progressive fatigue
- Shortness of breath
- Palpitations
- Weakness
- Glossitis
- Nausea, anorexia
- Headache
- Fainting
- Irritability, forgetfulness
- Pallor and slight jaundice

TEST RESULTS
- The Schilling test and a therapeutic trial of vitamin B_{12} injections distinguish folic acid deficiency anemia from pernicious anemia.
- Blood studies show macrocytosis, a decreased reticulocyte count, abnormal platelets, and a serum folate level of less than 4 mg/ml.

TREATMENT
- Folic acid supplements given orally (usually 1 to 5 mg/day) or parenterally (to patients who are severely ill, have malabsorption, or can't take oral medication) and elimination of contributing causes
- Well-balanced diet
- With combined vitamin B_{12} and folate deficiency, folic acid replenishment alone possibly aggravating neurologic dysfunction

NURSING CONSIDERATIONS
- Teach the patient to meet daily folic acid requirements by including a food from each food group in every meal. If the patient has a severe deficiency, explain that diet only reinforces folic acid supplementation and isn't therapeutic by itself. Urge compliance with the prescribed course of therapy. Advise the patient not to stop taking the supplements when he begins to feel better.
- Encourage the patient to avoid alcohol, nonherbal teas, antacids, and phosphates, which impair the absorption of B vitamins and iron.
- If the patient has glossitis, emphasize the importance of good oral hygiene. Suggest regular use of mild or diluted mouthwash and a soft toothbrush.
- Watch fluid and electrolyte balance, particularly in the patient who has severe diarrhea and is receiving parenteral fluid replacement therapy.
- Because anemia causes severe fatigue, schedule regular rest periods un-

til the patient can resume normal activity.

- To prevent folic acid deficiency anemia, emphasize the importance of a well-balanced diet high in folic acid. Identify alcoholics with poor dietary habits, and try to arrange for appropriate counseling. Tell women who aren't breast-feeding to use commercially prepared formulas.

Idiopathic thrombocytopenic purpura

Idiopathic thrombocytopenic purpura (ITP) is a platelet deficiency that occurs when the immune system destroys the body's own platelets. ITP may be acute, as in postviral thrombocytopenia, or chronic, as in essential thrombocytopenia or autoimmune thrombocytopenia.

Alert *Acute ITP usually affects children ages 2 to 6; chronic ITP mainly affects adults younger than age 50, especially women ages 20 to 40.*

The prognosis for acute ITP is excellent; nearly four out of five patients recover without treatment. The prognosis for chronic ITP is good; remissions lasting weeks or years are common, especially among women.

CAUSES
- Drug reactions
- Immunization with a live virus vaccine
- Immunologic disorders
- Viral infection

PATHOPHYSIOLOGY
ITP occurs when circulating immunoglobulin (Ig) G molecules react with host platelets, which are then destroyed in the spleen and, to a lesser degree, in the liver. Normally, the life span of platelets in circulation is 7 to 10 days. In ITP, platelets survive 3 days or less. This can cause complications, such as hemorrhage, cerebral hemorrhage, and purpuric lesions of vital organs (such as the brain and kidney).

CLINICAL FINDINGS
- Nosebleeds
- Oral bleeding
- Hemorrhage into the skin, mucous membranes, and other tissues, causing red discoloration of skin (purpura)
- Small purplish hemorrhagic spots on skin (petechiae)
- Excessive menstrual bleeding

TEST RESULTS
- Blood studies reveal:
- platelet count less than 20,000/mm³
- prolonged bleeding time
- abnormal size and appearance of platelets
- decreased hemoglobin level (if bleeding occurred).
- Bone marrow studies show abundant megakaryocytes (platelet precursor cells) and a circulating platelet survival time of only several hours to a few days.
- Humoral tests measure platelet-associated IgG that may help establish the diagnosis; half the patients have elevated IgG.

TREATMENT
For acute ITP
- Glucocorticoids to prevent further platelet destruction
- Immunoglobulin to prevent platelet destruction

- Plasmapheresis
- Platelet pheresis

For chronic ITP
- Corticosteroids to suppress phagocytic activity and enhance platelet production
- Splenectomy (when splenomegaly accompanies the initial thrombocytopenia)
- Blood and blood component transfusions and vitamin K to correct anemia and coagulation defects

Alternative treatments
- Immunosuppressants to help stop platelet destruction
- High-dose I.V. immunoglobulin
- Immunoabsorption apheresis using staphylococcal protein A columns

NURSING CONSIDERATIONS
- Teach the patient to observe for petechiae, ecchymoses, and other signs of recurrence.
- Monitor patients receiving immunosuppressants for signs of bone marrow depression, infection, mucositis, GI ulcers, and severe diarrhea or vomiting.
- Tell the patient to avoid aspirin and ibuprofen.

Iron deficiency anemia

Iron deficiency anemia is a disorder of oxygen transport in which hemoglobin synthesis is deficient. A common disease worldwide, iron deficiency anemia affects 10% to 30% of adults in the United States. Iron deficiency anemia occurs most commonly in premenopausal women, infants (particularly premature or low-birth-weight

infants), children, and adolescents (especially girls). The prognosis after replacement therapy is favorable.

CAUSES
- Blood loss due to drug-induced GI bleeding (from anticoagulants, aspirin, or steroids) or heavy menses, hemorrhage from trauma, peptic ulcers, cancer, increased laboratory blood samples in chronically ill patients, sequestration in patients on dialysis, or varices
- Inadequate dietary intake of iron (less than 1 to 2 mg/day), as in prolonged nonsupplemented breast-feeding or bottle-feeding of infants or during periods of stress, such as rapid growth, in children and adolescents
- Intravascular hemolysis-induced hemoglobinuria or paroxysmal nocturnal hemoglobinuria
- Iron malabsorption, as in chronic diarrhea, partial or total gastrectomy, and malabsorption syndromes, such as celiac disease and pernicious anemia
- Mechanical trauma to red blood cells (RBCs) caused by a prosthetic heart valve or vena cava filters
- Pregnancy, which diverts maternal iron to the fetus for erythropoiesis

PATHOPHYSIOLOGY
Iron deficiency anemia occurs when the supply of iron is inadequate for optimal RBC formation, resulting in smaller (microcytic) cells with less color (hypochromic) on staining. Body stores of iron, including plasma iron, become depleted, and the concentration of serum transferrin, which binds with and transports iron, decreases. Insufficient iron stores lead to a depleted RBC mass with subnormal hemoglobin concentration and, in turn, subnormal oxygen-carrying capacity

of the blood. This depletion can lead to complications, such as infection, pneumonia, pica, bleeding, or an over-dosage of iron supplements.

CLINICAL FINDINGS

Because iron deficiency anemia progresses gradually, many patients exhibit only symptoms of an underlying condition. They tend not to seek medical treatment until anemia is severe.

Advanced stages

- Dyspnea on exertion, fatigue, listlessness, pallor, inability to concentrate, irritability, headache, and a susceptibility to infection due to decreased oxygen-carrying capacity of the blood caused by decreased hemoglobin level
- Increased cardiac output and tachycardia due to decreased oxygen perfusion
- Coarsely ridged, spoon-shaped (koilonychia), brittle, and thin nails due to decreased capillary circulation
- Sore, red, and burning tongue due to papillae atrophy
- Sore, dry skin in the corners of the mouth due to epithelial changes

TEST RESULTS

Blood studies (serum iron, total iron-binding capacity, ferritin levels) and iron stores in bone marrow may confirm iron deficiency anemia. However, the results of these tests can be misleading because of complicating factors, such as infection, pneumonia, blood transfusion, or iron supplements. Characteristic blood test results include:

- low hemoglobin level (males, less than 12 g/dl; females, less than 10 g/dl)
- low hematocrit (males, less than 47; females, less than 42)
- low serum iron with high binding capacity level
- low serum ferritin level
- low RBC count, with microcytic and hypochromic cells (in early stages, RBC count possibly normal, except in infants and children)
- decreased mean corpuscular hemoglobin level in severe anemia
- depleted or absent iron stores (by specific staining) and hyperplasia of normal precursor cells (by bone marrow studies).

TREATMENT

The first priority of treatment is to determine the underlying cause of anemia. Only then can iron replacement therapy begin. Possible treatments include:

- oral preparation of iron (treatment of choice) or a combination of iron and ascorbic acid (enhances iron absorption)
- parenteral iron (for the patient who's noncompliant with oral dose, needing more iron than can be given orally, with malabsorption preventing adequate iron absorption, or for a maximum rate of hemoglobin regeneration).

Because total-dose I.V. infusion of supplemental iron is painless and requires fewer injections, it's usually preferred to I.M. administration. Considerations include:

- total-dose infusion of iron dextran (InFeD) in normal saline solution given over 1 to 8 hours (pregnant and elderly patients with severe anemia)
- I.V. test dose of 0.5 ml given first (to minimize the risk of an allergic reaction).

NURSING CONSIDERATIONS

- Advise the patient not to stop therapy even if he feels better.

- Tell the patient he may take iron supplements with a meal to decrease gastric irritation. Advise him to avoid milk, milk products, and antacids because they interfere with iron absorption; however, vitamin C can increase absorption.
- Warn the patient that iron supplements may result in dark green or black stools and can cause constipation.
- Instruct the patient to drink liquid supplemental iron through a straw to prevent staining his teeth.
- Tell the patient to report bothersome adverse reactions, such as nausea, vomiting, and diarrhea.
- If the patient receives I.V. iron, monitor the infusion rate carefully, and observe for an allergic reaction. Stop the infusion and begin supportive treatment immediately if the patient shows signs of an adverse reaction. Also, watch for dizziness and headache and for thrombophlebitis around the I.V. site.
- Use the Z-track injection method when administering iron I.M. to prevent skin discoloration, scarring, and irritating iron deposits in the skin.
- Because an iron deficiency may recur, advise regular checkups and blood studies.

Pernicious anemia

Pernicious anemia, the most common type of megaloblastic anemia, is caused by vitamin B_{12} malabsorption.

Alert *The onset of pernicious anemia typically occurs from ages 50 to 60, and the incidence increases with age.*

If not treated, pernicious anemia is fatal. Its manifestations subside with treatment, but some neurologic deficits may be permanent.

CAUSES
- Genetic predisposition (suggested by familial incidence)
- Immunologically related diseases, such as thyroiditis, myxedema, and Graves' disease (significantly higher incidence in these patients)
- Older age (progressive loss of vitamin B_{12} absorption)

Alert *Elderly patients commonly have a dietary deficiency of vitamin B_{12} in addition to or instead of poor absorption.*

- Partial gastrectomy (iatrogenic induction)

PATHOPHYSIOLOGY
Pernicious anemia is characterized by decreased production of hydrochloric acid in the stomach and a deficiency of intrinsic factor, which is normally secreted by the parietal cells of the gastric mucosa and is essential for vitamin B_{12} absorption in the ileum. The resulting vitamin B_{12} deficiency inhibits cell growth, particularly of red blood cells (RBCs), leading to production of few, deformed RBCs with poor oxygen-carrying capacity. It also causes neurologic damage by impairing myelin formation and permanent central nervous system (CNS) symptoms (if the patient isn't treated within 6 months of appearance of symptoms). Other possible complications include hypokalemia (first week of treatment), gastric polyps, and stomach cancer.

CLINICAL FINDINGS
Characteristically, pernicious anemia has an insidious onset, but eventually causes an unmistakable triad of symptoms.
- Weakness due to tissue hypoxia

- Sore tongue due to atrophy of the papillae
- Numbness and tingling in the extremities

Other common manifestations may include:
- pale appearance of lips and gums
- faintly jaundiced sclera and pale to bright yellow skin due to hemolysis-induced hyperbilirubinemia
- high susceptibility to infection, especially of the genitourinary tract
- nausea, vomiting, anorexia, weight loss, flatulence, diarrhea, and constipation from disturbed digestion due to gastric mucosal atrophy and decreased hydrochloric acid production
- gingival bleeding and tongue inflammation (may hinder eating and intensify anorexia)
- neuritis; weakness in extremities
- peripheral numbness and paresthesia
- disturbed position sense
- lack of coordination, ataxia, impaired fine finger movement
- positive Babinski's and Romberg's signs
- light-headedness
- altered vision, taste, and hearing; optic muscle atrophy
- loss of bowel and bladder control and, in males, impotence, due to demyelination (initially affects peripheral nerves but gradually extends to the spinal cord) caused by vitamin B_{12} deficiency
- irritability, poor memory, headache, depression, and delirium (some symptoms are temporary, but irreversible CNS changes may have occurred before treatment)
- low hemoglobin level due to widespread destruction of RBCs caused by increasingly fragile cell membranes
- palpitations, wide pulse pressure, dyspnea, orthopnea, tachycardia, premature beats and, eventually, heart failure due to compensatory increased cardiac output.

TEST RESULTS

Laboratory screening must rule out other anemias with similar symptoms but different treatments, such as folic acid deficiency anemia and vitamin B_{12} deficiency resulting from malabsorption due to GI disorders, gastric surgery, radiation, or drug therapy.

A family history of pernicious anemia is an indicator in addition to these test results:
- hemoglobin level of 4 to 5 g/mm^3
- low RBC count
- mean corpuscular volume greater than 120 mm^3 due to increased amounts of hemoglobin in larger-than-normal RBCs
- serum vitamin B_{12} less than 0.1 mcg/ml
- bone marrow aspiration showing erythroid hyperplasia (crowded red bone marrow), with more megaloblasts but few normally developing RBCs
- gastric analysis showing absence of free hydrochloric acid after histamine or pentagastrin injection
- Schilling test reveals little or no excretion of radiolabeled vitamin B_{12} into the urine (definitive test for pernicious anemia)
- serologic findings including intrinsic factor antibodies and antiparietal cell antibodies.

TREATMENT
- Early parenteral vitamin B_{12} replacement (can reverse pernicious anemia, minimize complications, and possibly prevent permanent neurologic damage)
- Concomitant iron and folic acid replacement to prevent iron deficiency

anemia (rapid cell regeneration increasing the patient's iron and folate requirements)
● After initial response, decreasing vitamin B_{12} dosage to monthly self-administered maintenance dose (must be given for life)
● Bed rest for extreme fatigue until hemoglobin level rises
● Blood transfusions for dangerously low hemoglobin level
● Digoxin (Lanoxin), diuretic, and low-sodium diet (if patient is in heart failure)
● Antibiotics to combat infections

NURSING CONSIDERATIONS
● Provide patient and family teaching to promote compliance with lifelong vitamin B_{12} replacement even after symptoms subside.
● If the patient has severe anemia, plan activities, rest periods, and necessary diagnostic tests to conserve his energy. Monitor pulse rate often; tachycardia means his activities are too strenuous.
● To ensure accurate Schilling test results, make sure that all urine over a 24-hour period is collected and that the specimens are uncontaminated.
● Warn the patient to guard against infections, and tell him to report signs of infection promptly.
● Provide a well-balanced diet, including foods high in vitamin B_{12} (meat, liver, fish, eggs, and milk). Offer between-meal snacks, and encourage the family to bring favorite foods from home.
● Because a sore mouth and tongue make eating and talking painful, avoid giving the patient irritating foods. Supply a pad and pencil or some other aid to facilitate nonverbal communication. Swab the patient's mouth with tap water or warm saline solution.

● Warn the patient with a sensory deficit not to use a heating pad because it may cause burns.
● If the patient is incontinent, establish a regular bowel and bladder routine. After the patient is discharged, a home health care nurse should follow up on this schedule and make adjustments as needed.
● If neurologic damage causes behavioral problems, assess the patient's mental and neurologic status often; if necessary, give tranquilizers, as ordered, and apply a jacket restraint at night.
● To prevent pernicious anemia, emphasize the importance of vitamin B_{12} supplements for patients who have had extensive gastric resections or who follow strict vegetarian diets.

Polycythemia vera

Polycythemia vera is a chronic disorder characterized by increased red blood cell (RBC) mass, erythrocytosis, leukocytosis, thrombocytosis, and increased hemoglobin level, with normal or increased plasma volume. This disease is also known as *primary polycythemia, erythremia, polycythemia rubra vera, splenomegalic polycythemia,* and *Vaquez-Osler disease.* It usually occurs from ages 40 to 60, most commonly among Jewish males of European ancestry. It seldom affects children and doesn't appear to be familial.

The prognosis depends on the age at diagnosis, the type of treatment used, and complications. Mortality is high if polycythemia is untreated, associated with leukemia, or associated with myeloid metaplasia (presence of marrowlike tissue and ectopic hematopoiesis in extramedullary sites, such as the liver and spleen, and nucleated erythrocytes in blood).

CAUSES

The cause of polycythemia vera is unknown, but is probably related to multipotential stem cell defect.

PATHOPHYSIOLOGY

In polycythemia vera, uncontrolled and rapid cellular reproduction and maturation cause proliferation or hyperplasia of all bone marrow cells (panmyelosis).

Increased RBC mass makes the blood abnormally viscous and inhibits blood flow to the microcirculation. Diminished blood flow and thrombocytosis set the stage for intravascular thrombosis.

CLINICAL FINDINGS

- Feeling of fullness in the head or headache due to altered blood volume, as in hypovolemia and hyperviscosity
- Dizziness due to hypervolemia and hyperviscosity
- Ruddy cyanosis (plethora) of the nose and clubbing of the digits due to thrombosis in smaller vessels
- Painful pruritus due to abnormally high concentrations of mast cells in the skin and their releases of heparin and histamine

TEST RESULTS

- Blood studies reveal:
- increased RBC mass
- increased blood histamine levels
- decreased serum iron concentration
- increased uric acid level.
- Arterial blood gas analysis reveals normal arterial oxygen saturation in association with splenomegaly.

- Urine studies reveal decreased or absent urinary erythropoietin.
- Bone marrow biopsy shows excess production of myeloid stem cells.

TREATMENT

- Phlebotomy to reduce RBC mass
- Myelosuppressive therapy with radioactive phosphorus (^{32}P) to suppress erythropoiesis, possibly increasing the risk of leukemia, or hydroxyurea

NURSING CONSIDERATIONS
For phlebotomy

- Explain the procedure, and reassure the patient that it will relieve distressing symptoms. Check blood pressure, pulse rate, and respiratory rate. During phlebotomy, make sure that the patient is lying down comfortably to prevent vertigo and syncope. Stay alert for tachycardia, clamminess, or complaints of vertigo. If these effects occur, the procedure should be stopped.
- Immediately after phlebotomy, check blood pressure and pulse rate. Have the patient sit up for about 5 minutes before allowing him to walk; this prevents vasovagal attack or orthostatic hypotension. Also, have the patient drink 24 oz (710 ml) of juice or water.
- Tell the patient to watch for and report signs or symptoms of iron deficiency (pallor, weight loss, asthenia [weakness], and glossitis).
- Keep the patient active and ambulatory to prevent thrombosis. If bed rest is absolutely necessary, prescribe a daily program of active and passive range-of-motion exercises.
- Watch for such complications as hypervolemia, thrombocytosis, and signs or symptoms of an impending stroke (decreased sensation, numb-

ness, transitory paralysis, fleeting blindness, headache, and epistaxis).
● Regularly examine the patient closely for bleeding. Tell him which are the most common bleeding sites, such as the nose, gingiva, and skin, so he can check for bleeding. Advise him to report abnormal bleeding promptly.
● To compensate for increased uric acid production, give additional fluids, administer allopurinol, and alkalinize urine to prevent uric acid calculi.
● If the patient has symptomatic splenomegaly, suggest or provide small, frequent meals, followed by a rest period, to prevent nausea and vomiting.
● Report acute abdominal pain immediately; it may signal splenic infarction, renal calculi, or abdominal organ thrombosis.

During myelosuppressive treatment

● Monitor complete blood count (CBC) and platelet count before and during therapy. Warn the outpatient who develops leukopenia that his resistance to infection is low; advise him to avoid crowds and watch for symptoms of infection. If leukopenia develops in a hospitalized patient who needs reverse isolation, follow facility guidelines. If thrombocytopenia develops, tell the patient to watch for signs of bleeding (blood in urine, nosebleeds, and black stools).
● Tell the patient about possible reactions (nausea, vomiting, and risk of infection) to alkylating agents. Alopecia may follow the use of busulfan (Busulfex) and cyclophosphamide (Cytoxan); sterile hemorrhagic cystitis may follow the use of cyclophosphamide (forcing fluids can prevent it). Watch for and report all reactions. If nausea and vomiting occur, begin antiemetic therapy and adjust the patient's diet.

During ^{32}P treatment

● Explain the procedure to relieve anxiety. Tell the patient he may require repeated phlebotomies until ^{32}P takes effect. Take a blood sample for CBC and platelet count before beginning treatment. (Use of ^{32}P requires radiation precautions to prevent contamination.)
● Have the patient lie down during I.V. administration (to facilitate the procedure and prevent extravasation) and for 15 to 20 minutes afterward.

Thalassemia

Thalassemia, a hereditary group of hemolytic anemias, is characterized by defective synthesis in the polypeptide chains of the protein component of hemoglobin. Consequently, red blood cell (RBC) synthesis is also impaired.

Alert *Thalassemia is most common in people of Mediterranean ancestry (especially Italian and Greek) but also occurs in people whose ancestors originated in Africa, southern China, southeast Asia, and India.*

In beta-thalassemia, the most common form of this disorder, synthesis of the beta polypeptide chain is defective. It occurs in three clinical forms: major, intermedia, and minor. The severity of the resulting anemia depends on whether the patient is homozygous or heterozygous for the thalassemic trait. The prognosis varies:
● Thalassemia major—Patients seldom survive to adulthood.
● Thalassemia intermedia—Children develop normally into adulthood, although puberty is usually delayed.

- Thalassemia minor—Patients have normal life span.

CAUSES
- Heterozygous inheritance of the same gene (thalassemia minor)
- Homozygous inheritance of the partially dominant autosomal gene (thalassemia major or thalassemia intermedia)

PATHOPHYSIOLOGY
Total or partial deficiency of beta polypeptide chain production impairs hemoglobin synthesis and results in continual production of fetal hemoglobin, lasting even past the neonatal period. Normally, immunoglobulin synthesis switches from gamma- to beta-polypeptides at the time of birth. This conversion doesn't happen in thalassemic infants. Their red cells are hypochromic and microcytic. Complications can include pathologic fractures due to expansion of the marrow cavities with thinning of the long bones, cardiac arrhythmias and, heart failure.

CLINICAL FINDINGS
Signs and symptoms of thalassemia major, also known as *Cooley's anemia, Mediterranean disease,* and *erythroblastic anemia,* include:
- in healthy infant at birth, during second 6 months of life, develops severe anemia, bone abnormalities, failure to thrive, and life-threatening complications
- pallor and yellow skin and sclera in infants ages 3 to 6 months
- splenomegaly or hepatomegaly, with abdominal enlargement; frequent infections; bleeding tendencies (especially nose bleeds); and anorexia

- small body, large head (characteristic features), and possible mental retardation
- possible features similar to Down syndrome in infants because of thickened bone at the base of the nose from bone marrow hyperactivity.

Signs and symptoms of thalassemia intermedia include:
- some degree of anemia, jaundice, and splenomegaly
- possibly signs of hemosiderosis due to increased intestinal absorption of iron.

Signs of thalassemia minor include:
- mild anemia (usually produces no symptoms and is commonly overlooked; should be differentiated from iron deficiency anemia).

TEST RESULTS
Diagnosis of thalassemia major includes:
- low RBC count and hemoglobin level, microcytosis, and high reticulocyte count
- elevated bilirubin and urinary and fecal urobilinogen levels
- low serum folate level reflecting increased folate use by hypertrophied bone marrow
- peripheral blood smear showing target cells, microcytes, pale nucleated RBCs, and marked anisocytosis
- thinning and widening of the marrow space on skull and long bone X-rays due to overactive bone marrow
- granular appearance of bones of skull and vertebrae, areas of osteoporosis in long bones, and deformed (rectangular or biconvex) phalanges
- significantly increased fetal hemoglobin level and slightly increased hemoglobin A_2 level on quantitative hemoglobin studies

- excluding iron deficiency anemia (also produces hypochromic microcytic RBCs).

Diagnosis of thalassemia intermedia includes:
- hypochromic microcytic RBCs (less severe than in thalassemia major).

Diagnosis of thalassemia minor includes:
- hypochromic microcytic RBCs
- significantly increased hemoglobin A_2 level and moderately increased fetal hemoglobin level on quantitative hemoglobin studies.

TREATMENT

Treatment of thalassemia major is essentially supportive and includes:
- prompt treatment with appropriate antibiotics for infections
- folic acid supplements to help maintain folic acid levels despite increased requirements
- transfusions of packed RBCs to increase hemoglobin level (used judiciously to minimize iron overload)
- splenectomy and bone marrow transplantation (effectiveness hasn't been confirmed)
- no treatment for thalassemia intermedia and thalassemia minor
- no iron supplements (contraindicated in all forms of thalassemia).

NURSING CONSIDERATIONS
- During and after RBC transfusions for thalassemia major, watch for adverse reactions — shaking chills, fever, rash, itching, and hives.
- Stress the importance of good nutrition, meticulous wound care, periodic dental checkups, and other measures to prevent infection.
- For a young patient, discuss with his parents various options for healthy physical and creative outlets. Such a child must avoid strenuous athletic activity because of increased oxygen demand and the tendency toward pathologic fractures, but he may participate in less stressful activities.
- Teach parents to watch for signs of hepatitis and iron overload — always possible with frequent transfusions.
- Because parents may have questions about the vulnerability of future offspring, refer them for genetic counseling. Also, refer adult patients with thalassemia minor and thalassemia intermedia for genetic counseling; they need to recognize the risk of transmitting thalassemia major to their children if they have children with another person who has thalassemia. If such people choose to have children, all their children should be evaluated for thalassemia by age 1. Be sure to tell people with thalassemia minor that their condition is benign.

von Willebrand's disease

von Willebrand's disease is a hereditary bleeding disorder, occurring more often in females and characterized by a prolonged bleeding time, a moderate deficiency of clotting factor VIII (antihemophilic factor), and impaired platelet function. This disease commonly causes bleeding from the skin or mucosal surfaces and, in females, excessive uterine bleeding. Bleeding may range from mild and asymptomatic to severe, potentially fatal, hemorrhage. The prognosis is usually good.

CAUSES
von Willebrand's disease is caused by inherited autosomal dominant trait.

Recently, an acquired form has been identified in patients with cancer and immune disorders.

PATHOPHYSIOLOGY

A possible mechanism is that mild to moderate deficiency of factor VIII and defective platelet adhesion prolong coagulation time. Specifically, this results from a deficiency of von Willebrand's factor (vWF), which stabilizes the factor VIII molecule and is needed for proper platelet function.

Defective platelet function is characterized in vivo by decreased agglutination and adhesion at the bleeding site and in vitro by reduced platelet retention when blood is filtered through a column of packed glass beads, and diminished ristocetin-induced platelet aggregation.

CLINICAL FINDINGS

- Easy bruising
- Epistaxis (nosebleed)
- Bleeding from the gums
- Petechiae (rarely)
- Hemorrhage after laceration or surgery (in severe forms)
- Menorrhagia (in severe forms)
- GI bleeding (in severe forms)
- Excessive postpartum bleeding (uncommon)
- Massive soft tissue hemorrhage and bleeding into joints (rare)

TEST RESULTS

- Prolonged bleeding time is greater than 6 minutes.
- Partial thromboplastin time is slightly prolonged (greater than 45 seconds).
- Blood studies reveal normal platelet count and clot retraction, absent or low factor VIII, absent or low factor VIII–related antigens, and low factor VIII activity.

- Ristocetin coagulation factor assay shows defective in vitro platelet aggregation.

TREATMENT

- Infusion of cryoprecipitate or blood fractions rich in factor VIII to shorten bleeding time and replace factor VIII
- Parenteral or intranasal desmopressin (DDAVP) to increase serum levels of vWF

NURSING CONSIDERATIONS

- The care plan should include local measures to control bleeding and patient teaching to prevent bleeding, unnecessary trauma, and complications.
- After surgery, monitor bleeding time for 24 to 48 hours, and watch for signs of new bleeding.
- During a bleeding episode, elevate and apply cold compresses and gentle pressure to the bleeding site.
- Refer parents of affected children for genetic counseling.
- Advise the patient to consult the physician after even minor trauma and before surgery to determine if replacement of blood components is necessary.
- Tell the patient to watch for signs of hepatitis within 6 weeks to 6 months after transfusion.
- Warn against using aspirin and other drugs that impair platelet function.

8

IMMUNE SYSTEM

The immune system is responsible for safeguarding the body from disease-causing microorganisms. It's part of a complex system of host defenses.

Host defenses may be innate or acquired. Innate defenses include physical and chemical barriers, the complement complex, and cells, such as phagocytes (cells programmed to destroy foreign cells, such as bacteria) and natural killer lymphocytes.

Physical barriers, such as the skin and mucous membranes, prevent invasion by most organisms. Chemical barriers include lysozymes (found in such body secretions as tears, mucus, and saliva) and hydrochloric acid in the stomach. Lysozymes destroy bacteria by removing cell walls. Hydrochloric acid breaks down food and destroys pathogens carried by food or swallowed mucus.

Organisms that penetrate this first line of defense simultaneously trigger the inflammatory and immune responses, some innate and others acquired.

Acquired immunity comes into play when the body encounters a cell or cell product that it recognizes as foreign, such as a bacterium or virus. The two types of immunity provided by cells are humoral (provided by B lymphocytes) and cell-mediated (provided by T lymphocytes). All cells involved in the inflammatory and immune responses arrive from a single type of stem cell in the bone marrow. B cells mature in the marrow, and T cells migrate to the thymus, where they mature.

The inflammatory response is the immediate local response to tissue injury, whether from trauma or infection. It involves the action of polymorphonuclear leukocytes, basophils and mast cells, platelets and, to some extent, monocytes and macrophages.

The environment contains thousands of pathogenic microorganisms. Normally, our host defense system protects us from these harmful invaders. When this network of safeguards breaks down, however, the result is an altered immune response or immune system failure.

Acquired immunodeficiency syndrome

Human immunodeficiency virus (HIV) infection may cause acquired immunodeficiency syndrome (AIDS). Although it's characterized by gradual destruction of cell-mediated (T cell) immunity, it also affects humoral immunity and even autoimmunity because of the central role of the CD4+ (helper) T lymphocyte in immune reactions. The resulting immunodeficiency makes the patient susceptible to opportunistic infections, cancers, and other abnormalities that define AIDS.

This syndrome was first described by the Centers for Disease Control and Prevention (CDC) in 1981. Because transmission is similar, AIDS shares epidemiologic patterns with hepatitis B and sexually transmitted diseases (STDs).

Depending on individual variations and the presence of cofactors that influence disease progression, the time from acute HIV infection to the appearance of symptoms (mild to severe) to the diagnosis of AIDS and, eventually, to death varies greatly. Current combination drug therapy in conjunction with treatment and prophylaxis of common opportunistic infections can delay the natural progression and prolong survival.

CAUSES

The HIV-1 retrovirus is the primary etiologic agent. Transmission occurs by contact with infected blood or body fluids and is associated with identifiable high-risk behaviors. It's disproportionately represented in:
- homosexual and bisexual men
- I.V. drug users
- recipients of contaminated blood or blood products (dramatically decreased since mid-1985)
- heterosexual partners of persons in the former groups
- neonates of infected women.

PATHOPHYSIOLOGY

The natural history of AIDS begins with infection by the HIV retrovirus, which is detectable only by laboratory tests, and ends with death. Over twenty years of data strongly suggest that HIV isn't transmitted by casual household or social contact. The HIV virus may enter the body by any of several routes involving the transmission of blood or body fluids, for example:
- direct inoculation during intimate sexual contact, especially associated with the mucosal trauma of receptive rectal intercourse
- transfusion of contaminated blood or blood products (a risk diminished by routine testing of all blood products)
- sharing contaminated needles
- transplacental or postpartum transmission from an infected mother to her fetus (by cervical or blood contact at delivery and in breast milk).

HIV strikes helper T cells bearing the CD4+ antigen. Normally a receptor for major histocompatibility complex molecules, the antigen serves as a receptor for the retrovirus and allows it to enter the cell. Viral binding also requires the presence of a coreceptor (believed to be the chemokine receptor CCR5) on the cell surface. The virus also may infect CD4+ antigen-bearing cells of the GI tract, uterine cervix, and neuroglia.

Like other retroviruses, HIV copies its genetic material in a reverse manner compared with other viruses and cells. Through the action of reverse transcriptase, HIV produces deoxyribonucleic acid (DNA) from its viral ribonucleic acid (RNA). Transcription is commonly poor, leading to mutations, some of which make HIV resistant to antiviral drugs. The viral DNA enters

OPPORTUNISTIC INFECTIONS IN AIDS

This chart shows the complicating infections that may occur in acquired immunodeficiency syndrome (AIDS).

MICROBIOLOGICAL AGENT	ORGANISM	CONDITION
Protozoa	Pneumocystis carinii Cryptosporidium Toxoplasma gondii Histoplasma	P. carinii pneumonia Cryptosporidiosis Toxoplasmosis Histoplasmosis
Fungi	Candida albicans Cryptococcus neoformans	Candidiasis Cryptococcosis
Viruses	Herpes Cytomegalovirus (CMV)	Herpes simplex 1 and 2 CMV retinitis
Bacteria	Mycobacterium tuberculosis M. avium-intracellulare	Tuberculosis Mycobacteriosis

Other opportunistic conditions include:
◆ Kaposi's sarcoma
◆ wasting disease
◆ AIDS dementia complex.

the nucleus of the cell and is incorporated into the host cell's DNA, where it's transcribed into more viral RNA. If the host cell reproduces, it duplicates the HIV DNA along with its own and passes it on to the daughter cells. Thus, if activated, the host cell carries this information and, if activated, replicates the virus. Viral enzymes, proteases, arrange the structural components and RNA into viral particles that move out to the periphery of the host cell, where the virus buds and emerges from the host cell. Thus, the virus is now free to travel and infect other cells.

HIV replication may lead to cell death or it may become latent. HIV infection leads to profound pathology, either directly through destruction of CD4+ cells, other immune cells, and neuroglial cells or indirectly through the secondary effects of CD4+ T-cell dysfunction and resulting immunosuppression.

The HIV infectious process takes three forms:
● immunodeficiency as inopportunistic infections and unusual cancers (see *Opportunistic infections in AIDS*)
● autoimmunity (lymphoid interstitial pneumonitis, arthritis, hypergammaglobulinemia, and production of autoimmune antibodies)
● neurologic dysfunction (AIDS dementia complex, HIV encephalopathy, and peripheral neuropathies).

CLINICAL FINDINGS

HIV infection manifests in many ways. After a high-risk exposure and inoculation, the infected person usually experiences a mononucleosis-like syndrome, which may be attributed to flu or another virus and then may remain asymptomatic for years. In this latent stage, the only sign of HIV infection is laboratory evidence of sero-conversion.

When symptoms appear, they may take many forms, including:

- persistent generalized lympha-denopathy secondary to impaired function of CD4+ cells
- nonspecific symptoms, including weight loss, fatigue, night sweats, fevers related to altered function of CD4+ cells, immunodeficiency, and infection of other CD4+ antigen-bearing cells
- neurologic symptoms resulting from HIV encephalopathy and infection of neuroglial cells
- opportunistic infection or cancer related to immunodeficiency.

Alert *In children, HIV infection has a mean incubation time of 17 months. Signs and symptoms resemble those in adults, except for findings related to STDs. Children have a high incidence of opportunistic bacterial infections: otitis media, sepsis, chronic salivary gland enlargement, lymphoid interstitial pneumonia, Mycobacterium avium-intracellulare complex function, and pneumonias, including Pneumocystis carinii.*

TEST RESULTS

The CDC has developed an HIV/AIDS classification matrix defining AIDS as an illness characterized by one or more indicator diseases, coexisting with laboratory evidence of HIV infection and other possible causes of immunosuppression. Diagnosis of AIDS includes one or more of the following:

- confirmed presence of HIV infection
- CD4+ T-cell count of less than 200 cells/mm^3
- the presence of one or more conditions specified by the CDC as Categories A, B, or C. (See *Conditions associated with AIDS,* page 312.)

TREATMENT

No cure has yet been found for AIDS. Primary therapy includes the use of various combinations of different types of antiretroviral agents. The primary goals of antiretroviral therapy are maximal suppression of HIV viral load, restoration and preservation of immunologic function, improving the quality of life, and reducing morbidity and mortality. To reduce drug resistance and accomplish the goals of therapy, potent regimens using a minimum of three drugs are recommended for most patients. These regimens are commonly referred to as highly active antiretroviral therapy or HAART.

The antiretroviral drug classes include:

- protease inhibitors to block replication of virus particles formed through the action of viral protease (reducing the number of new virus particles produced)
- nucleoside reverse-transcriptase inhibitors to interfere with the copying of viral RNA into DNA by the enzyme reverse transcriptase
- nucleotide reverse transcriptase inhibitors, which act similarly to nucleoside reverse-transcriptase inhibitors
- nonnucleoside reverse-transcriptase inhibitors to interfere with the action of reverse transcriptase by binding directly to enzymes
- fusion inhibitors to prevent HIV from entering healthy T cells by attaching themselves to proteins on the surface of T cells or proteins on the surface of HIV.

Additional treatment may include:

- immunomodulatory agents to boost the immune system weakened by AIDS and retroviral therapy
- human granulocyte colony-stimulating growth factor to stimulate neutrophil production (Retroviral ther-

CONDITIONS ASSOCIATED WITH AIDS

The Centers for Disease Control and Prevention (CDC) lists acquired immunodeficiency syndrome (AIDS)-associated diseases under three categories. Periodically, the CDC adds to these lists.

CATEGORY A
◆ Persistent generalized lymph node enlargement
◆ Acute primary human immunodeficiency virus (HIV) infection with accompanying illness
◆ History of acute HIV infection

CATEGORY B
◆ Bacillary angiomatosis
◆ Oropharyngeal or persistent vulvovaginal candidiasis, fever, or diarrhea lasting longer than 1 month
◆ Idiopathic thrombocytopenic purpura
◆ Pelvic inflammatory disease, especially with a tubulo-ovarian abscess
◆ Peripheral neuropathy

CATEGORY C
◆ Candidiasis of the bronchi, trachea, lungs, or esophagus
◆ Invasive cervical cancer
◆ Disseminated or extrapulmonary coccoidiomycosis
◆ Extrapulmonary cryptococcosis
◆ Chronic interstitial cryptosporidiosis

◆ Cytomegalovirus (CMV) disease affecting organs other than the liver, spleen, or lymph nodes
◆ CMV retinitis with vision loss
◆ Encephalopathy related to HIV
◆ Herpes simplex infection with chronic ulcers or herpetic bronchitis, pneumonitis, or esophagitis
◆ Disseminated or extrapulmonary histoplasmosis
◆ Chronic intestinal isopsoriasis
◆ Kaposi's sarcoma
◆ Burkitt's lymphoma or its equivalent
◆ Immunoblastic lymphoma or its equivalent
◆ Primary brain lymphoma
◆ Disseminated or extrapulmonary *Mycobacterium avium* complex or *M. kansasii*
◆ Pulmonary or extrapulmonary *M. tuberculosis*
◆ Disseminated or extrapulmonary infection with another species of *Mycobacterium*
◆ *Pneumocystis carinii* pneumonia
◆ Recurrent pneumonia
◆ Progressive multifocal leukoencephalopathy
◆ Recurrent *Salmonella* septicemia
◆ Toxoplasmosis of the brain
◆ Wasting disease caused by HIV

---

apy causes anemia, so patients may receive epoetin alfa [Epogen].)
● anti-infective and antineoplastic agents to combat opportunistic infections and associated cancers (some prophylactically to help resist opportunistic infections)
● supportive therapy, including nutritional support, fluid and electrolyte replacement therapy, pain relief, and psychological support.

NURSING CONSIDERATIONS
● Advise health care workers and the public to use precautions in all situations that risk exposure to blood, body fluids, and secretions. Diligent practice of standard precautions can prevent the inadvertent transmission of AIDS and other infectious diseases transmitted by similar routes.
● Recognize that a diagnosis of AIDS is profoundly distressing because of the disease's social impact and discouraging prognosis. The patient may lose his job and financial security as well as the support of his family and friends. Do your best to help the patient cope with an altered body image, the emotional burden of serious ill-

ness, and the threat of death. Encourage and assist the patient in learning about AIDS societies and support programs.

Allergic rhinitis

Allergic rhinitis is a reaction to airborne (inhaled) allergens. Depending on the allergen, the resulting rhinitis and conjunctivitis may occur seasonally (hay fever) or year-round (perennial allergic rhinitis). Allergic rhinitis is the most common atopic allergic reaction, affecting more than 20 million Americans. It's most prevalent in young children and adolescents but can occur in all age-groups.

CAUSES
- Immunoglobulin (Ig) E–mediated type I hypersensitivity response to an environmental antigen (allergen) in a genetically susceptible person

Common triggers
- Perennial allergens and irritants
  - Animal dander
  - Cigarette smoke
  - Dust mite excreta, fungal spores, and molds
  - Feather pillows
- Windborne pollens
  - Spring — oak, elm, maple, alder, birch, and cottonwood
  - Summer — grasses, sheep sorrel, and English plantain
  - Autumn — ragweed and other weeds

PATHOPHYSIOLOGY
During primary exposure to an allergen, T cells recognize the foreign allergens and release chemicals that instruct B cells to produce specific anti-bodies called IgE. IgE antibodies attach themselves to mast cells. Mast cells with attached IgE can remain in the body for years, ready to react when they next encounter the same allergen.

The second time the allergen enters the body, it comes into direct contact with the IgE antibodies attached to the mast cells. This action stimulates the mast cells to release chemicals, such as histamine, which initiate a response that causes tightening of the smooth muscles in the airways, dilation of small blood vessels, increased mucus secretion in the nasal cavity and airways, and itching. These reactions can lead to complications, such as sinus and middle ear infections, due to swelling of the turbinates and mucous membranes and nasal polyps, which may result from edema and infection and can increase nasal obstruction.

CLINICAL FINDINGS
Seasonal allergic rhinitis
- Paroxysmal sneezing
- Profuse watery rhinorrhea
- Nasal obstruction or congestion
- Pruritus of the nose and eyes
- Pale, cyanotic, and edematous nasal mucosa
- Red and edematous eyelids and conjunctivae
- Excessive lacrimation
- Headache or sinus pain
- Itching in the throat and malaise

Perennial allergic rhinitis
- Chronic nasal obstruction
- Obstruction can extend to eustachian tube obstruction, particularly in children

In both
- Dark circles, which may appear under the patient's eyes ("allergic shin-

ers") because of venous congestion in the maxillary sinuses

- Severity of signs and symptoms that may vary from season to season and from year to year

To distinguish between allergic rhinitis and other disorders of the nasal mucosa, remember these differences:

- In chronic vasomotor rhinitis, eye symptoms are absent, rhinorrhea is mucoid, and seasonal variation is absent.
- In infectious rhinitis (the common cold), the nasal mucosa is beet red; nasal secretions contain polymorphonuclear, not eosinophilic, exudate; and signs and symptoms include fever and sore throat. This condition isn't a recurrent seasonal phenomenon.
- In rhinitis medicamentosa, which results from excessive use of nasal sprays or drops, nasal drainage and mucosal redness and swelling disappear when such medication is withheld.
- In children, differential diagnosis should rule out a nasal foreign body, such as a bean or button.

TEST RESULTS

- Microscopic examination of sputum and nasal secretions reveals large numbers of eosinophils.
- Blood chemistry shows normal or elevated IgE.
- Skin testing paired with tested responses to environmental stimuli pinpoints the responsible allergens.

TREATMENT

- Controlling symptoms by eliminating the environmental antigen, if possible, and providing drug therapy and immunotherapy
- Antihistamines to block histamine effects but commonly produce anticholinergic adverse effects, such as sedation, dry mouth, nausea, dizziness, blurred vision, and nervousness (Some antihistamines, such as fexofenadine [Allegra], produce fewer adverse effects and are less likely to cause sedation.)
- Inhaled intranasal steroids that produce local anti-inflammatory effects with minimal systemic adverse effects; commonly used intranasal steroids including beclomethasone (Beconase AQ), flunisolide (Nasarel), and fluticasone (Flonase) usually aren't effective for acute exacerbations; nasal decongestants and oral antihistamines possibly needed instead
- Use of intranasal steroids regularly, as prescribed, for optimal effectiveness (Cromolyn sodium [Nasalcrom] may help prevent allergic rhinitis. But this drug may take up to 4 weeks to produce a satisfactory effect and must be taken regularly during allergy season.)
- Long-term management including immunotherapy, or desensitization with injections of extracted allergens, administered before or during allergy season or perennially; seasonal allergies requiring particularly close dosage regulation

NURSING CONSIDERATIONS

- Before desensitization injections, assess the patient's symptom status. Afterward, watch for adverse reactions, including anaphylaxis and severe localized erythema.
- Keep epinephrine and emergency resuscitation equipment available, and observe the patient for 30 minutes after the injection. Instruct the patient to call the physician if a delayed reaction should occur.

The following protocol is recommended for allergic rhinitis:

- Monitor the patient's compliance with prescribed drug treatment regimens. Also carefully note changes in the control of his symptoms or signs of drug misuse.
- To reduce environmental exposure to airborne allergens, suggest that the patient sleep with the windows closed, avoid the countryside during pollination seasons, use air conditioning to filter allergens and minimize moisture and dust, and eliminate dust-collecting items, such as wool blankets, deep-pile carpets, and heavy drapes, from the home.
- In severe and resistant cases, suggest that the patient consider drastic changes in lifestyle such as relocation to a pollen-free area either seasonally or year-round.

✳ Life-threatening
Anaphylaxis

Anaphylaxis is an acute, potentially life-threatening type I (immediate) hypersensitivity reaction marked by the sudden onset of rapidly progressive urticaria (vascular swelling in skin accompanied by itching) and respiratory distress. With prompt recognition and treatment, the prognosis is good. However, a severe reaction may precipitate vascular collapse, leading to systemic shock and, sometimes, death. The reaction typically occurs within minutes but can occur up to 1 hour after reexposure to the antigen.

CAUSES
The cause of anaphylaxis is usually the ingestion of or other systemic exposure to sensitizing drugs or other substances. Substances may include:
- Allergen extracts

- Diagnostic chemicals, such as sulfobromophthalein sodium, sodium dehydrocholate, and radiographic contrast media
- Enzymes such as L-asparaginase
- Food additives containing sulfite
- Food proteins, such as those in legumes, nuts, berries, seafood, and egg albumin
- Hormones
- Insect venom
- Local anesthetics
- Penicillin or other antibiotics (induce anaphylaxis in 1 to 4 of every 10,000 patients treated; most likely after parenteral administration or prolonged therapy and in patients with an inherited tendency to food or drug allergy, or atopy)
- Polysaccharides
- Salicylates
- Serums (usually horse serum)
- Sulfonamides
- Vaccines

PATHOPHYSIOLOGY
Anaphylaxis requires previous sensitization or exposure to the specific antigen, resulting in immunoglobulin (Ig) E production by plasma cells in the lymph nodes and enhancement by helper T cells (see *Understanding anaphylaxis,* pages 316 and 317). IgE antibodies then bind to membrane receptors on mast cells in connective tissue and to basophils.

On reexposure, the antigen binds to adjacent IgE antibodies or cross-linked IgE receptors, activating a series of cellular reactions that trigger mast cell degranulation. With degranulation, powerful chemical mediators, such as histamine, eosinophil chemotactic factor of anaphylaxis, and platelet-activating factor, are released from the mast cells. IgG or IgM enters

(Text continues on page 318.)

UNDERSTANDING ANAPHYLAXIS

An anaphylactic reaction requires previous sensitization or exposure to the specific antigen. What happens in anaphylaxis is described here.

1. RESPONSE TO THE ANTIGEN

Immunoglobulin (Ig) M and IgG recognize the antigen as a foreign substance and attach to it.

Destruction of the antigen by the complement cascade begins but remains unfinished, either because of insufficient amounts of the protein catalyst or because the antigen inhibits certain complement enzymes. The patient has no signs and symptoms at this stage.

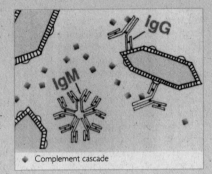

◆ Complement cascade

2. RELEASED CHEMICAL MEDIATORS

The antigen's continued presence activates IgE on basophils. The activated IgE promotes the release of mediators, including histamine, serotonin, and leukotrienes. The sudden release of histamine causes vasodilation and increases capillary permeability. The patient begins to have signs and symptoms, including sudden nasal congestion, itchy and watery eyes, flushing, sweating, weakness, and anxiety.

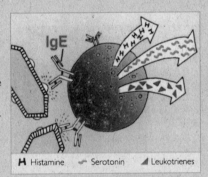

H Histamine   ⬿ Serotonin   ◢ Leukotrienes

3. INTENSIFIED RESPONSE

The activated IgE also stimulates mast cells in connective tissue along the venule walls to release more histamine and eosinophil chemotactic factor of anaphylaxis (ECF-A). These substances produce disruptive lesions that weaken the venules. Now, red and itchy skin, wheals, and swelling appear, and signs and symptoms worsen.

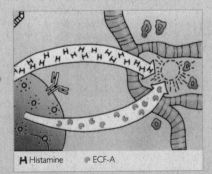

H Histamine   ● ECF-A

4. DISTRESS

In the lungs, histamine causes endothelial cells to burst and endothelial tissue to tear away from surrounding tissue. Fluids leak into the alveoli, and leukotrienes prevent the alveoli from expanding, thus reducing pulmonary compliance. Tachypnea, crowing, accessory muscle use, and cyanosis signal respiratory distress. Resulting neurologic signs and symptoms include changes in the patient's level of consciousness, severe anxiety and, possibly, seizures.

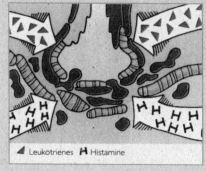

◢ Leukotrienes **H** Histamine

5. DETERIORATION

Meanwhile, basophils and mast cells begin to release prostaglandins and bradykinin along with histamine and serotonin. These substances increase vascular permeability, causing fluids to leak from the vessels. Shock, confusion, cool and pale skin, generalized edema, tachycardia, and hypotension signal rapid vascular collapse.

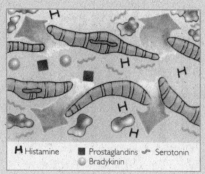

H Histamine ■ Prostaglandins ∿ Serotonin
◉ Bradykinin

6. FAILED COMPENSATORY MECHANISMS

Damage to the endothelial cells causes basophils and mast cells to release heparin. Additional substances are also released to neutralize the other mediators. Eosinophils release arylsulfatase B to neutralize the leukotrienes, phospholipase D to neutralize heparin, and cyclic adenosine monophosphate (AMP) and the prostaglandins E_1 and E_2 to increase the metabolic rate. But these events can't reverse anaphylaxis. Hemorrhage, disseminated intravascular coagulation, and cardiopulmonary arrest result.

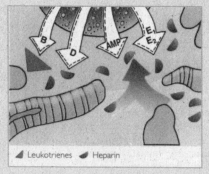

◢ Leukotrienes ◢ Heparin

into the reaction and activates the complement cascade, leading to the release of complement fractions.

At the same time, two other chemical mediators, bradykinin and leukotrienes, induce vascular collapse by stimulating contraction of certain groups of smooth muscles and increasing vascular permeability. These substances, together with the other chemical mediators, cause vasodilation, smooth muscle contraction, enhanced vascular permeability, and increased mucus production. Continued release, along with the spread of these mediators through the body by way of the basophils in the circulation, triggers the systemic responses. Also, increased vascular permeability leads to decreased peripheral resistance and plasma leakage from the circulation to the extravascular tissues. Consequent reduction of blood volume causes hypotension, hypovolemic shock, and cardiac dysfunction.

CLINICAL FINDINGS
- Sudden physical distress within seconds or minutes after exposure to an allergen
- Delayed or persistent reaction possibly occurring up to 24 hours later
- Severity inversely related to the interval between exposure to the allergen and the onset of symptoms

The first symptoms include:
- feeling of impending doom or fright due to activation of IgE and subsequent release of chemical mediators
- sweating due to release of histamine and vasodilation
- sneezing, shortness of breath, nasal pruritus, urticaria, and angioedema (swelling of nerves and blood vessels) secondary to histamine release and increased capillary permeability.

Systemic manifestations may include:
- hypotension, shock, and sometimes cardiac arrhythmias due to increased vascular permeability and subsequent decrease in peripheral resistance and leakage of plasma fluids
- nasal mucosal edema, profuse watery rhinorrhea, itching, nasal congestion, and sudden sneezing attacks due to histamine release, vasodilation, and increased capillary permeability
- edema of the upper respiratory tract, resulting in hypopharyngeal and laryngeal obstruction, due to increased capillary permeability and mast cell degranulation
- hoarseness, stridor, wheezing, and accessory muscle use secondary to bronchiole smooth muscle contraction and increased mucus production
- severe stomach cramps, nausea, diarrhea, and urinary urgency and incontinence resulting from smooth muscle contraction of the intestines and bladder.

TEST RESULTS
- No single diagnostic test can identify anaphylaxis.
- Test results that may provide some clues to the patient's risk of anaphylaxis are skin tests showing hypersensitivity to a specific allergen and elevated serum IgE levels.

TREATMENT
- Immediate administration of epinephrine 1:1,000 aqueous solution to reverse bronchoconstriction and cause vasoconstriction, I.M. or subcutaneously if the patient hasn't lost consciousness and is normotensive, or I.V. if the reaction is severe (repeating dosage every 5 to 20 minutes as needed)

- Tracheostomy or endotracheal intubation and mechanical ventilation to maintain a patent airway
- Oxygen therapy to increase tissue perfusion
- Longer-acting epinephrine, corticosteroids, and diphenhydramine (Benadryl) to reduce the allergic response (long-term management)
- Albuterol mini-nebulizer treatment
- Cimetidine (Tagamet) or other histamine-2 receptor antagonist
- Aminophylline to reverse bronchospasm
- Volume expanders to maintain and restore circulating plasma volume
- I.V. vasopressors, such as norepinephrine (Levophed) and dopamine (Intropin), to stabilize blood pressure
- Cardiopulmonary resuscitation to treat cardiac arrest

NURSING CONSIDERATIONS

- To prevent anaphylaxis, teach the patient to avoid exposure to known allergens. In addition, every patient prone to anaphylaxis should wear a medical identification bracelet identifying his allergies.
- If a patient must receive a drug to which he's allergic, prevent a severe reaction by making sure that he receives careful desensitization with gradually increasing doses of the antigen or advance administration of steroids. Of course, a person with a known allergic history should receive a drug with a high anaphylactic potential only after cautious pretesting for sensitivity. Closely monitor the patient during testing, and make sure that you have resuscitative equipment and epinephrine ready. When the patient needs a drug with a high anaphylactic potential (particularly parenteral drugs), make sure that he receives each dose under close medical observation.
- Closely monitor a patient undergoing diagnostic tests that use radiographic contrast media, such as excretory urography, cardiac catheterization, and angiography.

Ankylosing spondylitis, also called *rheumatoid spondylitis* or *Marie-Strümpell disease,* primarily affects the sacroiliac, apophyseal, and costocervical joints and the adjacent ligamentous or tendinous attachments to bone. It usually occurs as a primary disorder, but it may also occur secondary to reactive arthritis, such as in Reiter syndrome, psoriatic arthritis, or inflammatory bowel disease.

The disorder affects more men than women. Progressive disease is well recognized in men, but commonly overlooked or missed in women, who have more peripheral joint involvement.

CAUSES

- Circulating immune complexes and human leukocyte antigen (HLA)-B27 (the histocompatibility antigen) suggesting immune system activity in 90% of patients
- Exact cause unknown
- Familial tendency

PATHOPHYSIOLOGY

Ankylosing spondylitis is an inflammatory disease that progressively restricts spinal movement. It begins in the sacroiliac and gradually progresses to the lumbar, thoracic, and cervical spine. Bone and cartilage deterioration

CLINICAL FINDINGS

● Intermittent low back pain that's most severe in the morning or after inactivity and relieved by exercise (one of the first findings)
● Mild fatigue
● Fever
● Anorexia and weight loss
● With symmetrical or asymmetrical peripheral arthritis, pain occurring in the shoulders, hips, knees, and ankles
● Pain over the symphysis pubis
● Stiffness and limited range of motion (ROM) of the lumbar spine
● Pain and limited expansion of the chest resulting from costovertebral and sternomanubrial joint involvement
● Limited ROM resulting from hip deformity
● Kyphosis of the spine in advanced disease caused by chronic stooping to relieve discomfort
● Redness and inflammation of the eyes from iritis
● Warmth, swelling, and tenderness of affected joints
● Aortic murmur caused by regurgitation and cardiomegaly
● Decrease in vital capacity to 70% or less of predicted volume when upper lobe pulmonary fibrosis present

TEST RESULTS

Diagnosis requires meeting established criteria. (See *Diagnosing primary ankylosing spondylitis.*)

The following test results may support the diagnosis:
● Serum findings include positive HLA-B27 antigen test in about 95% of patients with primary ankylosing spondylitis and up to 80% of patients with secondary disease. The absence of rheumatoid factor helps to rule out rheumatoid arthritis, which produces similar symptoms.

leads to fibrous tissue formation and eventual fusion of the spine or peripheral joints. An autoimmune correlation is possible.

In primary disease, sacroiliitis is usually bilateral and symmetrical. In secondary disease, it's commonly unilateral and asymmetrical. The patient may also have extra-articular disease, such as acute anterior iritis (in about 25% of patients), proximal root aortitis, and heart block and apical pulmonary fibrosis.

Rarely, disease progression can impose severe physical restrictions on activities of daily living and occupational functions. Atlantoaxial subluxation is a rare complication of primary ankylosing spondylitis.

- Erythrocyte sedimentation rate and serum alkaline phosphatase and creatine kinase levels may be slightly elevated in active disease.
- Serum immunoglobulin A levels may be elevated.
- X-ray studies define characteristic changes. These changes may not appear for up to 3 years after the disease's onset. They include bilateral sacroiliac involvement (the hallmark of the disease), blurring of the joints' bony margins in early disease, patchy sclerosis with superficial bony erosions, eventual squaring of vertebral bodies, and "bamboo spine" with complete ankylosis.

TREATMENT

No treatment reliably stops disease progression. Treatment is symptomatic and can include:
- management to delay further deformity, including stressing the importance of good posture, stretching and deep breathing exercises, and braces and lightweight supports
- heat, warm showers, bath, ice, and nerve stimulation to relieve symptoms
- nonsteroidal anti-inflammatory drugs to control pain and inflammation
- etanercept (Enbrel), a tumor necrosis factor blocker, and infliximab (Remicade), a monoclonal antibody, to reduce the signs and symptoms associated with ankylosing spondylitis
- hip replacement surgery with severe hip involvement, which affects about 15% of patients
- spinal wedge osteotomy to separate and reposition the vertebrae with severe spinal involvement. (Only for selected patients because of the possibility of spinal cord damage and a lengthy recuperation.)

NURSING CONSIDERATIONS

- Consider the patient's limited ROM when planning self-care activities.
- Give analgesics, apply heat locally, and massage as indicated to promote mobility and comfort.
- Have the patient perform active ROM exercises to prevent restricted, painful movement.
- Pace periods of exercise and rest to help the patient achieve comfortable energy levels and oxygenation of lungs.
- Assess the patient's respiratory status. Breathing may be compromised because of severe kyphosis.
- If treatment includes surgery, ensure proper body alignment and positioning.
- Because ankylosing spondylitis is a chronic, progressively crippling condition, involve other caregivers, such as a social worker, visiting nurse, and dietitian.
- To minimize deformities, advise the patient to avoid physical activity that places stress on the back such as lifting heavy objects.
- Teach the patient to stand upright; to sit upright in a high, straight-backed chair; and to avoid leaning over a desk.
- Instruct the patient to sleep in a prone position on a hard mattress and to avoid using pillows under the neck or knees.
- Advise the patient to avoid prolonged walking, standing, sitting, or driving; to perform regular stretching and deep-breathing exercises; and to swim regularly if possible.
- Teach the patient muscle-strengthening exercises to increase muscle flexibility.

- Instruct the patient to have his height measured every 3 to 4 months to detect kyphosis.
- Encourage a nutritious diet and weight maintenance.
- Suggest that the patient seek vocational counseling if work requires standing or prolonged sitting at a desk.
- Tell the patient to contact the local arthritis agency or the Ankylosing Spondylitis Association for additional information and support.

Latex allergy

Latex allergy is a hypersensitivity reaction to products that contain natural latex, a substance found in an increasing number of products at home and at work. It's derived from the sap of a rubber tree, not synthetic latex. The hypersensitivity reactions can range from local dermatitis to a life-threatening anaphylactic reaction.

CAUSES
- Exposure to latex proteins (found in natural rubber products) that produce a true latex allergy
- More frequent exposure leading to a higher risk in populations, including:
- Medical and dental professionals
- Patients with spina bifida or other conditions that require multiple surgeries involving latex material
- Workers in latex companies
- Those in frequent contact with latex-containing products (at risk)
- Other individuals at risk, including patients with a history of:
- Asthma or other allergies, especially to bananas, avocados, tropical fruits, or chestnuts

- Frequent intermittent urinary catheterization
- Multiple intra-abdominal or genitourinary surgeries

PATHOPHYSIOLOGY
A true latex allergy is an immunoglobulin (Ig) E–mediated immediate hypersensitivity reaction. Mast cells release histamine and other secretory products. Vascular permeability increases and vasodilation and bronchoconstriction occur.

Chemical sensitivity dermatitis is a type IV delayed hypersensitivity reaction to the chemicals used in processing rather than the latex itself. In a cell-mediated allergic reaction, sensitized T lymphocytes are triggered, stimulating the proliferation of other lymphocytes and mononuclear cells. This results in tissue inflammation and contact dermatitis. Like anaphylaxis, a true latex allergy may lead to respiratory obstruction, systemic vascular collapse, and death.

CLINICAL FINDINGS
- Hypotension due to vasodilation and increased vascular permeability
- Tachycardia secondary to hypotension
- Urticaria and pruritus due to histamine release
- Difficulty breathing, bronchospasm, wheezing, and stridor secondary to bronchoconstriction
- Angioedema from increased vascular permeability and loss of water to tissues

TEST RESULTS
- Radioallergosorbent test shows specific IgE antibodies to latex. It's the safest test for use in patients with a history of type I hypersensitivity.

- Patch test results in hives with itching or redness as a positive response.

TREATMENT
- Prevention of exposure, including using latex-free products to decrease possible exacerbation of hypersensitivity
- Drug therapy, such as corticosteroids, antihistamines, and histamine-2 receptor antagonists before and after possible exposure to latex to depress immune response and block histamine release

If the patient is experiencing an acute emergency, treatment includes:
- immediate administration of epinephrine 1:1,000 aqueous solution to reverse bronchoconstriction and cause vasoconstriction, I.M. or subcutaneously if the patient hasn't lost consciousness and is normotensive, or I.V. if the reaction is severe (repeating dosage every 5 to 20 minutes as needed)
- tracheostomy or endotracheal intubation and mechanical ventilation to maintain a patent airway
- oxygen therapy to increase tissue perfusion
- volume expanders to maintain and restore circulating plasma volume
- I.V. vasopressors, such as norepinephrine (Levophed) and dopamine (Intropin), to stabilize blood pressure
- cardiopulmonary resuscitation to treat cardiac arrest
- longer-acting epinephrine, corticosteroids, and diphenhydramine (Benadryl) to reduce the allergic response (long-term management)
- drugs to reverse bronchospasm, including aminophylline and albuterol.

NURSING CONSIDERATIONS
- Make sure that items that aren't available latex-free, such as stethoscopes and blood pressure cuffs, are wrapped in cloth before they come in contact with a hypersensitive patient's skin.
- Place the patient in a private room or with another patient who requires a latex-free environment.
- When adding medication to an I.V. bag, inject the drug through the spike port, not the rubber latex port.
- Advise the patient to wear an identification tag mentioning his latex allergy.
- Teach the patient and his family how to use an epinephrine autoinjector.
- Teach the patient to be aware of all latex-containing products and to use vinyl or silicone products instead. Advise him that Mylar balloons don't contain latex.

Lupus erythematosus

Lupus erythematosus is a chronic inflammatory disorder of the connective tissues that appears in two forms: discoid lupus erythematosus, which affects only the skin, and systemic lupus erythematosus (SLE), which affects multiple organ systems as well as the skin and can be fatal. SLE is characterized by recurring remissions and exacerbations, which are especially common during the spring and summer.

The prognosis improves with early detection and treatment but remains poor for patients who develop cardiovascular, renal, or neurologic complications or severe bacterial infections.

CAUSES
The exact cause of SLE remains a mystery, but available evidence points to interrelated immunologic, environ-

mental, hormonal, and genetic factors. These may include:

- Abnormal estrogen metabolism
- Exposure to sunlight or ultraviolet light
- Immunization
- Physical or mental stress
- Pregnancy
- Streptococcal or viral infections
- Treatment with certain drugs, such as procainamide (Pronestyl), hydralazine (Apresoline), anticonvulsants and, less frequently, penicillins, sulfa drugs, and hormonal contraceptives

PATHOPHYSIOLOGY

Autoimmunity is believed to be the prime mechanism involved in SLE. The body produces antibodies against components of its own cells, such as the antinuclear antibody (ANA), and immune complex disease follows. Patients with SLE may produce antibodies against many different tissue components, such as red blood cells (RBCs), neutrophils, platelets, lymphocytes, or almost any organ or tissue in the body. Possible complications of SLE include concomitant infections, urinary tract infections (UTIs), renal failure, and osteonecrosis of the hip from long-term steroid use.

CLINICAL FINDINGS

The onset of SLE may be acute or insidious and produces no characteristic clinical pattern. (See *Signs of systemic lupus erythematosus*.)

Clinical findings relate to tissue injury and subsequent inflammation and necrosis resulting from the invasion by immune complexes. They commonly include:

- fever
- weight loss
- malaise
- fatigue

SIGNS OF SYSTEMIC LUPUS ERYTHEMATOSUS

Diagnosing systemic lupus erythematosus (SLE) is difficult because it commonly mimics other diseases; symptoms may be vague and vary greatly among patients.

For these reasons, the American Rheumatism Association issued a list of criteria for classifying SLE to be used primarily for consistency in epidemiologic surveys. Usually, four or more of these signs are present at some time during the course of the disease:

- ◆ malar or discoid rash
- ◆ photosensitivity
- ◆ oral or nasopharyngeal ulcerations
- ◆ nonerosive arthritis (of two or more peripheral joints)
- ◆ pleuritis or pericarditis
- ◆ profuse proteinuria (more than 0.5 g/day) or excessive cellular casts in urine
- ◆ seizures or psychoses
- ◆ hemolytic anemia, leukopenia, lymphopenia, or thrombocytopenia
- ◆ anti–double-stranded deoxyribonucleic acid or positive findings of antiphospholipid antibodies (elevated immunoglobulin [Ig] G or IgM anticardiolipin antibodies, positive test result for lupus anticoagulant, or false-positive serologic test results for syphilis)
- ◆ abnormal antinuclear antibody titer.

- rashes
- polyarthralgia
- joint involvement, similar to rheumatoid arthritis (although the arthritis of lupus is usually nonerosive)
- skin lesions, most commonly an erythematous rash in areas exposed to light (the classic butterfly rash over the nose and cheeks occurs in less than 50% of patients) or a scaly, papular rash (mimics psoriasis), especially in sun-exposed areas

- vasculitis (especially in the digits), possibly leading to infarctive lesions, necrotic leg ulcers, or digital gangrene
- Raynaud's phenomenon (about 20% of patients)
- patchy alopecia and painless ulcers of the mucous membranes
- pulmonary abnormalities, such as pleurisy, pleural effusions, pneumonitis, pulmonary hypertension and, rarely, pulmonary hemorrhage
- cardiac involvement, such as pericarditis, myocarditis, endocarditis, and early coronary atherosclerosis
- microscopic hematuria, pyuria, and urine sediment with cellular casts due to glomerulonephritis, possibly progressing to kidney failure (particularly when untreated)
- UTIs, possibly due to heightened susceptibility to infection
- seizure disorders and mental dysfunction
- central nervous system (CNS) involvement, such as emotional instability, psychosis, and organic brain syndrome
- headaches, irritability, and depression (common)
- lymph node enlargement (diffuse or local and nontender)
- abdominal pain
- nausea, vomiting, diarrhea, constipation
- irregular menstrual periods or amenorrhea during the active phase of SLE.

TEST RESULTS
- Complete blood count with differential possibly shows anemia and a decreased white blood cell (WBC) count.
- Blood studies reveal a decreased platelet count and an elevated erythrocyte sedimentation rate, and serum electrophoresis may show hypergammaglobulinemia.
- ANA and lupus erythematosus cell tests show positive results in active SLE.
- Anti–double-stranded deoxyribonucleic acid antibody—the most specific test for SLE—correlates with disease activity, especially renal involvement, and helps monitor response to therapy; it may be low or absent in remission.
- Urine studies possibly show RBCs and WBCs, urine casts and sediment, and significant protein loss (more than 0.5 g/24 hours).
- Serum complement blood studies show decreased serum complement (C3 and C4) levels indicating active disease.
- Chest X-ray possibly shows pleurisy or lupus pneumonitis.
- Electrocardiography possibly shows a conduction defect with cardiac involvement or pericarditis.
- Kidney biopsy determines the disease stage and extent of renal involvement.
- Lupus anticoagulant and anticardiolipin tests are possibly positive in some patients (usually in patients prone to antiphospholipid syndrome of thrombosis, abortion, and thrombocytopenia).

TREATMENT
- Nonsteroidal anti-inflammatory compounds, including aspirin, to control arthritis symptoms
- Topical corticosteroid creams, such as triamcinolone (Aristocort), for acute skin lesions
- Intralesional corticosteroids or antimalarials, such as hydroxychloroquine (Plaquenil), to treat joint pain or arthritis, skin rashes, mouth ulcers, fatigue, and fever

- Systemic corticosteroids to reduce systemic symptoms of SLE, for acute generalized exacerbations, or for serious disease related to vital organ systems, such as pleuritis, pericarditis, lupus nephritis, vasculitis, and CNS involvement
- High-dose steroids and cytotoxic therapy, such as cyclophosphamide (Cytoxan), to treat diffuse proliferative glomerulonephritis
- Immunosuppressives, such as azathioprine (Imuran), to restrain the overactive immune system and can be used for those patients whose kidneys or CNSs are affected
- Methotrexate (Trexall) for its anti-inflammatory and immunosuppressive effects (Due to its potential toxicities, it should be only used in patients who are unresponsive to other therapies.)
- Antihypertensive drugs and dietary changes to minimize effects of renal involvement
- Dialysis or kidney transplantation for renal failure

NURSING CONSIDERATIONS
- Watch for constitutional symptoms, such as joint pain or stiffness, weakness, fever, fatigue, and chills. Observe for dyspnea, chest pain, and edema of the extremities. Note the size, type, and location of skin lesions. Check urine for hematuria, scalp for hair loss, and skin and mucous membranes for petechiae, bleeding, ulceration, pallor, and bruising.
- Provide a balanced diet. Renal involvement may mandate a low-sodium, low-protein diet.
- Urge the patient to get plenty of rest. Schedule diagnostic tests and procedures to allow adequate rest. Explain all tests and procedures. Tell the patient that several blood samples are needed initially, and then periodically, to monitor progress.
- Apply heat packs to relieve joint pain and stiffness. Encourage regular exercise to maintain full range of motion (ROM) and prevent contractures. Teach ROM exercises as well as body alignment and postural techniques. Arrange for physical therapy and occupational counseling as appropriate.
- Explain the expected benefit of prescribed medications. Watch for adverse effects, especially when the patient is taking high doses of corticosteroids.
- Advise the patient receiving cyclophosphamide to maintain adequate hydration. If prescribed, give mesna (Mesnex) to prevent hemorrhagic cystitis and ondansetron (Zofran) to prevent nausea and vomiting.
- Monitor the patient's vital signs, intake and output, weight, and laboratory reports. Check pulse rates and observe for orthopnea. Check stools and GI secretions for blood.
- Observe for hypertension, weight gain, and other signs of renal involvement.
- Assess the patient for signs of neurologic damage, such as personality change, paranoid or psychotic behavior, ptosis, or diplopia. Take seizure precautions. If Raynaud's phenomenon is present, warm and protect the patient's hands and feet.
- Refer the patient to the Lupus Foundation of America and the Arthritis Foundation as necessary.

Rheumatoid arthritis

Rheumatoid arthritis (RA) is a chronic, systemic inflammatory disease that primarily attacks peripheral joints and the surrounding muscles, tendons, ligaments, and blood vessels. Partial remissions and unpredictable exacerbations mark the course of this potentially crippling disease. RA strikes women three times more often than men.

Alert *RA can occur at any age. The peak onset period for women is ages 30 to 60.*

This disease usually requires lifelong treatment and, sometimes, surgery. (See *Drug therapy for rheumatoid arthritis,* pages 328 and 329.) In most patients, it follows an intermittent course and allows normal activity between flares, although 10% of affected people have total disability from severe joint deformity, associated extra-articular symptoms, such as vasculitis, or both. The prognosis worsens with the development of nodules, vasculitis, and high titers of rheumatoid factor (RF).

CAUSES

The cause of the chronic inflammation characteristic of RA isn't known. Possible theories include:

- abnormal immune activation (occurring in a genetically susceptible individual) leading to inflammation, complement activation, and cell proliferation within joints and tendon sheaths
- development of an immunoglobulin (Ig) M antibody against the body's own IgG (also called RF); RF aggregates into complexes, generates inflammation, causing eventual cartilage damage and triggering other immune responses
- possible infection (viral or bacterial), hormone action, or lifestyle factors influencing onset.

PATHOPHYSIOLOGY

If not arrested, the inflammatory process in the joints occurs in four stages. In the first stage, synovitis develops from congestion and edema of the synovial membrane and joint capsule. Infiltration by lymphocytes, macrophages, and neutrophils continues the local inflammatory response. These cells, as well as fibroblast-like synovial cells, produce enzymes that help to degrade bone and cartilage.

In the second stage, pannus — thickened layers of granulation tissue — covers and invades cartilage and eventually destroys the joint capsule and bone.

In the third stage, fibrous ankylosis — fibrous invasion of the pannus and scar formation — occludes the joint space. Bone atrophy and misalignment causes visible deformities and disrupts the articulation of opposing bones, which causes muscle atrophy and imbalance and, possibly, partial dislocations (subluxations).

In the last stage, fibrous tissue calcifies, resulting in bony ankylosis and total immobility.

Complications of RA include fibrosis and ankylosis, soft tissue contractures, joint deformities, Sjögren's syndrome, destruction of C2, spinal cord compression, temporomandibular joint disease, infection, osteoporosis, myositis (inflammation of voluntary muscles), cardiopulmonary lesions, lymphadenopathy, and peripheral neuritis.

CLINICAL FINDINGS

RA usually develops insidiously and initially causes nonspecific signs and symptoms, most likely related to the initial inflammatory reactions before the inflammation of the synovium, including:

DRUG THERAPY FOR RHEUMATOID ARTHRITIS

This flowchart identifies the major pathophysiologic events in rheumatoid arthritis and shows where in this chain of events the major drug therapies act to control the disease.

```
            ┌──────────────────────────────────┐
            │      Stimulus for initiation      │
            └──────────────────────────────────┘
                            ↓
            ┌──────────────────────────────────┐
            │     Antigen-antibody response     │
            │     Immunoglobulin production     │
            └──────────────────────────────────┘
                            ↓
            ┌──────────────────────────────────┐
            │  Production of rheumatoid factor  │─────
            └──────────────────────────────────┘
┌──────────┐                ↓
│ Steroids │───────────────✳
└──────────┘                ↓
            ┌──────────────────────────────────┐
            │ Immune complex formation and      │◄────
            │ deposition                        │
            └──────────────────────────────────┘
┌──────────────────┐        ↓
│ Gold preparations│───────✳
└──────────────────┘        ↓
            ┌──────────────────────────────────┐
            │ Inflammatory response in synovium │
            │ Increased blood flow and          │
            │ capillary permeability            │
            └──────────────────────────────────┘
┌──────────────┐  ┌──────────┐    ┆
│ Aspirin      │  │ Steroids │───✳
│ Nonsteroidal │  └──────────┘    ┆
│ anti-        │─────────────────✳
│ inflammatory │                  ┆         ┌──────────────────┐
│ drugs(NSAIDs)│                 ✳◄──────────│ Biologic disease │
└──────────────┘                            │ response modifiers│
                                            └──────────────────┘
```

Edema	Lysosomal enzyme release	

Synovial hypoxia	Synovial destruction	

Aspirin
NSAIDs

Joint fusion	Joint swelling	Loss of joint spaces	Rheumatoid nodules

Key: ✳ = treatment

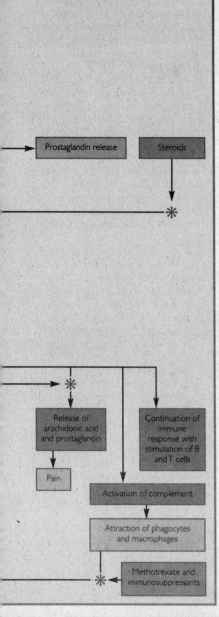

Prostaglandin release

Steroids

*

*

Release of
arachidonic acid
and prostaglandin

Continuation of
immune
response with
stimulation of B
and T cells

Pain

Activation of complement

Attraction of phagocytes
and macrophages

Methotrexate and
immunosuppressants

*

- fatigue
- malaise
- anorexia and weight loss
- persistent low-grade fever
- lymphadenopathy
- vague articular symptoms.

As the disease progresses, signs and symptoms include:

- specific localized, bilateral, and symmetric articular symptoms, frequently in the fingers at the proximal interphalangeal, metacarpophalangeal, and metatarsophalangeal joints, possibly extending to the wrists, knees, elbows, and ankles from inflammation of the synovium
- stiffening of affected joints after inactivity, especially on arising in the morning, due to progressive synovial inflammation and destruction
- spindle-shaped fingers from marked edema and congestion in the joints
- joint pain and tenderness, at first only with movement but eventually even at rest, due to prostaglandin release, edema, and synovial inflammation and destruction
- feeling of warmth at joint from inflammation
- diminished joint function and deformities as synovial destruction continues
- flexion deformities or hyperextension of metacarpophalangeal joints, subluxation of the wrist, and stretching of tendons pulling the fingers to the ulnar side (ulnar drift), or characteristic swan-neck or boutonnière deformity from joint swelling and loss of joint space
- carpal tunnel syndrome from synovial pressure on the median nerve causing paresthesia in the fingers.

Extra-articular findings may include:

- gradual appearance of rheumatoid nodules — subcutaneous, round or oval, nontender masses (20% of RF-positive patients), usually on elbows, hands, or Achilles tendon from destruction of the synovium
- vasculitis possibly leading to skin lesions, leg ulcers, and multiple systemic complications from infiltration of immune complexes and subsequent tissue damage and necrosis in the vasculature
- pericarditis, pulmonary nodules or fibrosis, pleuritis, or inflammation of the sclera and overlying tissues of the eye from immune complex invasion and subsequent tissue damage and necrosis
- peripheral neuropathy with numbness or tingling in the feet or weakness and loss of sensation in the fingers from infiltration of the nerve fibers
- stiff, weak, or painful muscles secondary to limited mobility and decreased use.

TEST RESULTS

- X-rays show bone demineralization and soft-tissue swelling (early stages), cartilage loss and narrowed joint spaces and, finally, cartilage and bone destruction and erosion, subluxations, and deformities (later stages).
- RF titer is positive in 75% to 80% of patients (titer of 1:160 or higher).
- Synovial fluid analysis shows increased volume and turbidity but decreased viscosity and elevated white blood cell count (usually greater than 10,000/mm^3).
- Serum protein electrophoresis possibly shows elevated serum globulin level.
- Erythrocyte sedimentation rate and C-reactive protein levels shows elevations in 85% to 90% of patients, which may be useful to monitor response to therapy because elevation frequently parallels disease activity.
- Complete blood count usually shows moderate anemia, slight leukocytosis, and slight thrombocytosis.

TREATMENT

Medications used for pain relief and to reduce inflammation include:
- salicylates, particularly aspirin
- nonsteroidal anti-inflammatory drugs, such as etodolac (Lodine), ibuprofen (Motrin), and indomethacin (Indocin)
- corticosteroids, such as prednisone, in low doses, for anti-inflammatory effects; in higher doses for immunosuppressive effect on T cells.

Disease modifying antirheumatic drugs (DMARDs) are used to slow the course of the disease, promote remission, and prevent progressive joint destruction. These include:
- azathioprine (Imuran), cyclosporine (Neoral), and methotrexate (Trexall) are given in early disease for immunosuppression, suppressing T and B lymphocyte proliferation causing destruction of the synovium
- antimalarials, such as hydroxychloroquine (Plaquenil), sulfasalazine (Azulfidine), gold salts, and leflunomide (Arava), are given to reduce acute and chronic inflammation.

Biological response modifiers intercept cytokines that cause inflammation. Drugs in this category include:
- tumor necrosis factor inhibitors, such as etanercept (Enbrel), infliximab (Remicade), and adalimumab (Humira), for patients who don't have an adequate response to DMARDs
- Anakinra (Kineret), in an interleukin-1 inhibitor.

Other treatments

- Synovectomy (removal of destructive, proliferating synovium, usually in the wrists, knees, and fingers) to possibly halt or delay the course of the disease.
- Osteotomy (cutting of bone or excision of a wedge of bone) to realign joint surfaces and redistribute stress.
- Tendon transfers to prevent deformities or relieve contractures.
- Joint reconstruction or total joint arthroplasty, including metatarsal head and distal ulnar resectional arthroplasty, and insertion of a Silastic prosthesis between metacarpophalangeal and proximal interphalangeal joints in severe disease.
- Arthrodesis (joint fusion) for stability and relief from pain (sacrifices joint mobility).

NURSING CONSIDERATIONS

- Assess all joints carefully. Look for deformities, contractures, immobility, and the inability to perform activities of daily living.
- Monitor the patient's vital signs, and note weight changes, sensory disturbances, and his level of pain. Administer analgesics, as ordered, and watch for adverse effects.
- Provide meticulous skin care. Check for rheumatoid nodules as well as pressure ulcers and skin breakdown due to immobility, vascular impairment, corticosteroid treatment, or improper splinting. Use lotion or cleaning oil, not soap, for dry skin.
- Explain all diagnostic tests and procedures. Tell the patient to expect multiple blood samples to allow firm diagnosis and accurate monitoring of therapy.
- Monitor the duration, not the intensity, of morning stiffness because duration more accurately reflects the severity of the disease. Encourage the patient to take hot showers or baths at bedtime or in the morning to reduce the need for pain medication.
- Apply splints carefully and correctly. Observe for pressure ulcers if the patient is in traction or wearing splints.
- Explain the nature of the disease. Make sure that the patient and his family understand that RA is a chronic disease that requires major changes in lifestyle. Emphasize that there are no miracle cures, despite claims to the contrary.
- Encourage a balanced diet, but make sure that the patient understands that special diets won't cure RA. Stress the need for weight control because obesity adds further stress to joints.
- Urge the patient to perform activities of daily living, such as dressing and feeding himself (supply easy-to-open cartons, lightweight cups, and unpackaged silverware). Allow the patient enough time to calmly perform these tasks.
- Provide emotional support. Remember that the patient with chronic illness easily becomes depressed, discouraged, and irritable. Encourage the patient to discuss his fears concerning dependency, sexuality, body image, and self-esteem. Refer him to an appropriate social service agency as needed.
- Discuss sexual aids, such as alternative positions, pain medication, and moist heat to increase mobility.
- Before discharge, make sure that the patient knows how and when to take prescribed medication and how to recognize possible adverse effects.
- Teach the patient how to stand, walk, and sit correctly. Tell him to sit in chairs with high seats and armrests;

he'll find it easier to get up from a chair if his knees are lower than his hips. If he doesn't own a chair with a high seat, recommend putting blocks of wood under the legs of a favorite chair. Suggest an elevated toilet seat.

● Instruct the patient to pace daily activities, resting for 5 to 10 minutes out of each hour and alternating sitting and standing tasks. Adequate sleep is important and so is correct sleeping posture. He should sleep on his back on a firm mattress and should avoid placing a pillow under his knees, which encourages flexion deformity.

● Teach him to avoid putting undue stress on joints by using the largest joint available for a given task, avoiding positions of flexion and promoting positions of extension, holding objects parallel to the knuckles as briefly as possible, always using his hands toward the center of his body, sliding — not lifting — objects whenever possible, and supporting weak or painful joints as much as possible. Enlist the aid of an occupational therapist to teach how to simplify activities and protect arthritic joints. Stress the importance of shoes with proper support.

● Suggest dressing aids — long-handled shoehorn, reacher, elastic shoelaces, zipper-pull, and button-hook — and helpful household items, such as easy-to-open drawers, hand-held shower nozzle, handrails, and grab bars. The patient who has trouble maneuvering fingers into gloves should wear mittens. Tell him to dress while in a sitting position as often as possible.

● Refer the patient to the Arthritis Foundation for more information on coping with the disease.

Vasculitis

Vasculitis includes a broad spectrum of disorders characterized by inflammation and necrosis of blood vessels. Its clinical effects depend on the vessels involved and reflect tissue ischemia caused by blood flow obstruction. The prognosis is also variable. For example, hypersensitivity vasculitis is usually a benign disorder limited to the skin, but more extensive polyarteritis nodosa can be rapidly fatal. Vasculitis can occur at any age, except for mucocutaneous lymph node syndrome, which occurs only during childhood. Vasculitis may be a primary disorder or occur secondary to other disorders, such as rheumatoid arthritis or systemic lupus erythematosus.

CAUSES

Vasculitis has been associated with a history of serious infectious disease, such as hepatitis B or bacterial endocarditis, and high-dose antibiotic therapy.

PATHOPHYSIOLOGY

How vascular damage develops in vasculitis isn't well understood. Current theory holds that it's initiated by excessive circulating antigen, which triggers the formation of soluble antigen–antibody complexes. These complexes can't be cleared effectively by the reticuloendothelial system, so they're deposited in blood vessel walls (type III hypersensitivity). Increased vascular permeability associated with release of vasoactive amines by platelets and basophils exacerbates this process. The deposited complexes activate the complement cascade, resulting in chemotaxis of neutrophils, which release lysosomal enzymes. In turn, these enzymes cause vessel damage and necrosis, which may precipitate thrombosis, occlusion, hemorrhage, and ischemia.

Another mechanism that may contribute to vascular damage is the cell-mediated (T-cell) immune response. In this response, circulating antigen triggers lymphocytes to release soluble mediators, which attracts macrophages. The macrophages release intracellular enzymes, which cause vascular damage. Macrophages can also transform into the epithelioid and multinucleated giant cells that typify the granulomatous vasculitides. Phagocytosis of immune complexes by macrophages enhances granuloma formation. Renal, cardiac, and hepatic involvement may be fatal if vasculitis is left untreated. Complications can include renal failure, renal hypertension, glomerulitis, fibrous scarring of the lung tissue, stroke, and GI bleeding.

CLINICAL FINDINGS AND TEST RESULTS

Clinical effects of vasculitis and confirming laboratory procedures depend on the blood vessels involved. (See *Types of vasculitis,* pages 334 and 335.)

TREATMENT

- In primary vasculitis, treatment may involve the removal of an offending antigen or the use of anti-inflammatory or immunosuppressant drugs. For example, antigenic drugs, food, and other environmental substances should be identified and eliminated, if possible.
- Drug therapy in primary vasculitis commonly involves low-dose cyclophosphamide (Cytoxan) with daily corticosteroids.

- In rapidly fulminant vasculitis, the cyclophosphamide dosage may be increased daily for the first 2 to 3 days, followed by the regular dose. Prednisone should be given in divided doses for 7 to 10 days, with consolidation to a single morning dose by 2 to 3 weeks.
- When the vasculitis appears to be in remission or when prescribed cytotoxic drugs take full effect, corticosteroids are tapered down to a single daily dose. Finally, an alternate-day schedule of steroids may continue for 3 to 6 months before slow discontinuation of steroids.
- In secondary vasculitis, treatment focuses on the underlying disorder.

NURSING CONSIDERATIONS

- Assess patients with Wegener's granulomatosis for dry nasal mucosa. Instill nose drops to lubricate the mucosa and help diminish crusting, or irrigate the nasal passages with warm normal saline solution.
- Monitor the patient's vital signs. Use a Doppler ultrasonic flowmeter, if available, to auscultate blood pressure in the patient with Takayasu's arteritis, whose peripheral pulses are generally difficult to palpate.
- Monitor intake and output, and check for edema daily. Keep the patient well hydrated (3 qt [3 L] daily) to reduce the risk of hemorrhagic cystitis associated with cyclophosphamide therapy.
- Provide emotional support to help the patient and his family cope with an altered body image.
- Teach the patient how to recognize adverse effects of drug therapy. Monitor the patient's white blood cell count during cyclophosphamide therapy to prevent severe leukopenia.

Types of vasculitis

Type	Vessels involved	Signs and symptoms
Polyarteritis nodosa	Small to medium arteries throughout body, with lesions that tend to be segmental, occur at bifurcations and branchings of arteries, spread distally to arterioles and, in severe cases, circumferentially involve adjacent veins	Hypertension, abdominal pain, myalgia, headache, joint pain, and weakness
Allergic granulomatosis angiitis (Churg-Strauss syndrome)	Small to medium arteries (including arterioles, capillaries, and venules), mainly of the lungs but also other organs	Resemblance to polyarteritis nodosa with hallmark of severe pulmonary involvement
Polyangiitis overlap syndrome	Small to medium arteries (including arterioles, capillaries, and venules) of the lungs and other organs	Combined symptoms of polyarteritis nodosa, allergic angiitis, and granulomatosis
Wegener's granulomatosis	Small to medium vessels of the respiratory tract and kidney	Fever, pulmonary congestion, cough, malaise, anorexia, weight loss, and mild to severe hematuria
Temporal arteritis	Medium to large arteries, most commonly branches of the carotid artery	Fever, myalgia, jaw claudication, vision changes, and headache (associated with polymyalgia rheumatica syndrome)
Takayasu's arteritis (aortic arch syndrome)	Medium to large arteries, particularly the aortic arch, its branches and, possibly, the pulmonary artery	Malaise, pallor, nausea, night sweats, arthralgia, anorexia, weight loss, pain or paresthesia distal to affected area, bruits, loss of distal pulses, syncope and, if a carotid artery is involved, diplopia and transient blindness; may progress to heart failure or stroke
Hypersensitivity vasculitis	Small vessels, especially of the skin	Palpable purpura, papules, nodules, vesicles, bullae, or ulcers or chronic or recurrent urticaria
Mucocutaneous lymph node syndrome (Kawasaki disease)	Small to medium vessels, primarily of the lymph nodes; may progress to involve coronary arteries	Fever; nonsuppurative cervical adenitis; edema; congested conjunctivae; erythema of oral cavity, lips, and palms; and desquamation of fingertips; may progress to arthritis, myocarditis, pericarditis, myocardial infarction, and cardiomegaly
Behcet's syndrome	Small vessels, primarily of the mouth and genitalia, but also of the eyes, skin, joints, GI tract, and central nervous system	Recurrent oral ulcers, eye lesions, genital lesions, and cutaneous lesions

DIAGNOSIS

History of symptoms; elevated erythrocyte sedimentation rate (ESR); leukocytosis; anemia; thrombocytosis; depressed C3 complement; rheumatoid factor more than 1:60; circulating immune complexes; tissue biopsy showing necrotizing vasculitis

History of asthma; eosinophilia; tissue biopsy showing granulomatous inflammation with eosinophilic infiltration

Possible history of allergy; eosinophilia; tissue biopsy showing granulomatous inflammation with eosinophilic infiltration

Tissue biopsy showing necrotizing vasculitis with granulomatous inflammation; leukocytosis; elevated ESR and immunoglobulin (Ig) A and IgG levels; low titer rheumatoid factor; circulating immune complexes; antineutrophil cytoplasmic antibody in more than 90% of patients

Decreased hemoglobin level; elevated ESR; tissue biopsy showing panarteritis with infiltration of mononuclear cells, giant cells within vessel wall, fragmentation of internal elastic lamina, and proliferation of intima

Decreased hemoglobin level; leukocytosis; positive lupus erythematosus cell preparation and elevated ESR; arteriography showing calcification and obstruction of affected vessels; tissue biopsy showing inflammation of adventitia and intima of vessels, and thickening of vessel walls

History of exposure to antigen, such as a microorganism or drug; tissue biopsy showing leukocytoclastic angiitis, usually in postcapillary venules, with infiltration of polymorphonuclear leukocytes, fibrinoid necrosis, and extravasation of erythrocytes

History of symptoms; elevated ESR; tissue biopsy showing intimal proliferation and infiltration of vessel walls with mononuclear cells; echocardiography necessary

History of symptoms

9

SENSORY SYSTEM

Through the sensory system, a person receives stimuli that facilitate interaction with the surrounding world. Afferent pathways connect specialized sensory receptors in the eyes, ears, nose, and mouth to the brain — the final station for continuous processing of sensory stimuli. Alterations in sensory function may lead to dysfunctions of sight and hearing as well as smell, taste, balance, and coordination.

Cataract

A cataract is a gradually developing opacity of the lens or lens capsule of the eye. Light shining through the cornea is blocked by this opacity, and a blurred image is cast onto the retina. As a result, the brain interprets a hazy image. Cataracts commonly occur bilaterally, and each progresses independently. Exceptions are traumatic cataracts, which are usually unilateral, and congenital cataracts, which may remain stationary. Cataracts are prevalent in people older than age 70, as part of the aging process. The prognosis is generally good; surgery improves vision in 95% of affected people.

CAUSES
- Aging (senile cataracts)
- Atopic dermatitis
- Complicated cataracts
- Congenital disorders
- Diabetes mellitus
- Drugs toxic to the lens:
  - Ergot alkaloids
  - Exposure to ultraviolet rays
  - Phenothiazines
  - Pilocarpine (Pilocar)
  - Prednisone (Deltasone)
  - Tamoxifen (Nolvadex)
- Exposure to ionizing radiation or infrared rays
- Foreign body injury
- Genetic abnormalities
- Glaucoma
- Hypoparathyroidism
- Maternal rubella during the first trimester of pregnancy
- Myotonic dystrophy
- Retinal detachment
- Retinitis pigmentosa
- Traumatic cataracts
- Uveitis

PATHOPHYSIOLOGY
Pathophysiology may vary with each form of cataract. Congenital cataracts are particularly challenging. (See *Congenital cataracts*.) Senile cataracts show evidence of protein aggregation, ox-

idative injury, and increased pigmentation in the center of the lens. In traumatic cataracts, phagocytosis of the lens or inflammation may occur when a lens ruptures. The mechanism of a complicated cataract varies with the disease process; for example, in diabetes, increased glucose in the lens causes it to absorb water.

Typically, cataract development goes through four stages:

- immature — the lens isn't totally opaque
- mature — the lens is completely opaque and vision loss is significant
- tumescent — the lens is filled with water; may lead to glaucoma
- hypermature — the lens proteins deteriorate, causing peptides to leak through the lens capsule; glaucoma may develop if intraocular fluid outflow is obstructed.

Complications of cataracts include blindness and glaucoma.

CLINICAL FINDINGS

- Gradual painless blurring and loss of vision due to lens opacity
- Milky white pupil due to lens opacity
- Blinding glare from headlights at night due to the inefficient reflection of light rays by the opacities
- Poor reading vision caused by reduced clarity of images
- Better vision in dim light than in bright light in patients with central opacity (As pupils dilate, patients can see around the opacity.)
- White area behind the pupil, which remains unnoticeable until the cataract is advanced.

Alert *Elderly patients with reduced vision may become depressed and withdraw from social activities rather than complain about reduced vision.*

CONGENITAL CATARACTS

Congenital cataracts may be caused by:
- chromosomal abnormalities
- metabolic disease (such as galactosemia)
- intrauterine nutritional deficiencies
- infection during pregnancy (such as rubella).

Congenital cataracts may not be apparent at birth unless the eye is examined by a funduscope.

If the cataract is removed within a few months of birth, the infant will be able to develop proper retinal fixation and cortical visual responses. After surgery, the child is likely to favor the normal eye; the brain suppresses the poor image from the affected eye, leading to underdeveloped vision (amblyopia) in that eye. Postoperatively, in the child with bilateral cataracts, vision develops equally in both eyes.

TEST RESULTS

- Indirect ophthalmoscopy and slit-lamp examination show a dark area in the normally homogeneous red reflex.
- Visual acuity test confirms vision loss.

TREATMENT

- Extracapsular cataract extraction to remove the anterior lens capsule, and cortex and intraocular lens (IOL) implant in the posterior chamber, typically performed by using phacoemulsification to fragment the lens with ultrasonic vibrations, then aspirating the pieces (see *Comparing methods of cataract removal,* pages 338 and 339)
- Intracapsular cataract extraction to remove the entire lens within the intact capsule by cryoextraction (An IOL may be placed in the anterior or posterior chamber after lens removal, or a

COMPARING METHODS OF CATARACT REMOVAL

Cataracts can be removed by extracapsular or intracapsular techniques.

EXTRACAPSULAR CATARACT EXTRACTION

The surgeon may use irrigation and aspiration or phacoemulsification.

To irrigate and aspirate, he makes an incision at the limbus, opens the anterior lens capsule with a cystotome, and exerts pressure from below to express the lens. He then irrigates and suctions the remaining lens cortex.

In phacoemulsification, he uses an ultrasonic probe to break the lens into minute particles and then aspirates the particles.

Irrigation and aspiration

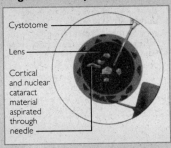

Cystotome

Lens

Cortical and nuclear cataract material aspirated through needle

Phacoemulsification

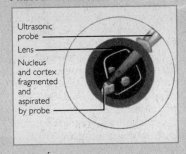

Ultrasonic probe

Lens

Nucleus and cortex fragmented and aspirated by probe

contact lens or aphakic glasses may be used to enhance vision.)

- Laser surgery after an extracapsular cataract extraction to restore visual acuity when a secondary membrane forms in the posterior lens capsule that has been left intact
- Discission (an incision) and aspiration
- Contact lenses or lens implantation after surgery to improve visual acuity, binocular vision, and depth perception

NURSING CONSIDERATIONS
Postoperatively

- Remind the patient to return for a checkup the next day and warn him to avoid activities that increase intraocular pressure such as straining.
- Urge the patient to protect the eye from accidental injury at night by wearing a plastic or metal shield with perforations; a shield or glasses should be worn for protection during the day.
- Before discharge, teach the patient to administer antibiotic ointment or eyedrops to prevent infection and steroids to reduce inflammation; combination steroid-antibiotic eyedrops can also be used.
- Advise the patient to immediately report a sharp pain in the eye uncontrolled by analgesics or clouding in the anterior chamber.
- Caution the patient about activity restrictions, and advise him that he'll receive his corrective reading glasses or lenses in several weeks.

mic emergency. Unless treated promptly, this acute form of glaucoma causes
blindness in 3 to 5 days.

INTRACAPSULAR CATARACT EXTRACTION

The surgeon makes a partial incision at the superior limbus arc. He then removes the lens using specially designed forceps or a cryoprobe, which adheres to the frozen lens to facilitate its removal.

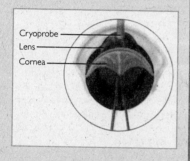

Cryoprobe
Lens
Cornea

Glaucoma

Glaucoma is a group of disorders
characterized by an abnormally high
intraocular pressure (IOP) that damages the optic nerve and other intraocular structures. Untreated, it leads to a
gradual loss of vision and, ultimately,
blindness. Glaucoma occurs in several
forms: chronic open-angle (primary),
acute angle-closure, congenital (inherited as an autosomal recessive trait),
and secondary to other causes. Chronic open-angle glaucoma is usually bilateral, with an insidious onset and a
slowly progressive course. Acute
angle-closure glaucoma typically has a
rapid onset, constituting an ophthal-

Glaucoma accounts for 12% of
new cases of blindness in the United
States. Blacks have the highest incidence of glaucoma, and it's the single
most common cause of blindness in
this group. The prognosis is good
with early treatment.

CAUSES

Chronic open-angle glaucoma

- Aging
- Diabetes mellitus
- Genetics
- Hypertension
- Severe myopia

Acute angle-closure glaucoma

- Drug-induced mydriasis (extreme dilation of the pupil)
- Emotional excitement, which can lead to hypertension

Secondary glaucoma

- Diabetes
- Infections
- Steroids
- Surgery
- Trauma
- Uveitis

PATHOPHYSIOLOGY

Chronic open-angle glaucoma results
from overproduction or obstruction of
the outflow of aqueous humor
through the trabecular meshwork or
Schlemm's canal, causing increased
IOP and damage to the optic nerve.
(See *Normal flow of aqueous humor,* page
340.) In secondary glaucoma, conditions such as trauma and surgery increase the risk of obstruction of intraocular fluid outflow caused by edema or other abnormal processes.

NORMAL FLOW OF AQUEOUS HUMOR

Aqueous humor, a transparent fluid produced by the ciliary epithelium of the ciliary body, flows from the posterior chamber through the pupil to the anterior chamber. It then flows peripherally and filters through the trabecular meshwork to Schlemm's canal, through which the fluid ultimately enters venous circulation.

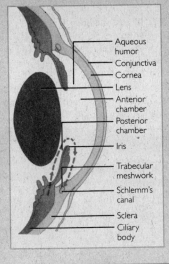

- Aqueous humor
- Conjunctiva
- Cornea
- Lens
- Anterior chamber
- Posterior chamber
- Iris
- Trabecular meshwork
- Schlemm's canal
- Sclera
- Ciliary body

Acute angle-closure glaucoma results from obstruction to the outflow of aqueous humor. Obstruction may be caused by anatomically narrow angles between the anterior iris and the posterior corneal surface, shallow anterior chambers, a thickened iris that causes angle closure on pupil dilation, or a bulging iris that presses on the trabeculae, closing the angle (peripheral anterior synechiae). Any of these may cause IOP to increase suddenly.

(See *Congenital glaucoma.*) Complications include blindness.

Alert *In older patients, partial closure of the angle may also occur, so that two forms of glaucoma may coexist.*

CLINICAL FINDINGS

Clinical manifestations of chronic open-angle glaucoma typically are bilateral and include:

- mild aching in the eyes caused by increased IOP
- loss of peripheral vision due to compression of retinal rods and nerve fibers
- halos around lights as a result of corneal edema
- reduced visual acuity, especially at night, not correctable with glasses.

Clinical manifestations of acute angle-closure glaucoma have a rapid onset, are usually unilateral, and include:

- inflammation
- red, painful eye caused by an abrupt elevation of IOP
- sensation of pressure over the eye due to increased IOP
- moderate pupillary dilation nonreactive to light
- cloudy cornea due to compression of intraocular components
- blurring and decreased visual acuity due to aberrant neural conduction
- photophobia due to abnormal IOP
- halos around lights due to corneal edema
- nausea and vomiting caused by increased IOP.

TEST RESULTS

- Pressure measurement tonometry using an applanation, Schiøtz, or pneumatic tonometer; fingertip tension estimates IOP. (On gentle palpation of closed eyelids, one eye feels

harder than the other in acute angle-closure glaucoma.)
- Slit-lamp examination reveals the eye's anterior structures, including the cornea, iris, and lens.
- Gonioscopy determines the angle of the eye's anterior chamber, enabling differentiation between chronic open-angle glaucoma and acute angle-closure glaucoma, revealing a normal angle in chronic open-angle glaucoma and an abnormal angle in acute angle-closure glaucoma. (See *Optic disk changes in chronic glaucoma,* page 342.)
- Ophthalmoscopy shows cupping of the optic disk in chronic open-angle glaucoma. A pale disk suggests acute angle-closure glaucoma.
- Perimetry or visual field tests detect loss of peripheral vision due to chronic open-angle glaucoma.
- Fundus photography monitors the disk for changes.

TREATMENT

Treatment of chronic open-angle glaucoma may include:
- beta-adrenergic blockers, such as timolol (Betimol,) or betaxolol (Betoptic) (a beta$_1$-receptor antagonist), to decrease aqueous humor production
- alpha agonists, such as brimonidine (Alphagan P) or apraclonidine (Iopidine), to reduce IOP
- carbonic anhydrase inhibitors, such as dorzolamide (Trusopt) or acetazolamide (Diamox), to decrease the formation and secretion of aqueous humor
- epinephrine to reduce IOP by improving aqueous outflow
- prostaglandins, such as latanoprost (Xalatan), to reduce IOP
- miotic eyedrops, such as pilocarpine (Isopto Carpine), to reduce IOP by facilitating the outflow of aqueous humor.

CONGENITAL GLAUCOMA

Congenital glaucoma, a rare disease, occurs when a congenital defect in the angle of the anterior chamber obstructs the outflow of aqueous humor. Congenital glaucoma is usually bilateral, with an enlarged cornea that may be cloudy and bulging. Symptoms in a neonate, although difficult to assess, may include tearing, pain, and photophobia.

Untreated, congenital glaucoma causes damage to the optic nerve and blindness. Surgical intervention (such as goniotomy, goniopuncture, trabeculotomy, or trabeculectomy) is necessary to reduce intraocular pressure and prevent vision loss.

When medical therapy fails to reduce IOP, the following surgical procedures may be performed:
- argon laser trabeculoplasty of the trabecular meshwork of an open angle to produce a thermal burn that changes the surface of the meshwork and increases the outflow of aqueous humor
- trabeculectomy to remove scleral tissue followed by a peripheral iridectomy to produce an opening for aqueous outflow under the conjunctiva, creating a filtering bleb.

Acute angle-closure glaucoma is an ocular emergency requiring immediate intervention to reduce high IOP, including:
- I.V. mannitol (20%) or oral glycerin (50%) to reduce IOP by creating an osmotic pressure gradient between the blood and intraocular fluid
- steroid drops to reduce inflammation
- acetazolamide to reduce IOP by decreasing the formation and secretion of aqueous humor

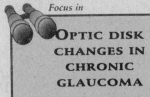

Focus in

OPTIC DISK CHANGES IN CHRONIC GLAUCOMA

Ophthalmoscopy and slit-lamp examination show cupping of the optic disk, which is characteristic of chronic glaucoma.

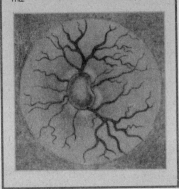

prevent an increase in IOP, resulting in disk changes and loss of vision.

● For the patient with acute angle-closure glaucoma, give medications as ordered and prepare him for laser iridotomy or surgery.

● Postoperative care after peripheral iridectomy includes cycloplegic eyedrops to relax the ciliary muscle and to decrease inflammation, thus preventing adhesions. *Note:* Cycloplegics must be used only in the affected eye. The use of these drops in the normal eye may precipitate an attack of acute angle-closure glaucoma in that eye, threatening the patient's residual vision.

● Following surgical filtering, postoperative care includes dilation and topical steroids to rest the pupil.

● Stress the importance of glaucoma screening for early detection and prevention. All people over age 35 should have an annual tonometric examination.

● pilocarpine to constrict the pupil, forcing the iris away from the trabeculae and allowing fluid to escape

● timolol to decrease IOP

● opioid analgesics to reduce pain, if needed

● laser iridotomy or surgical peripheral iridectomy, if drug therapy doesn't reduce IOP, to relieve pressure and preserve vision by promoting outflow of aqueous humor

● cycloplegic drops, such as apraclonidine, in the affected eye (only after laser peripheral iridectomy) to relax the ciliary muscle and reduce inflammation to prevent adhesions.

NURSING CONSIDERATIONS

● Stress the importance of compliance with prescribed drug therapy to

Hearing loss

Hearing loss, or deafness, results from a mechanical or nervous impediment to the transmission of sound waves. It is further defined as an inability to perceive the range of sounds audible to an individual with normal hearing. Types of hearing loss include congenital hearing loss, sudden deafness, noise-induced hearing loss, and presbycusis.

CAUSES

● Congenital hearing loss possibly transmitted as a dominant, autosomal dominant, autosomal recessive, or sex-linked recessive trait

- Hearing loss in neonates possibly resulting from trauma, toxicity, or infection during pregnancy or delivery; with predisposing factors, including:
  - congenital abnormalities of the ears, nose, or throat
  - maternal exposure to rubella or syphilis during pregnancy
  - prematurity or low birth weight
  - serum bilirubin levels above 20 mg/dl
  - trauma or prolonged fetal anoxia during delivery
  - use of ototoxic drugs during pregnancy
- Noise-induced hearing loss, which may be transient or permanent, commonly associated with workers subjected to constant industrial noise, military personnel, hunters, and rock musicians, and may follow:
  - brief exposure to extremely loud noise (greater than 90 dB)
  - prolonged exposure to loud noise (85 to 90 dB)
- Presbycusis, an otologic effect of aging, resulting from a loss of hair cells in the organ of Corti
- Sudden deafness (considered a medical emergency) in a person with no prior hearing impairment; causes and predisposing factors possibly including:
  - acute infections, especially mumps (most common cause of unilateral sensorineural hearing loss in children); other bacterial and viral infections, such as rubella, rubeola, influenza, herpes zoster, and infectious mononucleosis; and *Mycoplasma* infections
  - blood dyscrasias (leukemia, hypercoagulation)
  - head trauma or brain tumors
  - metabolic disorders (diabetes mellitus, hypothyroidism, hyperlipoproteinemia)
  - neurologic disorders (multiple sclerosis, neurosyphilis)
  - ototoxic drugs (tobramycin [Nebcin], streptomycin, quinine, gentamicin, furosemide [Lasix], ethacrynic acid [Edecrin])
  - vascular disorders (hypertension, arteriosclerosis)

Pathophysiology

The major forms of hearing loss are classified as:

- conductive loss — interrupted passage of sound from the external ear to the junction of the stapes and oval window caused by wax, or otitis media or externa
- sensorineural loss — impaired cochlea or acoustic (eighth cranial) nerve dysfunction causing failure of transmission of sound impulses within the inner ear or brain
- mixed loss — combined dysfunction of conduction and sensorineural transmission.

Hearing loss may be partial or total and is calculated from this American Medical Association formula: Hearing is 1.5% impaired for every decibel that the pure tone average exceeds 25 dB.

Clinical findings

At birth, congenital hearing loss may not be apparent, but a deficient response to auditory stimuli generally becomes obvious within 2 to 3 days.

Other clinical features include:

- impaired speech development
- loss of perception of certain frequencies (around 4,000 Hz)
- tinnitus
- inability to understand the spoken word.

   Alert A deaf infant's behavior can appear normal and mislead the parents as well as the professional, especially if *the infant has autosomal recessive deafness and is the first child of carrier parents.*

TEST RESULTS
- Audiologic examination provides evidence of hearing loss and possible causes.
- Weber's, Rinne, and specialized audiologic tests differentiate between conductive and sensorineural hearing loss.

TREATMENT
Therapy for congenital hearing loss not treatable with surgery consists of:
- identifying the underlying cause
- developing the patient's ability to communicate
- giving phototherapy and exchange transfusions for hyperbilirubinemia
- aggressively immunizing children against rubella to reduce the risk of maternal exposure during pregnancy; educating pregnant patients about the dangers of exposure to drugs, chemicals, or infection; and monitoring carefully during labor and delivery to prevent fetal anoxia.

Treatment of sudden deafness includes:
- prompt identification of the underlying cause
- prevention, necessitating educating patients and health care professionals about recognizing and treating sudden deafness.

For patients with noise-induced hearing loss, treatment includes:
- overnight rest, usually restoring normal hearing in those who have been exposed to noise levels greater than 90 dB for several hours
- reduction of exposure to loud noises, generally preventing high-frequency hearing loss

- speech and hearing rehabilitation, following repeated exposure to noise; hearing aids are seldom helpful.

For patients with presbycusis, treatment includes:
- amplifying sound, such as with a hearing aid, may help some patients but many patients are intolerant of loud noise.

NURSING CONSIDERATIONS
- When speaking to a patient who can read lips, stand directly in front of him, with the light on your face, and speak slowly and distinctly. If possible, speak to him at eye level. Approach the patient within his visual range, and elicit his attention by raising your arm or waving; touching him may startle him.
- Make other personnel aware of the patient's disability and his established method of communication. Explain all diagnostic tests and facility procedures in a way the patient understands.
- When addressing an older patient, speak slowly and distinctly in a low tone; avoid shouting.
- Provide emotional support and encouragement to the patient learning to use a hearing aid. Teach him how the hearing aid works and how to maintain it.
- Refer a child with suspected hearing loss to an audiologist or otolaryngologist for further evaluation. Any child who fails a language screening examination should be referred to a speech pathologist for language evaluation. The child with a mild language delay may be involved with a home language enrichment program.
- To help prevent hearing loss, watch for signs of hearing impairment in patients receiving ototoxic drugs. Emphasize the danger of excessive exposure to noise; stress the danger to

pregnant patients of exposure to drugs, chemicals, or infection (especially rubella); and encourage the use of protective devices in a noisy environment.

Macular degeneration

Macular degeneration — atrophy or degeneration of the macular disk — is the most common cause of legal blindness in adults age 50 and older. Commonly affecting both eyes, it accounts for about 12% of blindness in the United States and for about 17% of new cases of blindness. It's also one of the causes of severe irreversible and unpreventable loss of central vision in elderly people.

Two types of age-related macular degeneration occur. The dry, or atrophic, form is characterized by atrophic pigment epithelial changes and typically causes mild, gradual vision loss. The wet, exudative form rapidly causes severe vision loss. It's characterized by the subretinal formation of new blood vessels (neovascularization) that cause leakage, hemorrhage, and fibrovascular scar formation.

CAUSES
- Unknown
- Risk factors:
- Aging
- Family history
- Gender (females more likely to develop the disorder)
- History of cigarette smoking
- Nutrition (low levels of certain nutrients, such as antioxidants, and minerals such as zinc)
- Obesity
- Race (more common in whites)

PATHOPHYSIOLOGY
Macular degeneration results from hardening and obstruction of retinal arteries, which probably reflect normal degenerative changes. The formation of new blood vessels in the macular area obscures central vision. Underlying pathologic changes occur primarily in the retinal pigment epithelium, Bruch's membrane, and choriocapillaries in the macular region.

The dry form develops as yellow extracellular deposits, or drusen, accumulate beneath the pigment epithelium of the retina; they may be prominent in the macula. Drusen are common in elderly people. Over time, drusen grow and become more numerous. Vision loss occurs as the retinal pigment epithelium detaches and becomes atrophic.

Exudative macular degeneration develops as new blood vessels in the choroid project through abnormalities in Bruch's membrane and invade the potential space underneath the retinal pigment epithelium. As these vessels leak, fluid in the retinal pigment epithelium increases, resulting in blurry vision.

Possible complications are visual impairment progressing to blindness and nystagmus (if the macular degeneration is bilateral).

CLINICAL FINDINGS
- Changes in central vision due to neovascularization such as a blank spot (scotoma) in the center of a page when reading
- Distorted appearance of straight lines caused by relocation of retinal receptors
- Worsening intermittent blurred vision

TEST RESULTS

● Indirect ophthalmoscopy shows gross macular changes, opacities, hemorrhage, neovascularization, retinal pallor, or retinal detachment.
● I.V. fluorescein angiography sequential photographs show leaking vessels as fluorescein dye flows into the tissues from the subretinal neovascular net.
● Amsler grid test reveals central visual field loss.

TREATMENT

● Laser photocoagulation and photodynamic therapy are two procedures that seal leaking blood vessels in the eye. They reduce the incidence of severe vision loss in patients with subretinal neovascularization (exudative form).
● There's currently no cure for the atrophic form.

NURSING CONSIDERATIONS

● Inform patients with bilateral central vision loss about the visual rehabilitation services available to them.
● Special devices, such as low-vision optical aids, are available to improve quality of life in patients with good peripheral vision.
● Help the patient identify ways to modify his home to maintain safety.

Ménière's disease

Ménière's disease, an inner ear disease that results from a labyrinthine dysfunction (also known as *endolymphatic hydrops*), causes severe vertigo, sensorineural hearing loss, and tinnitus.

Alert Ménière's disease usually affects adults ages 30 to 60, is slightly more common in males than in females, and rarely occurs in children. Usually, only one ear is involved. After multiple attacks over several years, residual tinnitus and hearing loss can be incapacitating.

CAUSES

● Unknown
● May be associated with:
– Autonomic nervous system dysfunction
– Family history
– Head trauma
– Immune disorder
– Middle ear infection
– Migraine headaches
– Premenstrual edema

PATHOPHYSIOLOGY

Ménière's disease may result from overproduction or decreased absorption of endolymph — the fluid contained in the labyrinth of the ear. Accumulated endolymph dilates the semicircular canals, utricle, and saccule and causes degeneration of the vestibular and cochlear hair cells. Overstimulation of the vestibular branch of cranial nerve VIII impairs postural reflexes and stimulates the vomiting reflex. (See *Normal vestibular function.*) Perception of sound is impaired as a result of this excessive cranial nerve stimulation, and injury to sensory receptors for hearing may affect auditory acuity.

This condition may also stem from autonomic nervous system dysfunction that produces a temporary constriction of blood vessels supplying the inner ear.

Complications include continued tinnitus and hearing loss.

CLINICAL FINDINGS

● Sudden severe spinning, whirling vertigo, lasting from 10 minutes to several hours, due to increased endolymph (Attacks may occur several times per year, or remissions may last as long as several years.)

- Tinnitus caused by altered firing of sensory auditory neurons (may have residual tinnitus between attacks)
- Hearing impairment due to sensorineural loss (Hearing may be normal between attacks, but repeated attacks may progressively cause permanent hearing loss.)
- Feeling of fullness or blockage in the affected ear preceding an attack, a result of changing sensitivity of pressure receptors
- Severe nausea, vomiting, sweating, and pallor during an acute attack due to autonomic dysfunction
- Nystagmus due to asymmetry and intensity of impulses reaching the brain stem
- Loss of balance and falling to the affected side due to vertigo

TEST RESULTS

- Audiometric testing shows a sensorineural hearing loss and loss of discrimination and recruitment.
- Electronystagmography shows normal or reduced vestibular response on the affected side.
- Cold caloric testing reveals an impaired oculovestibular reflex.
- Electrocochleography shows an increased ratio of summating potential to action potential.
- Brain stem evoked-response audiometry test rules out an acoustic neuroma, a brain tumor, and vascular lesions in the brain stem.
- Computed tomography scan and magnetic resonance imaging rule out acoustic neuroma as a cause of symptoms.

NORMAL VESTIBULAR FUNCTION

The semicircular canals and vestibule of the inner ear are responsible for equilibrium and balance. Each of the three semicircular canals lies at a 90-degree angle to the others. When the head is moved, endolymph inside each semicircular canal moves in an opposite direction. The movement stimulates hair cells, which send electrical impulses to the brain through the vestibular portion of cranial nerve VIII. Head movement also causes movement of the vestibular otoliths (crystals of calcium salts) in their gel medium, which tugs on hair cells, initiating the transmission of electrical impulses to the brain through the vestibular nerve. Together, these two organs help detect the body's present position as well as a change in direction or motion.

TREATMENT

During an acute attack, treatment may include:

- lying down to minimize head movement, and avoiding sudden movements and glaring lights to reduce dizziness
- promethazine (Phenergan) or prochlorperazine (Compazine) to relieve nausea and vomiting
- atropine to control an attack by reducing autonomic nervous system function
- dimenhydrinate (Dramamine) to control vertigo and nausea
- central nervous system depressants, such as lorazepam (Ativan) or diazepam (Valium) during an acute attack, to reduce excitability of vestibular nuclei
- antihistamines, such as meclizine (Antivert) or diphenhydramine (Benadryl), to reduce dizziness and vomiting.

Long-term management may include:

- diuretics, such as triamterene (Dyrenium) or acetazolamide (Diamox), to reduce endolymph pressure
- vasodilators to dilate blood vessels supplying the inner ear
- sodium restriction to reduce endolymphatic hydrops
- avoidance of caffeine, monosodium glutamate, and alcohol in the diet because they may make symptoms worse
- antihistamines or mild sedatives to prevent attacks
- systemic streptomycin to produce chemical ablation of the sensory neuroepithelium of the inner ear and thereby control vertigo in patients with bilateral disease for whom no other treatment can be considered.

In Ménière's disease that persists despite medical treatment or produces incapacitating vertigo, the following surgical procedures may be performed:

- endolymphatic drainage and shunt procedures to reduce pressure on the hair cells of the cochlea and prevent further sensorineural hearing loss
- vestibular nerve resection in patients with intact hearing to reduce vertigo and prevent further hearing loss
- labyrinthectomy for relief of vertigo in patients with incapacitating symptoms and poor or no hearing because destruction of the cochlea results in a total loss of hearing in the affected ear
- cochlear implantation to improve hearing in patients with profound deafness due to Ménière's disease.

NURSING CONSIDERATIONS

If the patient is in the health care facility during an attack of Ménière's disease:

- Advise him against reading and exposure to glaring lights.
- Keep the side rails of the patient's bed up to prevent falls. Tell him not to get out of bed or walk without assistance.
- Instruct the patient to avoid sudden position changes and any tasks that vertigo makes hazardous.
- Before surgery, if the patient is vomiting, record fluid intake and output and characteristics of vomitus. Administer antiemetics as ordered, and give small amounts of fluid frequently.
- After surgery, record intake and output carefully. Tell the patient to expect dizziness and nausea for 1 or 2 days after surgery. Give prophylactic antibiotics and antiemetics as ordered.

Otosclerosis

The most common cause of chronic, progressive, conductive hearing loss, otosclerosis is the slow formation of spongy bone in the otic capsule, particularly at the oval window. It occurs in at least 10% of people of European descent and is three times as prevalent in females as in males; onset is usually between ages 15 and 30. Occurring unilaterally at first, the disorder may progress to bilateral conductive hearing loss. With surgery, the prognosis is good.

CAUSES

- Autosomal dominant trait
- Pregnancy

PATHOPHYSIOLOGY

In otosclerosis, the normal bone of the otic capsule is gradually replaced with a highly vascular spongy bone. This spongy bone immobilizes the footplate of the normally mobile stapes, disrupting the conduction of vibrations from the tympanic membrane to the cochlea. Because the sound pressure vibrations aren't transmitted to the fluid of the inner ear, the result is conductive hearing loss. If the inner ear becomes involved, sensorineural hearing loss may develop.

CLINICAL FINDINGS

* Progressive hearing loss, which starts unilaterally and may become bilateral without evidence of a middle ear infection
* Bilateral conductive hearing loss due to the disruption of the conduction of vibrations from the tympanic membrane to the cochlea
* Tinnitus due to overstimulation of cranial nerve VIII afferents
* Ability to hear a conversation better in a noisy environment than in a quiet one (paracusis of Willis) as a result of masking effects

TEST RESULTS

* Otoscopic examination shows a normal-appearing tympanic membrane. Occasionally, the tympanic membrane may appear pinkish orange (Schwartze's sign) as a result of vascular and bony changes in the middle ear.
* Rinne test reveals bone conduction lasting longer than air conduction; normally, the reverse is true. As otosclerosis progresses, bone conduction also deteriorates.
* Audiometric testing reveals hearing loss ranging from 60 dB in early stages to total loss.
* Weber's test detects sounds lateralizing to the more affected ear.

Alert Audiometric testing should be performed in late adolescence, when otosclerosis and noise-induced hearing may start to occur.

TREATMENT

* Prevention of infection with prophylactic antibiotics
* Stapedectomy (removal of the stapes) and insertion of a prosthesis to restore partial or total hearing
* Stapedotomy (creation of a small hole in the footplate of the stapes) and insertion of a wire and piston as a prosthesis to help restore hearing
* Hearing aid (air conduction aid with molded ear insertion receiver) if surgery isn't possible, to permit hearing of conversation in normal surroundings

NURSING CONSIDERATIONS

* During the first 24 hours after surgery, keep the patient lying flat, with the affected ear facing upward (to maintain the position of the graft). Enforce bed rest with bathroom privileges for 48 hours. Keep the side rails up and assist him with ambulation. Assess for pain and vertigo.
* Tell the patient that his hearing won't return until edema subsides and packing is removed.
* Before discharge, instruct the patient to avoid loud noises and sudden pressure changes until healing is complete (usually 6 months). Advise the patient not to blow his nose for at least 1 week to prevent contaminated

air and bacteria from entering the eustachian tube.

- Stress the importance of protecting the ears against cold; avoiding activities that cause dizziness, and avoiding contact with anyone who has an upper respiratory tract infection. Teach the patient and his family how to change the external ear dressing and care for the incision. Emphasize the need to complete the prescribed antibiotic regimen and return for scheduled follow-up care.

10

INTEGUMENTARY SYSTEM

The integumentary system, the largest and heaviest body system, includes the skin—the integument, or external covering of the body—and the epidermal appendages, including the hair, nails, and sebaceous, eccrine, and apocrine glands. It protects the body against injury and invasion of microorganisms, harmful substances, and radiation; regulates body temperature; serves as a reservoir for food and water; and synthesizes vitamin D.

Acne

Acne is a chronic inflammatory disease of the sebaceous glands. It's usually associated with a high rate of sebum secretion and occurs on areas of the body that have sebaceous glands, such as the face, neck, chest, back, and shoulders. There are two types of acne: inflammatory, in which the hair follicle is blocked by sebum, causing bacteria to grow and eventually rupture the follicle; and noninflammatory, in which the follicle doesn't rupture but remains dilated.

Alert *Acne vulgaris develops in 80% to 90% of adolescents or young adults, primarily between ages 15 and 18.*

Although the lesions can appear as early as age 8, acne primarily affects adolescents.

Although the severity and overall incidence of acne are usually greater in males, it tends to start at an earlier age and lasts longer in females.

The prognosis varies and depends on the severity and underlying causes; with treatment, the prognosis is usually good.

CAUSES
- Multifactorial
- Possible causes of acne include:
- blockage of the pilosebaceous ducts (hair follicles)
- increased activity of sebaceous glands.
- Factors that may predispose an individual to acne include:
- androgen stimulation
- certain drugs, including corticosteroids, corticotropin, androgens, iodides, bromides, phenytoin (Dilantin), isoniazid (Nydrazid), and lithium (Eskalith)
- cobalt irradiation
- cosmetics
- emotional stress
- exposure to heavy oils, greases, or tars
- heredity

- hormonal contraceptive use (Many females experience acne flare-ups during their first few menses after starting or stopping hormonal contraceptives.)
- hyperalimentation
- trauma or rubbing from tight clothing
- tropical climate.

PATHOPHYSIOLOGY

Androgens stimulate sebaceous gland growth and the production of sebum, which is secreted into dilated hair follicles that contain bacteria. The bacteria, usually *Propionibacterium acnes* and *Staphylococcus epidermis,* are normal skin flora that secrete lipase. This enzyme interacts with sebum to produce free fatty acids, which provoke inflammation. Hair follicles also produce more keratin, which joins with the sebum to form a plug in the dilated follicle. Complications of acne may include acne conglobate, scarring (when acne is severe), impaired self-esteem, abscesses, or secondary bacterial infections.

CLINICAL FINDINGS

The acne plug may appear as:
- a closed comedo, or whitehead (not protruding from the follicle and covered by the epidermis)
- an open comedo, or blackhead (protruding from the follicle and not covered by the epidermis; melanin or pigment of the follicle causes the black color).

Rupture or leakage of an enlarged plug into the epidermis produces:
- inflammation
- characteristic acne pustules, papules or, in severe forms, acne cysts or abscesses (chronic, recurring lesions producing acne scars).

In females, signs and symptoms may include increased severity just before or during menstruation when estrogen levels are at the lowest.

TEST RESULTS

There are no specific tests to confirm a diagnosis of acne vulgaris.

TREATMENT

Topical treatments of acne include:
- application of antibacterial agents and azelaic acid to stop or slow bacteria growth and decrease inflammation
- antibacterial agents applied alone or with tretinoin (Retin-A; retinoic acid), which dry and peel the skin opening blocked follicles and moving the sebum up to the skin level
- application of adapalene (Differin) to decrease comedo formation.

Systemic therapy consists primarily of:
- antibiotics, usually tetracycline, to decrease bacterial growth
- culture to identify a possible secondary bacterial infection (Look for exacerbation of pustules or abscesses while on tetracycline or erythromycin drug therapy.)
- oral isotretinoin (Accutane) to inhibit sebaceous gland function and keratinization (Because of its severe adverse affects, a 16- to 20-week course of isotretinoin is limited to patients with severe papulopustular or cystic acne not responding to conventional therapy. Because this drug is known to cause birth defects, the manufacturer, with U.S. Food and Drug Administration approval, recommends the following precautions: pregnancy testing before dispensing; dispensing only a 30-day supply; repeat pregnancy testing throughout the treatment period; effective contraception during treatment; and informed consent. Because of its effects on the liver, a serum triglyceride level should

be drawn before and periodically during treatment.)
- for females only, antiandrogens: birth control pills, such as norgestimate/ethinyl estradiol (Ortho Tri-Cyclen) or spironolactone
- cleaning face gently with bare hands and patting dry using a mild cleanser
- surgery to remove comedones and to open and drain pustules
- dermabrasion to smooth skin with severe acne scarring
- bovine collagen injections into the dermis beneath the scarred area to fill in affected areas and even out the skin surface.

NURSING CONSIDERATIONS

- Check the patient's drug history because certain medications, such as hormonal contraceptives, may cause an acne flare-up.
- Try to identify predisposing factors that may be eliminated or modified.
- Try to identify eruption patterns (seasonal or monthly).
- Explain the causes of acne to the patient and his family. Make sure they understand that the prescribed treatment is more likely to improve acne than a strict diet and fanatical scrubbing with soap and water. Provide written instructions regarding treatment.
- Describe the importance of not picking lesions (irritating the skin exacerbates breakouts) and of practicing good personal hygiene to prevent secondary infections.
- Instruct the patient receiving tretinoin to apply it at least 30 minutes after washing his face and at least 1 hour before bedtime. Warn against using it around the eyes or lips. After treatments, the skin should look pink and dry. If it appears red or starts to peel,

the preparation may have to be weakened or applied less often. Advise the patient to avoid exposure to sunlight or to use a sunscreen. If the prescribed regimen includes tretinoin and benzoyl peroxide, avoid skin irritation by using one preparation in the morning and the other at night.
- Instruct the patient to take tetracycline on an empty stomach and not to take it with antacids or milk because it interacts with their metallic ions and is then poorly absorbed.
- Tell the patient who's taking isotretinoin to avoid vitamin A supplements, which can worsen any adverse effects. Also, teach the patient how to deal with the dry skin and mucous membranes that usually occur during treatment. Tell the female patient about the severe risk of teratogenicity. Monitor liver function and lipid level.
- Inform the patient that acne takes a long time to clear — even years for complete resolution. Encourage continued local skin care even after acne clears.
- Explain the adverse effects of all drugs.
- Pay special attention to the patient's perception of his physical appearance, and offer emotional support.

Burns

Burns are classified as first-degree, second-degree superficial, second-degree deep partial thickness, third-degree full-thickness, and fourth-degree. A first-degree burn is limited to the epidermis. The most common example of a first-degree burn is sunburn, which results from overexposure to the sun. In a second-degree burn, the epidermis and part of the dermis are damaged. A third-degree burn damages the epidermis and dermis, and vessels and tissue are visible. In fourth-degree burns, the damage extends through deeply charred subcutaneous tissue to muscle and bone. Severe burns require immediate pain management and commonly result in permanent disability requiring lengthy periods of rehabilitation.

In victims younger than age 4 and older than age 60, there's a higher incidence of complications and thus a higher mortality. Immediate, aggressive burn treatment increases the patient's chance for survival. Later, supportive measures and strict sterile technique can minimize infection. Survival and recovery from a major burn are more likely when the burn wound is reduced to less than 20% of the total body surface area (BSA). (See *Using the Rule of Nines and the Lund-Browder chart,* pages 356 and 357.)

CAUSES
Friction and excessive exposure to sunlight may cause burns. Thermal burns, the most common type, typically result from:
- automobile accidents
- clothes that have caught on fire
- improper handling of firecrackers
- improper handling of gasoline
- parental abuse (in children or elderly people)
- playing with matches
- residential fires
- scalding and kitchen accidents.

Chemical burns result from contact, ingestion, inhalation, or injection of:
- acids
- alkalis
- vesicants.

Electrical burns result from:
- chewing on electrical cords
- contact with faulty electrical wiring or high-voltage power lines.

PATHOPHYSIOLOGY
The injuring agent denatures cellular proteins. Some cells die because of traumatic or ischemic necrosis. Loss of collagen cross-linking also occurs with denaturation, creating abnormal osmotic and hydrostatic pressure gradients, which cause the movement of intravascular fluid into interstitial spaces. Cellular injury triggers the release of mediators of inflammation, contributing to local and, in the case of major burns, systemic increases in capillary permeability. Specific pathophysiologic events depend on the cause and classification of the burn. (See *Classifications of burns.*)

First-degree burns
A first-degree burn causes localized injury or destruction to the skin (epidermis only) by direct (such as chemical spill) or indirect (such as sunlight) contact. The barrier function of the skin remains intact, and these burns aren't life-threatening.

Second-degree superficial partial-thickness burns
Second-degree superficial partial-thickness burns involve destruction to the epidermis and some dermis. Thin-walled, fluid-filled blisters develop within a few minutes of the injury. As these blisters break, the nerve endings become exposed to the air. Because pain and tactile responses remain intact, subsequent treatments are very painful. The barrier function of the skin is lost.

CLASSIFICATIONS OF BURNS

The depth of skin and tissue damage determines the burn classification. This illustration shows the four degrees of burn classifications.

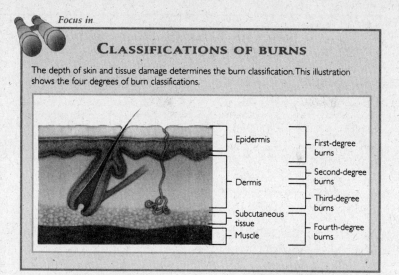

Epidermis

Dermis

Subcutaneous tissue

Muscle

First-degree burns

Second-degree burns

Third-degree burns

Fourth-degree burns

Second-degree deep partial-thickness burns

Second-degree deep partial-thickness burns involve destruction of the epidermis and dermis, producing blisters and mild to moderate edema and pain. The hair follicles are still intact, so hair will grow again. Compared with second-degree superficial partial-thickness burns, there's less pain sensation with this burn because the sensory neurons have undergone extensive destruction. The areas around the burn injury remain very sensitive to pain. The barrier function of the skin is lost.

Third- and fourth-degree burns

A major burn affects every body system and organ. A third-degree burn extends through the epidermis and dermis and into the subcutaneous tissue layer. A fourth-degree burn involves muscle, bone, and interstitial tissues. Within only hours, fluids and protein shift from capillary to intersti-

tial spaces, causing edema. There's an immediate immunologic response to a burn injury, making burn wound sepsis a potential threat. Finally, an increase in calorie demand after a burn injury increases the metabolic rate.

Possible complications of burns include loss of function (burns to face, hands, feet, and genitalia), total occlusion of circulation in an extremity (due to edema from circumferential burns), airway obstruction (neck burns) or restricted respiratory expansion (chest burns), pulmonary injury (from smoke inhalation or pulmonary embolism), acute respiratory distress syndrome (due to left-sided heart failure or myocardial infarction), greater damage than indicated by the surface burn (electrical and chemical burns), or internal tissue damage along the conduction pathway (electrical burns). Burns can also lead to infections, dehydration, cardiac arrhythmias (due to electrical shock and fluid shifts), hy-

(Text continues on page 358.)

USING THE RULE OF NINES AND THE LUND-BROWDER CHART

You can quickly estimate the extent of an adult patient's burn by using the Rule of Nines. This method divides an adult's body surface area into percentages. To use this method, mentally transfer your patient's burns to the body chart shown below; then add up the corresponding percentages for each burned body section. The total, an estimate of the extent of your patient's burn, enters into the formula to determine his initial fluid replacement needs.

You can't use the Rule of Nines for infants and children because their body section percentages differ from those of adults. For example, an infant's head accounts for about 17% of the total body surface area compared with 7% for an adult. Instead, use the Lund-Browder chart.

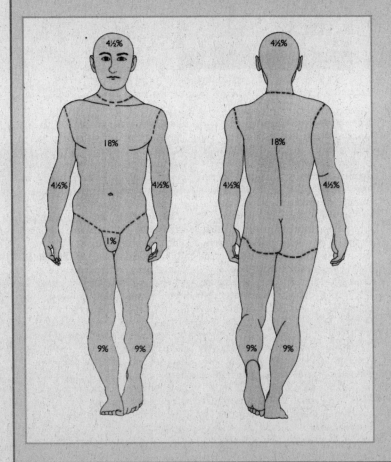

Lund-Browder chart

To determine the extent of an infant's or child's burns, use the Lund-Browder chart shown here.

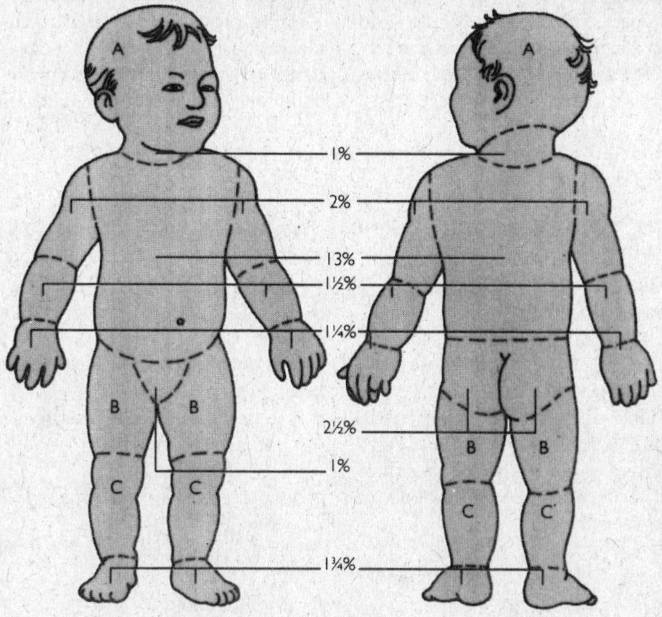

Relative percentages of areas affected by growth

At birth	0 to 1 year	1 to 4 years	5 to 9 years	10 to 15 years	Adult
A: Half of head					
9½%	8½%	6½%	5½%	4½%	3½%
B: Half of thigh					
2¾%	3¼%	4%	4¼%	4½%	4¾%
C: Half of leg					
2½%	2½%	2¾%	3%	3¼%	3½%

potension (secondary to shock or hypovolemia), burn shock (due to fluid shifts out of the vascular compartments, possibly leading to kidney damage and renal failure), and stroke, heart attack, or pulmonary embolism (due to formation of blood clots resulting from slower blood flow). In addition, patients with burns can develop peptic ulcer disease or ileus (due to decreased blood supply in the abdominal area), disseminated intravascular coagulation (more severe burn states), pain, depression, and financial burden (due to psychological component of disfigurement).

CLINICAL FINDINGS

- Localized pain and erythema, usually without blisters in the first 24 hours (first-degree burn)
- Chills, headache, localized edema, and nausea and vomiting (more severe first-degree burn)
- Thin-walled, fluid-filled blisters appearing within minutes of the injury, with mild to moderate edema and pain (second-degree superficial partial-thickness burn)
- White, waxy appearance to damaged area (second-degree deep partial-thickness burn)
- White, brown, or black leathery tissue and visible thrombosed vessels due to destruction of skin elasticity (dorsum of hand most common site of thrombosed veins), without blisters (third-degree burn)
- Silver-colored, raised area, usually at the site of electrical contact (electrical burn)
- Singed nasal hairs, mucosal burns, voice changes, coughing, wheezing, soot in mouth or nose, and darkened sputum (with smoke inhalation and pulmonary damage)

TEST RESULTS

There are no specific tests results related to the diagnosis of burns, but diagnosis involves determining the size and classifying the wound. The following methods are used to determine size:

- percentage of BSA covered by the burn using the Rule of Nines chart
- Lund-Browder chart (more accurate because it allows BSA changes with age); correlation of the burn's depth and size to estimate its severity. (See *Using the Rule of Nines and the Lund-Browder chart,* pages 356 and 357.)

Major burns include:
- third-degree burns over more than 10% of BSA
- second-degree burns over more than 25% of adult BSA (over 20% in children)
- burns of hands, face, feet, or genitalia
- burns complicated by fractures or respiratory damage
- electrical burns
- all burns in poor-risk patients.

Moderate burns include:
- third-degree burns over 2% to 10% of BSA
- second-degree burns over 15% to 25% of adult BSA (10% to 20% in children).

Minor burns include:
- third-degree burns over less than 2% of BSA
- second-degree burns over less than 15% of adult BSA (10% in children).

TREATMENT

Initial burn treatments are based on the type of burn and may include:
- immersing the burned area in cool water (55° F [12.8° C]) or applying cool compresses (minor burns)

- administering pain medication as needed or anti-inflammatory medications
- covering the area with an antimicrobial agent and a nonstick bulky dressing (after debridement); prophylactic tetanus injection as needed
- preventing hypoxia by maintaining an open airway; assessing airway, breathing, and circulation; checking for smoke inhalation immediately on receipt of the patient; assisting with endotracheal intubation; and giving 100% oxygen (first immediate treatment for moderate and major burns)
- controlling active bleeding
- covering partial-thickness burns over 30% of BSA or full-thickness burns over 5% of BSA with a clean, dry, sterile bed sheet (Because of drastic reduction in body temperature, don't cover large burns with saline-soaked dressings.)
- removing smoldering clothing (first soaking in saline solution if clothing is stuck to the patient's skin), rings, and other constricting items
- immediate I.V. therapy to prevent hypovolemic shock and maintain cardiac output (lactated Ringer's solution or a fluid replacement formula; additional I.V. lines may be needed)
- antimicrobial therapy (for all patients with major burns)
- complete blood count, electrolyte, glucose, blood urea nitrogen, and serum creatinine levels; arterial blood gas analysis; typing and crossmatching; urinalysis for myoglobinuria and hemoglobinuria
- closely monitoring intake and output, frequently checking vital signs (every 15 minutes), and possibly inserting an indwelling urinary catheter
- using a nasogastric tube to decompress the stomach and avoid aspiration of stomach contents

- irrigating the wound with copious amounts of normal saline solution (chemical burns)
- surgical intervention, including skin grafts and more thorough surgical cleaning (major burns).

NURSING CONSIDERATIONS

- Don't treat the burn wound for a patient being transferred to a specialty facility within 4 hours. Wrap the patient in a sterile sheet and blanket for warmth, elevate the burned extremity, and prepare the patient for transport.

Upon discharge or during prolonged care:

- Ensure increased calorie intake in response to the increased metabolic rate to promote healing and recovery.
- Teach the patient and give complete discharge instructions for home care; stress the importance of keeping the dressing clean and dry, elevating the burned extremity for the first 24 hours, and having the wound rechecked in 1 to 2 days.
- Stress the importance of taking pain medication as needed, especially before dressing changes.

Dermatitis

Dermatitis is an inflammation of the skin that occurs in several forms: seborrheic, nummular, hand or foot, contact, localized neurodermatitis (lichen simplex chronicus), exfoliative, and stasis. (See *Types of dermatitis,* pages 360 to 362.)

NURSING CONSIDERATIONS

- Warn the patient that drowsiness is possible with the use of antihistamines. If nocturnal itching interferes

(Text continues on page 362.)

TYPES OF DERMATITIS

TYPE	CAUSE	CLINICAL FINDINGS	TREATMENT
Seborrheic dermatitis A subacute skin disease affecting the scalp, face, and occasionally other areas that's characterized by lesions covered with yellow or brownish gray scales	◆ Unknown; stress, immunodeficiency, and neurologic conditions may be predisposing factors; related to the yeast *Pityrosporum ovale* (normal flora)	◆ Eruptions in areas with many sebaceous glands (usually scalp, face, chest, axillae, and groin) and in skin folds ◆ Itching, redness, and inflammation of affected areas; lesions possibly appearing greasy; fissures possible ◆ Indistinct, occasionally yellowish scaly patches from excess stratum corneum (Dandruff may be a mild seborrheic dermatitis.)	◆ Removal of scales with frequent washing and shampooing with selenium sulfide suspension (most effective), zinc pyrithione, ketoconazole 2%, or tar and salicylic acid shampoo ◆ Application of topical corticosteroids and antifungals to involved area
Nummular dermatitis A chronic form of dermatitis characterized by inflammation in coin-shaped, scaling, or vesicular patches; usually pruritic	◆ Possibly precipitated by stress, dry skin, irritants, or scratching	◆ Round, nummular (coin-shaped), red lesions, usually on arms and legs, with distinct borders of crusts and scales ◆ Possible oozing and severe itching ◆ Summertime remissions common, with wintertime recurrence	◆ Elimination of known irritants ◆ Measures to relieve dry skin: increased humidification, limited frequency of baths, use of bland soap and bath oils, and application of emollients ◆ Application of wet dressings in acute phase ◆ Topical corticosteroids (occlusive dressings or intralesional injections) for persistent lesions ◆ Tar preparations and antihistamines to control itching ◆ Antibiotics for secondary infection

TYPE	CAUSE	CLINICAL FINDINGS	TREATMENT
Contact dermatitis Typically, sharply demarcated inflammation of the skin resulting from contact with an irritating chemical or atopic allergen (a substance producing an allergic reaction in the skin) and irritation of the skin resulting from contact with concentrated substances to which the skin is sensitive, such as perfumes, soaps, or chemicals	◆ Mild irritants: chronic exposure to detergents or solvents ◆ Strong irritants: damage on contact with acids or alkalis ◆ Allergens: sensitization after repeated exposure	◆ Mild irritants and allergens: erythema and small vesicles that ooze, scale, and itch ◆ Strong irritants: blisters and ulcerations ● Classic allergic response: clearly defined lesions, with straight lines following points of contact ◆ Severe allergic reaction: marked erythema, blistering, and edema of affected areas	◆ Elimination of known allergens and decreased exposure to irritants, wearing protective clothing such as gloves, and washing immediately after contact with irritants or allergens ◆ Topical anti-inflammatory agents (including corticosteroids), systemic corticosteroids for edema and bullae, antihistamines, and local application of Burow's solution (for blisters)
Hand or foot dermatitis A skin disease characterized by inflammatory eruptions of the hands or feet	◆ In many cases unknown but may result from irritant or allergic contact ◆ Excessively dry skin a common contributing factor ◆ Half of patients atopic	◆ Redness and scaling of the palms or soles ◆ May produce painful fissures ◆ Some cases present with blisters (dyshidrotic eczema)	◆ Same as for nummular dermatitis ◆ Severe cases possibly requiring systemic steroids
Localized neurodermatitis (lichen simplex chronicus, essential pruritus) Superficial inflammation of the skin characterized by itching and papular eruptions that appear on thickened, hyperpigmented skin	◆ Chronic scratching or rubbing of a primary lesion or insect bite or other skin irritation ◆ May be psychogenic	◆ Intense, sometimes continual scratching ◆ Thick, sharp-bordered, possibly dry, scaly lesions with raised papules and accentuated skin lines (lichenification) ◆ Usually affects easily reached areas, such as ankles, lower legs, anogenital area, back of neck, and ears ◆ One or several lesions present; asymmetric distribution	◆ Scratching must stop, after which lesions disappear in about 2 weeks ◆ Fixed dressings or Unna's boot to cover affected areas ◆ Topical corticosteroids under occlusion or by intralesional injection ◆ Antihistamines and open wet dressings ◆ Emollients ◆ Patient informed about underlying cause

(continued)

TYPE	CAUSE	CLINICAL FINDINGS	TREATMENT
Exfoliative dermatitis Severe skin inflammation characterized by redness and widespread erythema and scaling, covering virtually the entire skin surface	◆ Preexisting skin lesions progressing to exfoliative stage, such as in contact dermatitis, drug reaction, lymphoma, leukemia, or atopic dermatitis ◆ May be idiopathic	◆ Generalized dermatitis, with acute loss of stratum corneum, erythema, and scaling ◆ Sensation of tight skin ◆ Hair loss ◆ Possible fever, sensitivity to cold, shivering, gynecomastia, and lymphadenopathy	◆ Hospitalization, with protective isolation and hygienic measures to prevent secondary bacterial infection ◆ Open wet dressings, with colloidal baths ◆ Bland lotions over topical corticosteroids ◆ Maintenance of constant environmental temperature to prevent chilling or overheating ◆ Careful monitoring of renal and cardiac status ◆ Systemic antibiotics and steroids
Stasis dermatitis A condition usually caused by impaired circulation and characterized by eczema of the legs with edema, hyperpigmentation, and persistent inflammation	◆ Secondary to peripheral vascular diseases affecting the legs, such as recurrent thrombophlebitis and resultant chronic venous insufficiency	◆ Varicosities and edema common, but obvious vascular insufficiency not always present ◆ Usually affects the lower leg just above internal malleolus or sites of trauma or irritation ◆ Early signs: dusky red deposits of hemosiderin in skin, with itching and dimpling of subcutaneous tissue ◆ Later signs: edema, redness, and scaling of large areas of legs ◆ Possible fissures, crusts, and ulcers	◆ Measures to prevent venous stasis: avoidance of prolonged sitting or standing, use of support stockings, weight reduction in obesity, and leg elevation ◆ Corrective surgery for underlying cause ◆ After ulcer develops, encourage rest periods with legs elevated, open wet dressings, Unna's boot (zinc gelatin dressing provides continuous pressure to affected areas), and antibiotics for secondary infection after wound culture

with sleep, suggest methods for inducing natural sleep, such as drinking a glass of warm milk, to prevent overuse of sedatives.

● Assist the patient in scheduling daily skin care. Keep his fingernails short to limit excoriation and secondary infections caused by scratching.

● Apply cool, moist compresses to relieve itching and burning.

Pressure ulcers

Pressure ulcers, commonly called *pressure sores* or *bedsores,* are localized areas of cellular necrosis that commonly occur in the skin and subcutaneous tissue over bony prominences. These ulcers may be superficial, caused by local skin irritation with subsequent surface maceration, or deep, originating in underlying tissue. Deep lesions typically go undetected until they penetrate the skin, but by then, they have usually caused subcutaneous damage. (See *Staging pressure ulcers,* pages 364 and 365.)

Most pressure ulcers develop over five body locations: sacral area, greater trochanter, ischial tuberosity, heel, and lateral malleolus. Collectively, these areas account for 95% of all pressure ulcer sites. Patients who have contractures are at an increased risk for developing pressure ulcers because of the added pressure on the tissue and the alignment of the bones.

> **Alert** *Age also has a role in the incidence of pressure ulcers. Muscle is lost with aging, and skin elasticity decreases. Both of these factors increase the risk of developing pressure ulcers.*

Partial-thickness ulcers usually involve the dermis and epidermis; with treatment, these wounds heal within a few weeks. Full-thickness ulcers also involve the dermis and epidermis, but in these wounds, the damage is more severe and complete. There may also be damage to the deeper tissue layers. Ulcers of the subcutaneous tissue and muscle may require several months to heal. If the damage has affected the bone in addition to the skin layers, osteomyelitis may occur, which will prolong healing time.

CAUSES
- Constant moisture on the skin causing tissue maceration
- Friction or shearing forces causing damage to the epidermal and upper dermal skin layers
- Immobility and decreased level of activity
- Impaired hygiene status, such as with urinary or fecal incontinence, leading to skin breakdown
- Malnutrition (associated with pressure ulcer development)
- Medical conditions, such as diabetes and orthopedic injuries
- Psychological factors, such as depression and chronic emotional stresses

PATHOPHYSIOLOGY
A pressure ulcer is caused by an injury to the skin and its underlying tissues. The pressure exerted on the area causes ischemia and hypoxemia to the affected tissues because of decreased blood flow to the site. As the capillaries collapse, thrombosis occurs, which subsequently leads to tissue edema and progression to tissue necrosis. Ischemia also adds to an accumulation of waste products at the site, which in turn leads to the production of toxins. The toxins further break down the tissue and eventually lead to cell death.

Complications of pressure ulcers include progression of the pressure ulcer to a more severe state (greatest risk); secondary infections such as sepsis; loss of limb from bone involvement; or osteomyelitis.

CLINICAL FINDINGS
- Blanching erythema, varying from pink to bright red depending on the patient's skin color; in dark-skinned people, purple discoloration or a darkening of normal skin color (first clini-

STAGING PRESSURE ULCERS

The staging system described here is based on the recommendations of the National Pressure Ulcer Advisory Panel (NPUAP) (Consensus Conference, 1991) and the Agency for Health Care Policy and Research (*Clinical Practice Guidelines for Treatment of Pressure Ulcers*, 1992). The stage I definition was updated by the NPUAP in 1997.

STAGE I

A stage I pressure ulcer is an observable pressure-related alteration of intact skin. The indicators, compared with the adjacent or opposite area on the body, may include changes in one or more of the following factors: skin temperature (warmth or coolness), tissue consistency (firm or boggy feel), or sensation (pain or itching). The ulcer appears as a defined area of persistent redness in lightly pigmented skin; in darker skin, the ulcer may appear with persistent red, blue, or purple hues.

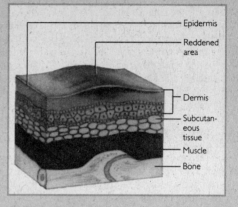

Epidermis
Reddened area
Dermis
Subcutaneous tissue
Muscle
Bone

STAGE II

A stage II pressure ulcer is characterized by partial-thickness skin loss involving the epidermis or dermis. The ulcer is superficial and appears as an abrasion, blister, or shallow crater.

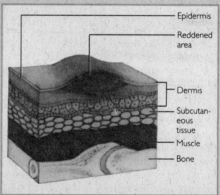

Epidermis
Reddened area
Dermis
Subcutaneous tissue
Muscle
Bone

cal sign) (When the examiner presses a finger on the reddened area, the "pressed on" area whitens and color returns within 1 to 3 seconds if capillary refill is good.)

- Pain at the site and surrounding area
- Localized edema due to the inflammatory response
- Increased body temperature due to the initial inflammatory response (in

STAGE III

A stage III pressure ulcer is characterized by full-thickness skin loss involving damage or necrosis of subcutaneous tissue, which may extend down to, but not through, the underlying fascia. The ulcer appears as a deep crater with or without undermining of adjacent tissue.

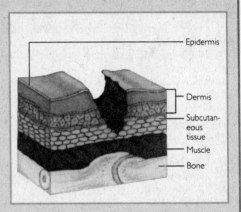

- Epidermis
- Dermis
- Subcutaneous tissue
- Muscle
- Bone

STAGE IV

Full-thickness skin loss with extensive destruction, tissue necrosis, or damage to muscle, bone, or support structures (for example, tendon or joint capsule) characterizes a stage IV pressure ulcer. Tunneling and sinus tracts also may be associated with stage IV pressure ulcers.

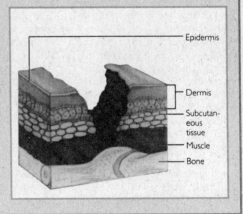

- Epidermis
- Dermis
- Subcutaneous tissue
- Muscle
- Bone

more severe cases, cool skin due to more severe damage or necrosis)
- Nonblanching erythema (more severe cases) ranging from dark red to purple or cyanotic; indicates deeper dermal involvement
- Blisters, crusts, or scaling as the skin deteriorates and the ulcer progresses
- Usually dusky red appearance, doesn't bleed easily, and is warm to the touch and possibly mottled (deep

ulcer originating at the bony prominence below the skin surface)
- Possible foul-smelling, purulent drainage from the ulcerated lesion
- Eschar tissue on and around the lesion due to the necrotic tissue that prevents healthy tissue growth

TEST RESULTS
- Wound culture reveals exudate or evidence of infection.
- Elevated white blood cell count indicates infection.
- Laboratory tests reveal an elevated erythrocyte sedimentation rate.
- Total serum protein and serum albumin levels show severe hypoproteinemia.

TREATMENT
- Repositioning of the patient every 2 hours, or more often if indicated, with support of pillows
- Movement and range-of-motion (ROM) exercises to promote circulation
- Foam, gel, or air mattress to aid in healing by reducing pressure on the ulcer site and reducing the risk of more ulcers
- Foam, gel, or air mattress on chairs and wheelchairs as indicated
- Nutritional assessment and dietary consult as indicated; nutritional supplements, such as vitamin C and zinc, for the malnourished patient; monitoring serum albumin and protein markers and body weight
- Adequate fluid intake and increased fluids for a dehydrated patient
- Meticulous skin care and hygiene practices
- Stage II — covering the ulcer with transparent film, polyurethane foam, or hydrocolloid dressing
- Stage II or IV — loosely filling the wound with saline- or gel-moistened gauze, managing exudate with an absorbent dressing (moist gauze or foam), and covering with a secondary dressing
- Clean, bulky dressing for certain types of ulcers such as decubiti
- Surgical debridement for deeper wounds (stage III or IV) as indicated

NURSING CONSIDERATIONS
- Assess the skin of the bedridden or high-risk patient for possible changes in color, turgor, temperature, and sensation. Assess the patient for pain. Examine an existing ulcer for any change in size or degree of damage. When using pressure relief aids or topical agents, explain their function to the patient.
- Prevent pressure ulcers by repositioning the bedridden patient at least every 2 hours around the clock. To minimize the effects of a shearing force, use a footboard and raise the head of the bed to an angle not exceeding 60 degrees. Also, use a draw or pull sheet to turn the patient or to pull him up. Keep the patient's knees slightly flexed for short periods. Perform passive ROM exercises, or encourage the patient to do active exercises, if possible.
- To prevent pressure ulcers in immobilized patients, use pressure relief aids on their beds.
- Provide meticulous skin care. Keep the skin clean and dry without the use of harsh soaps. Gently massaging the skin around the affected area — not on it — promotes healing. Thoroughly rub moisturizing lotions into the skin to prevent maceration of the skin surface.
- Change bedding frequently for patients who are diaphoretic or incontinent, or who have large amounts of drainage from wounds, suture lines,

or drain sites. Use a fecal incontinence bag for incontinent patients.

- Clean open lesions with a 3% solution of hydrogen peroxide or normal saline solution. Dressings, if needed, should be porous and lightly taped to healthy skin. Debridement of necrotic tissue may be necessary to allow healing. One method is to apply open wet dressings and allow them to dry on the ulcer. Removal of the dressings mechanically debrides exudate and necrotic tissue. Other methods include surgical debridement with a fine scalpel blade and chemical debridement using proteolytic enzyme agents.
- Encourage adequate intake of nutritious food and fluids to maintain body weight and promote healing. Consult with the dietitian to provide a diet that promotes granulation of new tissue. Encourage the debilitated patient to eat frequent, small meals that provide protein- and calorie-rich supplements. Assist the weakened patient with his meals.

Scleroderma

Scleroderma (also known as *systemic sclerosis*) is an uncommon disease of diffuse connective tissue characterized by inflammatory and then degenerative and fibrotic changes in the skin, blood vessels, synovial membranes, skeletal muscles, and internal organs (especially the esophagus, intestinal tract, thyroid, heart, lungs, and kidneys). There are several forms of scleroderma, including diffuse systemic sclerosis, localized, linear, chemically induced localized, eosinophilia-myalgia syndrome, toxic oil syndrome, and graft-versus-host disease.

Scleroderma is three to four times more common in females than in males, especially between ages 30 and 50. The peak incidence of occurrence is in 50- to 60-year-olds.

Scleroderma usually progresses slowly. When the condition is limited to the skin, the prognosis is usually favorable. However, about 30% of patients with scleroderma die within 5 years of onset due to infection or by kidney or heart failure.

CAUSES

The cause of scleroderma is unknown, but some possible causes include:
- anticancer agents, such as bleomycin (Blenoxane), or nonopioid analgesics such as pentazocine (Talwin)
- fibrosis due to an abnormal immune system response
- systemic exposure to silica dust or polyvinyl chloride
- underlying vascular cause with tissue changes initiated by persistent perfusion.

PATHOPHYSIOLOGY

Scleroderma usually begins in the fingers and extends proximally to the upper arms, shoulders, neck, and face. The skin atrophies, edema and infiltrates containing $CD4^+$ T cells surround the blood vessels, and inflamed collagen fibers become edematous (losing strength and elasticity), and degenerative. The dermis becomes tightly bound to the underlying structures, resulting in atrophy of the affected dermal appendages and destruction of the distal phalanges by osteoporosis. As the disease progresses, this atrophy can affect other areas. For example, in some patients, muscles and joints become fibrotic. Complications of scleroderma include compromised circulation due to abnormal thickening of the arterial intima, possibly causing slowly healing ulcerations on fingertips or toes leading to gangrene. Also, the patient may experience decreased food intake and weight loss as a result of GI symptoms, arrhythmias and dyspnea due to cardiac and pulmonary fibrosis, and malignant hypertension due to renal involvement, called renal crisis (may be fatal if untreated; advanced disease).

CLINICAL FINDINGS
● Skin thickening, commonly limited to the distal extremities and face, but which can also involve internal organs (limited systemic sclerosis)
● CREST syndrome (a benign subtype of limited systemic sclerosis): Calcinosis, Raynaud's phenomenon, Esophageal dysfunction, Sclerodactyly, and Telangiectasia
● Generalized skin thickening and involvement of internal organs (diffuse systemic sclerosis)
● Patchy skin changes with a teardrop-like appearance known as *morphea* (localized scleroderma)
● Band of thickened skin on the face or extremities that severely damages underlying tissues, causing atrophy and deformity (linear scleroderma)

Alert *Atrophy and deformity with scleroderma are most common in childhood.*

● Raynaud's phenomenon (blanching, cyanosis, and erythema of the fingers and toes when exposed to cold or stress); progressive phalangeal resorption may shorten the fingers (early symptoms)
● Pain, stiffness, and swelling of fingers and joints (later symptoms)
● Taut, shiny skin over the entire hand and forearm due to skin thickening

● Tight and inelastic facial skin, causing a masklike appearance and "pinching" of the mouth; contractures with progressive tightening
● Thickened skin over proximal limbs and trunk (diffuse systemic sclerosis)
● Frequent reflux, heartburn, dysphagia, and bloating after meals due to GI dysfunction
● Abdominal distention, diarrhea, constipation, and malodorous floating stool

TEST RESULTS
● Laboratory test results reveal slightly elevated erythrocyte sedimentation rate, positive rheumatoid factor in 25% to 35% of patients, and positive antinuclear antibody.
● Urinalysis shows proteinuria, microscopic hematuria, and casts (with renal involvement).
● Hand X-rays reveal terminal phalangeal tuft resorption, subcutaneous calcification, and joint space narrowing and erosion.
● Chest X-rays show bilateral basilar pulmonary fibrosis.
● GI X-rays reveal distal esophageal hypomotility and stricture, duodenal loop dilation, small-bowel malabsorption pattern, and large diverticula.
● Pulmonary function studies show decreased diffusion and vital capacity.
● Electrocardiogram shows nonspecific abnormalities related to myocardial fibrosis.
● Skin biopsy reveals changes consistent with disease progression, such as marked thickening of the dermis and occlusive vessel changes.

TREATMENT
There's no cure for scleroderma. Treatment, which aims to preserve normal body functions and minimize complications, may include:

- immunosuppressants, such as cyclosporine (Neoral) or chlorambucil (Leukeran)
- vasodilators and antihypertensives, such as nifedipine (Procardia), prazosin (Minipress), or topical nitroglycerin; digital sympathectomy; or rarely, cervical sympathetic blockade to treat Raynaud's phenomenon
- digital plaster cast to immobilize the area, minimize trauma, and maintain cleanliness; possible surgical debridement for chronic digital ulceration
- antacids (to reduce total acid level in GI tract), omeprazole (Prilosec), a proton pump inhibitor (to block the formation of gastric acid), periodic dilation, and a soft, bland diet for esophagitis with stricture
- broad-spectrum antibiotics to treat small-bowel involvement to counteract the bacterial overgrowth in the duodenum and jejunum related to hypomotility
- short-term benefit from vasodilators, such as nifedipine or hydralazine (Apresoline), to decrease contractility and oxygen demand and to cause vasodilation (for pulmonary hypertension)
- angiotensin-converting enzyme inhibitor to preserve renal function (early intervention in renal crisis)
- physical therapy to maintain function and promote muscle strength, heat therapy to relieve joint stiffness, and patient teaching to make performance of daily activities easier.

NURSING CONSIDERATIONS

- Assess motion restrictions, pain, vital signs, intake and output, respiratory function, and daily weight.
- Because of compromised circulation, warn against fingerstick blood tests.

- Remember that air conditioning may aggravate Raynaud's phenomenon.
- Help the patient and her family adjust to the patient's new body image and to the limitations and dependence that these changes cause.
- Teach the patient to avoid fatigue by pacing activities and organizing schedules to include necessary rest.
- Encourage the patient and her family to express their feelings, and help them cope with their fears and frustrations by offering information about the disease, its treatment, and relevant diagnostic tests.
- Direct the patient to seek out support groups, which can be found in every state. Instruct her to call 1-800-722-HOPE (4673) or go to *www.scleroderma.org* to determine the closest location.

MUSCULOSKELETAL SYSTEM

The musculoskeletal system is a complex system of bones, joints, muscles, ligaments, tendons, and other tissues that gives the body form and shape. It also protects vital organs, makes movement possible, stores calcium and other minerals in the bony matrix for mobilization if deficiency occurs, and provides sites for hematopoiesis (blood cell production) in the marrow.

Bone fracture

When a force exceeds the compressive or tensile strength of the bone (the ability of the bone to hold together), a fracture will occur. (For an explanation of the terms used to identify fractures, see *Classifying fractures*.)

An estimated 25% of the population has traumatic musculoskeletal injury each year, and a significant number of these involve fractures.

The prognosis varies with the extent of disability or deformity, amount of tissue and vascular damage, adequacy of reduction and immobilization, and the patient's age, health, and nutritional status.

Alert *Children's bones usually heal rapidly and without deformity.*

However, epiphyseal plate fractures in children are likely to cause deformity because they interfere with normal bone growth. In elderly people, underlying systemic illness, impaired circulation, or poor nutrition may cause slow or poor healing.

Causes
- Automobile accidents
- Bone tumors
- Falls
- Medications that cause iatrogenic osteoporosis (such as steroids)
- Metabolic illnesses (such as hypoparathyroidism or hyperparathyroidism)
- Sports
- Use of drugs that impair judgment or mobility
- Young age (immaturity of bone)

Alert *The highest incidence of bone fractures occurs in young males ages 15 to 24 (tibia, clavicle, and lower humerus) and are usually the result of trauma. In elderly people, upper femur, upper humerus, forearm, wrist, vertebrae, and pelvis fractures are commonly associated with osteoporosis.*

Pathophysiology
When a bone is fractured, the periosteum and blood vessels in the cortex, marrow, and surrounding soft tissue

CLASSIFYING FRACTURES

One of the best-known systems for classifying fractures uses a combination of terms that describe general classification, fragment position, and fracture line — such as *simple*, *nondisplaced*, and *oblique* — to describe fractures.

GENERAL CLASSIFICATION OF FRACTURES

◆ Simple (closed) — Bone fragments don't penetrate the skin.
◆ Compound (open) — Bone fragments penetrate the skin.
◆ Incomplete (partial) — Bone continuity isn't completely interrupted.
◆ Complete — Bone continuity is completely interrupted.

CLASSIFICATION BY FRAGMENT POSITION

◆ Comminuted — The bone breaks into small pieces.
◆ Impacted — One bone fragment is forced into another.
◆ Angulated — Fragments lie at an angle to each other.
◆ Displaced — Fracture fragments separate and are deformed.
◆ Nondisplaced — The two sections of bone maintain essentially normal alignment.

◆ Overriding — Fragments overlap, shortening the total bone length.
◆ Segmental — Fractures occur in two adjacent areas with an isolated central segment.
◆ Avulsed — Fragments are pulled from the normal position by muscle contractions or ligament resistance.

CLASSIFICATION BY FRACTURE LINE

◆ Linear — The fracture line runs parallel to the bone's axis.
◆ Longitudinal — The fracture line extends in a longitudinal (but not parallel) direction along the bone's axis.
◆ Oblique — The fracture line crosses the bone at about a 45-degree angle to the bone's axis.
◆ Spiral — The fracture line crosses the bone at an oblique angle, creating a spiral pattern.
◆ Transverse — The fracture line forms a right angle with the bone's axis.

---

are disrupted. A hematoma forms between the broken ends of the bone and beneath the periosteum, and granulation tissue eventually replaces the hematoma.

Damage to bone tissue triggers an intense inflammatory response in which cells from surrounding soft tissue and the marrow cavity invade the fracture area, and blood flow to the entire bone is increased. Osteoblasts in the periosteum, endosteum, and marrow produce osteoid (collagenous, young bone that hasn't yet calcified, also called *callus*), which hardens along the outer surface of the shaft and over the broken ends of the bone. Osteoclasts reabsorb material from previously formed bones and osteo-

blasts to rebuild bone. Osteoblasts then transform into osteocytes (mature bone cells).

Possible complications of bone fracture are permanent deformity and dysfunction if bones fail to heal (nonunion) or if they heal improperly (malunion), aseptic necrosis (not caused by infection) of bone segments due to impaired circulation, and hypovolemic shock as a result of blood vessel damage (especially with a fractured femur). The patient can also develop muscle contractures or compartment syndrome (see *Recognizing compartment syndrome, page 372*), renal calculi from decalcification due to prolonged immobility, and fat embolism due to disruption of marrow or activation of the sympathetic nervous system after the trauma (may lead to respiratory or central nervous system distress).

CLINICAL FINDINGS

● Deformity due to unnatural alignment
● Swelling due to vasodilation and infiltration by inflammatory leukocytes and mast cells
● Muscle spasm
● Tenderness
● Impaired sensation distal to the fracture site due to pinching or severing of neurovascular elements by the trauma or by bone fragments
● Limited range of motion
● Crepitus, or "clicking" sounds on movement caused by shifting bone fragments
● Severe pain after numbness dissipates

TEST RESULTS

● X-rays of the suspected fracture and the joints above and below confirm the diagnosis.

TREATMENT

For arm or leg fracture, emergency treatment consists of:
● splinting the limb above and below the suspected fracture to immobilize it
● applying a cold pack to reduce pain and edema
● elevating the limb to reduce pain and edema.

Alert *The acronym RICE is useful to help remember treatment for a fracture in the first 24 hours:*
R *Rest*
I *Ice*
C *Compression*
E *Elevation*

Treatment in severe bone fracture that causes blood loss includes:
● direct pressure to control bleeding
● fluid replacement as soon as possible to prevent or treat hypovolemic shock.

After confirming a fracture, treatment begins with a reduction. Closed reduction involves:
● manual manipulation
● local anesthetic (such as lidocaine)
● analgesic (such as morphine I.M.)
● muscle relaxant (such as diazepam [Valium] I.V.) or a sedative (such as midazolam [Versed]) to facilitate the muscle stretching necessary to realign the bone.

When closed reduction is impossible, open reduction by surgery involves:

immobilization of the fracture by means of rods, plates, or screws and application of a plaster cast
- tetanus prophylaxis
- prophylactic antibiotics
- surgery to repair soft tissue damage
- thorough wound debridement
- physical therapy after cast removal to restore limb mobility.

When a splint or cast fails to maintain the reduction, immobilization requires skin or skeletal traction, using a series of weights and pulleys. This may involve:
- elastic bandages and sheepskin coverings to attach traction devices to the patient's skin (skin traction)
- pin or wire inserted through the bone distal to the fracture and attached to a weight to allow more prolonged traction (skeletal traction).

NURSING CONSIDERATIONS
- Watch for signs of shock in the patient with a severe open fracture of a large bone such as the femur.
- Monitor vital signs, and be especially alert for rapid pulse, decreased blood pressure, pallor, and cool, clammy skin — all of which may indicate that the patient is in shock.
- Administer I.V. fluids as ordered.
- Offer reassurance to the frightened patient.
- Ease pain with analgesics.
- Help the patient set realistic goals for recovery.
- If the bone fracture requires long-term immobilization with traction, reposition the patient often to increase comfort and prevent pressure ulcers. Assist with active range-of-motion exercises to prevent muscle atrophy. Encourage deep breathing and coughing to avoid hypostatic pneumonia.
- Urge adequate fluid intake to prevent urinary stasis and constipation.

Watch for signs of renal calculi (flank pain, nausea, and vomiting).
- Provide good cast care, and support the cast with pillows. Observe for skin irritation near cast edges, and check for foul odors or discharge. Tell the patient to report signs or symptoms of impaired circulation (skin coldness, numbness, tingling, or discoloration) immediately. Warn him not to get the cast wet and not to insert foreign objects under the cast.
- Encourage the patient to start moving around as soon as he's able. Help him to walk. Demonstrate how to use crutches properly.
- After cast removal, refer the patient to a physical therapist to restore limb mobility.

Carpal tunnel syndrome

Carpal tunnel syndrome, a form of repetitive stress injury, is the most common nerve entrapment syndrome. It usually occurs in women ages 30 to 60 (posing a serious occupational health problem). However, men who are also employed as assembly-line workers and packers and who repeatedly use poorly designed tools are just as likely to develop this disorder. Any strenuous use of the hands — sustained grasping, twisting, or flexing — aggravates this condition.

CAUSES
Carpal tunnel syndrome is mostly idiopathic, but it may also result from:
- acromegaly
- amyloidosis
- benign tumor
- diabetes mellitus

THE
CARPAL TUNNEL

The carpal tunnel is clearly visible in this palmar view and cross section of a right hand. Note the blood vessels and median nerve flexor tendons of the fingers passing through the tunnel on their way from the forearm to the hand.

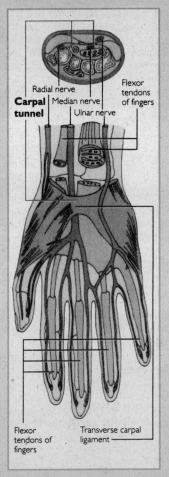

Radial nerve

Carpal tunnel

Median nerve

Ulnar nerve

Flexor tendons of fingers

Flexor tendons of fingers

Transverse carpal ligament

- flexor tenosynovitis (commonly associated with rheumatic disease)
- hypothyroidism
- multiple myeloma
- nerve compression
- obesity
- other conditions that increase fluid pressure in the wrist, including alterations in the endocrine or immune systems
- pregnancy
- repetitive stress injury
- rheumatoid arthritis
- wrist dislocation or sprain, including Colles' fracture followed by edema.

PATHOPHYSIOLOGY

The carpal bones and the transverse carpal ligament form the carpal tunnel. (See *The carpal tunnel*.) Inflammation or fibrosis of the tendon sheaths that pass through the carpal tunnel usually causes edema and compression of the median nerve. This compression neuropathy causes sensory and motor changes in the median distribution of the hands, initially impairing sensory transmission to the thumb, index finger, second finger, and inner aspect of the third finger. Continued use of the affected wrist may increase tendon inflammation, compression, and neural ischemia, causing a decrease in wrist function.

Untreated carpal tunnel syndrome can produce permanent nerve damage with loss of movement and sensation.

CLINICAL FINDINGS

- Weakness, pain, burning, numbness, or tingling in one or both hands
- Paresthesia affecting the thumb, forefinger, middle finger, and half of the fourth finger
- Inability to make a fist

- Atrophic nails
- Dry and shiny skin
- Symptoms typically worse at night and in the morning because of vasodilation and venous stasis
- Pain possibly spreading to the forearm and, in severe cases, as far as the shoulder
- Pain relieved by shaking or rubbing the hands vigorously or dangling the arms at the side
- Decreased sensation to light touch or pinpricks in the affected fingers
- Muscle atrophy occurring in about half of all cases of carpal tunnel syndrome (usually a late sign)

TEST RESULTS
- Tinel's sign reveals tingling over the median nerve on light percussion.
- Phalen's maneuver reproduces symptoms of carpal tunnel syndrome by having the patient hold her forearms vertically and allowing both hands to drop into complete flexion at the wrists for 1 minute.
- Compression test provokes pain and paresthesia along the distribution of the median nerve by applying a blood pressure cuff and inflating it above systolic pressure on the forearm for 1 to 2 minutes.
- Electromyography detects a median nerve motor conduction delay of more than 5 milliseconds.
- Laboratory tests identify underlying disease.

TREATMENT
- Conservative treatment should be tried first, including resting the hands by splinting the wrist in neutral extension for 1 to 2 weeks.
- Nonsteroidal anti-inflammatory drugs may provide symptomatic relief.
- Injection of the carpal tunnel with hydrocortisone and lidocaine may provide significant but temporary relief.
- If a definite link has been established between the patient's occupation and the development of repetitive stress injury, she may have to seek other work.
- Correction of an underlying disorder.
- Surgical decompression of the nerve by resecting the entire transverse carpal tunnel ligament or by using endoscopic surgical techniques. Neurolysis (freeing of the nerve fibers) may also be necessary.

NURSING CONSIDERATIONS
- Administer mild analgesics as needed. Encourage the patient to use her hands as much as possible. Assist with eating and bathing as needed.
- Teach the patient how to apply and remove a splint. Tell her not to make it too tight. Show her how to perform daily gentle range-of-motion exercises without the splint. Make sure the patient knows how to do these exercises before she's discharged.
- After surgery, monitor vital signs and regularly check the color, sensation, and motion of the affected hand.
- Advise the patient who's about to be discharged to exercise her hands occasionally in warm water. If the arm is in a sling, tell her to remove the sling several times per day to do exercises for her elbow and shoulder.
- Suggest occupational counseling for the patient who has to change jobs because of repetitive stress injury.

Clubfoot

Clubfoot, also called *talipes,* is the most common congenital disorder of the lower extremities. It's marked primarily by a deformed talus and shortened Achilles tendon, which give the foot a characteristic clublike appearance. In talipes equinovarus, the foot points downward (equinus) and turns inward (varus), while the front of the foot curls toward the heel (forefoot adduction).

Clubfoot occurs in about 1 per 1,000 live births, is usually bilateral, and is twice as common in boys as in girls. It may be associated with other birth defects, such as myelomeningocele, spina bifida, and arthrogryposis. Clubfoot is correctable with prompt treatment.

CAUSES

A combination of genetic and environmental factors in utero appears to cause clubfoot, including:
- arrested development during the 9th and 10th weeks of embryonic life, when the feet are formed (children without a family history of clubfoot)
- heredity (The mechanism of transmission is undetermined; the sibling of a child born with clubfoot has 1 chance in 35 of being born with the same anomaly, and a child of a parent with clubfoot has 1 chance in 10.)
- muscle abnormalities leading to variations in length and tendon insertions
- secondary to paralysis, poliomyelitis, or cerebral palsy (older children), in which case treatment includes management of the underlying disease.

PATHOPHYSIOLOGY

Abnormal development of the foot during fetal growth leads to abnormal muscles and joints and contracture of soft tissue. The condition called *apparent clubfoot* results when a fetus maintains a position in utero that gives his feet a clubfoot appearance at birth; it can usually be corrected manually. Another form of apparent clubfoot is inversion of the feet, resulting from the denervation type of progressive muscular atrophy and progressive muscular dystrophy. Possible complications of talipes equinovarus include chronic impairment (neglected clubfoot).

CLINICAL FINDINGS

Talipes equinovarus varies greatly in severity. Deformity may be so extreme that the toes touch the inside of the ankle, or it may be only vaguely apparent.

Every case includes:
- deformed talus
- shortened Achilles tendon
- shortened and flattened calcaneus bone of the heel
- shortened, underdeveloped calf muscles and soft-tissue contractures at the site of the deformity (depending on degree of the varus deformity)
- foot is tight in its deformed position, resisting manual efforts to push it back into normal position
- no pain, except in elderly, arthritic patients with secondary deformity.

TEST RESULTS

Early diagnosis of clubfoot is usually no problem because the deformity is obvious. In subtle deformity, however, true clubfoot must be distinguished from apparent clubfoot (metatarsus varus or pigeon toe), usually by X-rays showing superimposition of the talus and calcaneus and a ladder-like appearance of the metatarsals (true clubfoot).

TREATMENT

Treatment for clubfoot is done in three stages:
- correcting the deformity
- maintaining the correction until the foot regains normal muscle balance
- observing the foot closely for several years to prevent the deformity from recurring.

Clubfoot deformities are usually corrected in this order:
- forefoot adduction
- varus (or inversion)
- equinus (or plantar flexion).

Trying to correct all three deformities at once only results in a mis-shapen, rocker-bottomed foot.

NURSING CONSIDERATIONS

The primary concern in clubfoot is early recognition, preferably in neonates.
- Look for any exaggerated attitudes in an infant's feet. Make sure you recognize the difference between true clubfoot and apparent clubfoot. Don't use excessive force in trying to manipulate a clubfoot. The foot with apparent clubfoot moves easily.
- Stress to parents the importance of prompt treatment. Clubfoot demands immediate therapy and orthopedic supervision until growth is completed.
- After casting, elevate the child's feet with pillows. Check the toes every 1 to 2 hours for temperature, color, sensation, motion, and capillary refill time; watch for edema. Before a child in a clubfoot cast is discharged, teach parents to recognize circulatory impairment.
- Insert plastic petals over the top edges of a new cast while it's still wet

to keep urine from soaking and soft-ening the cast. This is done as follows: Cut a plastic sheet into strips long enough to cover the outside of the cast, and tuck them about a finger length beneath the cast edges. Using overlapping strips of tape, tack the corner of each petal to the outside of the cast. When the cast is dry, petal the edges with adhesive tape to keep out plaster crumbs and prevent skin irritation. Perform good skin care under the cast edges every 4 hours, washing and carefully drying the skin. (Don't rub the skin with alcohol, and don't use oils or powders, which tend to macerate the skin.)
- If the child is old enough to walk, caution parents not to let the foot part of the cast get soft and thin from wear. If it does, much of the correction may be lost.
- When the wedging method of shaping the cast is being used, check circulatory status frequently; it may be impaired by increased pressure on tissues and blood vessels. The equinus (posterior release) correction especially places considerable strain on ligaments, blood vessels, and tendons.
- After surgery, elevate the child's feet with pillows to decrease swelling and pain. Report any signs of discomfort or pain immediately. Try to locate the source of pain; it may result from cast pressure rather than from the incision. If bleeding occurs under the cast, circle the location and mark the time on the cast. If bleeding spreads, report it to the physician.
- Explain to the older child and his parents that surgery can improve clubfoot with good function but can't totally correct it; the affected calf muscle will remain slightly underdeveloped.
- Emphasize the need for long-term orthopedic care to maintain correc-

tion. Teach parents the prescribed exercises that the child can do at home. Urge them to make the child wear the corrective shoes ordered and the splints during naps and at night. Make sure they understand that treatment for clubfoot continues during the entire growth period. Correcting this defect permanently takes time and patience.

Developmental dysplasia of the hip

Developmental dysplasia of the hip (DDH), an abnormality of the hip joint present from birth, is the most common disorder affecting the hip joints in children younger than age 3. About 85% of affected infants are females.

DDH can be unilateral or bilateral. This abnormality occurs in three forms of varying severity:
- Unstable dysplasia — the hip is positioned normally but can be dislocated by manipulation.
- Subluxation (or incomplete dislocation) — the femoral head rides on the edge of the acetabulum.
- Complete dislocation — the femoral head is totally outside the acetabulum.

CAUSES

Although the causes of DDH aren't clear, it's more likely to occur in the following circumstances:
- dislocation after breech delivery (malposition in utero, 10 times more common than after cephalic delivery)
- elevated maternal relaxin, hormone secreted by the corpus luteum during pregnancy that causes relaxation of the pubic symphysis and cervical dila-

tion (may promote relaxation of the joint ligaments, predisposing the infant to DDH)
- large neonates and twins (more common).

PATHOPHYSIOLOGY

The precise cause of congenital dislocation is unknown. Excessive or abnormal movement of the joint during a traumatic birth may cause dislocation. Displacement of bones within the joint may damage joint structures, including articulating surfaces, blood vessels, tendons, ligaments, and nerves. This may lead to ischemic necrosis because of the disruption of blood flow to the joint. If corrective treatment isn't begun until after age 2, DDH may cause degenerative hip changes, abnormal acetabular development, lordosis (abnormally increased concave curvature of the lumbar and cervical spine), joint malformation, sciatic nerve injury (paralysis), avascular necrosis of the femoral head, soft-tissue damage, and permanent disability.

CLINICAL FINDINGS

- No gross deformity or pain (in neonates)
- Hip riding above the acetabulum, causing the level of the knees to be uneven (complete dysplasia)
- Limited abduction on the dislocated side (as the child grows older and begins to walk)
- Swaying from side to side ("duck waddle" due to uncorrected bilateral dysplasia)
- Limping due to uncorrected unilateral dysplasia

Observations during physical examination of the relaxed child that strongly suggest DDH include:

- extra fold of skin over the thigh on the affected side, when the child is placed on his back or lies prone
- buttock fold on the affected side higher with the child lying prone (also restricted abduction of the affected hip). (See *Ortolani's and Trendelenburg's signs of DDH*.)

TEST RESULTS

- X-rays show the location of the femur head and a shallow acetabulum. They're also used to monitor disease or treatment progress.
- Sonography and magnetic resonance imaging assess reduction.

TREATMENT

The earlier an infant receives treatment for DDH, the better the chances are for normal development. Treatment varies with the patient's age.

In infants younger than age 3 months, treatment includes:
- gentle manipulation to reduce the dislocation, followed by a splint-brace or harness to hold the hips in a flexed and abducted position to maintain the reduction
- splint-brace or harness worn continuously for 2 to 3 months, then a night splint for another month to tighten and stabilize the joint capsule in correct alignment.

If treatment doesn't begin until after age 3 months, it may include:
- bilateral skin traction (in infants) or skeletal traction (in children who have started walking) to try to reduce the dislocation by gradually abducting the hips
- Bryant's traction or divarication traction (both extremities placed in traction, even if only one is affected, to help maintain immobilization) for children younger than age 3 and

ORTOLANI'S AND TRENDELENBURG'S SIGNS OF DDH

A positive Ortolani's or Trendelenburg's sign confirms developmental dysplasia of the hip (DDH).

ORTOLANI'S SIGN

◆ Place the infant on his back, with the hip flexed and in abduction. Adduct the hip while pressing the femur downward. This will dislocate the hip.
◆ Then abduct the hip while moving the femur upward. A click or a jerk (produced by the femoral head moving over the acetabular rim) indicates subluxation in an infant younger than 1 month. The sign indicates subluxation or complete dislocation in an older infant.

TRENDELENBURG'S SIGN

◆ When the child rests his weight on the side of the dislocation and lifts his other knee, the pelvis drops on the normal side because abductor muscles in the affected hip are weak.
◆ However, when the child stands with his weight on the normal side and lifts the other knee, the pelvis remains horizontal.

weighing less than 35 lb (15.9 kg) for 2 to 3 weeks
- gentle closed reduction under general anesthesia to further abduct the hips, followed by a spica cast for 3 months (if traction fails)
- in children older than age 18 months, open reduction and pelvic or femoral osteotomy to correct bony deformity followed by immobilization in a spica cast for 6 to 8 weeks
- in children ages 6 to 12 months, immobilization in a spica cast for approximately 3 months.

In children ages 2 to 5, treatment is difficult and includes skeletal traction and subcutaneous adductor tenotomy (surgical cutting of the tendon).

Treatment begun after age 5 rarely restores satisfactory hip function.

NURSING CONSIDERATIONS

- Teach parents how to correctly splint or brace the child's hips as ordered. Stress the need for frequent checkups.
- Listen sympathetically to the parents' expressions of anxiety and fear. Explain possible causes of developmental hip dislocation, and give reassurance that early, prompt treatment will probably result in complete correction.
- During the child's first few days in a cast or splint-brace, he may be prone to irritability because of the unaccustomed restricted movement. Encourage the parents to stay with the child as much as possible and to calm and reassure him.
- Assure parents that the child will adjust to this restriction and return to normal sleeping, eating, and playing behavior in a few days.
- Instruct parents to remove braces and splints while bathing the infant but to replace them immediately afterward. Stress good hygiene; parents should bathe and change the child frequently and wash the perineum with warm water and soap at each diaper change.

If treatment requires a spica cast:
- When transferring the child immediately after casting, use your palms to avoid making dents in the cast. Such dents predispose the patient to pressure sores. Remember that the cast needs 24 to 48 hours to dry naturally. Don't use heat to make it dry faster because heat also makes it more fragile.

- Immediately after the cast is applied, use a plastic sheet to protect it from moisture around the perineum and buttocks. Cut the sheet into strips long enough to cover the outside of the cast, and tuck them about a finger length beneath the cast edges. Using overlapping strips of tape, tack the corner of each petal to the outside of the cast. Remove the plastic under the cast every 4 hours; then wash, dry, and retuck it. Disposable diapers folded lengthwise over the perineum may also be used.
- Position the child either on a Bradford frame elevated on blocks, with a bedpan under the frame, or on pillows to support the child's legs. Be sure to keep the cast dry, and change the child's diapers often.
- Wash and dry the skin under the cast edges every 2 to 4 hours. Don't use oils or powders; they can macerate the skin.
- Turn the child every 2 hours during the day and every 4 hours at night. Check color, sensation, and motion of the infant's legs and feet. Be sure to examine all toes. Notify the physician of dusky, cool, or numb toes.
- Shine a flashlight under the cast every 4 hours to check for objects and crumbs. Check the cast daily for odors, which may herald infection.
- If the child complains of itching, he may benefit from diphenhydramine (Benadryl), or you may aim a hair dryer set on cool at the cast edges to relieve itching. Don't scratch or probe under the cast. Investigate any persistent itching.
- Provide adequate nutrition and maintain adequate fluid intake to avoid renal calculi and constipation, both complications of inactivity.

- If the child is restless, apply a jacket restraint to keep him from falling out of bed or off the frame.
- Provide adequate stimuli to promote growth and development. If the child's hips are abducted in a froglike position, tell parents that he may be able to fit on a tricycle that the parent can push (if the child is unable to pedal) or an electric child's car. Encourage parents to let the child sit at a table by seating him on pillows on a chair, to put him on the floor for short periods of play, and to let him play with other children his age.
- Tell parents to watch for signs that the child is outgrowing the cast (cyanosis, cool extremities, or pain).
- Tell the parents that treatment may be prolonged and requires patience.

The patient in Bryant's traction may be cared for at home if the parents are taught traction application and maintenance:
- Encourage the parents to cuddle and hold the child and to encourage him to interact with siblings and friends.
- Maintain skin integrity and check circulation at least every 2 hours.
- Feed the child carefully to avoid aspiration and choking.
- If necessary, refer the child and parents to a child life specialist to ensure continued developmental progress.

Gout

Gout, also called *gouty arthritis,* is a metabolic disease marked by urate deposits that cause painful arthritic joints. It's found mostly in the foot, especially the great toe, ankle, and midfoot, but may affect any joint. Gout follows an intermittent course, and patients may be totally free from symptoms for years between attacks. The prognosis is good with treatment.

Alert *Primary gout usually occurs in men after age 30 and in postmenopausal women; secondary gout occurs in elderly people.*

CAUSES
- Exact cause of primary gout unknown
- Genetic defect in purine metabolism, causing overproduction of uric acid (hyperuricemia), retention of uric acid, or both

In secondary gout, which develops during the course of another disease (such as obesity, diabetes mellitus, hypertension, sickle cell anemia, and renal disease), the cause may be:
- breakdown of nucleic acid causing hyperuricemia
- result of drug therapy, especially after the use of hydrochlorothiazide or pyrazinamide, which decrease urate excretion (ionic form of uric acid).

PATHOPHYSIOLOGY
When uric acid becomes supersaturated in blood and other body fluids, it crystallizes and forms a precipitate of urate salts that accumulates in connective tissue throughout the body; these deposits are called *tophi.* The presence of the crystals triggers an acute inflammatory response when neutrophils begin to ingest the crystals. Tissue damage begins when the neutrophils release their lysosomes (see chapter 8, Immune system). The lysosomes not only damage the tissues but also perpetuate the inflammation.

In asymptomatic gout, serum urate levels increase but don't crystallize or produce symptoms. As the disease progresses, it may cause hypertension or urate kidney stone formation.

The first acute attack strikes suddenly and peaks quickly. Although it generally involves only one or a few joints, this initial attack is extremely painful. Affected joints appear hot, tender, inflamed, dusky red, or cyanotic. The metatarsophalangeal joint of the great toe usually becomes inflamed first (podagra), then the instep, ankle, heel, knee, or wrist joints. Sometimes a low-grade fever is present. Mild acute attacks typically subside quickly but tend to recur at irregular intervals. Severe attacks may persist for days or weeks.

Intercritical periods are the symptom-free intervals between gout attacks. Most patients have a second attack within 6 months to 2 years, but some attacks, common in those who are untreated, tend to be longer and more severe than initial attacks. Such attacks are also polyarticular, invariably affecting joints in the feet and legs, and sometimes accompanied by fever. A migratory attack sequentially strikes various joints and the Achilles tendon and is associated with either subdeltoid or olecranon bursitis.

Eventually, chronic polyarticular gout sets in. This final, unremitting stage of the disease is marked by persistent painful polyarthritis, with large tophi in cartilage, synovial membranes, tendons, and soft tissue. Tophi form in the fingers, hands, knees, feet, ulnar sides of the forearms, helices of the ears, Achilles tendons and, rarely, in internal organs, such as the kidneys and myocardium. The skin over the tophus may ulcerate and release a chalky, white exudate that's composed primarily of uric acid crystals.

Complications of gout may include eventual erosions, deformity, and disability due to chronic inflammation and tophi that cause secondary joint degeneration. Patients can also develop hypertension; albuminuria (in some patients) and kidney involvement, with tubular damage from aggregates of urate crystals; progressively poorer excretion of uric acid; and chronic renal dysfunction.

CLINICAL FINDINGS
- Joint pain due to uric acid deposits and inflammation
- Redness and swelling in joints due to uric acid deposits and irritation
- Tophi in the great toe, ankle, and pinna of the ear due to urate deposits
- Elevated skin temperature from inflammation

TEST RESULTS
- Needle aspiration reveals needle-like monosodium urate crystals in synovial fluid. Tissue sections show tophaceous deposits.
- Blood studies reveal hyperuricemia (uric acid greater than 420 µmol/mmol of creatinine)
- Urine studies reveal elevated 24-hour urine uric acid (usually higher in secondary than in primary gout).
- X-rays are initially normal; in chronic gout, damage of articular cartilage and subchondral bone. Outward displacement of the overhanging margin from the bone contour characterizes gout.

TREATMENT
- Immobilization and protection of the inflamed, painful joints
- Local application of heat or cold
- Increased fluid intake (to 3 qt [3 L] per day, if not contradicted by other conditions, to prevent kidney stone formation)
- Concomitant treatment with colchicine (oral or I.V.) every hour for 8 hours to inhibit phagocytosis of uric

acid crystals by neutrophils, until the pain subsides or nausea, vomiting, cramping, or diarrhea develops (in acute inflammation)

- Nonsteroidal anti-inflammatory drugs (NSAIDs) for pain and inflammation

Alert *An older patient is at risk for GI bleeding associated with the use of NSAIDs. Encourage the patient to take these drugs with meals, and monitor the patient's stools for occult blood.*

Treatment for chronic gout aims to decrease serum uric acid levels, including:

- maintenance dosage of allopurinol (Zyloprim) to suppress uric acid formation or control uric acid levels, preventing further attacks (use cautiously in patients with renal failure)
- colchicine to prevent recurrent acute attacks until uric acid returns to its normal level (doesn't affect uric acid level)
- uricosuric agents (probenecid and sulfinpyrazone [Anturane]) to promote uric acid excretion and inhibit uric acid accumulation (of limited value in patients with renal impairment)
- dietary restrictions, primarily avoiding alcohol and purine-rich foods.

NURSING CONSIDERATIONS

- Encourage bed rest, but use a bed cradle to keep bedcovers off extremely sensitive, inflamed joints.
- Give pain medication as needed, especially during acute attacks. Apply hot or cold packs to inflamed joints according to what the patient finds effective. Administer anti-inflammatory medication and other drugs as ordered. Watch for adverse effects. Be alert for GI disturbances with colchicine.

- Urge the patient to drink plenty of fluids (up to 2 qt [2 L] per day) to prevent kidney stone formation. When encouraging fluids, record intake and output accurately. Be sure to monitor serum uric acid levels regularly. Alkalinize urine with sodium bicarbonate or other agent, if ordered.
- Watch for acute gout attacks 24 to 96 hours after surgery. Even minor surgery can precipitate an attack. Before and after surgery, administer colchicine, as ordered, to help prevent gout attacks.
- Tell the patient to avoid high-purine foods, such as anchovies, liver, sardines, kidneys, sweetbreads, lentils, and alcoholic beverages — especially beer and wine — which raise the urate level. Explain the principles of a gradual weight reduction diet to the obese patient. Such a diet features foods containing moderate amounts of protein and very little fat.
- Advise the patient receiving allopurinol, probenecid, and other drugs to immediately report any adverse effects, such as drowsiness, dizziness, nausea, vomiting, urinary frequency, or dermatitis. Warn the patient taking probenecid or sulfinpyrazone to avoid aspirin or other salicylate. Their combined effect causes urate retention.
- Inform the patient that long-term colchicine therapy is essential during the first 3 to 6 months of treatment with uricosuric drugs or allopurinol.

Herniated nucleus pulposus

Herniated nucleus pulposus, also called *ruptured* or *slipped disk* and *herniated disk,* occurs when all or part of the nucleus pulposus — the soft, gelatinous, central portion of an intervertebral disk—is forced through the disk's weakened or torn outer ring (anulus fibrosus).

Herniated disk usually occurs in adults (mostly men) under age 45. About 90% of herniated disks are lumbar or lumbosacral; 8%, cervical; and 1% to 2%, thoracic. Patients with a congenitally small lumbar spinal canal or with osteophyte formation along the vertebrae may be more susceptible to nerve root compression and more likely to have neurologic symptoms.

CAUSES
- Intervertebral joint degeneration
  - *Alert In older patients whose disks have begun to degenerate, even minor trauma may cause herniation.*
- Severe trauma or strain

PATHOPHYSIOLOGY
An intervertebral disk has two parts: the soft center called the *nucleus pulposus* and the tough, fibrous surrounding ring called the *anulus fibrosus*. The nucleus pulposus acts as a shock absorber, distributing the mechanical stress applied to the spine when the body moves.

Physical stress, usually a twisting motion, can tear or rupture the anulus fibrosus so that the nucleus pulposus herniates into the spinal canal. When this happens, the extruded disk may impinge on spinal nerve roots as they exit from the spinal canal or on the spinal cord itself, resulting in back pain and other signs of nerve root irritation. The vertebrae move closer together and in turn exert pressure on the nerve roots as they exit between the vertebrae. Pain and possibly sensory and motor loss follow. A herniated disk can also follow intervertebral

joint degeneration; minor trauma may cause herniation.

Complications of herniated disc are neurologic deficits (most common) and bowel and bladder problems (with lumbar herniations).

Herniation occurs in three steps:
- Protrusion—the nucleus pulposus presses against the anulus fibrosus.
- Extrusion—the nucleus pulposus bulges forcibly through the anulus fibrosus, pushing against the nerve root.
- Sequestration—the anulus fibrosis gives way as the disk's core bursts and presses against the nerve root. (See *How a herniated disk develops*.)

CLINICAL FINDINGS
- Severe lower-back pain that radiates to the buttocks, legs, and feet, usually unilaterally
- When herniation follows trauma, pain starting suddenly, subsiding in a few days, and then recurring at shorter intervals and with progressive intensity; sciatic pain follows, beginning as a dull pain in the buttocks
- Valsalva's maneuver, coughing, sneezing, or bending intensifying the pain; commonly accompanied by muscle spasms
- Sensory and motor loss in the area innervated by the compressed spinal nerve root and, in later stages, weakness and atrophy of leg muscles

TEST RESULTS
- Straight-leg-raising test is positive if the patient complains of posterior leg (sciatic) pain, not back pain. The test involves the patient lying in a supine position while the examiner places one hand on the patient's ilium to stabilize the pelvis and the other hand under the ankle and then slowly raises the patient's leg.

HOW A HERNIATED DISK DEVELOPS

These illustrations show how herniation of an intervertebral disk develops.

Normal vertebra and intervertebral disk

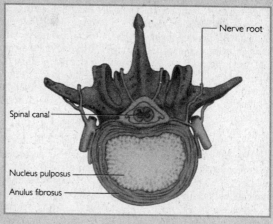

- Nerve root
- Spinal canal
- Nucleus pulposus
- Anulus fibrosus

Physical stress, from severe trauma or strain, or intervertebral joint degeneration may cause herniation. Herniation occurs in three stages: protrusion, extrusion, and sequestration.

Protrusion

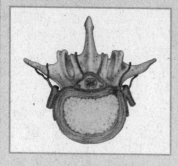

Extrusion and sequestration

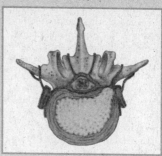

● Lasègue's sign is positive if the patient displays resistance and pain as well as loss of ankle or knee-jerk reflex, which indicates spinal root compression. The test involves the patient lying flat while the thigh and knee are flexed to a 90-degree angle.

● X-rays of the spine are essential to rule out other abnormalities but may not diagnose herniated disk because marked disk prolapse can be present despite a normal X-ray.
● A thorough check of the patient's peripheral vascular status — including

posterior tibial and dorsalis pedis pulses and skin temperature of extremities — helps rule out ischemic disease, another cause of leg pain or numbness.

- Myelography, computed tomography scans, and magnetic resonance imaging (MRI) provide the most specific diagnostic information, showing spinal canal compression by herniated disk material. MRI is the method of choice to confirm the diagnosis and determine the exact level of herniation.

TREATMENT

Unless neurologic impairment progresses rapidly, treatment is initially conservative and may consist of:
- several weeks of bed rest (possibly with pelvic traction)
- nonsteroidal anti-inflammatory drugs
- heat application
- an exercise program
- epidural corticosteroids, short-term oral corticosteroids, nerve root blocks, or physical therapy for pain control
- muscle relaxants, such as diazepam (Valium), methocarbamol (Robaxin), or cyclobenzaprine (Flexeril), to relieve associated muscle spasms.

A herniated disk that fails to respond to conservative treatment may necessitate surgery, including:
- laminectomy involving excision of a portion of the lamina and removal of the nucleus pulposus of the protruding disk
- spinal fusion to overcome segmental instability if laminectomy doesn't alleviate pain and disability (Laminectomy and spinal fusion are sometimes performed concurrently to stabilize the spine.)
- microdiskectomy to remove fragments of nucleus pulposus.

NURSING CONSIDERATIONS

- If the patient requires myelography, question him carefully about allergies to iodides, iodine-containing substances, or seafood because such allergies may indicate sensitivity to the test's radiopaque dye. Reinforce previous explanations of the need for this test, and tell the patient to expect some discomfort. Assure him that he'll receive a sedative before the test, if needed, to keep him as calm and comfortable as possible. After the test, urge the patient to remain in bed with his head elevated and to drink plenty of fluids. Monitor intake and output. Watch for seizures and allergic reactions.
- During conservative treatment, watch for any deterioration in neurologic status (especially during the first 24 hours after admission), which may indicate an urgent need for surgery. Use antiembolism stockings as prescribed, and encourage the patient to move his legs as allowed. Provide high-topped sneakers to prevent footdrop. Work closely with the physical therapy department to ensure a consistent regimen of leg- and back-strengthening exercises. Give plenty of fluids to prevent renal stasis, and remind the patient to deep-breathe and to use blow bottles or an incentive spirometer to preclude pulmonary complications. Provide good skin care. Assess for bowel function. Use a fracture bedpan for the patient on complete bed rest.
- After laminectomy, microdiskectomy, or spinal fusion, enforce bed rest as ordered. If a blood drainage system (closed drainage system or Jackson-Pratt drain) is in use, check the tubing frequently for kinks and a secure vacuum. Empty the drainage system at the end of each shift, and record the

amount and color of drainage. Report colorless moisture on dressings (possible cerebrospinal fluid leakage) or excessive drainage immediately. Observe neurovascular status of legs (color, motion, temperature, and sensation).

● Monitor vital signs, and check for bowel sounds and abdominal distention. Use logrolling technique to turn the patient. Administer analgesics, as ordered, especially 30 minutes before initial attempts at sitting or walking. Give the patient assistance during his first attempt to walk. Provide a straight-backed chair for limited sitting.

● Teach the patient who has undergone spinal fusion how to wear a brace. Assist with straight-leg-raising and toe-pointing exercises as ordered. Before discharge, teach proper body mechanics — bending at the knees and hips (never at the waist), standing straight, and carrying objects close to the body. Advise the patient to lie down when tired and to sleep on his side (never on his abdomen) on an extra-firm mattress or a bed board. Urge maintenance of proper weight to prevent lordosis caused by obesity.

● If the patient requires chemonucleolysis, make sure he isn't allergic to meat tenderizers (chymopapain is a similar substance). Such an allergy contraindicates the use of this enzyme, which can produce severe anaphylaxis in a sensitive patient. After chemonucleolysis, enforce bed rest as ordered. Administer analgesics and apply heat as needed. Urge the patient to cough and deep-breathe. Assist with special exercises, and tell the patient to continue these exercises after discharge.

● Tell the patient who must receive a muscle relaxant about possible adverse effects, especially drowsiness.

Warn him to avoid activities that require alertness until he has built up a tolerance to the drug's sedative effects.

● Provide emotional support. During periods of frustration and depression, assure the patient of his progress and offer encouragement.

Muscular dystrophy

Muscular dystrophy is a group of congenital disorders characterized by progressive symmetric wasting of skeletal muscles without neural or sensory defects. Paradoxically, some wasted muscles tend to enlarge (pseudohypertrophy) because connective tissue and fat replace muscle tissue, giving a false impression of increased muscle strength.

The four main types of muscular dystrophy are:
● Duchenne's, or pseudohypertrophic; 50% of all cases
● Becker's, or benign pseudohypertrophic
● Landouzy-Dejerine, or facioscapulohumeral
● limb-girdle.

The prognosis varies with the form of disease. Duchenne's muscular dystrophy strikes during early childhood and is usually fatal during the second decade of life. It affects males, 13 to 33 per 100,000 persons. Patients with Becker's muscular dystrophy can live into their 40s; it mostly affects males, 1 to 3 per 100,000 persons. Facioscapulohumeral and limb-girdle muscular dystrophies usually don't shorten life expectancy, and they affect both sexes equally.

CAUSES

- Autosomal dominant disorder (facioscapulohumeral muscular dystrophy)
- Autosomal recessive disorder (limb-girdle muscular dystrophy)
- Various genetic mechanisms typically involving an enzymatic or metabolic defect
- X-linked recessive disorders due to defects in the gene coding, mapped genetically to the Xp21 locus, for the muscle protein dystrophin, which is essential for maintaining muscle cell membrane; muscle cells deteriorating or dying without it (Duchenne's and Becker's muscular dystrophies)

PATHOPHYSIOLOGY

Abnormally permeable cell membranes allow leakage of a variety of muscle enzymes, particularly creatine kinase. This metabolic defect, which causes the muscle cells to die, is present from fetal life onward. The absence of progressive muscle wasting at birth suggests that other factors compound the effect of dystrophin deficiency. The specific trigger is unknown, but phagocytosis of the muscle cells by inflammatory cells causes scarring and loss of muscle function.

As the disease progresses, skeletal muscle becomes almost totally replaced by fat and connective tissue. The skeleton eventually becomes deformed, causing progressive immobility. Cardiac and smooth muscle of the GI tract typically become fibrotic. No consistent structural abnormalities are seen in the brain.

Possible complications of Duchenne's muscular dystrophy are weakened cardiac and respiratory muscles leading to tachycardia, electrocardiographic abnormalities, and pulmonary complications and death commonly due to sudden heart failure, respiratory failure, or infection.

CLINICAL FINDINGS

In Duchenne's muscular dystrophy:
- insidious onset between ages 3 and 5
- initial effect on legs, pelvis, and shoulders
- waddling gait, toe-walking, and lumbar lordosis due to muscle weakness
- difficulty climbing stairs; frequent falls
- enlarged, firm calf muscles
- confined to wheelchair (usually by ages 9 to 12).

In Becker's (benign pseudohypertrophic) muscular dystrophy, clinical findings are similar to those of Duchenne's muscular dystrophy but with slower progression.

In facioscapulohumeral (Landouzy-Dejerine) muscular dystrophy:
- weakened face, shoulder, and upper arm muscles (initial sign)
- pendulous lip and absent nasolabial fold
- inability to pucker the mouth or to whistle
- abnormal facial movements and absence of facial movements when laughing or crying
- diffuse facial flattening leading to a masklike expression
- inability to raise the arms above the head.

In limb-girdle muscular dystrophy:
- weakness in upper arms and pelvis first
- lumbar lordosis with abdominal protrusion
- winging of the scapulae
- waddling gait
- inability to raise the arms.

TEST RESULTS

● Electromyography shows short, weak bursts of electrical activity in affected muscles.

● Muscle biopsy reveals a combination of muscle cell degeneration and regeneration. In later stages, it reveals fat and connective tissue deposits.

● Immunologic and molecular biological techniques (now available in specialized medical centers) facilitate accurate prenatal and postnatal diagnosis of Duchenne's and Becker's muscular dystrophies. (They replace muscle biopsy and elevated serum creatine kinase levels in diagnosis.)

TREATMENT

No treatment can stop the progressive muscle impairment.

NURSING CONSIDERATIONS

● When respiratory involvement occurs in Duchenne's muscular dystrophy, encourage coughing, deep-breathing exercises, and diaphragmatic breathing. Teach parents how to recognize early signs of respiratory complications.

● Encourage and assist with active and passive range-of-motion exercises to preserve joint mobility and prevent muscle atrophy.

● Advise the patient to avoid long periods of bed rest and inactivity; if necessary, limit television viewing and other sedentary activities.

● Refer the patient for physical therapy. Splints, braces, and surgery to correct contractures; trapeze bars; overhead slings; and a wheelchair can help preserve mobility. A footboard or high-topped sneakers and a foot cradle increase comfort and prevent footdrop.

● Because inactivity may cause constipation, encourage adequate fluid intake, increase dietary bulk, and obtain an order for a stool softener. The patient is prone to obesity due to reduced physical activity; help him and his family plan a low-calorie, high-protein, high-fiber diet.

● Always allow the patient plenty of time to perform even simple physical tasks because he's likely to be slow and awkward.

● Encourage communication among family members to help them deal with the emotional strain this disorder produces. Provide emotional support to help the patient cope with continual changes in body image.

● Help the child with Duchenne's muscular dystrophy maintain peer relationships and realize his intellectual potential by encouraging his parents to keep him in a regular school as long as possible.

● If necessary, refer adult patients for sexual counseling. Refer those who must acquire new job skills for vocational rehabilitation. (Contact the Department of Labor and Industry in your state for more information.) For information on social services and financial assistance, refer these patients and their families to the Muscular Dystrophy Association.

● Refer family members for genetic counseling.

Osteoarthritis

Osteoarthritis (also referred to as degenerative joint disease), the most common form of arthritis, is a chronic condition causing the deterioration of joint cartilage and the formation of reactive new bone at the margins and subchondral areas of the joints. It usually affects weight-bearing joints (knees, feet, hips, lumbar vertebrae). Osteoarthritis is widespread (affecting more than 60 million persons in the United States) and is most common in women. Typically, its earliest symptoms manifest during middle age and progress from there.

Disability depends on the site and severity of involvement and can range from minor limitation of finger movement to severe disability in persons with hip or knee involvement. The rate of progression varies, and joints may remain stable for years in an early stage of deterioration.

CAUSES

The primary defect in idiopathic and secondary osteoarthritis is loss of articular cartilage due to functional changes in chondrocytes (cells responsible for the formation of the proteoglycans, glycoproteins that act as cementing material in the cartilage, and collagen).

Idiopathic osteoarthritis, a normal part of aging, results from many factors, including:

* chemical (drugs that stimulate the collagen-digesting enzymes in the synovial membrane such as steroids)
* mechanical (repeated stress on the joint)
* metabolic (endocrine disorders such as hyperparathyroidism) and genetic (decreased collagen synthesis).

Secondary osteoarthritis usually follows an identifiable predisposing event that leads to degenerative changes, such as:

* trauma (most common cause)
* congenital deformity
* obesity.

PATHOPHYSIOLOGY

Osteoarthritis occurs in synovial joints. The joint cartilage deteriorates, and reactive new bone forms at the margins and subchondral areas of the joints. The degeneration results from damage to the chondrocytes. Cartilage softens with age, narrowing the joint space. Mechanical injury erodes articular cartilage, leaving the underlying bone unprotected. This causes sclerosis, or thickening and hardening of the bone underneath the cartilage.

Cartilage flakes irritate the synovial lining, which becomes fibrotic and limits joint movement. Synovial fluid may be forced into defects in the bone, causing cysts. New bone, called *osteophyte* (bone spur), forms at joint margins as the articular cartilage erodes, causing gross alteration of the bony contours and enlargement of the joint.

Complications of osteoarthritis include irreversible joint changes and node formation (nodes eventually become red, swollen, and tender, causing numbness and loss of finger dexterity), subluxation of the joint, decreased joint range of motion (ROM), joint contractures, pain (can be debilitating in later stages), and loss of independence in activities of daily living.

CLINICAL FINDINGS

Symptoms, which increase with poor posture, obesity, and occupational stress, include:

* deep, aching joint pain due to degradation of the cartilage, inflammation, and bone stress, particularly after exercise or weight bearing (the most common symptom, usually relieved by rest)
* stiffness in the morning and after exercise (relieved by rest)
* crepitus, or "grating" of the joint during motion, due to cartilage damage

- Heberden's nodes (bony enlargements of the distal interphalangeal joints) due to repeated inflammation
- altered gait from contractures due to overcompensation of the muscles supporting the joint
- decreased ROM due to pain and stiffness
- joint enlargement due to stress on the bone and disordered bone growth
- localized headaches (may be a direct result of cervical spine arthritis).

TEST RESULTS

- Arthroscopy shows bone spurs and narrowing of joint space.
- Blood studies reveal increased erythrocyte sedimentation rate (with extensive synovitis).

X-rays of the affected joint help confirm the diagnosis but may be normal in the early stages. X-rays may require many views and typically show:

- narrowing of joint space or margin
- cystlike bony deposits in joint space and margins; sclerosis of the subchondral space
- joint deformity due to degeneration or articular damage
- bony growths at weight-bearing areas
- joint fusion.

TREATMENT

- Weight loss to reduce stress on the joint (see *Specific care for arthritic joints*)
- Balance of rest and exercise
- Medications, including aspirin, fenoprofen (Nalfon), ibuprofen (Motrin), indomethacin (Indocin), and other nonsteroidal anti-inflammatory drugs; propoxyphene (Darvon); and celecoxib (Celebrex)

SPECIFIC CARE FOR ARTHRITIC JOINTS

In the patient with osteoarthritis, specific care depends on the affected joint.
◆ Hand: Apply hot soaks and paraffin dips to relieve pain as ordered.
◆ Lumbar and sacral spine: Recommend a firm mattress or bed board to decrease morning pain.
◆ Cervical spine: Check the cervical collar for constriction; watch for redness with prolonged use.
◆ Hip: Use moist heat pads to relieve pain, and administer antispasmodic drugs as ordered. Assist with range-of-motion (ROM) and strengthening exercises, always making sure the patient gets the proper rest afterward. Check crutches, cane, braces, and walker for proper fit, and teach the patient to use them correctly. For example, the patient with unilateral joint involvement should use an orthopedic appliance (such as a cane or walker) on the unaffected side. Advise the use of cushions when sitting and the use of an elevated toilet seat.
◆ Knee: Assist with prescribed ROM exercises, exercises to maintain muscle

tone, and progressive resistance exercises to increase muscle strength. Provide elastic supports or braces, if needed.

To minimize the long-term effects of osteoarthritis, teach the patient to:
◆ plan for adequate rest during the day, after exertion, and at night
◆ take medication exactly as prescribed and report adverse effects immediately
◆ avoid overexertion, take care to stand and walk correctly, minimize weight-bearing activities, and be especially careful when stooping or picking up objects
◆ always wear well-fitting supportive shoes and not let the heels become too worn down
◆ install safety devices at home such as guard rails in the bathroom
◆ perform ROM exercises as gently as possible
◆ maintain proper body weight to lessen strain on joints
◆ avoid percussive activities.

- Support or stabilization of joint with crutches, braces, cane, walker, cervical collar, or traction to reduce stress
- Intra-articular injections of corticosteroids (every 4 to 6 months) to possibly delay node development in the hands (if used too frequently, may accelerate arthritic progression by depleting the normal ground substance of the cartilage)

Surgical treatment, reserved for patients with severe disability or uncontrollable pain, may include:
- arthroplasty (partial or total replacement of deteriorated part of joint with prosthetic appliance)
- arthrodesis (surgical fusion of bones, primarily in spine [laminectomy])
- osteoplasty (scraping and lavage of deteriorated bone from the joint)
- osteotomy (change in alignment of bone to relieve stress by excision of a wedge of bone or cutting of bone).

NURSING CONSIDERATIONS

- Promote adequate rest, particularly after activity. Plan rest periods during the day, and provide for adequate sleep at night. Moderation is the key — teach the patient to pace daily activities.
- Assist with physical therapy, and encourage the patient to perform gentle, isometric ROM exercises.
- If the patient needs surgery, provide appropriate preoperative and postoperative care.
- Provide emotional support and reassurance to help the patient cope with limited mobility. Explain that osteoarthritis isn't a systemic disease.

Osteomyelitis

Osteomyelitis is a bone infection characterized by progressive inflammatory destruction after formation of new bone. It may be chronic or acute. It commonly results from a combination of local trauma — usually trivial but causing a hematoma — and an acute infection originating elsewhere in the body. Although osteomyelitis typically remains localized, it can spread through the bone to the marrow, cortex, and periosteum. Acute osteomyelitis is usually a blood-borne disease and most commonly affects rapidly growing children. Chronic osteomyelitis, which is rare, is characterized by draining sinus tracts and widespread lesions.

Alert Osteomyelitis occurs more commonly in children (especially boys) than in adults — usually as a complication of an acute localized infection. Typical sites in children are the lower end of the femur and the upper ends of the tibia, humerus, and radius. The most common sites in adults are the pelvis and vertebrae, generally after surgery or trauma.

The incidence of chronic and acute osteomyelitis is declining, except in drug abusers.

With prompt treatment, the prognosis for acute osteomyelitis is good; for chronic osteomyelitis, the prognosis remains poor.

CAUSES

The most common pyogenic organism in osteomyelitis is *Staphylococcus aureus*.

Others include:
- *Escherichia coli*
- *Pasteurella multocida* (part of the normal mouth flora of cats and dogs)
- pneumococcus

- *Proteus vulgaris*
- *Pseudomonas aeruginosa*
- *Streptococcus pyogenes.*

PATHOPHYSIOLOGY

Typically, the pyogenic organisms find a culture site in a hematoma from recent trauma or in a weakened area, such as the site of local infection (for example, furunculosis), and travel through the bloodstream to the metaphysis, the section of a long bone that's continuous with the epiphysis plates, where the blood flows into sinusoids. (See *Avoiding osteomyelitis*, page 394.)

Possible complications of osteomyelitis include amputation (of an arm or leg when resistant chronic osteomyelitis causes severe, unrelenting pain and decreases function); weakened bone cortex, predisposing the bone to pathologic fracture; and arrested growth of an extremity (in children with severe disease).

CLINICAL FINDINGS

Clinical features of chronic and acute osteomyelitis are generally the same and may include:
- rapid onset of acute osteomyelitis, with sudden pain in the affected bone and tenderness, heat, swelling, erythema, guarding of the affected region of the limb, and restricted movement
- chronic infection persisting intermittently for years, flaring after minor trauma or persisting as drainage of pus from an old pocket in a sinus tract
- accompanying fever and tachycardia
- dehydration (in young patients)
- irritability and poor feeding (in infants).

TEST RESULTS

- White blood cell count shows leukocytosis.
- Blood studies reveal elevated erythrocyte sedimentation rate.
- Blood cultures show the causative organism.
- Magnetic resonance imaging delineates bone marrow from soft tissue, facilitating the diagnosis.
- X-rays may not show bone involvement until the disease has been active for 2 to 3 weeks.
- Bone scans detect early infection.

TREATMENT

Treatment for acute osteomyelitis should begin before definitive diagnosis and includes:
- large doses of antibiotics I.V. (usually a penicillinase-resistant penicillin, such as nafcillin or oxacillin) after blood cultures are taken
- early surgical drainage to relieve pressure and abscess formation
- immobilization of the affected body part by cast, traction, or bed rest to prevent failure to heal or recurrence
- supportive measures, such as analgesics for pain and I.V. fluids to maintain hydration
- incision and drainage, followed by a culture of the drainage (if an abscess or sinus tract forms).

Antibiotic therapy to control infection may include:
- systemic antibiotics
- intracavitary instillation of antibiotics through closed-system continuous irrigation with low intermittent suction
- limited irrigation with a blood drainage system with suction
- packed, wet, antibiotic-soaked dressings.

Chronic osteomyelitis treatment may include:

AVOIDING OSTEOMYELITIS

Bones are essentially isolated from the body's natural defense system after an organism gets through the periosteum. They're limited in their ability to replace necrotic tissue caused by infection, which may lead to chronic osteomyelitis.

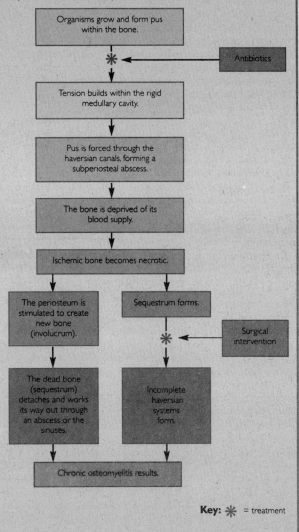

Organisms grow and form pus within the bone.

※ ← Antibiotics

Tension builds within the rigid medullary cavity.

Pus is forced through the haversian canals, forming a subperiosteal abscess.

The bone is deprived of its blood supply.

Ischemic bone becomes necrotic.

The periosteum is stimulated to create new bone (involucrum).

Sequestrum forms.

※ ← Surgical intervention

The dead bone (sequestrum) detaches and works its way out through an abscess or the sinuses.

Incomplete haversian systems form.

Chronic osteomyelitis results.

Key: ※ = treatment

surgery, usually required to remove dead bone and promote drainage (Prognosis remains poor even after surgery.)

● hyperbaric oxygen to stimulate normal immune mechanisms

● skin, bone, and muscle grafts to fill in dead space and increase the blood supply.

NURSING CONSIDERATIONS

● Use strict aseptic technique when changing dressings and irrigating wounds. If the patient is in skeletal traction for compound fractures, cover insertion points of pin tracks with small, dry dressings, and tell him not to touch the skin around the pins and wires.

● Administer I.V. fluids to maintain adequate hydration as needed. Provide a diet high in protein and vitamin C.

● Assess daily the patient's vital signs, wound appearance, and any new pain, which may indicate secondary infection.

● Carefully monitor suctioning equipment. Monitor the amount of solution instilled and suctioned.

● Support the affected limb with firm pillows. Keep the limb level with the body; don't let it sag. Provide good skin care. Turn the patient gently every 2 hours, and watch for signs of developing pressure ulcers. Report any signs of pressure ulcer formation immediately.

● Provide good cast care. Support the cast with firm pillows, and smooth rough cast edges by petaling with pieces of adhesive tape or moleskin. Check circulation and drainage; if a wet spot appears on the cast, circle it with a marking pen and note the time of appearance (on the cast). Be aware of how much drainage is expected. Check the circled spot at least every 4 hours. Report any enlargement immediately.

● Protect the patient from mishaps, such as jerky movements and falls, which may threaten bone integrity. Report sudden pain, crepitus, or deformity immediately. Watch for any sudden malposition of the limb, which may indicate fracture.

● Provide emotional support and appropriate diversions. Before discharge, teach the patient how to protect and clean the wound and how to recognize signs of recurring infection (increased temperature, redness, localized heat, and swelling). Stress the need for follow-up examinations. Instruct the patient to seek prompt treatment for possible sources of recurrence — blisters, boils, styes, and impetigo.

Osteoporosis

Osteoporosis is a metabolic bone disorder in which the rate of bone resorption accelerates while the rate of bone formation slows, causing a loss of bone mass. Bones affected by this disease lose calcium and phosphate salts and become porous, brittle, and abnormally vulnerable to fractures. Osteoporosis may be primary or secondary to an underlying disease, such as Cushing's syndrome or hyperthyroidism. It primarily affects the weight-bearing vertebrae. Only when the condition is advanced or severe, as in secondary disease, do similar changes occur in the skull, ribs, and long bones. Usually, the femoral heads and pelvic acetabula are selectively affected. Osteoporosis is more common in women who are white and who have a family history of osteoporosis.

Primary osteoporosis is commonly called *postmenopausal osteoporosis* because it usually develops in postmenopausal women.

CAUSES

The cause of primary osteoporosis is unknown, but contributing factors include:

- declining gonadal and adrenal function
- faulty protein metabolism due to relative or progressive estrogen deficiency (Estrogen stimulates osteoblastic activity and limits the osteoclastic-stimulating effects of parathyroid hormones.)
- mild but prolonged negative calcium balance due to inadequate dietary intake of calcium (may be an important contributing factor)
- sedentary lifestyle.

The many causes of secondary osteoporosis include:

- alcoholism
- cigarette smoking
- endocrine disorders, such as hyperthyroidism, hyperparathyroidism, Cushing's syndrome, and diabetes mellitus (Plasma calcium and phosphate concentrations are maintained by the endocrine system.)
- lactose intolerance
- malabsorption
- malnutrition
- medications (aluminum-containing antacids, corticosteroids, anticonvulsants)
- osteogenesis imperfecta
- prolonged therapy with steroids or heparin (Heparin promotes bone resorption by inhibiting collagen synthesis or enhancing collagen breakdown.)
- scurvy

- Sudeck's atrophy (localized to hands and feet, with recurring attacks)
- total immobilization or disuse of a bone (as in hemiplegia).

PATHOPHYSIOLOGY

In normal bone, the rates of bone formation and resorption are constant; replacement follows resorption immediately, and the amount of bone replaced equals the amount of bone resorbed. Osteoporosis develops when the remodeling cycle is interrupted and new bone formation falls behind resorption.

When bone is resorbed faster than it forms, the bone becomes less dense. Men have approximately 30% greater bone mass than women, which may explain why osteoporosis develops later in men.

Possible complications of osteoporosis include spontaneous fractures as the bones lose volume and become brittle and weak, and shock, hemorrhage, or fat embolism (fatal complications of fractures).

CLINICAL FINDINGS

Osteoporosis is typically discovered suddenly, such as when:

- a postmenopausal woman bends to lift something, hears a snapping sound, and then feels a sudden pain in her lower back
- vertebral collapse causes back pain that radiates around the trunk (most common presenting feature) and is aggravated by movement or jarring.

In another common pattern, osteoporosis can develop insidiously, showing:

- increasing deformity, kyphosis, loss of height, decreased exercise tolerance, and a markedly aged appearance

- spontaneous wedge fractures, pathologic fractures of the neck and femur, Colles' fractures of the distal radius after a minor fall, and hip fractures (common as bone is lost from the femoral neck).

TEST RESULTS
- Dual- or single-photon absorptiometry shows reduced bone mass of the extremities, hips, and spine.
- X-rays show typical degeneration in the lower thoracic and lumbar vertebrae. Vertebral bodies may appear flattened and may look denser than normal; bone mineral loss is evident only in later stages.
- Computed tomography scan assesses spinal bone loss.
- Blood studies reveal normal serum calcium, phosphorus, and alkaline phosphatase levels and possibly elevated parathyroid hormone levels.
- Bone biopsy shows thin, porous, but otherwise normal-looking bone.

TREATMENT
Treatment to control bone loss, prevent fractures, and control pain may include:
- physical therapy emphasizing gentle exercise and activity and regular, moderate weight-bearing exercise to slow bone loss and possibly reverse demineralization (The mechanical stress of exercise stimulates bone formation.)
- supportive devices such as a back brace
- surgery, if indicated, for pathologic fractures
- hormone replacement therapy with estrogen and progesterone to slow bone loss and prevent occurrence of fractures
- analgesics and local heat to relieve pain.

Other medications include:
- bisphosphonates (alendronate [Fosamax], ibandronate [Boniva], risedronate [Actonel]) to increase bone density and restore lost bone
- calcium and vitamin D supplements to support normal bone metabolism
- calcitonin (Miacalcin) to reduce bone resorption and slow the decline in bone mass
- raloxifene (Evista) to decrease bone loss and decrease the risk of spinal fractures
- vitamin C, calcium, and protein to support skeletal metabolism (through a balanced diet rich in nutrients).

Other measures include:
- early mobilization after surgery or trauma
- decreased alcohol and tobacco consumption
- careful observation for signs of malabsorption (fatty stools, chronic diarrhea)
- prompt, effective treatment of the underlying disorder (to prevent secondary osteoporosis).

NURSING CONSIDERATIONS
- Check the patient's skin daily for redness, warmth, and new sites of pain, which may indicate new fractures. Encourage activity; help the patient walk several times daily. As appropriate, perform passive range-of-motion exercises or encourage the patient to perform active exercises. Make sure the patient regularly attends scheduled physical therapy sessions.
- Impose safety precautions. Keep the side rails of the patient's bed in a raised position. Move the patient gently and carefully at all times. Explain to the patient's family and ancillary health care personnel how easily an

osteoporotic patient's bones can fracture.

● Make sure the patient and her family clearly understand the prescribed drug regimen. Tell them how to recognize significant adverse effects and to report them immediately. The use of bisphosphonates is associated with osteonecrosis of the jaw. The patient should have a dental examination with appropriate preventive dentistry before therapy begins.

● Tell the patient to report any new pain sites immediately, especially after trauma, no matter how slight. Advise the patient to sleep on a firm mattress and to avoid excessive bed rest. Make sure she knows how to wear her back brace.

● Thoroughly explain osteoporosis to the patient and her family. If they don't understand the nature of this disease, they may feel the fractures could have been prevented if they had been more careful.

● Teach the patient good body mechanics — to stoop before lifting anything and to avoid twisting movements and prolonged bending.

● Instruct the female patient taking estrogen about the proper technique for breast self-examination. Tell her to perform this examination at least once per month and to report any lumps immediately. Emphasize the need for regular gynecologic exams. Tell her to report abnormal bleeding promptly.

Paget's disease

Paget's disease, also called *osteitis deformans,* is a slowly progressive metabolic bone disease characterized by accelerated patterns of bone remodeling. An initial phase of excessive bone resorption (osteoclastic phase) is followed by a reactive phase of excessive abnormal bone formation (osteoblastic phase). Chronic accelerated remodeling eventually enlarges and softens the affected bones. The new bone structure, which is chaotic, fragile, and weak, causes painful deformities of external contour and internal structure. Paget's disease usually localizes in one or several areas of the skeleton (commonly, the lumbosacral spine, skull, pelvis, femur, and tibia are affected), but occasionally skeletal deformity is widely distributed.

In the United States, Paget's disease affects about 2.5 million people older than age 40 (mostly males). It can be fatal, particularly when it's associated with heart failure (widespread disease creates a continuous need for high cardiac output), bone sarcoma, or giant-cell tumors.

CAUSES

Although the exact cause of Paget's disease is unknown, one theory is that early viral infection causes a dormant skeletal infection that erupts many years later as Paget's disease.

Other possible causes include:
● autoimmune disease
● benign or malignant bone tumors
● estrogen deficiency
● vitamin D deficiency during the bone-developing years of childhood.

PATHOPHYSIOLOGY

Repeated episodes of accelerated osteoclastic resorption of spongy bone occur. The trabeculae diminish, and vascular fibrous tissue replaces marrow. This is followed by short periods of rapid, abnormal bone formation. The collagen fibers in this new bone are disorganized, and glycoprotein levels in the matrix decrease. The partially resorbed trabeculae thicken and enlarge because of excessive bone formation, and the bone becomes soft and weak. Complications of Paget's disease include blindness and hearing loss with tinnitus and vertigo (due to bony impingement on the cranial nerves), pathologic fractures, hypertension, renal calculi, hypercalcemia, gout, heart failure (due to the high blood flow demands of remodeling bones), respiratory failure (due to deformed thoracic bones), and malignant changes in involved bone (1% of the patients).

CLINICAL FINDINGS

Clinical effects of Paget's disease vary. Early stages may be asymptomatic. When signs and symptoms appear, they may include:
- usually severe and persistent pain intensifying with weight bearing, possibly with impaired movement due to impingement of abnormal bone on the spinal cord or sensory nerve root (Pain may also result from the constant inflammation accompanying cell breakdown.)
- characteristic cranial enlargement over frontal and occipital areas and possibly headaches, sensory abnormalities, and impaired motor function (with skull involvement)
- kyphosis (spinal curvature due to compression fractures of vertebrae)
- barrel chest
- asymmetrical bowing of the tibia and femur (commonly reduces height)
- waddling gait (from softening of pelvic bones)
- warm and tender disease sites susceptible to pathologic fractures after minor trauma
- slow and typically incomplete healing of pathologic fractures.

TEST RESULTS

- X-rays, computed tomography scan, and magnetic resonance imaging taken before overt symptoms develop show increased bone expansion and density.
- Radionuclide bone scan (more sensitive than an X-ray) clearly shows early Paget's lesions that reveal radioisotope concentrates in areas of active disease.
- Bone biopsy reveals the characteristic mosaic pattern.
- Blood studies show anemia, elevated serum alkaline phosphatase level (an index of osteoblastic activity and bone formation), and normal or elevated serum calcium level.
- A 24-hour urine study shows elevated level for hydroxyproline that reveals amino acids excreted by the kidneys and an index of osteoclastic hyperactivity.

TREATMENT

Primary treatment consists of drug therapy and includes one of the following medications:
- bisphosphonates (alendronate [Fosamax], pamidronate [Aredia], risedronate [Actonel]) to inhibit osteoclast-mediated bone resorption
- calcitonin (Miacalcin), a hormone, and etidronate (Didronel) to retard bone resorption and reduce serum alkaline phosphate and urinary hydroxyproline secretion (Calcitonin requires long-term maintenance therapy, but improvement is noticeable after the first few weeks of treatment; etidronate produces improvement after 1 to 3 months.)

Other treatment varies according to symptoms and includes:
- surgery to reduce or prevent pathologic fractures, correct secondary deformities, and relieve neurologic im-

pairment (Drug therapy with calcitonin or etidronate must precede surgery to decrease the risk of excessive bleeding from hypervascular bone.)
● joint replacement (difficult because bonding material [methyl methacrylate] doesn't set properly on pagetic bone)
● aspirin, indomethacin (Indocin), or ibuprofen (Motrin) to control pain.

NURSING CONSIDERATIONS
● To evaluate the effectiveness of analgesics, assess the patient's pain level daily. Watch for new areas of pain or restricted movements (which may indicate new fracture sites) and sensory or motor disturbances, such as difficulty in hearing, seeing, or walking.
● Monitor serum calcium and alkaline phosphatase levels.
● If the patient is confined to prolonged bed rest, prevent pressure ulcers by providing good skin care. Reposition the patient frequently, and use a flotation mattress. Provide high-topped sneakers to prevent footdrop.
● Monitor intake and output. Encourage adequate fluid intake to minimize renal calculi formation.
● Demonstrate how to inject calcitonin properly and rotate injection sites. Warn the patient that adverse effects may occur (nausea, vomiting, local inflammatory reaction at injection site, facial flushing, itching of hands, and fever). Reassure him that these adverse effects are usually mild and infrequent.
● To help the patient adjust to the changes in lifestyle imposed by this disease, teach him how to pace activities and, if necessary, how to use assistive devices. Encourage him to follow a recommended exercise program, avoiding both immobilization

and excessive activity. Suggest a firm mattress or a bed board to minimize spinal deformities. Warn against imprudent use of analgesics because diminished sensitivity to pain resulting from analgesic use may make the patient unaware of new fractures. To prevent falls at home, advise the removal of throw rugs and other obstacles.
● Emphasize the importance of regular checkups, including the eyes and ears.
● Tell the patient who's receiving etidronate to take this medication with fruit juice 2 hours before or after meals (milk or other high-calcium fluids impair absorption), to divide daily dosage to minimize adverse effects, and to watch for and report stomach cramps, diarrhea, fractures, and new or increased bone pain.
● Help the patient and family make use of community support resources, such as a visiting nurse or home health agency. For more information, refer them to the Paget Foundation.

☀ Life-threatening

Rhabdomyolysis

Rhabdomyolysis, the breakdown of muscle tissue, may cause myoglobinuria, in which varying amounts of muscle protein (myoglobin) appear in urine. Rhabdomyolysis usually follows major muscle trauma, especially a muscle crush injury. Long-distance running, certain severe infections, and exposure to electric shock can cause extensive muscle damage and excessive release of myoglobin. The prognosis is good if contributing causes are stopped or if the disease is checked before damage has progressed to an irreversible stage. Left unchecked, it can cause renal failure.

CAUSES
- Anesthetic agents (halothane) causing intraoperative rigidity
- Cardiac arrhythmias
- Electrolyte disturbances
- Excessive muscular activity associated with status epilepticus, electroconvulsive therapy, or high-voltage electrical shock
- Familial tendency
- Heatstroke
- Infection
- Strenuous exertion

PATHOPHYSIOLOGY
Muscle trauma that compresses tissue causes ischemia and necrosis. The ensuing local edema further increases compartment pressure and tamponade; pressure from severe swelling causes blood vessels to collapse, leading to tissue hypoxia, muscle infarction, neural damage in the area of the fracture, and release of myoglobin from the necrotic muscle fibers into the circulation.

Possible complications of rhabdomyolysis include renal failure, as myoglobin is trapped in renal capillaries or tubules, and amputation, if muscle necrosis is substantial.

CLINICAL FINDINGS
- Tenderness, swelling, and muscle weakness due to muscle trauma and pressure
- Dark, reddish brown urine from myoglobin

TEST RESULTS
- Urine studies reveal urine myoglobin level greater than 0.5 mg/dl (evident with only 200 g of muscle damage).

- Blood studies reveal elevated serum potassium, phosphate, creatinine, and creatine kinase levels.
- Hypocalcemia in early stages and hypercalcemia in later stages
- Computed tomography, magnetic resonance imaging, and bone scintigraphy detect muscle necrosis.
- Intracompartmental venous pressure measurements using a wick catheter, needle, or slit catheter inserted into the muscle may reveal increased intra-compartmental pressure, leading to decreased perfusion and tissue damage.

TREATMENT
- Treating the underlying disorder
- Preventing renal failure
- Bed rest
- Anti-inflammatory agents
- Corticosteroids (in extreme cases)
- Analgesics for pain
- Immediate fasciotomy and debridement (if compartment venous pressure is greater than 25 mm Hg)

NURSING CONSIDERATIONS
- Administer I.V. fluids and diuretics, as ordered, to reduce nephrotoxicity.
- To prevent rhabdomyolysis caused by physical exertion (such as long-distance running), recommend prolonged, low-intensity training as opposed to short bursts of intense exercise.

12

REPRODUCTIVE SYSTEM

The reproductive system must function properly to ensure survival of the species. The male reproductive system produces sperm and delivers them to the female reproductive tract. The female reproductive system produces the ovum. If a sperm fertilizes an ovum, this system also nurtures and protects the embryo and developing fetus and delivers it at birth. The functioning of the reproductive system is determined not only by anatomic structure but also by complex hormonal, neurologic, vascular, and psychogenic factors.

Anatomically, the main distinction between the male and the female is the presence of conspicuous external genitalia in the male. In contrast, the major reproductive organs of the female lie within the pelvic cavity.

Abnormal uterine bleeding

Abnormal uterine bleeding refers to abnormal endometrial bleeding without recognizable organic lesions. Abnormal uterine bleeding is the indication for almost 25% of gynecologic surgical procedures. The prognosis varies with the cause. Correction of hormonal imbalance or structural abnormality yields a good prognosis.

CAUSES

Abnormal uterine bleeding usually results from an imbalance in the hormonal-endometrial relationship in which persistent and unopposed stimulation of the endometrium by estrogen occurs. Disorders that cause sustained high estrogen levels include:
- anovulation (women in their late 30s or early 40s)
- immaturity of the hypothalamic-pituitary-ovarian mechanism (postpubertal teenagers)
- obesity (because enzymes present in peripheral adipose tissue convert the androgen androstenedione to estrogen precursors)
- polycystic ovary syndrome.
  Other causes of abnormal uterine bleeding include:
- coagulopathy, such as thrombocytopenia or leukemia (rare)
- drug-induced coagulopathy
- endometriosis
- trauma (foreign object insertion or direct trauma).

PATHOPHYSIOLOGY

Irregular bleeding is associated with hormonal imbalance and anovulation (failure of ovulation to occur). When progesterone secretion is absent but estrogen secretion continues, the endometrium proliferates and becomes hypervascular. When ovulation doesn't occur, the endometrium is randomly broken down and exposed vascular channels cause prolonged and excessive bleeding. In most cases of abnormal uterine bleeding, the endometrium shows no pathologic changes. However, in chronic unopposed estrogen stimulation (as from a hormone-producing ovarian tumor), the endometrium may show hyperplastic or malignant changes.

Possible complications include iron deficiency anemia (blood loss of more than 1.6 L over a short time), hemorrhagic shock or right-sided heart failure (rare), and endometrial adenocarcinoma due to chronic estrogen stimulation.

CLINICAL FINDINGS

- Metrorrhagia (episodes of vaginal bleeding between menses)
- Hypermenorrhea (heavy or prolonged menses, longer than 8 days, also incorrectly termed *menorrhagia*)
- Chronic polymenorrhea (menstrual cycle less than 18 days) or oligomenorrhea (infrequent menses)
- Fatigue due to anemia
- Oligomenorrhea and infertility due to anovulation

TEST RESULTS

Abnormal uterine bleeding may be caused by anovulation. Diagnosis of anovulation is based on:
- history of abnormal bleeding, bleeding in response to a brief course of progesterone, absence of ovulatory cycle body temperature changes, and low serum progesterone levels
- diagnostic studies ruling out other causes of excessive vaginal bleeding, such as organic, systemic, psychogenic, and endocrine causes, including certain cancers, polyps, pregnancy, and infection
- dilatation and curettage (D&C) or endometrial biopsy to rule out endometrial hyperplasia and cancer in women over age 35
- hemoglobin level and hematocrit to determine the need for blood transfusion or iron supplementation.

TREATMENT

- High-dose estrogen-progestogen combination therapy (hormonal contraceptives) to control endometrial growth and reestablish a normal cyclic pattern of menstruation (usually given four times daily for 5 to 7 days even though bleeding usually stops in 12 to 24 hours; drug choice and dosage determined by patient's age and cause of bleeding); maintenance therapy with lower-dose combination hormonal contraceptives
- Endometrial biopsy to rule out endometrial adenocarcinoma (patients age 35 and older)
- Progestogen therapy (alternative in many women, such as those susceptible to such adverse effects of estrogen as thrombophlebitis)
- I.V. estrogen followed by progesterone or combination hormonal contraceptives if the patient is young (more likely to be anovulatory) and severely anemic (if oral drug therapy is ineffective)
- D&C (short-lived treatment and not clinically useful, but an important diagnostic tool) with hysteroscopy as a useful adjunct

- Iron supplementation or transfusions of packed cells or whole blood, as indicated, in response to anemia caused by recurrent or excessive bleeding
- Explaining the importance of following the prescribed hormonal therapy; explaining D&C or endometrial biopsy procedure and purpose (if ordered)
- Stressing the need for regular checkups to assess the effectiveness of treatment

NURSING CONSIDERATIONS

- If a patient complains of abnormal bleeding, tell her to record the dates of the bleeding and the number of sanitary napkins she saturates per day. This helps to assess the pattern and the amount of bleeding. Instruct the patient not to use tampons.
- Instruct the patient to report abnormal bleeding immediately to help rule out major hemorrhagic disorders such as those that occur in abnormal pregnancy.
- To prevent abnormal bleeding due to organic causes and for early detection of malignancy, encourage the patient to have a Papanicolaou test and a pelvic examination annually.
- Offer reassurance and support. The patient may be particularly anxious about excessive or frequent blood loss and passage of clots. Suggest that she minimize blood flow by avoiding strenuous activity and by lying down with her feet elevated.

Benign prostatic hyperplasia

Although most men age 50 and older have some prostatic enlargement, in benign prostatic hyperplasia (BPH) — also known as *benign prostatic hypertrophy* — the prostate gland enlarges enough to compress the urethra and cause overt urinary obstruction. (See *Prostatic enlargement.*) Depending on the size of the enlarged prostate, the age and health of the patient, and the extent of obstruction, BPH is treated symptomatically or surgically. BPH is common, affecting up to 50% of men age 50 and older and 75% of men age 80 and older.

CAUSES

- The main cause of BPH may be age-associated changes in hormone activity. Androgenic hormone production decreases with age, causing an imbalance in androgen and estrogen levels and high levels of dihydrotestosterone, the main prostatic intracellular androgen.
- Other causes include:
- arteriosclerosis
- inflammation
- metabolic or nutritional disturbances.

PATHOPHYSIOLOGY

Regardless of the cause, BPH begins with nonmalignant changes in periurethral glandular tissue. The growth of the fibroadenomatous nodules (masses of fibrous glandular tissue) progresses to compress the remaining normal gland (nodular hyperplasia). The hyperplastic tissue is mostly glandular, with some fibrous stroma and smooth muscle. As the prostate enlarges, it may extend into the bladder and obstruct urinary outflow by compressing or distorting the prostatic urethra. There are periodic increases in sympathetic stimulation of the smooth muscle of the prostatic urethra and bladder neck. Progressive

PROSTATIC ENLARGEMENT

As the prostate gland enlarges, the urethra becomes compressed, causing overt urinary obstruction.

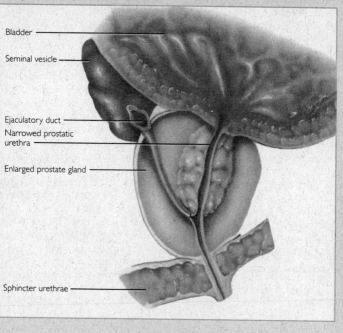

Bladder

Seminal vesicle

Ejaculatory duct

Narrowed prostatic urethra

Enlarged prostate gland

Sphincter urethrae

bladder distention may also cause a pouch to form in the bladder that retains urine when the rest of the bladder empties. This retained urine may lead to calculus formation or cystitis.

As BPH worsens, a common complication is complete urinary obstruction after infection or while using decongestants, tranquilizers, alcohol, antidepressants, or anticholinergics. Other complications include infection, hydronephrosis, renal insufficiency and, if untreated, renal failure, urinary calculi, hemorrhage, and shock.

CLINICAL FINDINGS

Clinical findings of BPH depend on the extent of prostatic enlargement and the lobes affected. Characteristically, the condition starts with a group of symptoms known as *prostatism* that include:

- reduced urinary stream caliber and force
- urinary hesitancy
- difficulty starting micturition (resulting in straining, a feeling of incomplete voiding, and an interrupted stream).

As the obstruction increases, it causes:

- frequent urination with nocturia
- sense of urgency
- dribbling
- urine retention
- incontinence
- possible hematuria
- visible midline mass above the symphysis pubis (This is a sign of an incompletely emptied bladder.)
- enlarged prostate with rectal palpation.

TEST RESULTS

- Excretory urography rules out urinary tract obstruction, hydronephrosis (distention of the renal pelvis and calices due to obstruction of the ureter and consequent retention of urine), calculi or tumors, and filling and emptying defects in the bladder.
- Alternatively, if the patient isn't cooperative, cystoscopy rules out other causes of urinary tract obstruction (neoplasm, calculi).
- Blood studies reveal elevated blood urea nitrogen and serum creatinine levels, suggesting renal dysfunction.
- Blood studies also reveal elevated prostate-specific antigen (PSA). Prostatic carcinoma must be ruled out.
- Urinalysis and urine cultures show hematuria, pyuria, and, with bacterial count more than $100,000/mm^3$, urinary tract infection (UTI).
- Cystourethroscopy for severe symptoms (definitive diagnosis) shows prostate enlargement, bladder wall changes, and a raised bladder. (It's done only immediately before surgery to help determine the best procedure.)

TREATMENT

Conservative therapy includes:
- prostate massages
- sitz baths
- fluid restriction to prevent bladder distention
- antimicrobials to treat infection
- regular ejaculation to help relieve prostatic congestion
- alpha-adrenergic blockers, such as alfuzosin (Uroxatral), prazosin (Minipress), tamsulosin (Flomax), and terazosin (Hytrin), to improve urine flow rates to relieve bladder outlet obstruction by preventing contractions of the prostatic capsule and bladder neck
- dutasteride (Avodart) or finasteride (Proscar) to possibly reduce the size of the prostate in some patients
- continuous drainage with an indwelling urinary catheter to alleviate urine retention (high-risk patients).

Surgery is the only effective therapy to relieve acute urine retention, hydronephrosis, severe hematuria, recurrent UTIs, and other intolerable symptoms. The following procedures involve open surgical removal:
- transurethral resection (if the prostate weighs less than 2 oz [56.7 g]); tissue removed with a wire loop and electric current using a resectoscope
- suprapubic (transvesical) resection (most common and useful for prostatic enlargement remaining within the bladder)
- retropubic (extravesical) resection allowing direct visualization (potency and continence usually maintained)
- balloon dilatation of the urethra and prostatic stents to maintain urethral patency (occasionally)
- laser excision to relieve prostatic enlargement
- nerve-sparing surgical techniques to reduce common complications such as erectile dysfunction.

NURSING CONSIDERATIONS

- Monitor and record the patient's vital signs, intake and output, and daily weight, watching closely for signs of postobstructive diuresis (such as increased urine output and hypotension) that may lead to serious dehydration, reduced blood volume, shock, electrolyte loss, and anuria.
- Insert an indwelling urinary catheter for urine retention (usually difficult in a patient with BPH). Using a catheter coudé may make insertion easier.
- If the catheter can't be passed transurethrally, assist with suprapubic cystostomy under local anesthetic (watching for rapid bladder decompression).

After prostatic surgery, interventions may include the following:

- Maintain patient comfort, watch for and prevent postoperative complications, observe for immediate dangers of prostatic bleeding (shock, hemorrhage), check the catheter often (every 15 minutes for the first 2 to 3 hours) for patency and urine color, and check dressings for bleeding.
- Postoperatively, many urologists insert a three-way catheter and establish continuous bladder irrigation. Keep the catheter open at a rate sufficient to maintain clear, light-pink returns; watch for fluid overload from absorption of the irrigating fluid into systemic circulation; observe an indwelling regular catheter closely (if used); and irrigate a catheter with stopped drainage caused by clots with 80 to 100 ml of normal saline solution, as ordered, maintaining strict sterile technique.
- Watch for septic shock (most serious complication of prostatic surgery); immediately report severe chills, sudden fever, tachycardia, hypotension, or other signs of shock; start rapid infusion of I.V. antibiotics as ordered; watch for signs and symptoms of a pulmonary embolus, heart failure, and renal failure; and monitor vital signs, central venous pressure, and arterial pressure continuously. (Supportive care in the intensive care unit may be needed.)
- Administer belladonna and opium suppositories or other anticholinergics, as ordered, to relieve painful bladder spasms that commonly occur after transurethral resection.
- After an open procedure, take patient comfort measures, such as providing suppositories (except after perineal prostatectomy), analgesic medication to control incisional pain, and frequent dressing changes. Suppositories and rectal temperatures are sometimes contraindicated following open prostatic procedures — confirm orders with the physician.
- Continue infusing I.V. fluids until the patient can drink sufficient fluids (2 to 3 qt [2 to 3 L] per day) to maintain adequate hydration.
- Administer stool softeners and laxatives, as ordered, to prevent straining. (Don't check for fecal impaction because a rectal examination may precipitate bleeding.)
- Reassure the patient that temporary frequency, dribbling, and occasional hematuria will likely occur after the catheter is removed.
- Reinforce prescribed limits on activity, such as lifting, strenuous exercise, and long automobile rides that increase bleeding tendency; caution the patient to restrict sexual activity for several weeks after discharge.
- Instruct the patient about the prescribed oral antibiotic drug regimen and the indications for using gentle laxatives.

- Urge the patient to seek medical care immediately if he can't void or if he passes bloody urine or develops a fever.
- Encourage annual digital rectal examinations and screening for PSA to identify a possible malignancy.

Endometriosis

Endometriosis is the presence of endometrial tissue outside the lining of the uterine cavity. Ectopic tissue is generally confined to the pelvic area, usually around the ovaries, uterovesical peritoneum, uterosacral ligaments, and cul-de-sac, but it can appear anywhere in the body. (See *Common sites of endometriosis*.)

Active endometriosis may occur at any age, including adolescence. As many as 50% of infertile women may have endometriosis, although the true incidence in fertile and infertile women remains unknown.

Severe symptoms of endometriosis may have an abrupt onset or may develop over many years. Infertility occurs in 30% to 40% of women with the disorder. Endometriosis usually manifests during the menstrual years; after menopause, it tends to subside. Hormonal treatment of endometriosis (continuous use of hormonal contraceptives, danazol [Danocrine], and gonadotropin-releasing hormone [GnRH] antagonists) is potentially effective in relieving discomfort, although treatment for advanced stages of endometriosis usually isn't as successful because of impaired follicular development. However, nonsurgical treatment of endometriosis generally remains inadequate. Surgery appears to be the more effective way to enhance fertility, although definitive class I evidence doesn't currently exist. Pharmacologic and surgical treatment of endometriosis may help manage chronic pelvic pain.

CAUSES
The cause of endometriosis remains unknown. The main theories to explain this disorder (one or more are perhaps true for certain populations of women) include:
- coelomic metaplasia (repeated inflammation inducing metaplasia of mesothelial cells to the endometrial epithelium)
- genetic predisposition and depressed immune system (may predispose to endometriosis)
- lymphatic or hematogenous spread (extraperitoneal disease)
- retrograde menstruation with implantation at ectopic sites. (Retrograde menstruation alone may not be sufficient for endometriosis to occur because it also occurs in women with no clinical evidence of endometriosis.)

PATHOPHYSIOLOGY
The ectopic endometrial tissue responds to normal stimulation in the same way as the endometrium, but more unpredictably. The endometrial cells respond to estrogen and progesterone with proliferation and secretion. During menstruation, the ectopic tissue bleeds, which causes inflammation of the surrounding tissues. This inflammation causes fibrosis, leading to adhesions that produce pain and infertility.

Complications of endometriosis include infertility due to fibrosis, scarring, and adhesions (major complication); chronic pelvic pain; and ovarian carcinoma (rare).

COMMON SITES OF ENDOMETRIOSIS

Ectopic endometrial tissue can implant almost anywhere in the pelvic peritoneum. It can even invade distant sites such as the lungs.

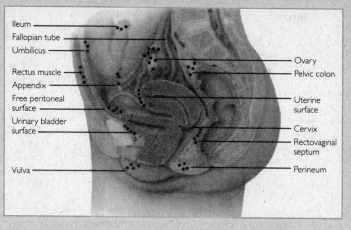

Labels (left): Ileum, Fallopian tube, Umbilicus, Rectus muscle, Appendix, Free peritoneal surface, Urinary bladder surface, Vulva

Labels (right): Ovary, Pelvic colon, Uterine surface, Cervix, Rectovaginal septum, Perineum

CLINICAL FINDINGS

- Dysmenorrhea, abnormal uterine bleeding, and infertility (classic symptoms)
- Pain that begins 5 to 7 days before menses and that peaks and lasts for 2 to 3 days (varies among patients); severity of pain not indicative of extent of disease

Other signs and symptoms depend on the location of the ectopic tissue and may include:

- infertility and profuse menses (ovaries and oviducts)
- deep-thrust dyspareunia (ovaries or cul-de-sac)
- suprapubic pain, dysuria, and hematuria (bladder)
- abdominal cramps, pain on defecation, constipation; bloody stools due to bleeding of ectopic endometrium in the rectosigmoid musculature (large bowel and appendix)
- bleeding from endometrial deposits in these areas during menses; pain on intercourse (cervix, vagina, and perineum).

TEST RESULTS

The only definitive way to diagnose endometriosis is through laparoscopy or laparotomy. Pelvic examination may suggest endometriosis or may be unremarkable. Findings suggestive of endometriosis include:

- multiple tender nodules on uterosacral ligaments or in the rectovaginal septum (in one-third of patients)
- ovarian enlargement in the presence of endometrial cysts on the ovaries.

Although laparoscopy is recommended to diagnose and determine the extent of disease, some clinicians recommend:

- empiric trial of GnRH agonist therapy to confirm or refute the impression of endometriosis before resorting to laparoscopy (controversial but may be cost-effective)
- biopsy at the time of laparoscopy (helpful to confirm the diagnosis), although in some instances diagnosis is confirmed by visual inspection.

TREATMENT

Treatment of endometriosis varies according to the stage of the disease and the patient's age and desire to have children. Conservative therapy for young women who want to have children includes:

- androgens such as danazol (Danocrine)
- progestins and continuous combined hormonal contraceptives (pseudopregnancy regimen) to relieve symptoms by causing a regression of endometrial tissue
- GnRH agonists to induce pseudomenopause (medical oophorectomy), causing remission of the disease (commonly used).

No pharmacologic treatment has been shown to cure the disease or be effective in all women. Some disadvantages of nonsurgical therapy include:

- adverse reaction to drug-induced menopause (including osteoporosis if used for more than 6 months), high expense of use for an extended duration, and possible recurrence of endometriosis after discontinuation of GnRH agonists
- high expense and weight gain when using danazol
- lowest fertility rates of any medical treatment for endometriosis when us-

ing continuous hormonal contraceptive pills
- weight gain and depressive symptoms when using progestin (but as effective as GnRH antagonists).

When ovarian masses are present, surgery must rule out cancer. Conservative surgery includes:

- laparoscopic removal of endometrial implants with conventional or laser techniques (no benefit shown for laser laparoscopy over electrocautery or suture methods)
- presacral neurectomy for central pelvic pain; effective in about 50% or fewer of appropriate candidates
- laparoscopic uterosacral nerve ablation (LUNA) also for central pelvic pain, although definitive studies supporting the efficacy of LUNA are lacking
- total abdominal hysterectomy with or without bilateral salpingo-oophorectomy; although success rates vary, it's unclear whether ovarian conservation is appropriate (treatment of last resort for women who don't want to have children or for extensive disease).

NURSING CONSIDERATIONS

- Minor gynecologic procedures are contraindicated immediately before and during menstruation.
- Advise adolescents to use sanitary napkins instead of tampons; this can help prevent retrograde flow in girls with a narrow vagina or small introitus.
- Because infertility is a possible complication, advise the patient who wants children not to postpone childbearing.
- Recommend an annual pelvic examination and Papanicolaou test to all patients.

Erectile dysfunction

Erectile dysfunction, or impotence, refers to a male's inability to attain or maintain penile erection sufficient to complete intercourse. The patient with primary impotence has never achieved a sufficient erection. Secondary impotence is more common but no less disturbing than the primary form; it implies that the patient has succeeded in completing intercourse in the past.

Transient periods of impotence aren't considered dysfunction and probably occur in half of adult males. Erectile disorder affects all age-groups but increases in frequency with age. The prognosis for erectile dysfunction depends on the severity and duration of the patient's impotence and the underlying causes.

CAUSES

Causes of erectile dysfunction include psychogenic factors (50% to 60% of cases), organic causes, or both psychogenic and organic factors in some patients. This complexity makes the isolation of the primary cause difficult.

Psychogenic causes of erectile dysfunction include:
- intrapersonal psychogenic causes reflecting personal sexual anxieties and generally involving guilt, fear, depression, or feelings of inadequacy resulting from previous traumatic sexual experience, rejection by parents or peers, exaggerated religious orthodoxy, abnormal mother-son intimacy, or homosexual experiences
- psychogenic factors reflecting a disturbed sexual relationship, possibly stemming from differences in sexual preferences between partners, lack of communication, insufficient knowledge of sexual function, or nonsexual personal conflicts
- situational impotence, a temporary condition in response to stress.

Organic causes include:
- chronic diseases that cause neurologic and vascular impairment, such as cardiopulmonary disease, diabetes, multiple sclerosis, or renal failure
- complications of surgery, particularly radical prostatectomy
- drug- or alcohol-induced dysfunction
- genital anomalies or central nervous system defects (rare)
- liver cirrhosis causing increased circulating estrogen as a result of reduced hepatic inactivation
- spinal cord trauma.

PATHOPHYSIOLOGY

Neurologic dysfunction results in lack of the autonomic signal and, in combination with vascular disease, interferes with arteriolar dilation. The blood is shunted around the sacs of the corpus cavernosum into medium-sized veins, which prevents the sacs from filling completely. Also, perfusion of the corpus cavernosum is initially compromised because of partial obstruction of small arteries, leading to loss of erection before ejaculation.

Psychogenic causes may exacerbate emotional problems in a circular pattern; anxiety causes fear of erectile dysfunction, which causes further emotional problems.

A complication of erectile dysfunction is severe depression (in patients with psychogenic or organic drug-induced erectile dysfunction), either causing the impotence or resulting from it. It may also place a strain on sexual relationships.

CLINICAL FINDINGS

Secondary erectile disorder is classified as:

- partial — inability to achieve or sustain a full erection
- intermittent — sometimes potent with the same partner
- selective — potent only with certain partners.

Some men lose erectile function suddenly, while others lose it gradually. If the cause isn't organic, erection may still be achieved through masturbation.

Immediately before a sexual encounter, patients with psychogenic impotence may:

- feel anxious
- perspire
- have palpitations
- lose interest in sexual activity.

TEST RESULTS

There are no test results that help support the diagnosis of erectile dysfunction, but such chronic diseases as diabetes and other vascular, neurologic, and urogenital problems must be ruled out. A detailed sexual history helps differentiate between organic and psychogenic factors and between primary and secondary impotence. Questions should include the following:

- Does the patient have intermittent, selective nocturnal or early morning erections?
- Can he achieve erections through other sexual activity?
- When did his dysfunction begin, and what was his life situation at that time?
- Did erectile problems occur suddenly or gradually?
- What prescription or nonprescription drugs is he taking?
- How often and how much alcohol does he drink?

Diagnosis also includes fulfilling the diagnostic criteria for the *Diagnostic and Statistical Manual of Mental Disorders,* Fourth Edition, Text Revision (*DSM-IV-TR*) diagnosis (when the disorder causes marked distress or interpersonal difficulty).

TREATMENT

Treatment for psychogenic impotence includes:

- sex therapy including both partners (The course and content of therapy depend on the specific cause of dysfunction and nature of the partner relationship.)
- teaching or helping the patient to improve verbal communication skills, eliminate unreasonable guilt, or reevaluate attitudes toward sex and sexual roles.

Treatment for organic impotence includes:

- reversing the cause, if possible
- psychological counseling to help the couple deal realistically with their situation and explore alternatives for sexual expression if reversing the cause isn't possible
- phosphodiesterase type 5 (PDE5) inhibitors, including sildenafil (Viagra), tadalafil (Cialis), or vardenafil (Levitra), to cause vasodilation within the penis (This may effectively manage erectile dysfunction in appropriate patients.)
- testosterone supplementation for hypogonadal men (This isn't given to men with prostate cancer.)
- prostaglandin E injected directly into the corpus cavernosum (This may induce an erection for 30 to 60 minutes in some men.)
- surgically inserted inflatable or noninflatable penile implants (used in

some patients with organic impotence).

NURSING CONSIDERATIONS

● When you identify a patient with impotence, help him feel comfortable about discussing his sexuality. Assess his sexual health during the initial history taking. When appropriate, refer him for further evaluation or treatment.

● Warn the patient taking a PDE5 inhibitor that use with nitrates or alpha-adrenergic blockers (other than tamsulosin [Flomax] at 0.4 mg once daily) is contraindicated because of the risk of a serious drop in blood pressure.

● After penile implant surgery, instruct the patient to avoid intercourse until the incision heals, usually in 6 weeks.

To help prevent impotence:

● Promote establishment of responsible health and sex education programs at primary, secondary, and college levels.

● Provide information about resuming sexual activity as part of discharge instructions for any patient with a condition that requires modification of daily activities. Such patients include those with cardiac disease, diabetes, hypertension, and chronic obstructive pulmonary disease as well as all postoperative patients.

Polycystic ovarian disease

Polycystic ovarian disease is a metabolic disorder characterized by multiple ovarian cysts. About 22% of the women in the United States have the disorder, and obesity is present in 50% to 80% of these women. Among those who seek treatment for infertility, more than 75% have some degree of polycystic ovarian disease, usually manifested by anovulation alone. Prognosis is good for ovulation and fertility with appropriate treatment.

CAUSES

The precise cause of polycystic ovarian disease is unknown. Theories include:

● abnormal enzyme activity triggering excess androgen secretion from the ovaries and adrenal glands

● endocrine abnormalities causing all of the signs and symptoms of polycystic ovarian disease: amenorrhea, polycystic ovaries on ultrasound, and hyperandrogenism (part of the Stein-Leventhal syndrome).

PATHOPHYSIOLOGY

A general feature of all anovulation syndromes is a lack of pulsatile release of gonadotropin-releasing hormone. Initial ovarian follicle development is normal. Many small follicles begin to accumulate because there's no selection of a dominant follicle. These follicles may respond abnormally to the hormonal stimulation, causing an abnormal pattern of estrogen secretion during the menstrual cycle. Endocrine abnormalities may be the cause of polycystic ovarian disease or cystic abnormalities; muscle and adipose tissue are resistant to the effects of insulin, and lipid metabolism is abnormal.

Possible complications of polycystic ovarian disease include malignancy due to sustained estrogenic stimulation of the endometrium, increased risk of cardiovascular disease, and type 2 diabetes mellitus due to insulin resistance.

Polycystic ovarian disease may also produce secondary amenorrhea, oligomenorrhea, and infertility.

CLINICAL FINDINGS

- Mild pelvic discomfort
- Lower back pain
- Dyspareunia
- Abnormal uterine bleeding secondary to disturbed ovulatory pattern
- Hirsutism
- Acne
- Male-pattern hair loss

TEST RESULTS

- History and physical examination show bilaterally enlarged polycystic ovaries and menstrual disturbance, usually dating back to menarche.
- Visualization of the ovary through ultrasound, laparoscopy, or surgery, commonly for another condition, may confirm ovarian cysts and reveal the disorder.
- Basal body temperature graphs and endometrial biopsy reveal slightly elevated urinary 17-ketosteroid levels and anovulation.
- Blood studies reveal elevated ratio of luteinizing hormone to follicle-stimulating hormone (usually 3:1 or greater) and elevated levels of testosterone and androstenedione.
- Unopposed estrogen action is revealed during the menstrual cycle as a result of anovulation.
- Direct visualization by laparoscopy rules out paraovarian cysts of the broad ligament, salpingitis, endometriosis, and neoplastic cysts.

TREATMENT

- Monitoring the patient's weight to maintain a normal body mass index to reduce risks associated with insulin resistance, which may cause spontaneous ovulation in some women

- Clomiphene (Clomid) to induce ovulation
- Medroxyprogesterone (Provera) for 10 days each month for a patient wanting to become pregnant
- Low-dose hormonal contraceptives to treat abnormal bleeding for the patient needing reliable contraception

NURSING CONSIDERATIONS

- Preoperatively, watch for signs of cyst rupture, such as increasing abdominal pain, distention, and rigidity; monitor vital signs for fever, tachypnea, or hypotension (possibly indicating peritonitis or intraperitoneal hemorrhage).
- Postoperatively, encourage frequent movement in bed and early ambulation, as ordered, to prevent pulmonary embolism.
- Provide emotional support, offering appropriate reassurance if the patient fears cancer or infertility.

Prostatitis

Prostatitis, or inflammation of the prostate gland, may be acute or chronic. Acute prostatitis most commonly results from gram-negative bacteria and is easy to recognize and treat. However, chronic prostatitis, the most common cause of recurrent urinary tract infections (UTIs) in men, is less easy to recognize. As many as 35% of men age 50 and older have chronic prostatitis. Granulomatous prostatitis (tuberculous prostatitis), nonbacterial prostatitis, and prostatodynia (painful prostate) are other classifications of the disease.

CAUSES

Bacterial prostatitis is caused by:

- *Escherichia coli* (80% of cases)
- *Klebsiella, Enterobacter, Proteus, Pseudomonas, Streptococcus,* or *Staphylococcus* organisms (20% of cases).

These organisms probably spread to the prostate by:
- an ascending urethral infection or through the bloodstream
- bacterial invasion from the urethra (chronic prostatitis)
- infrequent or excessive sexual intercourse
- invasion of rectal bacteria through lymphatics
- procedures, such as cystoscopy or catheterization (less commonly)
- reflux of infected bladder urine into prostate ducts.

Granulomatous prostatitis is caused by mycobacterium tuberculosis. The cause of nonbacterial prostatitis is unknown, but possible causes include infection by a protozoa or virus. The cause of prostatodynia is also unknown.

> **Alert** *Acute prostatitis is associated with benign prostatic hyperplasia in older men.*

PATHOPHYSIOLOGY

Spasms in the genitourinary tract or tension in the pelvic floor muscles may cause inflammation and nonbacterial prostatitis.

Bacterial prostatic infections can result from a previous or concurrent infection. The bacteria ascend from the infected urethra, bladder, lymphatics, or blood through the prostatic ducts and into the prostate. Infection stimulates an inflammatory response in which the prostate becomes larger, tender, and firm. Inflammation is usually limited to a few of the gland's excretory ducts.

Possible complications of prostatitis include UTI (common) and infected and abscessed testis (removed surgically).

CLINICAL FINDINGS

Acute prostatitis begins with:
- chills
- lower back pain, especially when standing, due to compression of the prostate gland
- perineal fullness
- suprapubic tenderness
- frequent and urgent urination
- dysuria, nocturia, and urinary obstruction due to the urethra being blocked by an enlarged prostate
- cloudy urine.

Signs of systemic infection include:
- fever
- myalgia
- fatigue
- arthralgia.

Signs and symptoms of chronic bacterial prostatitis may include:
- the same urinary symptoms as the acute form but to a lesser degree
- recurrent symptomatic cystitis.

Other possible signs include:
- evidence of UTI, such as urinary frequency, burning, and cloudy urine
- painful ejaculation
- bloody semen
- persistent urethral discharge
- sexual dysfunction.

TEST RESULTS

- Rectal examination finds evidence of acute prostatitis such as a very tender, warm, and enlarged prostate (characteristic).
- Rectal examination reveals a firm, irregularly shaped, and slightly enlarged prostate due to fibrosis (chronic bacterial prostatitis).
- Palpation shows a normal prostate gland by exclusion (nonbacterial prostatitis).

- Pelvic X-ray shows prostatic calculi.
- Urine culture identifies the causative infectious organism.
- Urine culture identifies no UTI or causative organism (nonbacterial prostatitis).

Firm diagnosis depends on a comparison of urine cultures of specimens obtained by the Meares-Stamey four-glass test. A significant increase in colony count in the prostatic specimens confirms prostatitis. This test requires four specimens:

- first specimen when the patient starts voiding (voided bladder one [VB1])
- second specimen midstream (VB2)
- third specimen after the patient stops voiding and the physician massages the prostate to produce secretions (expressed prostate secretions [EPS])
- final voided specimen (VB3).

TREATMENT

Systemic antibiotic therapy is the treatment of choice for acute prostatitis and may include:

- co-trimoxazole (Bactrim) orally for 30 days (for culture showing sensitivity)
- I.V. co-trimoxazole or I.V. gentamicin plus ampicillin until sensitivity test results are known (sepsis)
- parenteral therapy for 48 hours to 1 week; then oral agent for 30 more days (with favorable test results and clinical response)
- co-trimoxazole for at least 6 weeks (chronic prostatitis due to *E. coli*).

Supportive therapy includes:
- bed rest
- adequate hydration
- analgesics
- antipyretics
- sitz baths

- stool softeners as needed.

In symptomatic chronic prostatitis, treatment may include:
- instructing the patient to drink at least eight glasses of water daily
- regular careful massage of the prostate to relieve discomfort (Vigorous massage may cause secondary epididymitis or septicemia.)
- regular ejaculation to help promote drainage of prostatic secretions
- anticholinergics and analgesics to help relieve nonbacterial prostatitis symptoms
- alpha-adrenergic blockers and muscle relaxants to relieve pain
- continuous low-dose anabolic steroid therapy (effective in some men).

If drug therapy is unsuccessful, surgical treatment may include:
- transurethral resection of the prostate removing all infected tissue (not usually performed on young adults; may cause retrograde ejaculation and sterility)
- total prostatectomy (curative but may cause impotence and incontinence).

NURSING CONSIDERATIONS

- Ensure bed rest and adequate hydration. Provide stool softeners and administer sitz baths, as ordered.
- As necessary, prepare to assist with suprapubic needle aspiration of the bladder or a suprapubic cystostomy.
- Emphasize the need for strict adherence to the prescribed drug regimen. Instruct the patient to drink at least eight glasses of water per day. Have him report adverse drug reactions (rash, nausea, vomiting, fever, chills, and GI irritation).

13

CANCER

Cancer, also called *malignant neoplasia,* refers to a group of more than 100 different diseases that are characterized by deoxyribonucleic acid (DNA) damage that causes abnormal cell growth and development. In the United States, the most common forms of cancer are skin, prostate, breast, lung, and colorectal. Most of the numerous theories about carcinogenesis suggest that it involves initiation, promotion, and progression. *Initiation* refers to the damage to or mutation of DNA that occurs when the cell is exposed to an initiating substance or event (such as chemicals, virus, or radiation) during DNA replication (transcription). *Promotion* involves the mutated cell's exposure to factors (promoters) that enhance its growth, such as hormones (estrogen), food additives (nitrates), or drugs (nicotine). *Progression* is when the tumor invades, metastasizes, and becomes resistant to drugs; this step is irreversible.

Pathophysiologic changes

Cancer's characteristic features are rapid, uncontrollable proliferation of cells and independent spread from a primary site (site of origin) to other tissues where it establishes secondary foci (metastasis). This spread occurs through circulation in the blood or lymphatic fluid, by unintentional transplantation from one site to another during surgery, and by local extension. Thus, cancer cells differ from normal cells in terms of cell size, shape, number, differentiation, and purpose or function. In addition, cancer cells can travel to distant tissues and organ systems.

DIFFERENTIATION

Usually, cells become specialized during development. That is, the cells develop highly individualized characteristics that reflect their specific structure and functions in their corresponding tissue. For example, all blood cells are derived from a single stem cell that differentiates into red blood cells, white blood cells, platelets, monocytes, and lymphocytes. As the cells become more specialized, their reproduction and development slow down. Eventually, highly differentiated cells become unable to reproduce and some, skin cells for example, are programmed to die and be replaced.

UNDERSTANDING ANAPLASIA

Anaplasia refers to the loss of differentiation, a common characteristic of cancer cells. As differentiation is lost, the cancer cells no longer demonstrate the appearance and function of the original cell.

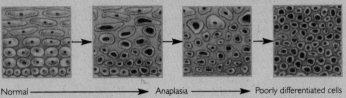

Normal ⟶ Anaplasia ⟶ Poorly differentiated cells

Cancer cells lose the ability to differentiate; that is, they enter a state, called *anaplasia,* in which they no longer appear or function like the original cell. (See *Understanding anaplasia.*)

Anaplasia occurs in varying degrees. The less the cells resemble the cell of origin, the more anaplastic they're said to be. As the anaplastic cells continue to reproduce, they lose the typical characteristics of the original cell. Some anaplastic cells begin functioning as another type of cell, possibly becoming a site for hormone production. For example, oat-cell lung cancer cells may produce antidiuretic hormone, which is produced by the hypothalamus but stored in and secreted by the posterior pituitary gland. When anaplasia occurs, cells of the same type in the same site exhibit many different shapes and sizes. Mitosis is abnormal and chromosome defects are common. The abnormal and uncontrolled cell proliferation of cancer cells is associated with numerous changes within the cancer cell itself. These changes affect the cell membrane, cytoskeleton, and nucleus.

Several important characteristics of the host affect tumor growth. These characteristics include age, gender, overall health status, and immune system function.

Alert *Age is an important factor affecting tumor growth. Relatively few cancers are found in children. Yet the incidence of cancer correlates directly with increasing age. This suggests that numerous or cumulative events are necessary for the initial mutation to continue, eventually forming a tumor.*

Between the initiating event and the emergence of a detectable tumor, some or all of the mutated cells may die. The survivors, if any, reproduce until the tumor reaches a diameter of 1 to 2 mm. New blood vessels form to support continued growth and proliferation. As the cells further mutate and divide more rapidly, they become more undifferentiated. The number of cancerous cells soon begins to exceed the number of normal cells. Eventually, the tumor mass extends, spreading into local tissues and invading the surrounding tissues. When the local tissue is blood or lymph, the tumor can gain access to the circulation. Once access is gained, tumor cells that detach or break off travel to distant sites in the body, where tumor cells can survive and form a new tumor in that secondary site. This process is called *metastasis*.

TUMOR CLASSIFICATION

Tumors are initially classified as benign or malignant depending on the specific features exhibited by the tumor. Typically, benign tumors are well differentiated; that is, their cells closely resemble those of the tissue of origin. Commonly encapsulated with well-defined borders, benign tumors grow slowly, usually displacing but not infiltrating surrounding tissues, and therefore causing only slight damage. Benign tumors don't metastasize.

Conversely, most malignant tumors are undifferentiated to varying degrees, having cells that may differ considerably from those of the tissue of origin. They're seldom encapsulated and are commonly poorly delineated. They rapidly expand in all directions, causing extensive damage as they infiltrate surrounding tissues. Most malignant tumors metastasize through the blood or lymph to secondary sites. Malignant tumors are further classified by tissue type, degree of differentiation (grading), and extent of the disease (staging). (See *Understanding TNM staging.*)

Grading

Histologically, malignant tumors are classified by their degree of differentiation. The greater their differentiation, the greater the tumor cells' similarity to the tissue of origin. Typically, a malignant tumor is graded on a scale of 1 to 4, in order of increasing clinical severity.

● Grade 1: Well differentiated; cells closely resemble the tissue of origin and maintain some specialized function.
● Grade 2: Moderately well differentiated; cells vary somewhat in size and shape with increased mitosis.

- Grade 3: Poorly differentiated; cells vary widely in size and shape with little resemblance to the tissue of origin; mitosis is greatly increased.
- Grade 4: Undifferentiated; cells exhibit no similarity to tissue of origin.

Staging

Malignant tumors are staged (classified anatomically) by the extent of the disease. The most commonly used method for staging is the TNM staging system, which evaluates Tumor size, Nodal involvement, and Metastatic progress. This classification system provides an accurate tumor description that's adjustable as the disease progresses. TNM staging enables reliable comparison of treatments and survival rates among large population groups; it also identifies nodal involvement and metastasis to other areas. (See *Understanding TNM staging,* page 419.)

TREATMENT

Cancer treatments include surgery, radiation therapy, chemotherapy, immunotherapy (also called *biotherapy*), and hormone therapy. Each may be used alone or in combination (called *multimodal therapy*), depending on the tumor's type, stage, localization, and responsiveness and on limitations imposed by the patient's clinical status.

Acute leukemia

Acute leukemia is one form of leukemia. Leukemia refers to a group of malignant disorders characterized by abnormal proliferation and maturation of lymphocytes and nonlymphocytic cells, leading to the suppression of normal cells. If untreated, acute leukemia is fatal, usually as a result of complications from leukemic cell infiltration of bone marrow or vital organs. With treatment, the prognosis varies. Two types of acute leukemia are acute lymphocytic leukemia (ALL) and acute myeloid leukemia (AML; also known as *acute nonlymphocytic leukemia* or *acute myeloblastic leukemia*).

ALL accounts for 80% of childhood leukemias. Treatment leads to remission in 81% of children, who survive an average of 5 years, and in 65% of adults, who survive an average of 2 years. Children between ages 2 and 8 who receive intensive therapy have the best survival rate.

AML is one of the most common leukemias in adults. Average survival time is only 1 year after diagnosis, even with aggressive treatment. Remissions lasting 2 to 10 months occur in 50% of children.

The patient's history usually reveals a sudden onset of high fever and abnormal bleeding, such as bruising after minor trauma, nosebleeds, gingival bleeding, and purpura. Fatigue and night sweats may also occur.

CAUSES

The exact cause of acute leukemia isn't known; 40% to 50% of patients have mutations in their chromosomes. Individuals with certain chromosomal disorders have a higher risk. People with Down syndrome, trisomy 13, and other heredity disorders have a higher incidence of leukemia.

Other risk factors include:
- certain viruses, such as human T-cell lymphotrophic virus
- cigarette smoking
- exposure to certain chemicals (such as benzene, which is present in cigarette smoke and gasoline)

WHAT HAPPENS IN LEUKEMIA

This illustration shows how white blood cells (agranulocytes and granulocytes) proliferate in the bloodstream in leukemia, overwhelming red blood cells (RBCs) and platelets.

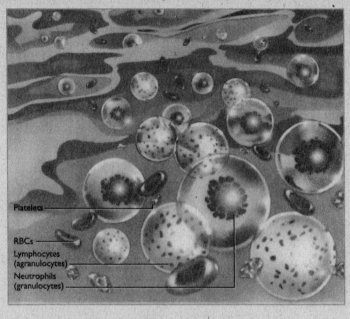

Platelets

RBCs

Lymphocytes
(agranulocytes)

Neutrophils
(granulocytes)

• exposure to large doses of ionizing radiation or drugs that depress the bone marrow.

PATHOPHYSIOLOGY

Immature hematopoietic cells undergo an abnormal transformation, giving rise to leukemic cells. Leukemic cells multiply and accumulate, crowding out other types of cells. Crowding prevents production of normal red blood cells and white blood cells (WBCs) and platelets, leading to pancytopenia—a reduction in the number of all cellular elements of the blood. (See *What happens in leukemia*.)

CLINICAL FINDINGS

Signs and symptoms of ALL and AML are similar. Effects of both leukemias are related to suppression of elements of the bone marrow and include:

• infection related to myelosuppression from treatment, direct invasion of the bone marrow, development of fistulas, or immunosuppression from hormonal release in response to chronic stress. Malnutrition and anemia further increase the patient's risk

of infection. Also, obstructions, effusions, and ulcerations may develop, creating a favorable environment for microbial growth.
- bleeding due to thrombocytopenia from bone marrow suppression. Even when the platelet count is normal, platelet function may be impaired in hematologic cancers.
- anemia due to cancer of the blood-forming cells, WBCs, or RBCs
- malaise and lethargy related to anemia, as there are fewer functional cells to maintain metabolism
- fever and night sweats resulting from bone marrow invasion and cellular proliferation within bone marrow
- pain due to infiltration of bone marrow
- paleness and weakness due to anemia
- weight loss due to generalized wasting of fat and protein, and decreased appetite.

TEST RESULTS
- Blood counts show thrombocytopenia and neutropenia; WBC differential determines cell type.
- Cerebrospinal fluid analysis reveals abnormal WBC invasion of the central nervous system.
- Bone marrow biopsy confirms the disease by showing a proliferation of immature WBCs. It's also used to determine whether the leukemia is lymphocytic or myeloid.
- Computed tomography scan shows which organs are affected.

TREATMENT
- Systemic chemotherapy to eradicate leukemic cells and induce remission
- Antibiotic, antifungal, and antiviral drugs

- Colony-stimulating factors such as filgrastim (Neupogen) to spur the growth of granulocytes, RBCs, and platelets
- Transfusions of platelets to prevent bleeding and RBCs to prevent anemia

Three-stage treatment of ALL
- Induction — usually vincristine, prednisone, and an anthracycline with or without asparaginase (Elspar) for adults
- Consolidation — high doses of chemotherapy designed to eliminate remaining leukemic cells
- Maintenance — lower doses of chemotherapy for up to 2 years (The goal is to eliminate stray leukemic cells that have evaded other drugs used in the induction and consolidation stages.)

Two-stage treatment of AML
- Induction — cytarabine (Cytosar-U) and an anthracycline
- Postremission — intensification, maintenance chemotherapy, or bone marrow transplantation

NURSING CONSIDERATIONS
Alert Because so many of these patients are children, be especially sensitive to their emotional needs and those of their families.
- Teach the patient and his family how to recognize infection (fever, chills, cough, sore throat) and abnormal bleeding (bruising, petechiae) and how to stop such bleeding (applying pressure and ice to the area).
- Encourage the patient to consume high-calorie, high-protein foods and beverages.
- Watch for signs and symptoms of meningeal leukemia (confusion, lethargy, headache).

- Prevent hyperuricemia, which may result from rapid chemotherapy-induced leukemic cell lysis. Give the patient about 2 qt (2 L) of fluids daily, and administer acetazolamide (Diamox), sodium bicarbonate tablets, and allopurinol (Zyloprim). Check urine pH often — it should be above 7.5.
- If the patient receives daunorubicin (Cerubidine) or doxorubicin (Adriamycin), watch for early signs of cardiotoxicity, such as arrhythmias, and signs of heart failure.
- Control infection by placing the patient in a private room and imposing reverse isolation, if necessary. Avoid using indwelling urinary catheters and giving I.M. injections.

Alert *A patient with a temperature over 101° F (38.3° C) and a decreased WBC count should receive prompt antibiotic therapy.*

- Discuss the option of home or hospice care as appropriate. Support groups such as the American Cancer Society may also be helpful.

Breast cancer

Breast cancer is the most common cancer in women. Although the disease may develop any time after puberty, 70% of cases occur in women older than age 50. Breast cancer ranks second among cancer deaths in women, behind cancer of the lung and bronchus.

CAUSES
The exact causes of breast cancer remain elusive. Scientists have discovered specific genes linked to approximately 5% of all cases of breast cancer (called BRCA1 and BRCA2), which confirms that the disease can be inherited from a person's mother or father. Those who inherit either of these genes have an 80% chance of developing breast cancer.

Other significant risk factors have been identified. These include:
- age
- alcohol use (one or more alcoholic beverages per day)
- being a premenopausal woman older than age 45
- benign breast disease
- colon, endometrial, or ovarian cancer
- early onset of menses or late menopause
- family history of breast cancer
- first pregnancy after age 30
- high-fat diet
- obesity
- nulligravida (never pregnant)
- postmenopausal progestin and estrogen therapy
- radiation exposure
- recent use of hormonal contraceptives.

PATHOPHYSIOLOGY
About one-half of all breast cancers develop in the upper outer quadrant.

Breast cancer is generally classified by the tissue of origin and the location of the lesion. *Lobular cancer* develops within the lobes. *Intraductal cancer,* the most common form, develops within the ducts. Less than 1% of breast cancers originate in the nonepithelial connective tissue. *Inflammatory cancer* (rare) grows rapidly and causes the overlying skin to become edematous, inflamed, and indurated. Paget's disease is the growth of cancerous cells within the breast ducts beneath the nipple.

Breast cancer is also classified as invasive or noninvasive. Invasive tumor cells, which make up 90% of all breast

HOW CANCER METASTASIZES

Cancer usually spreads through the bloodstream to other organs and tissues, as shown here.

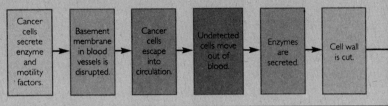

Cancer cells secrete enzyme and motility factors. → Basement membrane in blood vessels is disrupted. → Cancer cells escape into circulation. → Undetected cells move out of blood. → Enzymes are secreted. → Cell wall is cut.

cancers, break through the duct walls and encroach on other breast tissues. Noninvasive tumor cells remain confined to the duct in which they originated. Although growth rates vary, a lump may take up to 8 years to become palpable. Breast cancers can spread via the lymphatic system and bloodstream, through the right side of the heart to the lungs and, eventually, to the other breast, chest wall, liver, bone, and brain. (See *How cancer metastasizes.*)

CLINICAL FINDINGS
● Patient discovery of thickening of the breast tissue or a painless lump or mass in her breast related to cellular growth; palpation identifying a hard lump, mass, or thickening of breast tissue
● Inspection possibly revealing nipple retraction, scaly skin around the nipple, skin changes, erythema, and clear, milky, or bloody discharge related to tumor cell infiltration to surrounding tissues
● Edema in the arm indicating advanced nodal involvement
● Palpation of the cervical supraclavicular and axillary nodes possibly revealing lumps or enlargement

● Warm hot, pink area from inflammation and infiltration of surrounding tissues
● Pain related to advancement of tumor and subsequent pressure

TEST RESULTS
● Breast examination reveals breast lump.
● Mammography—the primary test for breast cancer—detects tumors.
● Fine-needle aspiration and excisional biopsy provide cells for histologic examination to confirm diagnosis.
● Hormone receptor assay pinpoints whether the tumor is estrogen- or progesterone-dependent so that appropriate therapy can be chosen.
● Ultrasonography distinguishes between a fluid-filled cyst and a solid mass.
● Chest X-ray pinpoints chest metastasis if present.
● Scans of the bone, brain, liver, and other organs detect distant metastasis if present.
● Ductoscopy reveals small intraductal lesions that aren't palpable or visible on mammography.
● Ductal lavage identifies cancerous cells in the milk ducts of the breast.

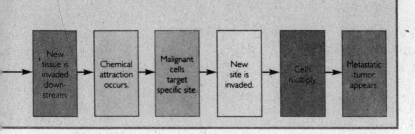

| New tissue is invaded downstream. | Chemical attraction occurs. | Malignant cells target specific site. | New site is invaded. | Cells multiply. | Metastatic tumor appears. |

TREATMENT

Treatment for breast cancer may include a combination of surgery, radiation, chemotherapy, and hormonal therapy.

● Lumpectomy for small, well-defined lesions (Through a small incision, the surgeon removes the tumor, surrounding tissue and, possibly, nearby lymph nodes. The patient usually undergoes radiation therapy afterward.)

● Partial mastectomy (The tumor is removed along with a wedge of normal tissue, skin, fascia, and axillary lymph nodes. Radiation therapy or chemotherapy is usually used after surgery to destroy undetected disease in other breast areas.)

● Total mastectomy involves removal of the breast tissue (This procedure is used if the cancer is confined to breast tissue and no lymph node involvement is detected. Chemotherapy or radiation therapy may follow.)

● Modified radical mastectomy to remove the entire breast, axillary lymph nodes, and the lining that covers the chest muscles (If the lymph nodes contain cancer cells, radiation therapy and chemotherapy follow.)

● Before or after tumor removal, radiation therapy to destroy a small, early-stage tumor without distant metastasis (It can also be used to prevent or treat local recurrence. Preoperative radiation therapy to the breast also 'sterilizes' the area, making the tumor more manageable surgically, especially in inflammatory breast cancer.)

● Cytotoxic drugs either as adjuvant therapy or primary therapy (Chemotherapy commonly involves a combination of drugs. A typical regimen makes use of cyclophosphamide [Cytoxan], methotrexate [Trexall], doxorubicin [Adriamycin], and fluorouracil [5-FU].)

● Hormone therapy to lower the levels of estrogen and other hormones suspected of nourishing breast cancer cells; antiestrogen therapy, with tamoxifen (Nolvadex) or raloxifene (Evista), for women at increased risk for developing breast cancer; other commonly used drugs include the antiandrogen aminoglutethimide (Cytadren), the androgen fluoxymesterone (Halotestin), and the progestin megestrol (Megace)

NURSING CONSIDERATIONS

● Provide teaching regarding the disorder, diagnosis, and treatment measures.

- Teach postoperative care if the patient has a mastectomy; deep breathing and coughing; position for comfort; prevention of thromboembolism; getting out of bed as soon as possible.
- Monitor incision and drainage; perform dressing changes and measure output from drains.
- Monitor vital signs and report changes in trends.
- Prevent lymphedema by instructing the patient in hand and arm exercises and avoiding activities that might cause infection of this area.
- Discuss reconstructive surgery as appropriate and breast prosthesis.
- Provide psychological and emotional support.

Alert *Explain phantom breast syndrome, a phenomenon in which a tingling or a pins-and-needles sensation is felt in the area of the amputated tissue, to the patient. Listen to concerns, offer support, and refer the patient to an appropriate organization, such as the American Cancer Society's Reach to Recovery, which offers caring and sharing groups to help breast cancer patients in the facility and at home.*

Cervical cancer

The third most common cancer of the female reproductive system, cervical cancer is classified as either microinvasive or invasive. Precursors to cervical cancer include minimal cervical dysplasia (squamous intraepithelial lenar), in which the lower third of the epithelium contains abnormal cells; and carcinoma in situ (cervical intraepithelial neoplasia) in which the full thickness of epithelium contains abnormally proliferating cells.

Dysplasia is curable 75% to 90% of the time with early detection and proper treatment. If untreated (and depending on the form in which it appears), it may progress to invasive cervical cancer.

CAUSES
The human papillomavirus (HPV) is accepted as the cause of virtually all cervical dysplasias and cervical cancers. Certain strains of the HPV (16, 18, 31) are associated with an increased risk of cervical cancer.

Several predisposing factors have been related to the development of cervical cancer:
- herpesvirus 2 and other bacterial or viral venereal infections
- intercourse at a young age (younger than age 16)
- multiple sexual partners.

PATHOPHYSIOLOGY
With invasive carcinoma, cancer cells penetrate the basement membrane and can spread directly to contiguous pelvic structures or disseminate to distant sites by lymphatic routes. Invasive carcinoma of the cervix accounts for 8,000 deaths annually in the United States alone. In almost all cases (95%), the histologic type is squamous cell carcinoma, which varies from well-differentiated cells to highly anaplastic spindle cells. Only 5% are adenocarcinomas. Invasive carcinoma usually occurs in patients between ages 30 and 50, though in rare cases it can occur in those younger than age 20.

CLINICAL FINDINGS
- Abnormal vaginal bleeding with persistent vaginal discharge and postcoital pain and bleeding related to cellular invasion and erosion of the cervical epithelium

- Pelvic pain secondary to pressure on surrounding tissues and nerves from cellular proliferation
- Vaginal leakage of urine and feces from fistulas due to erosion and necrosis of cervix
- Anorexia, weight loss, and anemia related to the hypermetabolic activity of cellular proliferation and increased tumor growth needs

TEST RESULTS
- Papanicolaou (Pap) smear reveals malignant cellular changes.
- Colposcopy identifies the presence and extent of early lesions.
- Biopsy confirms cell types.
- Computed tomography scan, nuclear imaging scan, and lymphangiography identify metastasis.

TREATMENT
- For preinvasive lesions, loop electrosurgical examination procedure, cryosurgery, laser destruction, conization (and frequent Pap test follow-up) or, rarely, hysterectomy
- Radical hysterectomy and radiation therapy (internal, external, or both) for invasive squamous cell carcinoma
- Radiation for all stages; surgery (preferable for some premenopausal women)

NURSING CONSIDERATIONS
- If the patient needs a biopsy, drape and prepare her as for a routine Pap test and pelvic examination. Explain to the patient she may feel pressure, minor abdominal cramps, or a pinch from the punch forceps.
- If the patient is having cryosurgery, warn her that she may experience abdominal cramps, headache, and sweating, but little pain. Also warn her she'll have profuse, watery discharge for days or weeks.

- Tell the patient to expect a discharge or spotting for about 1 week after excisional biopsy, cryosurgery, or laser therapy, and advise her not to douche, use tampons, or engage in sexual intercourse during this time. Tell her to watch for and report signs of infection. Stress the need for follow-up Pap tests and pelvic exams within 3 to 4 months after these procedures and periodically thereafter.

Alert After surgery, monitor vital signs and watch for complications such as bleeding, abdominal distention, severe pain, and breathing difficulties.
- Explain radiation therapy to the patient as appropriate.

Alert During radiation therapy, use safety precautions: time, distance, and shielding. Begin as soon as the radioactive source is in place. Inform the patient that she'll require a private room.
- If an implant is placed, encourage the patient to lie flat, with the head of the bed slightly elevated, and limit movements while in place. Monitor vital signs and watch for skin reaction, vaginal bleeding, abdominal discomfort, or evidence of dehydration. Limit time of exposure with the patient.
- Warn the patient to avoid persons with infections during radiation therapy as she'll have an increased susceptibility to infection.

Chronic lymphocytic leukemia

Chronic lymphocytic leukemia is the most benign and slowest progressing form of leukemia. This type of chronic leukemia occurs most commonly in elderly people, and more than one-half of the cases are male. According to the American Cancer Society, this type of leukemia accounts for about one-third of new adult cases annually. The prognosis is poor if anemia, thrombocytopenia, neutropenia, bulky lymphadenopathy, or severe lymphocytosis develops. Gross bone marrow replacement by abnormal lymphocytes is the most common cause of death, usually 4 to 5 years after diagnosis.

CAUSES
- Unknown
- Hereditary factors suspected

PATHOPHYSIOLOGY
Chronic lymphocytic leukemia is a generalized, progressive disease. It causes a proliferation and accumulation of relatively mature looking but immunologically inefficient lymphocytes. After these cells infiltrate, clinical signs appear.

CLINICAL FINDINGS
- Fever resulting from bone marrow invasion and cellular proliferation within bone marrow
- Bleeding tendencies secondary to thrombocytopenia
- Frequent infections related to deficient humoral immunity
- Fatigue related to anemia
- Enlargement of lymph nodes and hepatomegaly from infiltration by leukemic cells
- Splenomegaly secondary to increased numbers of lysed red blood cells being filtered

TEST RESULTS
- Lymph node biopsy distinguishes between benign and malignant tumors.

- Routine blood tests usually uncover the disease. In the early stages, the lymphocyte count is slightly elevated (greater than 20,000/mm^3). Although granulocytopenia is generally seen first, the lymphocyte count climbs (greater than 100,000/mm^3) as the disease progresses. A hemoglobin level lower than 11 g/dl, hypogammaglobulinemia, and depressed serum globulin levels are also evident.
- Bone marrow aspiration and biopsy shows lymphocytic invasion.

TREATMENT
- Systemic chemotherapy, using the alkylating drugs chlorambucil (Leukeran) or cyclophosphamide (Cytoxan), with presence of autoimmune hemolytic anemia or thrombocytopenia
- Prednisone for refractory disease
- Local radiation to reduce organ size and help to relieve symptoms when obstruction or organ impairment or enlargement occurs
- Radiation therapy for enlarged lymph nodes, painful bony lesions, or massive splenomegaly
- Allopurinol (Zyloprim) to prevent hyperuricemia

NURSING CONSIDERATIONS
- Provide patient teaching about chemotherapy, signs of infection to report to the physician, signs of thrombocytopenia and preventive measures to avoid bleeding (avoiding aspirin, soft toothbrush), and what to do if bleeding occurs (ice, pressure).

Alert If the patient will be discharged, tell him to avoid coming in contact with obviously ill people, especially children with common contagious childhood diseases.
- Emphasize the need for adequate rest and a high-calorie, high-protein diet.

- Teach the patient signs and symptoms of recurrence (swollen lymph nodes in the neck, axillae, and groin; increased abdominal size or discomfort), and tell him to notify his physician immediately if he detects any of them.
- Monitor the patient for pallor, petechiae, and bruising.
- Provide emotional support for the patient.
- If the patient is to return to his home, provide appropriate referrals such as home or hospice care.

Colorectal cancer

Colorectal cancer accounts for 10% to 15% of all new cancer cases in the United States. It occurs equally in both sexes and is the third most common cause of cancer. It strikes most commonly in people older than age 50. Because colorectal cancer progresses slowly and remains localized for a long time, early detection is key to recovery. Unless the tumor metastasizes, the 5-year survival rate is 80% for rectal cancer and 85% for colon cancer.

CAUSES

The primary risk factor for colorectal cancer is age. Several disorders and preexisting conditions are also linked to colorectal cancer, including:
- alcohol consumption
- colorectal polyps (the larger the polyp, the greater the risk)
- Crohn's disease
- familial adenomatous polyposis, such as Gardner's syndrome and Peutz-Jeghers syndrome
- genetic abnormality

- genetic factors — deletions on chromosomes 17 and 18
- hereditary nonpolyposis colorectal carcinoma
- high-fat, low-fiber diet
- obesity
- other pelvic cancers treated with abdominal radiation
- physical inactivity
- smoking
- Turcot's syndrome
- ulcerative colitis.

Alert Recent studies suggest that estrogen replacement therapy and nonsteroidal anti-inflammatory drugs, such as aspirin, may reduce the risk of colorectal cancer.

PATHOPHYSIOLOGY

Malignant colorectal tumors are almost always adenocarcinomas. About one-half of these are sessile lesions of the rectosigmoid area; the rest are polypoid lesions. The stages of colorectal cancer reflect the extent of bowel-mucosa and bowel-wall infiltration, lymph node involvement, and metastasis.

CLINICAL FINDINGS
Tumor on right colon
- Black tarry stools secondary to tumor erosion and necrosis of the intestinal lining
- Anemia secondary to increased tumor growth needs and bleeding resulting from necrosis and ulceration of mucosa
- Abdominal aching, pressure, or cramps secondary to pressure from tumor
- Weakness, fatigue, anorexia, weight loss secondary to increased tumor growth needs
- Vomiting as disease progresses related to possible obstruction

Tumor on left colon

- Intestinal obstruction including abdominal distention, pain, vomiting, cramps, and rectal pressure related to increasing tumor size and ulceration of mucosa
- Dark red or bright red blood in stools secondary to erosion and ulceration of mucosa

TEST RESULTS

- Digital rectal examination detects 15% of colorectal cancers, specifically rectal and perianal lesions.
- Fecal occult blood test detects blood in stools.
- Proctoscopy or sigmoidoscopy detects lesion in the GI tract.
- Colonoscopy reveals lesion in the colon up to the ileocecal valve.
- Barium enema locates lesions not visible or palpable.
- Computed tomography scan helps to detect cancer spread.
- Carcinoembryonic antigen, a tumor marker, becomes elevated in about 70% of patients with colorectal cancer.
- Liver function studies reveal liver metastasis if present.

TREATMENT

- Surgical removal of the malignant tumor, adjacent tissues, and cancerous lymph nodes through laparoscopy or extensive surgery (A permanent colostomy is rarely needed.)
- Chemotherapy or chemotherapy in combination with radiation therapy given before or after surgery to most patients whose cancer has deeply perforated the bowel wall or has spread to the lymph nodes; drugs commonly used include oxaliplatin (Eloxatin) in combination with fluorouracil (5-FU) followed by leucovorin (for patients with metastatic carcinoma)

NURSING CONSIDERATIONS

- Prepare the patient for surgery as indicated and consult with the enterostomal therapist if the patient is to have a stoma postoperatively. Review postoperative care (coughing and deep breathing, placement of nasogastric tube, urinary catheter).
- Encourage the patient to discuss feelings; refer him to a home health agency for follow-up care and counseling.

> **Alert** *Anyone who has had colorectal cancer is at increased risk for another primary cancer. Instruct the patient to have yearly screening and testing and to maintain a high-fiber diet.*

Gastric cancer

Common throughout the world, gastric cancer affects all races. However, unexplained geographic and cultural differences in incidence occur; for example, mortality is high in Japan, Iceland, Chile, and Austria. In the United States, incidence has decreased 50% during the past 25 years, and the death rate from gastric cancer is one-third that of 30 years ago. Incidence is highest in men over age 40. The prognosis depends on the stage of the disease at the time of diagnosis; overall, the 5-year survival rate is about 15%.

CAUSES

This cancer is commonly associated with gastritis, chronic inflammation of the stomach, gastric ulcers, *Helicobacter pylori* bacteria, and gastric atrophy.

Predisposing factors include:
- dietary factors, including types of food preparations, physical properties of some foods, and certain methods of

food preservation (especially smoking, pickling, and salting)
- environmental influences, such as high-alcohol content and smoking
- genetic factors, implied by the fact that it's more common among people with type A blood than among those with type O; it's also more common in people with a family history of gastric cancer.

PATHOPHYSIOLOGY

According to gross appearance, gastric cancer can be classified as polypoid, ulcerating, ulcerating and infiltrating, or diffuse. The parts of the stomach affected by gastric cancer are the pylorus and antrum (50%), the lesser curvature (25%), the cardia (10%), the body of the stomach (10%) and the greater curvature (2% to 3%). Gastric cancer metastasizes rapidly to the regional lymph nodes, omentum, liver, and lungs by the following routes: walls of the stomach, duodenum, and esophagus; lymphatic system; adjacent organs; bloodstream; and peritoneal cavity.

CLINICAL FINDINGS

- Chronic dyspepsia and epigastric discomfort
- Weight loss caused by anorexia
- A feeling of fullness after eating due to the pressure of infiltrating cancer and result of metabolites released by the tumor
- Anemia and blood in stools due to ulceration and erosion of the cancer into the stomach lining
- Fatigue related to anemia
- Dysphagia if cancer is in the cardia of the stomach
- Vomiting possibly caused by pressure of the tumor on vagal nerves

TEST RESULTS

- Barium X-rays of the GI tract, with fluoroscopy, show changes such as a tumor filling defect in the outline of the stomach, loss of flexibility, and distensibility; and abnormal gastric mucosa with or without ulceration.
- Gastroscopy with fiber-optic endoscopy helps rule out other diffuse gastric mucosal abnormalities by allowing direct visualization and gastroscopic biopsy to evaluate gastric mucosal lesions.
- Endoscopy for biopsy and cytologic washings and photography with fiber-optic endoscopy determine the progress of the disease and the effect of treatment.
- Computed tomography, chest X-rays, liver and bone scans, and liver biopsy help rule out metastasis to specific organs.

TREATMENT

- Surgical removal of the tumor; the nature and extent of the lesion determines the appropriate type of surgery
- Chemotherapy for GI cancers to control symptoms and prolong survival; adenocarcinoma of the stomach responds to several drugs, including fluorouracil (5-FU), carmustine (BiCNU), doxorubicin (Adriamycin), cisplatin (Platinol-AQ), methotrexate (Trexall) and mitomycin (Mutamycin)
- Antiemetics to control nausea, which increases as cancer advances
- Sedatives and tranquilizers to control overwhelming anxiety
- Opioids to relieve severe and unremitting pain
- Radiation therapy to help eradicate cancer
- Antispasmodics and antacids to help relieve GI distress

NURSING CONSIDERATIONS

● Prepare the patient for surgery as indicated; discuss postoperative care, importance of changing position every 2 hours, deep breathing and coughing, incentive spirometry, and positioning (usually semi-Fowler's to facilitate breathing and drainage).

> **Alert** *After gastric surgery, don't irrigate or check placement of the nasogastric tube because this may cause pressure at the incision site and possible rupture.*

● To prevent vitamin B_{12} deficiency, the patient must take a replacement for the duration of his life as well as iron supplement after gastrectomy.

● During radiation therapy, encourage the patient to eat high-calorie, well-balanced meals.

● Provide dietary instruction as indicated; frequent small meals to prevent dumping syndrome.

> **Alert** *Some patients need pancreatin and sodium bicarbonate after meals to prevent or control steatorrhea and dyspepsia.*

● Provide wound care and observe for signs of infection.

● Provide support for the patient and his family; consult with home care and hospice as appropriate.

Hodgkin's disease

Hodgkin's disease causes painless, progressive enlargement of the lymph nodes, spleen, and other lymphoid tissue. This type of cancer has a higher incidence in men, is slightly more common in whites, and occurs most commonly in two age-groups: 15 to 35 and older than age 50. A family history increases the likelihood of acquiring the disease. Although the disease is fatal if untreated, recent advances have made Hodgkin's disease potentially curable, even in advanced stages. With appropriate treatment, about 90% of patients live at least 5 years.

CAUSES

The cause of Hodgkin's disease is unknown. It probably involves a virus. Many patients with Hodgkin's disease have had infectious mononucleosis, so an indirect relationship may exist between the Epstein-Barr virus and Hodgkin's disease. Another possible risk factor is occupational exposure to herbicides and other chemicals.

PATHOPHYSIOLOGY

Hodgkin's disease is characterized by painless, progressive enlargement of lymph nodes, spleen, and other lymphoid tissue resulting from proliferation of lymphocytes, histiocytes, and eosinophils. Patients also have distinct chromosome abnormalities in their lymph node cells.

CLINICAL FINDINGS

People with Hodgkin's disease can develop signs and symptoms of whole-body involvement, including:

● painless swelling of the lymph nodes, usually beginning in the neck and progressing to the axillary, inguinal, mediastinal, and mesenteric regions; enlargement of the lymph nodes, spleen, and other lymphoid tissues resulting from proliferation of lymphocytes, histiocytes, and rarely eosinophils

● Painless swelling of the face and neck due to enlargement of lymph nodes

● Nerve pain from pressure of the nodes on nerve endings

● Increased susceptibility to infection due to defective immune function

- Intermittent fever that can last for several days or weeks, night sweats, fatigue, weight loss and malaise related to a hypermetabolic state of cellular proliferation and defective immune function
- Back and neck pain with hyperreflexia related to epidural infiltration
- Extremity pain, nerve irritation, or absence of pulse due to obstruction or pressure of tumor in surrounding lymph nodes
- Pericardial friction rub, pericardial effusion, and jugular vein engorgement secondary to direct invasion from mediastinal lymph nodes

TEST RESULTS

These tests may be used to rule out other disorders that enlarge the lymph nodes:
- Lymph node biopsy confirms the presence of Reed-Sternberg cells, abnormal histiocyte (macrophage) proliferation, and nodular fibrosis and necrosis. It's also used to determine the extent of lymph node involvement.
- Bone marrow, liver, mediastinal, and spleen biopsy reveal the extent of lymph node involvement.
- Chest X-ray, abdominal computed tomography scan, lung and bone scans, lymphangiography, and laparoscopy show the extent and stage of the disease.
- Hematologic tests may show mild to severe normocytic anemia, normochromic anemia (in 50% of patients), and elevated, normal, or reduced white blood cell count and differential with neutrophilia, lymphocytopenia, monocytosis, or eosinophilia (in any combination). Elevated serum alkaline phosphatase levels indicate liver or bone involvement.

TREATMENT

Depending on the stage of the disease, the patient may receive chemotherapy, radiation therapy, or both. Correct treatment leads to longer survival and may cure many patients.
- Other treatments — autologous bone marrow or peripheral stem cell transplantation and immunotherapy, used in conjunction with chemotherapy and radiation therapy
- Chemotherapy — consisting of various combinations of drugs, including the well-known MOPP protocol (mechlorethamine [Mustargen], vincristine [Oncovin], procarbazine [Matulane], and prednisone) being the first to result in significant cures; another useful combination being doxorubicin (Adriamycin), bleomycin (Blenoxane), vinblastine, and dacarbazine (DTIC-Dome); antiemetics, sedatives, and antidiarrheals given with chemotherapy to prevent adverse GI effects

NURSING CONSIDERATIONS

- Watch for and promptly report adverse effects of radiation therapy and chemotherapy (particularly anorexia, nausea, vomiting, diarrhea, fever, and bleeding).
- Minimize adverse effects of radiation therapy by maintaining good nutrition (aided by eating small, frequent meals of favorite foods), drinking plenty of fluids, pacing activities to counteract therapy-induced fatigue, and keeping the skin in radiated areas dry.
- Provide emotional support and refer the patient to local chapters of the American Cancer Society for information, financial assistance, and supportive counseling.

Lung cancer

Although lung cancer is largely preventable, it remains the most common cause of cancer death in men and women. Lung cancer is divided into two major classes: small-cell and non–small-cell cancer. The most common type of lung cancer, accounting for almost 80% of cases, is non–small-cell cancer. Types of non–small-cell cancer include adenocarcinoma, squamous cell, and large-cell. Small-cell lung cancer accounts for 20% of all lung cancers. It starts in the hormonal cells in the lungs. Small-cell lung cancers include oat cell, intermediate, and combined (small-cell combined with squamous or adenocarcinoma). The prognosis for lung cancer is generally poor, depending on the extent of the cancer and the cells' growth rate. Only about 13% of patients survive 5 years after diagnosis.

CAUSES
- Repeated tissue trauma from inhalation of carcinogens or irritants:
  - Air pollution
  - Arsenic
  - Asbestos
  - Nickel
  - Radon
  - Tobacco smoke

PATHOPHYSIOLOGY
Almost all lung cancers start in the epithelium of the lungs. In normal lungs, the epithelium lines and protects the tissue below it. However, when exposed to irritants or carcinogens, the epithelium continuously replaces itself until the cells develop chromosomal changes and become dysplastic (altered in size, shape, and organization). Dysplastic cells don't function well as protectors, so underlying tissue gets exposed to irritants and carcinogens. Eventually, the dysplastic cells turn into neoplastic carcinoma and start invading deeper tissues.

CLINICAL FINDINGS
Because early-stage lung cancer usually produces no symptoms, this disease is usually in an advanced state at diagnosis. For example, epidermoid and small-cell carcinomas commonly produce smoker's cough, hoarseness, wheezing, dyspnea, hemoptysis, and chest pain. Adenocarcinoma and large-cell carcinoma produce fever, weakness, weight loss, anorexia, and shoulder pain. Gynecomastia may result from large-cell carcinoma.

Hypertrophic pulmonary osteoarthropathy (bone and joint pain from cartilage erosion due to abnormal production of growth hormone) may result from large-cell carcinoma and adenocarcinoma. Cushing's and carcinoid syndromes may result from small-cell carcinoma.

Hypercalcemia may result from epidermoid tumors.

Metastatic signs and symptoms depend on the location and effect of the lung cancer. These include:
- hemoptysis, atelectasis, pneumonitis, and dyspnea resulting from bronchial obstruction
- miosis, ptosis, exophthalmos, and reduced sweating resulting from cervical thoracic sympathetic nerve involvement
- piercing chest pain, increasing dyspnea, severe shoulder pain, pain radiating down the arm due to chest wall invasion
- dysphagia resulting from esophageal compression

- cough, hemoptysis, stridor, and pleural effusion resulting from local lymphatic spread
- pericardial effusion, tamponade, and arrhythmias which can occur from pericardial involvement
- dyspnea, shoulder pain, unilateral paralyzed diaphragm with paradoxical motion due to phrenic nerve involvement
- hoarseness and vocal cord paralysis from recurrent nerve invasion
- venous distention and edema of the face, neck, chest, and back due to vena caval obstruction.

TEST RESULTS
- Chest X-ray usually shows tumor size and location.
- Cytologic sputum analysis is 80% reliable and requires a specimen expectorated from the lungs and tracheobronchial tree.
- Bronchoscopy may reveal the tumor site; bronchoscopic washings provide material for cytologic and histologic study.
- Needle biopsy confirms the diagnosis in 80% of patients.
- Tissue biopsy of metastatic sites is used to assess the extent (stage) of the disease and determine prognosis and treatment.
- Thoracentesis allows chemical and cytologic examination of pleural fluid.
- Computed tomography (CT) scan may help to evaluate mediastinal and hilar lymph node involvement and the extent of the disease.
- Bone scan, CT brain scan, liver function studies, and gallium scans of the liver and spleen detects metastasis.

TREATMENT
Various combinations of surgery, radiation therapy, and chemotherapy may improve the patient's prognosis and prolong survival. Treatment depends on the stage of illness. Unfortunately, lung cancer is usually advanced at diagnosis.
- Surgery possibly involving partial lung removal (wedge resection, segmental resection, lobectomy, or radical lobectomy) or total lung removal (pneumonectomy) (Complete surgical resection is the only chance for a cure, but fewer than 25% of patients have disease that's responsive to surgery.)
- Preoperative radiation therapy possibly reducing the tumor's bulk, allowing surgical resection and improving the patient's response; also generally recommended for stage I and stage II lesions (if surgery is contraindicated) and for stage III disease confined to the involved hemothorax and the ipsilateral supraclavicular lymph nodes
- Chemotherapy—causing dramatic, although temporary, responses in patients with small-cell carcinoma; other types of lung cancer being fairly resistant to it; drug combinations including cyclophosphamide (Cytoxan), doxorubicin (Adriamycin), and vincristine; cyclophosphamide, doxorubicin, vincristine, and etoposide (VePesid); and etoposide, cisplatin (Platinol-AQ), cyclophosphamide, and doxorubicin (Unfortunately, patients usually relapse in 7 to 14 months.) (see *Chemotherapy's action in the cell cycle*, page 436)
- Gefitinib (Iressa), a drug that blocks growth factor receptor activity (approved for advanced non–small-cell lung cancer); given as monotherapy when other chemotherapeutic drugs fail and the recipient seems to be benefiting or had benefited from its use

NURSING CONSIDERATIONS
- Explain expected postoperative procedures, such as insertion of an in-

CHEMOTHERAPY'S ACTION IN THE CELL CYCLE

Some chemotherapeutic agents are cell-cycle specific, impairing cellular growth by causing changes in the cell during specific phases of the cell cycle. Other agents are cell-cycle non-specific, affecting the cell at any phase during the cell cycle. The illustration below shows where the cell-cycle-specific agents work to disrupt cancer cell growth.

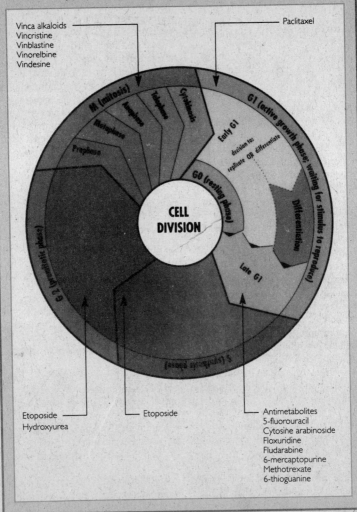

Vinca alkaloids
Vincristine
Vinblastine
Vinorelbine
Vindesine

Paclitaxel

Etoposide
Hydroxyurea

Etoposide

Antimetabolites
5-fluorouracil
Cytosine arabinoside
Floxuridine
Fludarabine
6-mercaptopurine
Methotrexate
6-thioguanine

dwelling catheter, use of an endotracheal tube or chest tube (or both), dressing changes, and I.V. therapy. Teach coughing, deep diaphragmatic breathing, and range-of-motion (ROM) exercises.

• Preoperatively, inform the patient he may take nothing by mouth beginning after midnight the night before surgery, that he'll shower with a soap-like antibacterial agent preoperatively, and he'll be given preoperative medications, such as a sedative and an anticholinergic to dry secretions.

After thoracic surgery:

• Maintain a patent airway, and monitor chest tubes to reestablish normal intrathoracic pressure and prevent postoperative and pulmonary complications.

• Suction the patient as needed, and encourage him to begin deep breathing and coughing as soon as possible.

• Monitor vital signs and monitor and record closed chest drainage. Position the patient on the surgical side to promote drainage and lung expansion.

• Watch for and report foul-smelling discharge and excessive drainage on dressing.

• To prevent pulmonary embolism, apply antiembolism stockings, sequential compression device, and encourage ROM exercises.

• If the patient is receiving chemotherapy and radiation, watch for possible adverse reactions. Provide antiemetics and antidiarrheals as needed. Schedule care activities to conserve energy.

• Provide soft, nonirritating foods that are high in protein, and encourage the patient to eat high-calorie between-meal snacks.

• Refer smokers who want to quit to local branches of the American Cancer Society or smoking-cessation programs.

Non-Hodgkin's lymphoma

Non-Hodgkin's lymphomas, also known as *malignant lymphomas,* are a heterogenous group of malignant diseases originating in the lymph glands and other lymphoid tissue. Nodular lymphomas have a better prognosis than the diffuse form of the disease, but in both, the prognosis is worse than in Hodgkin's disease. The incidence has increased 80% since the early 1970s. Non-Hodgkin's lymphomas are two to three times more common in males than in females and occur in all age-groups. They're about one to three times more common than Hodgkin's disease and cause twice as many deaths in children younger than age 15. An increased incidence occurs in whites and people of Jewish ancestry.

CAUSES
• Possibly viral source

PATHOPHYSIOLOGY
The malignant cells invade primarily the lymph nodes. Usually the first indication of malignant lymphoma is swelling of the lymph glands, enlarged tonsils and adenoids and painless, rubbery nodes in the cervical or supraclavicular areas. The disease may progress systemically, producing signs and symptoms related to the involved areas.

CLINICAL FINDINGS
• Swelling of the lymph glands, enlarged tonsils and adenoids, and pain-

less, rubbery nodes in the cervical supraclavicular areas due to infiltration of lymph nodes
- Dyspnea and coughing due to inflammation of cervical lymph nodes
- Fatigue, malaise, weight loss, fever, and night sweats due to a hypermetabolic state of cellular proliferation and defective immune function

TEST RESULTS
- Histologic evaluation of biopsied lymph nodes; of tonsils, bone marrow, liver, bowel, or skin; or of tissue removed during exploratory laparotomy confirm diagnosis.

TREATMENT
- Radiation therapy mainly in the early localized stage of the disease; total nodal irradiation generally effective for both nodular and diffuse histologies
- Chemotherapy, most effective with multiple combinations of antineoplastic drugs; for example, cyclophosphamide (Cytoxan), vincristine, doxorubicin (Adriamycin), and prednisone, which produce a complete remission in 70% to 80% of patients with nodular histology
- Monoclonal antibody therapy with rituximab (Rituxan) and radioimmunotherapy shows promise

NURSING CONSIDERATIONS
- Observe the patient who's receiving radiation or chemotherapy for anorexia, nausea, vomiting, or diarrhea. Plan small, frequent meals scheduled around treatment.
- If the patient can't tolerate oral feedings, administer I.V. fluids and, as ordered, give antiemetics and sedatives.
- Provide emotional support and refer the patient to the local chapter of

the American Cancer Society for information and counseling. Stress the need for continued treatment and follow-up care.

Ovarian cancer

Ovarian cancer is one of the leading causes of gynecological deaths in the United States. In women with previously treated breast cancer, ovarian cancer is more common than cancer at any other site and may be linked to mutations in the BRCA1 or BRCA2 gene. The prognosis varies with the histologic type and stage of the disease, but is generally poor because ovarian tumors produce few early signs and are usually advanced at diagnosis. Although about 46% of women with ovarian cancer survive for 5 years, the overall survival rate hasn't improved significantly.

CAUSES
- Familial tendency
- Infertility
- Irregular menses
- Nulliparity
- Ovarian dysfunction
- Possible exposure to asbestos, industrial pollutants, and talc

PATHOPHYSIOLOGY
Three main types of ovarian cancer exist. Primary epithelial tumors account for 90% of all ovarian cancers and include serous cystadenocarcinoma, mucinous cystadenocarcinoma, and endometrioid and mesonephric malignancies. Serous cystadenocarcinoma is the most common type and accounts for 50% of all cases. Germ cell tumors include endodermal sinus malignancies, embryonal carcinoma (a

rare ovarian cancer that appears in children), immature teratomas, and dysgerminoma. Sex cord (stromal) tumors include granulose cell tumors (which produce estrogen and may have feminizing effects), granulose-theca cell tumors, and the rare arrhenoblastomas (which produce androgen and have virilizing effects).

Primary epithelial tumors arise in the ovarian surface epithelium; germ cell tumors, in the ovum itself; and sex cord tumors, in the ovarian stroma. Ovarian tumors spread rapidly intraperitoneally by local extension or surface seeding and, occasionally, through the lymphatics and the bloodstream. Generally, extraperitoneal spread is through the diaphragm into the chest cavity, which may cause pleural effusions. Other metastasis is rare.

CLINICAL FINDINGS
* Vague abdominal discomfort, dyspepsia and other mild GI complaints from increasing size of tumor exerting pressure on nearby tissues
* Urinary frequency, constipation from obstruction resulting from increased tumor size
* Pain from tumor rupture, torsion, or infection
* Feminizing or masculinizing effects secondary to cellular type
* Ascites related to invasion and infiltration of the peritoneum
* Pleural effusions related to pulmonary metastasis

TEST RESULTS
* Abdominal ultrasound, computed tomography scan, or X-ray delineates tumor presence and size.
* Complete blood count may show anemia.

* Excretory urography reveals abnormal renal function and urinary tract abnormalities or obstruction.
* Chest X-ray reveals pleural effusion with distant metastasis.
* Barium enema shows obstruction and size of tumor.
* Lymphangiography reveals lymph node involvement.
* Liver function studies are abnormal with ascites.
* Paracentesis fluid aspiration reveals malignant cells.
* Tumor markers, such as carcinoembryonic antigen and human chorionic gonadotropin, are positive. (See *Common tumor cell markers,* page 440.)

TREATMENT
According to the staging of the disease and patient's age, treatment of ovarian cancer requires varying combinations of surgery, chemotherapy and, in some cases, radiation.
* Conservative treatment for young women or girls includes resection of the involved ovary, biopsies of the omentum and uninvolved ovary, peritoneal washings for cytologic examination of pelvic fluid, and careful follow-up, including periodic chest X-rays to rule out lung metastasis.
* Surgery may include total abdominal hysterectomy and removal of extensive metastasis as indicated. Bilateral salpingo-oophorectomy in a prepubertal girl necessitates hormone replacement therapy, beginning at puberty to induce the development of secondary sex characteristics.
* Chemotherapy extends survival time in most ovarian cancer patients, but it's largely palliative in advanced disease. Chemotherapeutic drugs include carboplatin (Paraplatin), docetaxel (Taxotere), cyclophosphamide (Cytoxan), doxorubicin (Adriamycin),

COMMON TUMOR CELL MARKERS

Tumor cell markers may be used to detect, diagnose, or treat cancer. Alone, however, they aren't sufficient for a diagnosis. Tumor cell markers may also be associated with other benign (nonmalignant) conditions. The chart below highlights some of the more commonly used tumor cell markers and their associated malignant and nonmalignant conditions.

MARKER	MALIGNANT CONDITIONS	NONMALIGNANT CONDITIONS
Alpha-fetoprotein	◆ Endodermal sinus tumor ◆ Liver cancer ◆ Ovarian germ cell cancer ◆ Testicular germ cell cancer (specifically embryonal cell carcinoma)	◆ Ataxia-telangiectasia ◆ Cirrhosis ◆ Hepatitis ◆ Pregnancy ◆ Wiskott-Aldrich syndrome
Carcinoembryonic antigen	◆ Bladder cancer ◆ Breast cancer ◆ Cervical cancer ◆ Colorectal cancer ◆ Kidney cancer ◆ Liver cancer ◆ Lung cancer ◆ Lymphoma ◆ Melanoma ◆ Ovarian cancer ◆ Pancreatic cancer ◆ Stomach cancer ◆ Thyroid cancer	◆ Inflammatory bowel disease ◆ Liver disease ◆ Pancreatitis ◆ Tobacco use
Human chorionic gonadotropin	◆ Choriocarcinoma ◆ Embryonal cell carcinoma ◆ Gestational trophoblastic disease ◆ Liver cancer ◆ Lung cancer ◆ Pancreatic cancer ◆ Specific dysgerminomas of the ovary ◆ Stomach cancer ◆ Testicular cancer	◆ Marijuana use ◆ Pregnancy
Prostatic acid phosphatase	◆ Prostate cancer	◆ Benign prostatic conditions
Prostate-specific antigen	◆ Prostate cancer	◆ Benign prostatic hyperplasia ◆ Prostatitis

paclitaxel (Taxol), cisplatin (Platinol-AQ), and topotecan (Hycamtin) given in combination.

● Radiation therapy generally isn't used for ovarian cancer because the resulting myelosuppression would limit the effectiveness of chemotherapy.

● Radioisotopes have been used as adjuvant therapy, but they cause small-bowel obstructions and stenosis.

Nursing considerations

- Before surgery, provide preoperative teaching and explain what to expect postoperatively: deep breathing and coughing, I.V. therapy, and range of motion.
- Postoperatively monitor vital signs, intake and output, and monitor dressings for bleeding. Monitor the patient for signs of infection.
- Provide abdominal support, and watch for abdominal distention. Reposition the patient often, and encourage her to walk shortly after surgery.
- Provide psychological support for the patient and her family and refer them to the American Cancer Society for information.

Prostate cancer

Prostate cancer is the most common cancer affecting men and the second cause of cancer death. Death rates in black men are more than twice as high as rates in white men. About 85% of these cancers originate in the posterior prostate gland; the rest grow near the urethra. Adenocarcinoma is the most common form.

Causes

- Age (more than 70% of all prostate cancer cases are diagnosed in men older than age 65)
- Diet high in saturated fats
- Ethnicity (Black men have the highest prostate cancer incidence in the world. The disease is common in North America and northwestern Europe and is rare in Asia and South America.)

Pathophysiology

Prostate cancer grows slowly. When primary lesions spread beyond the prostate gland, they invade the prostatic capsule and then spread along the ejaculatory ducts in the space between the seminal vesicles or perivesicular fascia. When prostate cancer is treated in its localized form, the 5-year survival rate is 70%; after metastasis, it's lower than 35%. Fatal prostate cancer usually results from widespread bone metastasis.

Clinical findings

Prostate cancer seldom produces signs and symptoms until it's advanced.

- Signs of advanced disease include a slow urine stream, urinary hesitancy, incomplete bladder emptying, and dysuria. These symptoms are due to obstruction caused by tumor progression. (See *Cancer's seven warning signs*, page 442.)

Test results

- Digital rectal examination (DRE) is performed to determine prostate location, size, and the presence of nodules.
- Biopsy of the prostate may distinguish between a benign or malignant mass.
- Blood tests may show elevated levels of prostate-specific antigen (PSA). Although an elevated PSA level occurs with metastasis, it also occurs with other prostate diseases.
- Transrectal prostatic ultrasonography may be used for patients with abnormal DRE and PSA findings.
- Bone scan and excretory urography determine the extent of the disease.
- Magnetic resonance imaging and computed tomography scans help define the tumor's extent.

TREATMENT

Therapy varies depending on the stage of the cancer and may include radiation, prostatectomy, and hormone therapy. Because most prostate cancers are androgen- or hormone-dependent, the main treatments are antiandrogens to suppress adrenal function or medical castration with estrogen or gonadotropin-releasing hormone analogs.

- Docetaxel (Taxotere) (chemotherapy drug)—for men with advanced prostate cancer that doesn't respond to hormone therapy; administered along with prednisone
- Chemotherapy with combinations of cyclophosphamide (Cytoxan), doxorubicin (Adriamycin), fluorouracil (5-FU), methotrexate (Trexall), estramustine (Emcyt), vinblastine, and cisplatin (Platinol) to reduce pain from metastasis (but hasn't helped patients live longer)

- Radical prostatectomy for localized lesions without metastasis; transurethral resection of the prostate to relieve an obstruction
- Radiation therapy possibly curing locally invasive lesions in early disease and relieving bone pain from metastatic skeletal involvement; used prophylactically to prevent tumor growth for patients with tumors in regional lymph nodes
- Radioactive 'seeds' implanted into the prostate to increase radiation to the area while minimizing exposure to surrounding tissues

NURSING CONSIDERATIONS

- Before prostatectomy discuss tube placement and dressing changes, and aftereffects of surgery, such as impotence and incontinence. Teach the patient to perform perineal exercises by squeezing his buttocks together and holding a few seconds, then relaxing.
- *Alert* *Regularly check the dressing, incision, and drainage systems for excessive bleeding; watch the patient for signs of bleeding (pallor, falling blood pressure, rising pulse rate) and infection.*
- Give antispasmodics, as ordered, to control postoperative bladder spasms. Give analgesics as needed.
- Provide catheter care. Check tubing of three-way catheter for kinks and blockages, especially if the patient reports pain. Warn him not to pull on the catheter.
- After transurethral prostatic resection, watch for signs of urethral stricture and abdominal distention. Irrigate the catheter as ordered.
- After perineal prostatic prostatectomy, avoid taking rectal temperatures or inserting rectal tubes. Provide pads to absorb urine leakage, a rubber ring for the patient to sit on, and sitz baths for pain and inflammation.

- After radiation therapy, watch for common adverse effects: proctitis, diarrhea, bladder spasms, and urinary frequency. Encourage the patient to drink at least 2 qt (2 L) of fluids daily to avoid cystitis, which is common in the first 2 to 3 weeks of treatment.

Skin cancer

Malignant melanoma is the most lethal skin cancer. It accounts for 1% to 2% of all malignant tumors, is slightly more common in women, is unusual in children, and occurs most commonly between ages 40 and 50. The incidence in younger age-groups is increasing because of increased sun exposure or, possibly, a decrease in the ozone layer.

CAUSES
Risk factors for developing melanoma are:
- blue eyes, Celtic or Scandinavian ancestry, fair skin, red hair, and susceptibility to sunburn; melanoma in Blacks is rare
- excessive exposure to sunlight
- family history of melanoma
- hormonal factors such as pregnancy
- increased nevi
- past history of melanoma
- tendency to freckle from the sun.

PATHOPHYSIOLOGY
An organelle in the melanocyte called a melanosome is responsible for producing melanin. One theory proposes that melanoma arises because the melanosome is abnormal or absent. This disease arises from melanocytes (cells that synthesize the pigment melanin). In addition to the skin, melanocytes are also found in the meninges, alimentary canal, respiratory tract, and lymph nodes.

Melanoma spreads through the lymphatic and vascular systems and metastasizes to the regional lymph nodes, skin, liver, lungs, and central nervous system. In most patients, superficial lesions are curable, but deeper lesions are more likely to metastasize. Common sites are the head and neck in men, the legs in women, and the backs of people exposed to excessive sunlight. Up to 70% of malignant melanomas arise from a preexisting nevus (circumscribed malformation of the skin) or mole. (See *Skin cancer*, page 444.)

CLINICAL FINDINGS
- Malignant melanoma with preexisting skin lesion or nevus that enlarges, changes color, becomes inflamed or sore, itches, ulcerates, bleeds, changes texture, or shows signs of surrounding pigment regression (When seeking to assess the malignant potential of a mole, look for asymmetry, an irregular border, color variation, and a diameter greater than 6 mm. Changes are secondary to malignant transformation of melanocytes in the basal layer of the epidermis or within the aggregated melanocytes of an existing nevus.)
- Red, white, and blue color over a brown or black background with an irregular, notched margin typically on areas of chronic irritation, caused by superficially spreading melanoma
- Polypoidal nodule with uniformly dark discoloration appearing as a blackberry but possibly flesh colored with flecks of pigment around base, due to nodular melanoma
- Large flat freckle of tan, brown, black, whitish, or slate color with ir-

Focus in

SKIN CANCER

TYPES OF SKIN CANCER

Any changes in an existing growth on the skin or a new growth that doesn't heal or ulcerates could indicate skin cancer or precancer — a collection of abnormal cells that may become cancerous without intervention. The key to successful treatment is early detection. Most early skin cancers can be removed in a simple outpatient surgical procedure. If left untreated, skin cancers can spread, leading to disability or even death.

Precancer

Actinic keratosis exhibits abnormal changes in keratinocytes that could someday become squamous cell carcinoma.

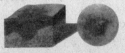

Dysplastic nevus exhibits abnormal growth of cells in a mole (melanocytes) that may someday become melanoma.

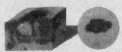

LESS SEVERE

Cancer

Basal cell carcinoma, the most common skin cancer, begins as a papule, enlarges, and develops a central crater. This cancer usually only spreads locally.

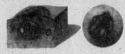

Squamous cell carcinoma begins as a firm, red nodule or scaly, crusted flat lesion. If not treated, this cancer can spread.

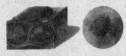

Malignant melanoma can arise on normal skin or from an existing mole. If not treated promptly, it can spread downward into other areas of the skin, lymph nodes, or internal organs.

The ABCDs of malignant melanoma

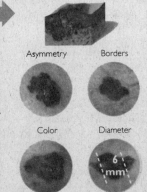

Asymmetry   Borders

Color   Diameter

MORE SEVERE

regularly scattered black nodules on surface, due to lentigo maligna melanoma

TEST RESULTS

● Excisional biopsy and full-depth punch biopsy with histologic examination distinguish malignant melanoma from a benign nevus, seborrheic keratosis, or pigmented basal cell epithelioma.

● Chest X-ray, gallium scan, bone scan, magnetic resonance imaging, and computed tomography scans of the chest, abdomen, or brain may detect metastasis, depending on the depth of tumor invasion.

TREATMENT

● Surgical resection of the tumor and a 3- to 5-cm margin; extent of resection depending on the size and location of the primary lesion (If a skin graft is needed to close a wide resection, plastic surgery provides excellent cosmetic repair. Surgical treatment may also include regional lymphadenectomy.)

● Deep primary lesions possibly requiring chemotherapy, usually with dacarbazine (DTIC-Dome) (For metastatic disease, chemotherapy with dacarbazine has been used with some success.)

● Immunotherapy with bacille Calmette-Guérin vaccine in advanced melanoma (In theory, this treatment combats cancer by boosting the body's disease-fighting systems.)

● Radiation therapy, usually reserved for metastatic disease, not prolonging survival but possibly reducing pain and tumor size

● Gene therapy

NURSING CONSIDERATIONS

● After diagnosis, review with the patient what to expect before and after surgery, what the wound will look like, and what type of dressing he'll have. Warn him that the donor site for a skin graft may be as painful as the tumor excision site, if not more so.

● After surgery, check dressings for signs of infection. If surgery included lymphadenectomy, minimize lymphedema by applying a compression stocking and instructing the patient to keep the extremity elevated.

● During chemotherapy, know what adverse effects to expect and take measures to minimize them. For example, give an antiemetic, as ordered, to reduce nausea and vomiting.

● Provide support and make referrals for home care, social services, and spiritual and financial assistance as needed.

Testicular cancer

Malignant testicular tumors primarily affect young to middle-aged men and are the most common solid tumor in this group. In children, testicular tumors are rare. The prognosis varies with the cell type and disease stage, but testicular cancer is considered curable. When treated with surgery and radiation, almost all patients with localized disease survive beyond 5 years. Testicular cancer is rare in nonwhite males and accounts for fewer than 1% of male cancer deaths.

CAUSES

The incidence is higher in men with cryptorchidism, even when surgically corrected, and in men whose mothers used diethylstilbestrol during pregnancy.

PATHOPHYSIOLOGY
Most testicular tumors originate in gonadal cells. About 40% are seminomas — uniform, undifferentiated cells resembling primitive gonadal cells. The remainder are nonseminomas — tumor cells showing various degrees of differentiation.

Testicular cancer spreads through the lymphatic system to the iliac, para-aortic, and mediastinal lymph nodes and may metastasize to the lungs, liver, viscera, and bone.

CLINICAL FINDINGS
- Firm, painless smooth testicular mass and occasional complaints of heaviness secondary to tumor growth
- Gynecomastia and nipple tenderness related to tumor production of chorionic gonadotropin or estrogen
- Urinary complaints related to ureteral obstruction
- Cough, hemoptysis, and shortness of breath from invasion of the pulmonary system

TEST RESULTS
- Transillumination of testicles reveals tumor that doesn't transilluminate.
- Surgical excision and biopsy reveals cell type.
- Excretory urography detects ureteral deviation from para-aortic node involvement.
- Serum alpha-fetoprotein and beta human chorionic gonadotropin levels as tumor markers are elevated.
- Lymphangiography, ultrasound, and abdominal computed tomography scan reveal mass and possible metastasis.

TREATMENT
The extent of surgery, radiation, and chemotherapy varies with tumor cell type and stage.
- Surgery including orchiectomy and retroperitoneal node dissection; most surgeons removing the testis, not the scrotum to allow for a prosthetic implant; hormone replacement therapy possible after bilateral orchiectomy
- Radiation of the retroperitoneal and homolateral iliac nodes following removal of a seminoma (All positive nodes receive radiation after removal of a nonseminoma. Patients with retroperitoneal extension receive prophylactic radiation to the mediastinal and supraclavicular nodes.)
- For tumors beyond stage 0, chemotherapy combinations including bleomycin (Blenoxane), etoposide (VePesid), and cisplatin (Platinol); etoposide and cisplatin; and cisplatin
- Chemotherapy and radiation followed by autologous bone marrow transplantation to help unresponsive patients

NURSING CONSIDERATIONS
- Reassure the patient that sterility and impotence need not follow unilateral orchiectomy, that synthetic hormones can restore hormonal balance.
- After orchiectomy, apply an ice pack for the first day to the scrotum and provide analgesics as ordered.

Alert Check the patient for signs and symptoms of excessive bleeding, swelling, and infection.

- Provide a scrotal athletic supporter to minimize pain during ambulation.
- Provide emotional support and refer the patient to the American Cancer Society for resources.

14

FLUIDS AND ELECTROLYTES

Electrolyte balance must remain in a narrow range for the body to function. The kidneys maintain chemical balance throughout the body by producing and eliminating urine. They regulate the volume, electrolyte concentration, and acid-base balance of body fluids; detoxify and eliminate wastes; and regulate blood pressure by regulating fluid volume. The skin and lungs also play a role in fluid and electrolyte balance. Sweating results in loss of sodium and water; every breath contains water vapor.

The kidneys maintain fluid balance in the body by regulating the amount and components of fluid inside and around the cells. The fluid inside each cell is called the *intracellular fluid* (ICF). ICF contains large amounts of potassium, magnesium, and phosphate ions. The fluid in the spaces outside the cells, called *extracellular fluid* (ECF), is constantly moving. Normally, ECF includes blood plasma and interstitial fluid (the fluid between cells in tissues). In some pathology states additional fluid accumulates (third spacing), where it isn't available to expand ICF if needed.

ECF is rapidly transported through the body by circulating blood and between blood and tissue fluids by fluid and electrolyte exchange across the capillary walls. ECF contains large amounts of sodium, chloride, and bicarbonate ions, plus such cell nutrients as oxygen, glucose, fatty acids, and amino acids. It also contains carbon dioxide, transported from the cells to the lungs for excretion, and other cellular products, transported from the cells to the kidneys for excretion.

Acid-base balance

Regulation of the extracellular fluid (ECF) environment involves the ratio of acid to base, measured clinically as pH. To regulate acid-base balance, the kidneys secrete hydrogen ions (acid), reabsorb sodium (acid) and bicarbonate ions (base), acidify phosphate salts, and produce ammonium ions (acid). This keeps the blood at its normal pH of 7.35 to 7.45.

The regulation of intracellular and extracellular electrolyte concentrations depends on balance between the intake of substances containing electrolytes and the output of electrolytes in urine, feces, and sweat. It also depends on transport of fluid and electrolytes between ECF and intracellular fluid (ICF). Fluid imbalance occurs when regulatory mechanisms can't compensate for abnormal intake and output at any level from the cell to the organism. Increased fluid volume in the interstitial spaces is called *edema*. Edema may be localized (obstruction of veins or lymphatic system or increased vascular permeability such as the swelling around an injury) or systemic (due to heart failure or renal disease). Edema results from abnormal expansion of the interstitial fluid or the accumulation of fluid in a third space, such as the peritoneum (ascites), pleural cavity (hydrothorax), or pericardial sac (pericardial effusion).

TONICITY

Many fluid and electrolyte disorders are classified according to how they affect osmotic pressure, or tonicity. Tonicity describes the relative concentrations of electrolytes (osmotic pressure) on both sides of a semipermeable membrane (the cell wall or the capillary wall). The word normal in this context refers to the usual electrolyte concentration of physiologic fluids. Normal saline has a sodium chloride concentration of 0.9%. Isotonic solutions have the same electrolyte concentration and therefore the same osmotic pressure as ECF. Hypertonic solutions have a greater than normal concentration of some essential electrolyte, usually sodium. Hypotonic solutions have a lower than normal concentration of some essential electrolyte, also usually sodium.

Isotonic alterations or disorders don't make the cells swell or shrink because osmosis doesn't occur. They occur when ICF and ECF have equal osmotic pressure, but there's a dramatic change in total-body fluid volume. Examples include blood loss from penetrating trauma or expansion of fluid volume if a patient receives too much normal saline solution.

Hypertonic alterations occur when the ECF is more concentrated than the ICF. Water flows out of the cell through the semipermeable cell membrane, causing cell shrinkage. This can occur when a patient is given hypertonic (greater than 0.9%) saline, when severe dehydration causes hypernatremia (high sodium concentration in blood), or when renal disease causes sodium retention.

When the ECF becomes hypotonic, osmotic pressure forces some ECF into the cells, causing them to swell. Overhydration is the most common cause; as water dilutes the ECF, it becomes hypotonic with respect to the ICF. Water moves into the cells until balance is restored. In extreme hypotonicity, cells may swell until they burst and die.

Pathophysiologic changes

Acidemia is an arterial pH of less than 7.35, which reflects a relative excess of acid in the blood. The hydrogen ion content in extracellular fluid (ECF) increases and the hydrogen ions move to the intracellular fluid (ICF). To keep the ICF electrically neutral, an equal amount of potassium leaves the cell, creating a relative hyperkalemia.

Acidosis is a systemic increase in hydrogen ion (H^+) concentration. If the lungs fail to eliminate carbon dioxide (CO_2) or if volatile (carbonic) or nonvolatile (lactic) acid products of metabolism accumulate, H+ concentration rises. Acidosis can also occur if persistent diarrhea causes loss of basic bicarbonate (HCO_3^-) anions or the kidneys fail to reabsorb HCO_3^- or secrete H+. (See *Interpreting ABG values*, pages 450 and 451.)

Alkalemia is arterial blood pH greater than 7.45, which reflects a relative excess of base in the blood. In alkalemia, an excess of H+ in the ICF forces them into the ECF. To keep the ICF electrically neutral, potassium moves from the ECF to the ICF, creating a relative hypokalemia.

Alkalosis is a body-wide decrease in H+ concentration. An excessive loss of CO_2 during hyperventilation, loss of nonvolatile acids during vomiting, or excessive ingestion of base may decrease H+ concentration.

BUFFER SYSTEMS

A buffer system consists of a weak acid (that doesn't readily release free H+) and a corresponding base, such as sodium bicarbonate. These buffers resist or minimize a change in pH when an acid or base is added to the buffered solution. Buffers work in seconds.

The four major buffers or buffer systems are:
- carbonic acid–bicarbonate system (the most important, works in lungs)
- hemoglobin (Hb)–oxyhemoglobin system (works in red blood cells), Hb binds free hydrogen, blood flows through lungs, hydrogen combines with CO_2
- other protein buffers (in ECF and ICF)
- phosphate system (primarily in ICF).

When primary disease processes alter either the acid or base component of the ratio, the lungs or kidneys (whichever isn't affected by the disease process) act to restore the ratio and normalize pH. Because the body's mechanisms that regulate pH occur in stepwise fashion over time, the body tolerates gradual changes in pH better than abrupt ones.

COMPENSATION BY THE KIDNEYS

If a respiratory disorder causes acidosis or alkalosis, the kidneys respond by altering their handling of H+ and HCO_3^- to return the pH to normal. Renal compensation begins hours to days after a respiratory alteration in pH. Despite this delay, renal compensation is powerful.
- Acidemia: the kidneys excrete excess H+, which may combine with phosphate or ammonia to form titratable acids in the urine. The net effect is to raise the concentration of HCO_3^- in the ECF and to restore acid-base balance.
- Alkalemia: the kidneys excrete excess HCO_3^-, usually with sodium ions. The net effect is to reduce the concentration of HCO_3^- in the ECF and to restore acid-base balance.

COMPENSATION BY THE LUNGS

If acidosis or alkalosis results from a metabolic or renal disorder, the respiratory system regulates the respiratory rate to return the pH to normal. The partial pressure of arterial carbon dioxide ($PaCO_2$) reflects CO_2 levels proportionate to blood pH. As the concentration of the gas increases, so does its partial pressure. Within minutes after the slightest change in $PaCO_2$, central chemoreceptors in the medulla that regulate the rate and depth of ventilation detect the change.

INTERPRETING ABG VALUES

This chart compares abnormal arterial blood gas (ABG) values and their significance for patient care.

DISORDER	pH	PACO$_2$ (MM HG)	HCO$_3^-$ (MEQ/L)
Normal	7.35 to 7.45	35 to 45	22 to 26
Respiratory acidosis	< 7.35	> 45	◆ Acute: may be normal ◆ Chronic: > 26
Respiratory alkalosis	> 7.45	< 35	◆ Acute: may be normal ◆ Chronic: < 22
Metabolic acidosis	< 7.35	< 35	< 22
Metabolic alkalosis	> 7.45	> 45	> 26

● Acidemia increases respiratory rate and depth to eliminate CO_2.
● Alkalemia decreases respiratory rate and depth to retain CO_2.

Calcium imbalance

Calcium plays an indispensable role in cell permeability, formation of bones and teeth, blood coagulation, transmission of nerve impulses, and normal muscle contraction. Nearly all (99%) of the body's calcium is found in the bones. The remaining 1% exists in ionized form in serum, and it's the maintenance of the 1% of ionized calcium in the serum that's critical to healthy neurologic function. The parathyroid glands regulate ionized calcium and determine its resorption into the bone, absorption from the GI mucosa, and excretion in urine and

stools. Severe calcium imbalance requires emergency treatment because an excess (hypercalcemia) can lead to cardiac arrhythmias and coma; deficit (hypocalcemia), tetany and seizures. (See *Controlling mineral balance*, pages 452 and 453.)

CAUSES
Hypercalcemia
● Adrenal insufficiency
● Hyperparathyroidism
● Hyperthyroidism
● Hypervitaminosis D
● Milk alkali syndrome
● Multiple fractures and prolonged immobilization
● Multiple myeloma
● Sarcoidosis
● Thiazide diuretics
● Tumors

Hypocalcemia
● Hypomagnesemia

◆ Renal: increased secretion and excretion of acid; compensation takes 24 hours to begin
◆ Respiratory: rate increases to expel carbon dioxide (CO_2)

◆ Renal: decreased hydrogen ion secretion and active secretion of bicarbonate (HCO_3^-) into urine

◆ Respiratory: lungs expel more CO_2 by increasing rate and depth of respirations

◆ Respiratory: hypoventilation is immediate but limited because of ensuing hypoxemia
◆ Renal: more effective but slow to excrete less acid and more base

● Hypoparathyroidism
● Inadequate intake of calcium and vitamin D
● Malabsorption or loss of calcium from the GI tract
● Overcorrection of acidosis
● Pancreatic insufficiency
● Renal failure
● Severe burns or infections

PATHOPHYSIOLOGY

Hypercalcemia may be caused by hyperparathyroidism, which increases serum calcium levels by promoting calcium absorption from the intestine, resorption from bone, and reabsorption from the kidneys. Hypervitaminosis D can promote increased absorption of calcium from the intestine. Tumors raise serum calcium levels by destroying bone or by releasing PTH or a PTH-like substance, osteoclast-activating factor, prostaglandins and, perhaps, a vitamin D-like sterol. Mul-

tiple fractures and prolonged immobilization release bone calcium and raise the serum calcium level. Multiple myeloma promotes loss of calcium from the bone. When calcium levels are greater than 3.2 mmol/L (13 mg/dl), calcification in kidneys, skin, vessels, lungs, heart, and stomach occurs and renal insufficiency may develop, especially if blood phosphate levels are normal or elevated due to impaired renal function. Severe hypercalcemia (serum levels that exceed 4.5 mmol/L or greater than 18 mg/dl) may produce cardiac arrhythmias and, eventually, coma.

Hypocalcemia caused by inadequate intake of calcium and vitamin D results in inhibited intestinal absorption of calcium. Hypoparathyroidism as a result of injury, disease, or surgery decreases or eliminates secretion of parathyroid hormone (PTH), which is necessary for calcium absorption and normal serum calcium levels. Malabsorption or loss of calcium from the GI tract can result from increased intestinal motility from severe diarrhea or laxative abuse. Malabsorption of calcium from the GI tract can also result from inadequate levels of vitamin D or PTH or a reduction in gastric acidity, which decreases the solubility of calcium salts. Severe burns or infections can lead to diseased and burned tissue trapping calcium from the extracellular fluid. Overcorrection of acidosis can lead to alkalosis, which causes decreased ionized calcium and induces symptoms of hypocalcemia. Pancreatic insufficiency may cause malabsorption of calcium and subsequent calcium loss in stools. In pancreatitis, participation of calcium ions in saponification contributes to calci-

(Text continues on page 454.)

CONTROLLING MINERAL BALANCE

Normally, the blood absorbs calcium from the digestive system and deposits it into the bones. In osteoporosis, blood levels of calcium are reduced because of dietary calcium deficiency, inability of the intestines to absorb calcium, or postmenopausal estrogen defi-

ciency. To maintain the blood calcium level as close to normal as possible, resorption from the bones increases, causing osteoporosis.

In addition to enhancing bone resorption, low calcium enhances the effects of two other factors: parathyroid hormone (PTH) and

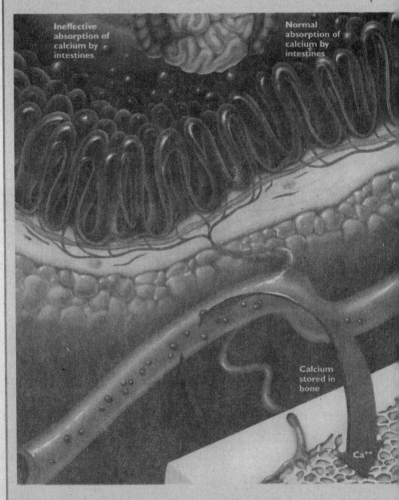

Ineffective
absorption of
calcium by
intestines

Normal
absorption of
calcium by
intestines

Calcium
stored in
bone

Ca++

vitamin D. PTH is produced by the parathyroid glands, which are buried in the thyroid gland. Vitamin D is supplied by the diet, produced in the skin as a reaction to sunlight, and processed into a highly potent form in the liver and kidneys. Both substances stimulate calcium absorption from the intestine and increase resorption from the bone. This results in an increased sacrifice of bone calcium to maintain normal levels of calcium in the blood.

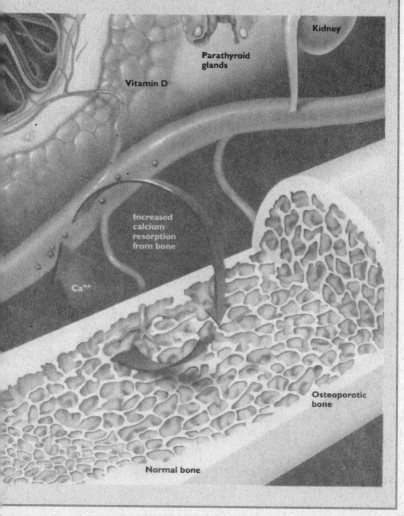

Kidney

Parathyroid glands

Vitamin D

Increased calcium resorption from bone

Ca++

Osteoporotic bone

Normal bone

um loss. Renal failure results in excessive excretion of calcium secondary to increased phosphate retention. Renal failure also results in loss of the active metabolite of vitamin D, which impairs calcium absorption. Hypomagnesemia causes decreased PTH secretion and blocks the peripheral action of that hormone.

CLINICAL FINDINGS
Hypercalcemia
- Drowsiness, lethargy, headaches, irritability, confusion, depression, or apathy due to decreased neuromuscular irritability (increased threshold)
- Weakness and muscle flaccidity due to depressed neuromuscular irritability and release of acetylcholine at the myoneural junction
- Bone pain and pathological fractures due to calcium loss from bones
- Heart block due to decreased neuromuscular irritability
- Anorexia, nausea, vomiting, constipation, and dehydration due to hyperosmolality
- Flank pain due to renal calculi formation

Hypocalcemia
Characteristic signs and symptoms of hypocalcemia are due to enhanced neuromuscular irritability. These include:
- periorbital paresthesia
- anxiety, irritability, and twitching
- carpopedal spasm
- tetany
- seizures
- hypotension and cardiac arrhythmias due to increased calcium influx.

Alert Although Chvostek's and Trousseau's signs are reliable indicators of hypocalcemia, they aren't specific.

TEST RESULTS
Hypercalcemia
- A serum calcium level above 5.5 mEq/L confirms hypercalcemia.

Alert However, because about half of serum calcium is bound to albumin, changes in serum protein must be considered when interpreting serum calcium levels.

- In patients with hypercalcemia, urine test results show an increase in urine calcium precipitation.
- In those with hypercalcemia, an electrocardiogram (ECG) reveals a shortened QT interval and heart block.

Hypocalcemia
- A serum calcium level below 4.5 mEq/L confirms hypocalcemia.
- In those with hypocalcemia, an ECG reveals lengthened QT interval, a prolonged ST segment, and arrhythmias.

TREATMENT
An acute imbalance requires immediate correction, followed by maintenance therapy and correction of the underlying cause.

Hypercalcemia
- Eliminating excess serum calcium through hydration with normal saline solution to promote calcium excretion in urine
- Loop diuretics, such as ethacrynic acid (Edecrin) and furosemide (Lasix), to promote calcium excretion

Alert Because thiazide diuretics inhibit calcium excretion, they're contraindicated in hypercalcemic patients.

- Corticosteroids, such as prednisone and hydrocortisone, to treat sarcoidosis, hypervitaminosis D, and certain tumors

- Calcitonin (Miacalcin) to help in certain instances
- Sodium phosphate solution administered by mouth or by retention enema to promote calcium deposits in bone and inhibit its absorption from the GI tract

Hypocalcemia
- For mild calcium deficit, nothing more than an adjustment in diet to allow adequate intake of calcium, vitamin D, and protein, possible with oral calcium supplements
- For acute hypocalcemia (emergent situation), immediate correction by I.V. administration of calcium gluconate or calcium chloride
- For chronic hypocalcemia, vitamin D supplements to facilitate GI absorption of calcium; forms include ergocalciferol (vitamin D_2), cholecalciferol (vitamin D_3), calcitriol, and dihydrotachysterol, a synthetic form of vitamin D_2

NURSING CONSIDERATIONS
Hypercalcemia
- Monitor serum calcium levels frequently. If the serum calcium level exceeds 5.7 mEq/L, watch for cardiac arrhythmias. Increase fluid intake to dilute calcium in serum and urine and to prevent renal damage and dehydration.
- If the patient is receiving normal saline solution diuresis therapy, monitor for signs of heart failure.
- Monitor intake and output and check urine for renal calculi and acidity.
- Monitor ECG and vital signs. If the patient is receiving a cardiac glycoside, watch for signs of toxicity.

Hypocalcemia
Alert If the patient is receiving massive transfusions of citrated blood or has chronic diarrhea, severe infection, or insufficient dietary intake of calcium or protein (common in elderly patients), monitor him for hypocalcemia.
- Monitor serum calcium levels every 12 to 24 hours; a calcium level below 4.5 mEq/L requires immediate attention. When giving calcium supplements, frequently check the pH levels; an alkalotic state that exceeds 7.45 pH inhibits calcium ionization. Check for Chvostek's and Trousseau's signs.
- Slowly administer I.V. calcium gluconate in dextrose 5% in water (never in saline solution, which encourages renal calcium loss).
- When administering calcium solutions, watch for anorexia, nausea, and vomiting, which are signs of overcorrection of hypercalcemia.
- To prevent hypocalcemia, advise patients (especially elderly ones) to eat foods rich in calcium, vitamin D, and protein, such as fortified milk and cheese, soybean products, and sardines.

Chloride imbalance

Hyperchloremia and hypochloremia are conditions of excessive or deficient or serum levels of the anion chloride. A predominantly extracellular anion, chloride accounts for two-thirds of all serum anions. Secreted by stomach mucosa as hydrochloric acid, chloride provides an acid medium conducive to digestion and activation of enzymes. It also participates in maintaining acid-base and body water balances, influences the osmolality or tonicity of extracellular fluid (ECF), plays a role in the exchange of oxygen (O_2) and carbon dioxide (CO_2) in red blood cells (RBCs), and helps activate salivary amylase (which, in turn, activates the digestive process).

CAUSES
Hyperchloremia
● Administering normal saline solution I.V. or by another route, such as orally or by nasogastric tube, saline enema, or irrigation
● Compensatory mechanisms for other metabolic abnormalities, such as metabolic acidosis, brain stem injury causing neurogenic hyperventilation, and hyperparathyroidism
● Excessive chloride intake or absorption, as in hyperingestion of ammonium chloride or ureterointestinal anastomosis, leading to hyperchloremia by allowing reabsorption of chloride by the bowel
● Hemoconcentration from dehydration

Hypochloremia
● Administration of dextrose I.V. without electrolytes, interfering with chloride absorption
● Excessive chloride loss resulting from prolonged diaphoresis or diarrhea as well as loss of hydrochloric acid in gastric secretions from gastric suctioning, gastric surgery, or vomiting
● Insufficient serum chloride levels resulting from decreased chloride intake or absorption, as in low dietary sodium intake, metabolic alkalosis, potassium deficiency, and sodium deficiency

PATHOPHYSIOLOGY
Chloride is mainly an extracellular anion; it accounts for two-thirds of all serum anions. Secreted by the stomach mucosa as hydrochloric acid, it provides an acid medium for digestion and enzyme activation. Chloride also helps maintain acid-base and water balances; influences the tonicity of ECF; facilitates exchange of O_2 and CO_2 in RBCs; and helps activate salivary amylase, which triggers the digestive process. Alterations in chloride levels produce effects throughout the body. (See *Hypochloremic alkalosis*.)

CLINICAL FINDINGS
Hyperchloremia
● Agitation, tachycardia, hypertension, pitting edema, and dyspnea result from associated ECF volume excess
● Hyperchloremia associated with excretion of base bicarbonate by the kidneys, inducing deep, rapid breathing; weakness; diminished cognitive ability; and ultimately, coma

Alert *Because of the natural affinity of sodium and chloride ions, chloride imbalance commonly produces signs and symptoms also associated with sodium imbalance.*

Hypochloremia
● Characteristic muscle weakness and twitching that mark hyponatremia because renal chloride loss always accompanies sodium loss, and sodium reabsorption isn't possible without chloride
● If chloride depletion results from metabolic alkalosis secondary to loss of gastric secretions, chloride is lost independently from sodium; typical signs and symptoms including muscle

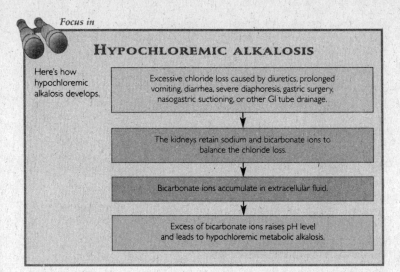

HYPOCHLOREMIC ALKALOSIS

Here's how hypochloremic alkalosis develops.

Excessive chloride loss caused by diuretics, prolonged vomiting, diarrhea, severe diaphoresis, gastric surgery, nasogastric suctioning, or other GI tube drainage.

↓

The kidneys retain sodium and bicarbonate ions to balance the chloride loss.

↓

Bicarbonate ions accumulate in extracellular fluid.

↓

Excess of bicarbonate ions raises pH level and leads to hypochloremic metabolic alkalosis.

hypertonicity, tetany, and shallow depressed breathing

TEST RESULTS
Hyperchloremia
● Hyperchloremia occurs when the serum chloride is greater than 108 mEq/L.
● Other supportive test results include a serum pH less than 7.35 and a serum CO_2 less than 22 mEq/L.

Hypochloremia
● Hypochloremia occurs when the serum chloride level is less than 98 mEq/L.
● Other supportive test results include a serum pH greater than 7.45 and a serum CO_2 greater than 32 mEq/L.

TREATMENT
With either kind of chloride imbalance, treatment must correct the underlying disorder.

Hyperchloremia
● I.V. sodium bicarbonate for severe hyperchloremic acidosis to raise serum bicarbonate level and permit renal excretion of the chloride anion because bicarbonate and chloride compete for combination with sodium
● Lactated Ringer's solution I.V. for mild hyperchloremia; converting to bicarbonate in the liver, thus increasing base bicarbonate to correct acidosis

Hypochloremia
● Correction of underlying condition causing excessive chloride loss
● Giving oral replacement (such as salty broth); or I.V. normal saline solution (if hypovolemia is present)
● Administration of a chloride-containing drug such as ammonium chloride to increase serum chloride levels
● Potassium chloride for metabolic alkalosis

NURSING CONSIDERATIONS

● Monitor for respiratory difficulty in patients with chloride imbalance.
● Monitor serum chloride levels and watch for signs of over-correction.
● Watch for excessive or continuous loss of gastric secretions as well as prolonged infusion of dextrose in water without saline, which can induce hypochloremia.

Alert *Watch for signs of metabolic acidosis. When administering I.V. fluids containing lactated Ringer's solution, monitor flow rate according to the patient's age, physical condition, and bicarbonate level, watching for irregularities.*

> ☀ **Life-threatening**
> ## *Fluid imbalance*

Disorders of fluid imbalance include hypervolemia and hypovolemia.

The expansion of extracellular fluid (ECF) volume, called *hypervolemia,* may involve the interstitial or intravascular space. Hypervolemia develops when excess sodium and water are retained in about the same proportions. It's always secondary to an increase in total-body sodium content, which causes water retention. Usually the body can compensate and restore fluid balance.

Water content of the human body progressively decreases from birth to old age. In the neonate, fluid accounts for as much as 75% of body weight; in adults, about 60% of body weight; and in elderly individuals, about 55%. Most of the decrease occurs in the first 10 years of life. *Hypovolemia,* or ECF volume deficit, is the isotonic loss of body fluids, that is, relatively equal losses of sodium and water.

Alert *Infants are at risk for hypovolemia because their bodies need to have a higher proportion of water to total body weight.*

CAUSES
Hypervolemia

● Conditions that increase the risk of sodium and water retention, including cirrhosis of the liver, corticosteroid therapy, heart failure, low dietary protein intake, nephrotic syndrome, and renal failure
● Fluid shift to the ECF compartment possibly following remobilization of fluid after burn treatment; hypertonic fluids, such as mannitol (Osmitrol) or hypertonic saline solution; and colloid oncotic fluids such as albumin
● Sources of excessive sodium and water intake including blood or plasma replacement; dietary intake of water, sodium chloride, or other salts; and parenteral fluid replacement with normal saline or lactated Ringer's solution

Hypovolemia

● Excessive fluid loss, reduced fluid intake, third-space fluid shift, and a combination of these factors causing ECF volume loss
● Fluid loss causes including abdominal surgery, diabetes mellitus with polyuria or diabetes insipidus, diarrhea or vomiting, excessive diuretic therapy, excessive use of laxatives, excessive perspiration, fever, fistulas, hemorrhage, nasogastric drainage, and renal failure with polyuria
● Fluid shift related to burns (during the initial phase), acute intestinal obstruction, acute peritonitis, crushing injury, hip or pelvic fracture (1.5 to 2 L of blood may accumulate in tissues around the fracture), pancreatitis, and pleural effusion

Focus in

FLUID MOVEMENT IN HYPONATREMIA

This illustration shows fluid movement in hyponatremia. When serum osmolality decreases because of decreased sodium concentration, fluid moves by osmosis from the extracellular area to the intracellular area.

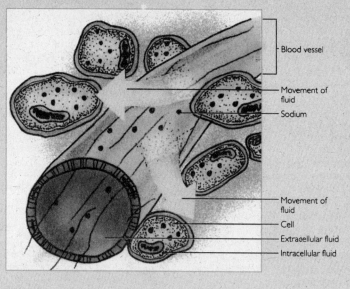

- Blood vessel
- Movement of fluid
- Sodium
- Movement of fluid
- Cell
- Extracellular fluid
- Intracellular fluid

- Possible causes of reduced fluid intake including dysphagia, coma, environmental conditions preventing fluid intake, and psychiatric illness

PATHOPHYSIOLOGY

Hypovolemia is an isotonic disorder. Fluid volume deficit decreases capillary hydrostatic pressure and fluid transport. Cells are deprived of normal nutrients that serve as substrates for energy production, metabolism, and other cellular functions. Decreased renal blood flow triggers the renin-angiotensin system to increase sodium and water reabsorption. The car-

diovascular system compensates by increasing heart rate, cardiac contractility, venous constriction, and systemic vascular resistance, thus increasing cardiac output and mean arterial pressure. Hypovolemia also triggers the thirst response, releasing more antidiuretic hormone (ADH) and producing more aldosterone. (See *Fluid movement in hyponatremia.*)

⬤ *Alert* *Elderly patients have diminished thirst sensitivity and physiologic response to hypovolemic states.*

When compensation fails, hypovolemic shock occurs in the following sequence:

- decreased intravascular fluid volume
- diminished venous return, which reduces preload and decreases stroke volume
- reduced cardiac output
- decreased mean arterial pressure
- impaired tissue perfusion
- decreased oxygen and nutrient delivery to cells
- multiple-organ-dysfunction syndrome.

In hypervolemia increased ECF volume causes the following sequence of events:
- circulatory overload
- increased cardiac contractility and mean arterial pressure
- increased capillary hydrostatic pressure
- shift of fluid to the interstitial space
- edema.

Elevated mean arterial pressure inhibits secretion of ADH and aldosterone and consequent increased urinary elimination of water and sodium. These compensatory mechanisms usually restore normal intravascular volume. If hypervolemia is severe or prolonged or the patient has a history of cardiovascular dysfunction, compensatory mechanisms may fail, and heart failure and pulmonary edema may ensue.

CLINICAL FINDINGS
Hypervolemia
- Rapid breathing due to fewer red blood cells per milliliter of blood (dilution causes a compensatory increase in respiratory rate to increase oxygenation)
- Dyspnea (labored breathing) due to increased fluid volume in pleural spaces
- Crackles (popping or bubbling sounds on auscultation) due to elevated hydrostatic pressure in pulmonary capillaries
- Rapid, bounding pulse due to increased cardiac contractility (from circulatory overload)
- Hypertension (unless heart is failing) due to circulatory overload (causes increased mean arterial pressure)
- Distended jugular veins due to increased blood volume and increased preload
- Moist skin (compensatory to increase water excretion through perspiration)
- Acute weight gain due to increased volume of total-body fluid from circulatory overload (best indicator of ECF volume excess)
- Edema (increased mean arterial pressure leads to increased capillary hydrostatic pressure, causing fluid shift from plasma to interstitial spaces)
- S_3 gallop (abnormal third heart sound due to rapid filling and volume overload of the ventricles during diastole)

Alert *Possible complications of hypervolemia include skin breakdown and acute pulmonary edema with hypoxemia.*

Hypovolemia
Signs and symptoms of hypovolemia depend on the amount of fluid loss. (See *Estimating fluid loss*.)

These may include:
- orthostatic hypotension due to increased systemic vascular resistance and decreased cardiac output
- tachycardia induced by the sympathetic nervous system to increase cardiac output and mean arterial pressure
- thirst to prompt ingestion of fluid (increased ECF osmolality stimulates the thirst center in the hypothalamus)
- flattened jugular veins due to decreased circulating blood volume

- sunken eyeballs due to decreased volume of total-body fluid and consequent dehydration of connective tissue and aqueous humor
- dry mucous membranes due to decreased body fluid volume (glands that produce fluids to moisten and protect the vascular mucous membranes fail, so they dry rapidly)
- diminished skin turgor due to decreased fluid in the dermal layer (making skin less pliant)
- rapid weight loss due to acute loss of body fluid

   Alert *In hypovolemic infants younger than age 4 months, the posterior and anterior fontanels are sunken when palpated. Between ages 4 and 18 months, the posterior fontanel is normally closed, but the anterior fontanel is sunken in hypovolemic infants.*

- decreased urine output due to decreased renal perfusion from renal vasoconstriction
- prolonged capillary refill time due to increased systemic vascular resistance.

   Alert *Possible complications of hypovolemia include shock, acute renal failure, and death.*

TEST RESULTS
Hypervolemia

No single diagnostic test confirms the disorder, but the following findings indicate hypervolemia:
- decreased serum potassium and blood urea nitrogen (BUN) levels due to hemodilution (Increased serum potassium and BUN levels usually indicate renal failure or impaired renal perfusion.)
- decreased hematocrit (HCT) due to hemodilution
- normal serum sodium (unless associated sodium imbalance is present; decreased cardiac output in patients

with cardiovascular dysfunction can trigger increased sodium resorption in the kidneys)
- low urine sodium excretion (usually less than 10 mEq/day because edematous patient is retaining sodium)
- increased hemodynamic values (including pulmonary artery, pulmonary

---

ESTIMATING FLUID LOSS

The following assessment parameters indicate the severity of fluid loss.

MINIMAL FLUID LOSS
Intravascular volume loss of 10% to 15% is regarded as minimal. Signs and symptoms include:
- slight tachycardia
- normal supine blood pressure
- positive postural vital signs, including a decrease in systolic 20 beats/minute
- increased capillary refill time (> 3 seconds)
- urine output greater than 30 ml/hour
- cool, pale skin on arms and legs
- anxiety.

MODERATE FLUID LOSS
Intravascular volume loss of about 25% is regarded as moderate. Signs and symptoms include:
- rapid, thready pulse
- supine hypotension
- cool truncal skin
- urine output of 10 to 30 ml/hour
- severe thirst
- restlessness, confusion, or irritability.

SEVERE FLUID LOSS
Intravascular volume loss of 40% or more is regarded as severe. Signs and symptoms include:
- marked tachycardia
- marked hypotension
- weak or absent peripheral pulses
- cold, mottled, or cyanotic skin
- urine output less than 10 ml/hour
- unconsciousness.

artery wedge, and central venous pressures).

Hypovolemia

No single diagnostic finding confirms hypovolemia, but the following test results are suggestive:

- increased BUN level (early sign)
- elevated serum creatinine level (late sign)
- increased serum protein and hemoglobin levels and HCT (unless caused by hemorrhage, when loss of blood elements causes subnormal values)
- rising blood glucose level
- elevated serum osmolality; except in hyponatremia, where serum osmolality is low
- serum electrolyte and arterial blood gas analysis may reflect associated clinical problems due to underlying cause of hypovolemia or treatment regimen.

If the patient has no underlying renal disorder, typical urinalysis findings include:

- urine specific gravity greater than 1.030
- increased urine osmolality
- urine sodium level less than 50 mEq/L.

TREATMENT

Hypervolemia

- Restricted sodium and water intake
- Preload reduction agents, such as morphine, furosemide (Lasix), and nitroglycerin, and afterload reduction agents, such as hydralazine (Apresoline) and captopril (Capoten) for pulmonary edema

Alert Carefully monitor I.V. fluid administration rate and patient response, especially in elderly patients or those with impaired cardiac or renal function, who are particularly vulnerable to acute pulmonary edema.

For severe hypervolemia or renal failure, the patient may undergo renal replacement therapy, including:

- hemodialysis or peritoneal dialysis
- continuous arteriovenous hemofiltration (allows removal of excess fluid from critically ill patients who may not need dialysis; the patient's arterial pressure serves as a natural pump, driving blood through the arterial line)
- continuous venovenous hemofiltration (similar to arteriovenous hemofiltration, but a mechanical pump is used when mean arterial pressure is less than 60 mm Hg).

Supportive measures include:

- oxygen administration to ensure sufficient tissue perfusion
- use of thromboembolic disease support hose to help mobilize edematous fluid
- bed rest with head of bed elevated to facilitate respiratory effort
- treatment of underlying condition that caused or contributed to hypervolemia.

Hypovolemia

- Oral fluids (may be adequate in mild hypovolemia if the patient is alert enough to swallow and can tolerate it)
- Parenteral fluids to supplement or replace oral therapy (moderate to severe hypovolemia; choice of parenteral fluid depends on type of fluids lost, severity of hypovolemia, and patient's cardiovascular, electrolyte, and acid-base status)
- Fluid resuscitation by rapid I.V. administration (severe volume depletion; depending on patient's condition, 100 to 500 ml of fluid over 15 minutes to 1 hour; fluid bolus may be given more quickly if needed)
- Blood or blood products (with hemorrhage)

- Antidiarrheals and antiemetics as needed to reduce fluid loss
- I.V. dopamine (Intropin) or norepinephrine (Levophed) to increase cardiac contractility and renal perfusion (if patient remains symptomatic after fluid replacement)
- Oxygen therapy to ensure sufficient tissue perfusion
- Autotransfusion (for some patients with hypovolemia caused by trauma)

NURSING CONSIDERATIONS
Hypervolemia
- If the patient is prone to hypervolemia, an infusion pump should be used with any infusions to prevent the administration of too much fluid.
- The patient's vital signs and hemodynamic status should be assessed to note his response to therapy. Signs of hypovolemia indicate overcorrection.

Alert Elderly, pediatric, and otherwise compromised patients are at higher risk for complications with therapy.

Hypovolemia
- The patient's mental status and vital signs should be monitored closely, including orthostatic blood pressure measurements when appropriate.
- If the blood pressure doesn't respond to interventions as expected, the patient should be reassessed for a bleeding site that may have been missed.

Magnesium imbalance

Magnesium is the second most common cation in intracellular fluid (ICF).

Approximately one-third of magnesium taken into the body is absorbed through the small intestine and eventually excreted in the urine; the remaining unabsorbed magnesium is excreted in stools.

Magnesium excess (hypermagnesemia) is common in patients with renal failure and excessive intake of magnesium-containing antacids.

Because many common foods contain magnesium, a dietary deficiency is rare. Hypomagnesemia generally follows impaired absorption, too-rapid excretion, or inadequate intake during total parenteral nutrition. It commonly coexists with other electrolyte imbalances, especially low calcium and potassium levels.

CAUSES
Hypermagnesemia results from the kidneys' inability to excrete magnesium that was either absorbed from the intestines or infused. Common causes of hypermagnesemia include:
- chronic renal insufficiency
- laxative use (magnesium sulfate, milk of magnesia, and magnesium citrate solutions), especially with renal insufficiency
- overcorrection of hypomagnesemia
- overuse of magnesium-containing antacids
- severe dehydration (resulting oliguria can cause magnesium retention).

Hypomagnesemia usually results from impaired absorption of magnesium in the intestines or excessive excretion in urine or stools. Possible causes include:
- decreased magnesium intake or absorption, as in malabsorption syndrome, chronic diarrhea, or postoperative complications after bowel resection; chronic alcoholism; prolonged diuretic therapy, nasogastric suctioning, or administration of parenteral fluids without magnesium salts; and starvation or malnutrition

excessive loss of magnesium, as in severe dehydration and diabetic acidosis; hyperaldosteronism and hypoparathyroidism, which result in hypokalemia and hypocalcemia; hyperparathyroidism and hypercalcemia; excessive release of adrenocortical hormones; and diuretic therapy.

PATHOPHYSIOLOGY

Magnesium is present in smaller quantity, but physiologically it's as significant as the other major electrolytes. The major function of magnesium is to enhance neuromuscular communication. Other functions include activating many enzymes in carbohydrate and protein metabolism; facilitating cell metabolism; facilitating sodium, potassium, and calcium transport across cell membranes; and facilitating protein transport.

Magnesium also stimulates parathyroid hormone (PTH) secretion, thus regulating ICF calcium levels. Therefore magnesium deficiency (hypomagnesemia) may result in transient hypoparathyroidism or interference with the peripheral action of PTH. Magnesium may also regulate skeletal muscles through its influence on calcium utilization by depressing acetylcholine release at synaptic junctions.

CLINICAL FINDINGS

Hypermagnesemia results in diminished reflexes, muscle weakness to flaccid paralysis due to suppression of acetylcholine release at the myoneural junction, blocking neuromuscular transmission and reducing cell excitability. Other symptoms include:
● respiratory distress secondary to respiratory muscle paralysis
● heart block and bradycardia due to decreased inward sodium current

● hypotension due to relaxation of vascular smooth muscle and reduction of vascular resistance by displacing calcium from the vascular wall surface.

Hypomagnesemia nearly always coexists with hypokalemia and hypocalcemia. Signs and symptoms include:
● hyperirritability, tetany, leg and foot cramps, positive Chvostek's and Trousseau's signs, confusion, delusions, and seizures due to alteration in neuromuscular transmission
● arrhythmias, vasodilation, and hypotension due to enhanced inward sodium current or concurrent effects of calcium and potassium imbalance.

TEST RESULTS

● Hypermagnesemia occurs when serum magnesium is greater than 2.5 mEq/L; elevated potassium and calcium levels may also exist.
● Hypomagnesemia occurs when serum magnesium levels are less than 1.5 mEq/L; low serum potassium and calcium levels also exist.

TREATMENT
Hypermagnesemia

● Increased fluid intake and loop diuretics (such as furosemide [Lasix]) with impaired renal function
● Calcium gluconate (10%), a magnesium antagonist, for temporary relief of symptoms in an emergency
● Peritoneal dialysis or hemodialysis if renal function fails or if excess magnesium can't be eliminated

Hypomagnesemia

● For mild cases, daily magnesium supplements I.M. or orally
● For severe cases, magnesium sulfate I.V. (10 to 40 mEq/L diluted in I.V. fluid

NURSING CONSIDERATIONS
Hypermagnesemia
● Frequently assess level of consciousness, muscle activity, and vital signs.

● Keep intake and output records. Provide sufficient fluids for adequate hydration and maintenance of renal function.

● Monitor and report electrocardiogram changes (peaked T waves, increased PR intervals, widened QRS complex).

● Advise patients, particularly elderly patients and patients with compromised renal function, not to abuse laxatives and antacids containing magnesium.

Hypomagnesemia
● Monitor serum electrolyte levels (including magnesium, calcium, and potassium) daily for mild deficits and every 6 to 12 hours during replacement therapy.

● Measure intake and output frequently.

● Monitor vital signs during I.V. therapy.

Alert Infuse magnesium replacement slowly and watch for bradycardia, heart block, and decreased respiratory rate. Have calcium gluconate I.V. available to reverse hypermagnesemia from overcorrection. In patients with torsades de pointes, elevated magnesium levels are therapeutic.

● Advise patients to eat foods high in magnesium, such as fish and green vegetables.

✳ Life-threatening
Metabolic acidosis
◆

Metabolic acidosis is an acid-base disorder characterized by excess acid and deficient bicarbonate (HCO_3^-) caused by an underlying nonrespiratory disorder. A primary decrease in plasma HCO_3^- causes pH to fall. It can occur with increased production of a nonvolatile acid (such as lactic acid), decreased renal clearance of a nonvolatile acid (as in renal failure), or loss of HCO_3^- (as in chronic diarrhea). Symptoms result from action of compensatory mechanisms in the lungs, kidneys, and cells.

Alert Metabolic acidosis is more prevalent among children, who are vulnerable to acid-base imbalance because their metabolic rates are rapid and ratios of water to total-body weight are low.

Severe or untreated metabolic acidosis can be fatal. The prognosis improves with prompt treatment of the underlying cause and rapid reversal of the acidotic state.

CAUSES
Metabolic acidosis usually results from excessive fat metabolism in the absence of usable carbohydrates. This can be caused by diabetic ketoacidosis, chronic alcoholism, malnutrition, or a low-carbohydrate, high-fat diet—all of which produce more ketoacids than the metabolic process can handle. Other causes include:

● anaerobic carbohydrate metabolism (decreased tissue oxygenation or perfusion—as in cardiac pump failure after myocardial infarction, pulmonary or hepatic disease, shock, or anemia—forces a shift from aerobic to anaerobic metabolism, causing a corresponding increase in lactic acid level)

● diarrhea, intestinal malabsorption, or loss of sodium bicarbonate from the intestines, causing HCO_3^- buffer system to shift to the acidic side (for example, Crohn's disease and ureteroenterostomy can also induce metabolic acidosis)

- inhibited secretion of acid due to hypoaldosteronism or the use of potassium-sparing diuretics
- salicylate intoxication (overuse of aspirin), exogenous poisoning or less commonly, Addison's disease (increased excretion of sodium and chloride and retention of potassium)
- underexcretion of metabolized acids or inability to conserve base due to renal insufficiency and failure (renal acidosis).

PATHOPHYSIOLOGY

As acid (hydrogen [H^+]) starts to accumulate in the body, chemical buffers (plasma HCO_3^- and proteins) in the cells and extracellular fluid (ECF) bind the excess H^+. Excess H^+ that the buffers can't bind decrease blood pH and stimulate chemoreceptors in the medulla to increase respiration. The consequent fall of partial pressure of arterial carbon dioxide ($PaCO_2$) frees H^+ to bind with HCO_3^-. Respiratory compensation occurs in minutes but isn't sufficient to correct the acidosis.

Healthy kidneys try to compensate by secreting excess H^+ into the renal tubules. These ions are buffered by either phosphate or ammonia and excreted into the urine in the form of weak acid. For each H^+ secreted into the renal tubules, the tubules reabsorb and return to the blood one sodium and one HCO_3^-.

The excess H^+ in ECF passively diffuse into cells. To maintain the balance of charge across the membranes, the cells release potassium ions. Excess H^+ change the normal balance of potassium, sodium, and calcium ions and thereby impair neural excitability.

CLINICAL FINDINGS

In mild acidosis, symptoms of the underlying disease may hide the direct clinical evidence. Signs and symptoms include:

- headache and lethargy progressing to drowsiness, central nervous system (CNS) depression, Kussmaul's respirations (as the lungs attempt to compensate by blowing off carbon dioxide), hypotension, stupor, and (if condition is severe and untreated) coma and death
- associated GI distress leading to anorexia, nausea, vomiting, diarrhea, and possibly dehydration
- warm, flushed skin due to a pH-sensitive decrease in vascular response to sympathetic stimuli
- fruity-smelling breath from fat catabolism and excretion of accumulated acetone through the lungs due to underlying diabetes mellitus.

In the metabolic acidosis of chronic renal failure, HCO_3^- is drawn from bone to buffer H^+; the results include:

- growth retardation in children
- bone disorders such as renal osteodystrophy.

TEST RESULTS

The following results confirm the diagnosis of metabolic acidosis:

- arterial pH less than 7.35 (as low as 7.10 in severe acidosis)
- $PaCO_2$ normal or less than 34 mm Hg as respiratory compensatory mechanisms take hold (HCO_3^- may be 22 mEq/L)

The following test results support the diagnosis of metabolic acidosis:

- urine pH less than 4.5 in the absence of renal disease (as the kidneys excrete acid to raise blood pH)
- serum potassium level greater than 5.5 mEq/L from chemical buffering

- glucose level greater than 150 mg/dl
- serum ketone bodies in diabetes
- elevated plasma lactic acid level in lactic acidosis
- anion gap greater than 14 mEq/L in high-anion-gap metabolic acidosis, lactic acidosis, ketoacidosis, aspirin overdose, alcohol poisoning, renal failure, or other conditions characterized by accumulation of organic acids, sulfates, or phosphates
- anion gap 12 mEq/L or less in normal anion gap metabolic acidosis from HCO_3^- loss, GI or renal loss, increased acid load (hyperalimentation fluids), rapid I.V. saline administration, or other conditions characterized by loss of HCO_3^-

TREATMENT

Treatment aims to correct the acidosis as quickly as possible by addressing both the symptoms and the underlying cause. Measures may include:
- sodium bicarbonate I.V. for severe high anion gap to neutralize blood acidity in patients with pH less than 7.20 and HCO_3^- loss; monitor plasma electrolytes, especially potassium, during sodium bicarbonate therapy (potassium level may fall as pH rises)
- I.V. lactated Ringer's solution to correct normal anion gap metabolic acidosis and ECF volume deficit
- evaluation and correction of electrolyte imbalances
- correction of the underlying cause (for example, in diabetic ketoacidosis, continuous low-dose I.V. insulin infusion)
- mechanical ventilation to maintain respiratory compensation if needed
- antibiotic therapy to treat infection
- dialysis for patients with renal failure or certain drug toxicities

- antidiarrheal agents for diarrhea-induced HCO_3^- loss
- monitor for secondary changes due to hypovolemia such as falling blood pressure (in diabetic acidosis).

NURSING CONSIDERATIONS
- Administer sodium bicarbonate according to arterial blood gas results as directed; frequently monitor vital signs, laboratory results, and level of consciousness because changes can occur rapidly.
- In diabetic acidosis, watch for secondary changes due to hypovolemia such as decreasing blood pressure.
- Record intake and output accurately to monitor renal function. Watch for signs of excessive serum potassium (weakness, flaccid paralysis, and arrhythmias, possibly leading to cardiac arrest). After treatment, check for overcorrection to hypokalemia.
- Because metabolic acidosis commonly causes vomiting, position the patient to prevent aspiration. Prepare for possible seizures with seizure precautions.

✴ Life-threatening

Metabolic alkalosis

Metabolic alkalosis occurs when low levels of acid or high bicarbonate (HCO_3^-) cause metabolic, respiratory, and renal responses, producing characteristic symptoms (most notably, hypoventilation). This condition is always secondary to an underlying cause. With early diagnosis and prompt treatment, prognosis is good, but untreated metabolic alkalosis may lead to coma and death.

CAUSES

Metabolic alkalosis results from loss of acid, retention of base, or renal mechanisms associated with low serum levels of potassium and chloride

● Alterations in extracellular electrolyte levels causing metabolic alkalosis include low chloride (as chloride diffuses out of the cell, hydrogen diffuses into the cell) and low plasma potassium causing increased hydrogen ion (H^+) excretion by the kidneys

● Critical acid loss caused by massive blood transfusions; chronic vomiting; Bartter's syndrome, Cushing's disease, and primary hyperaldosteronism (leading to sodium and chloride retention and urinary loss of potassium and hydrogen); use of certain diuretics (ethacrynic acid [Edecrin], furosemide [Lasix], and thiazides) and steroids; fistulas; and nasogastric (NG) tube drainage or lavage without adequate electrolyte replacement

● Excessive HCO_3^- retention causing chronic hypercapnia can result from excessive intake of absorbable alkali (as in milk alkali syndrome, commonly seen in patients with peptic ulcers); excessive intake of bicarbonate of soda or other antacids (usually for treatment of gastritis or peptic ulcer); excessive amounts of I.V. fluids with high concentrations of HCO_3^- or lactate; and respiratory insufficiency

PATHOPHYSIOLOGY

Chemical buffers in extracellular (ECF) and intracellular fluid bind HCO_3^- that accumulates in the body. Excess unbound HCO_3^- raises blood pH, which depresses chemoreceptors in the medulla, inhibiting respiration and raising partial pressure of arterial carbon dioxide ($Paco_2$). Carbon dioxide combines with water to form carbonic acid. Low oxygen levels limit respiratory compensation.

When the blood HCO_3^- rises to 28 mEq/L or more, the amount filtered by the renal glomeruli exceeds the reabsorptive capacity of the renal tubules. Excess HCO_3^- is excreted in the urine, and H^+ are retained. To maintain electrochemical balance, sodium ions (Na^+) and water are excreted with the HCO_3^-.

When H^+ levels in ECF are low, H^+ diffuse passively out of the cells and, to maintain the balance of charge across the cell membrane, extracellular potassium ions move into the cells. As intracellular H^+ levels fall, calcium ionization decreases, and nerve cells become more permeable to sodium ions. As Na^+ move into the cells, they trigger neural impulses, first in the peripheral nervous system and then in the central nervous system.

CLINICAL FINDINGS

Clinical features of metabolic alkalosis result from the body's attempt to correct the acid-base imbalance, primarily through hypoventilation. Signs and symptoms include:

● irritability, picking at bedclothes (carphology), twitching, and confusion due to decreased cerebral perfusion

● nausea, vomiting, and diarrhea (which aggravate alkalosis)

● cardiovascular abnormalities due to hypokalemia

● respiratory disturbances (such as cyanosis and apnea) and slow, shallow respirations

● diminished peripheral blood flow during repeated blood pressure checks may provoke carpopedal spasm in the hand (Trousseau's sign, a possible sign of impending tetany).

Alert *Uncorrected metabolic alkalosis may progress to seizures and coma.*

TEST RESULTS

- A blood pH greater than 7.45 and HCO_3^- greater than 26 mEq/L confirm diagnosis.
- $Paco_2$ greater than 45 mm Hg indicates attempts at respiratory compensation.
- Low potassium (less than 3.5 mEq/L), calcium (less than 8.9 mg/dl), and chloride (less than 98 mEq/L) indicate metabolic alkalosis.
- Urine pH above 7 confirms diagnosis.
- Alkaline urine after the renal compensatory mechanism begins to excrete HCO_3^- confirms diagnosis.
- Electrocardiogram may show low T wave, merging with a P wave, and atrial or sinus tachycardia.

TREATMENT

The goal of treatment is to correct the underlying cause of metabolic alkalosis. Possible treatments include:

- cautious use of ammonium chloride I.V. (rarely) or hydrochloric acid to restore ECF hydrogen and chloride levels
- potassium chloride (KCl) and normal saline solution (except in heart failure); usually sufficient to replace losses from gastric drainage
- discontinuation of diuretics and supplementary KCl (metabolic alkalosis from potent diuretic therapy)
- oral or I.V. acetazolamide (Diamox; enhances renal HCO_3^- excretion) to correct metabolic alkalosis without rapid volume expansion (acetazolamide also enhances potassium excretion, so potassium may be given before drug).

NURSING CONSIDERATIONS

- When administering ammonium chloride 0.9%, limit the infusion rate to 1 L in 4 hours; faster administration may cause hemolysis of red blood cells.
- Watch the patient closely for signs of muscle weakness, tetany, or decreased activity. Monitor vital signs frequently, and record intake and output to evaluate respiratory, fluid, and electrolyte status.
- Observe seizure precautions.
- To prevent metabolic alkalosis, warn patients against overusing alkaline agents. Irrigate NG tubes with isotonic saline solution instead of plain water to prevent loss of gastric electrolytes. Monitor I.V. fluid concentrations of HCO_3^- or lactate.

Phosphorus imbalance

Phosphorus exists primarily in inorganic combination with calcium in teeth and bones. In extracellular fluid, the phosphate ion supports several metabolic functions; utilization of B vitamins, acid-base homeostasis, bone formation, nerve and muscle activity, cell division, transmission of hereditary traits, and metabolism of carbohydrates, proteins, and fats. Renal tubular reabsorption of phosphate is inversely regulated by calcium levels— an increase in phosphorus causes a decrease in calcium. An imbalance causes hyperphosphatemia or hypophosphatemia. Hyperphosphatemia is most common in children, who tend to consume more phosphorus-rich foods and beverages than adults, and in children and adults with renal insufficiency. Incidence of hypo-

PARATHYROID HORMONE AND PHOSPHORUS

This illustration shows how parathyroid hormone (PTH) affects serum phosphorus (P) levels — by increasing phosphorus release from bone, increasing phosphorus absorption from the intestines, and decreasing phosphorus reabsorption in the renal tubules.

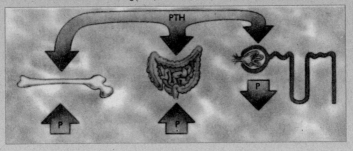

phosphatemia varies with the underlying cause. The prognosis for both conditions depends on the underlying cause.

CAUSES
Hyperphosphatemia
● Generally secondary to hypocalcemia, hypervitaminosis D, hypoparathyroidism, or renal failure (usually due to stress or injury)
● Overuse of laxatives with phosphates or phosphate enemas

Hypophosphatemia
● Chronic use of antacids containing aluminum hydroxide, diabetic acidosis, use of parenteral nutrition solution with inadequate phosphate content, renal tubular defects, and tissue damage in which phosphorus is released by injured cells
● Inadequate dietary intake; commonly related to malnutrition resulting from a prolonged catabolic state or chronic alcoholism
● Intestinal malabsorption, chronic diarrhea, hyperparathyroidism with resultant hypercalcemia, hypomagnesemia, or deficiency of vitamin D, which is necessary for intestinal phosphorus absorption

PATHOPHYSIOLOGY
The phosphate anion is involved in cellular metabolism as well as neuromuscular regulation and hematologic function. Phosphate reabsorption in the renal tubules is inversely related to calcium levels, which means that an increase in urinary phosphorous triggers calcium reabsorption and vice versa. (See *Parathyroid hormone and phosphorus*.)

CLINICAL FINDINGS
Hyperphosphatemia usually doesn't produce symptoms unless leading to hypocalcemia, with tetany and seizures.

Hypophosphatemia is associated with muscle weakness, tremor, and paresthesia due to deficiency of adenosine triphosphate.

TEST RESULTS

Hyperphosphatemia occurs when serum phosphate level is less than 4.5 mg/dl. Other test results include:
- serum calcium level less than 9 mg/dl
- urine phosphorus level less than 0.9 g/24 hours.

Hypophosphatemia occurs when serum phosphate level is less than 2.5 mg/dl; urine phosphate level is greater than 1.3 g/24 hours.

TREATMENT

- Phosphorus replacement with a high-phosphorus diet and oral administration of phosphate salt tablets or capsules
- For severe hyperphosphatemia, peritoneal dialysis or hemodialysis to lower the serum phosphorus level
- For severe hypophosphatemia, I.V. infusion of potassium phosphate

NURSING CONSIDERATIONS

- Carefully monitor calcium, magnesium, and phosphorus levels. Report any changes immediately.

Hyperphosphatemia

- Monitor intake and output. If urine output falls below 25 ml/hour or 600 ml/day, notify the physician immediately, because decreased output can seriously affect renal clearance of excess serum phosphorus.
- Watch for signs of hypocalcemia, such as muscle twitching and tetany, which commonly accompany hyperphosphatemia.

Hypophosphatemia

- Record intake and output accurately. Administer potassium phosphate slow I.V. to prevent overcorrection to hyperphosphatemia.
- To prevent recurrence, advise the patient to follow a high-phosphorus diet containing milk and milk products, kidney, liver, turkey, and dried fruits.

Potassium imbalance

Potassium, a cation that's the dominant cellular electrolyte, facilitates contraction of both skeletal and smooth muscles—including myocardial contraction—and figures prominently in nerve impulse conduction, acid-base balance, enzyme action, and cell-membrane function. Both hyperkalemia (potassium excess) and hypokalemia (potassium deficiency) can lead to muscle weakness and flaccid paralysis because both create an ionic imbalance in neuromuscular tissue excitability. Both conditions also diminish excitability and conduction rate of the heart muscle, which may lead to cardiac arrest.

CAUSES
Hyperkalemia

- Injuries or conditions that release cellular potassium or favor its retention, such as adrenal gland insufficiency, burns, crushing injuries, dehydration, diabetic acidosis, or failing renal function
- Kidneys' inability to excrete excessive amounts of potassium infused I.V or administered orally; from decreased urine output, renal dysfunction, or renal failure; or from the use of potassium-sparing diuretics such as triamterene (Dyrenium) by patients with renal disease

Hypokalemia

Because many foods contain potassium, hypokalemia rarely results from a dietary deficiency. Instead, potassium loss results from:

- Acid-base imbalances, which cause potassium shifting into cells without true depletion in alkalosis
- Certain drugs, especially potassium-wasting diuretics, steroids, and certain sodium-containing antibiotics (carbenicillin [Geocillin])
- Chronic renal disease, with tubular potassium wasting
- Cushing's syndrome, primary hyperaldosteronism, excessive ingestion of licorice, and severe serum magnesium deficiency
- Excessive GI or urinary losses, such as anorexia, dehydration, diarrhea, gastric suction, prolonged laxative use, or vomiting
- Hyperglycemia, causing osmotic diuresis and glycosuria
- Prolonged potassium-free I.V. therapy
- Trauma (burns, injury, or surgery), in which damaged cells release potassium, which enters serum or extracellular fluid (ECF) to be excreted in the urine

PATHOPHYSIOLOGY

Physiologic roles of potassium include maintaining cell electrical neutrality; facilitating cardiac muscle contraction and electrical conductivity; facilitating neuromuscular transmission of nerve impulses; and maintaining acid-base balance.

CLINICAL FINDINGS
Hyperkalemia

- Tachycardia changing to bradycardia, electrocardiogram (ECG) changes, and cardiac arrest due to hypopolarization and alterations in repolarization
- Nausea, diarrhea, and abdominal cramps due to decreased gastric motility
- Muscle weakness and flaccid paralysis due to inactivation of membrane sodium channels

Hypokalemia

- Dizziness, hypotension, arrhythmias, ECG changes, and cardiac arrest due to changes in membrane excitability
- Nausea, vomiting, anorexia, diarrhea, decreased peristalsis, and abdominal distention due to decreased bowel motility
- Muscle weakness, fatigue, and leg cramps due to decreased neuromuscular excitability

TEST RESULTS
Hyperkalemia

- Hyperkalemia occurs when serum potassium is greater than 5 mEq/L.
- Other supportive tests show metabolic acidosis.
- ECG changes include tented and elevated T waves, widened QRS complex, prolonged PR interval, flattened or absent P waves, depressed ST segment.

Hypokalemia

- Hypokalemia occurs when serum potassium is less than 3.5 mEq/L.

Alert Coexisting low serum calcium and magnesium levels not responsive to treatment for hypokalemia usually suggest hypomagnesemia.

- Other supportive tests include metabolic alkalosis.
- ECG changes include flattened T waves, elevated U waves, depressed ST segment.

TREATMENT
Hyperkalemia
- Rapid infusion of.10% calcium gluconate to decrease myocardial irritability and temporarily prevent cardiac arrest, but not correcting serum potassium excess (contraindicated in patients receiving a cardiac glycoside)
- As an emergency measure, sodium bicarbonate I.V. to increase pH and cause potassium to shift back into the cells
- Insulin and 10% glucose I.V. to move potassium from ECFs back into the cells. This may reverse severe symptoms long enough to treat the underlying cause.
- Sodium polystyrene sulfonate (Kayexalate) with 70% sorbitol to produce an exchange of sodium ions for potassium ions in the intestine
- Hemodialysis or peritoneal dialysis to help remove excess potassium

Hypokalemia
- Replacement therapy with potassium chloride (I.V. or by mouth)
- To prevent disorder, maintenance dose of potassium I.V. to patients who may not take anything by mouth

NURSING CONSIDERATIONS
- Monitor serum potassium and other electrolyte levels; monitor for overcorrection with electrolyte replacements. Assess intake and output.

Alert *Give I.V. potassium only after it's diluted in solution; potassium is irritating to vascular, subcutaneous, and fatty tissues and may cause phlebitis or tissue necrosis if it infiltrates. Infuse slowly (no more than 20 mEq/L/hour) to prevent hyperkalemia. Never administer by I.V. push or bolus; it may cause cardiac arrest.*
- Monitor for cardiac arrhythmias.

Hyperkalemia
- Administer sodium polystyrene sulfonate orally or rectally (by retention enema). Watch for signs of hypokalemia and hypoglycemia with repeated insulin and glucose treatment.

Hypokalemia
Alert *Remember that the kidneys excrete 80% to 90% of ingested potassium. Never give supplementary potassium to a patient whose urine output is less than 600 ml/day. Also, measure GI loss from suctioning or vomiting.*
- Carefully monitor the patient receiving a cardiac glycoside because hypokalemia may produce signs and symptoms of digoxin toxicity.
- To prevent hypokalemia, instruct patients to include foods rich in potassium in their diet; oranges, bananas, tomatoes, dark green leafy vegetables, milk, dried fruits, apricots, and peanuts.
- Monitor cardiac rhythm and be alert for arrhythmias.

✸ Life-threatening

Respiratory acidosis

Respiratory acidosis is an acid-base disturbance characterized by reduced alveolar ventilation. The patient's pulmonary system can't clear enough carbon dioxide (CO_2) from the body. This leads to hypercapnia (partial pressure of arterial carbon dioxide [$PaCO_2$] greater than 45 mm Hg) and acidosis (pH less than 7.35). Respiratory acidosis can be acute (due to a sudden failure in ventilation) or chronic (in long-term pulmonary disease). Any compromise in the essential components of breathing—ventilation, perfusion, and diffusion—may cause respiratory acidosis.

Prognosis depends on the severity of the underlying disturbance as well as the patient's general clinical condition. The prognosis is least optimistic for a patient with a debilitating disorder.

CAUSES

- Airway obstruction or parenchymal lung disease (interferes with alveolar ventilation)
- Asthma or chronic obstructive pulmonary disease (COPD)
- Cardiac arrest (acute)
- Central nervous system (CNS) trauma
- Chronic bronchitis
- Chronic metabolic alkalosis as respiratory compensatory mechanisms try to normalize pH by decreasing alveolar ventilation
- Drugs (alcohol, general anesthetics, hypnotics, opioids, and sedatives, including some "designer" drugs, such as 3,4-methylenedioxymethamphetamine or "ecstasy," decrease the sensitivity of the respiratory center)
- Extensive pneumonia
- Large pneumothorax
- Neuromuscular diseases, such as Guillain-Barré syndrome, myasthenia gravis, and poliomyelitis (respiratory muscles can't respond properly to respiratory drive)
- Pulmonary edema
- Severe acute respiratory distress syndrome (reduced pulmonary blood flow and poor exchange of CO_2 and oxygen between the lungs and blood)
- Sleep apnea
- Ventilation therapy (use of high-flow oxygen in patients with chronic respiratory disorders suppresses the patient's hypoxic drive to breathe; high positive end-expiratory pressure in the presence of reduced cardiac output may cause hypercapnia due to large increases in alveolar dead space)

PATHOPHYSIOLOGY

When pulmonary ventilation decreases, bicarbonate (HCO_3^-) is increased, and the CO_2 level rises in all tissues and fluids, including the medulla and cerebrospinal fluid. Retained CO_2 combines with water to form carbonic acid, which dissociates to release free hydrogen (H^+) and HCO_3^-. Increased $PaCO_2$ and free H^+ stimulate the medulla to increase respiratory drive and expel CO_2. As pH falls, 2,3-diphosphoglycerate accumulates in red blood cells, where it alters hemoglobin (Hb) so it releases oxygen. This reduced Hb, which is strongly alkaline, picks up H^+ and CO_2 and removes them from the serum.

As respiratory mechanisms fail, rising HCO_3^- stimulates the kidneys to retain HCO_3^- and sodium ions and excrete H^+. As a result, more sodium bicarbonate is available to buffer free H^+. Some hydrogen is excreted in the form of ammonium ion, neutralizing ammonia, which is an important CNS toxin.

As the H^+ concentration overwhelms compensatory mechanisms, H^+ move into the cells and potassium ions move out. Without enough oxygen, anaerobic metabolism produces lactic acid. Electrolyte imbalances and acidosis critically depress neurologic and cardiac functions.

CLINICAL FINDINGS

Clinical features vary according to the severity and duration of respiratory acidosis, the underlying disease, and the presence of hypoxemia. CO_2 and H^+ dilate cerebral blood vessels and increase blood flow to the brain, causing cerebral edema and depressing CNS activity. Possible signs and symptoms from cerebral edema and depressed CNS activity include restlessness, confusion, apprehension, somnolence, fine or flapping tremor (asterixis), coma, and headaches. Other clinical findings include:

- dyspnea and tachypnea
- papilledema
- depressed reflexes
- hypoxemia, unless the patient is receiving oxygen.

Respiratory acidosis may also cause cardiovascular abnormalities, including:

- tachycardia
- hypertension
- atrial and ventricular arrhythmias
- hypotension with vasodilation (bounding pulses and warm periphery, in severe acidosis).

Alert Possible complications of respiratory acidosis include profound CNS and cardiovascular deterioration due to dangerously low blood pH (less than 7.15); myocardial depression (leading to shock and cardiac arrest); and elevated $Paco_2$ despite optimal treatment (in chronic lung disease).

TEST RESULTS

- Arterial blood gas (ABG) analysis shows $Paco_2$ greater than 45 mm Hg; pH less than 7.35; and normal HCO_3^- in the acute stage. An elevated HCO_3^- in the chronic stage confirms the diagnosis.
- Chest X-ray commonly shows such causes as heart failure, pneumonia, COPD, and pneumothorax.
- Potassium level greater than 5 mEq/L confirms diagnosis.
- Blood studies reveal a low serum chloride level, confirming diagnosis.

- Acidic urine pH is revealed as the kidneys excrete H^+ to return blood pH to normal.
- Drug screening may confirm suspected drug overdose.

TREATMENT

Effective treatment of respiratory acidosis requires correction of the underlying source of alveolar hypoventilation. Treatment of pulmonary causes of respiratory acidosis includes:

- removal of a foreign body from the airway and positioning of patient to maximize air exchange
- artificial airway through endotracheal intubation or tracheotomy and mechanical ventilation (if the patient can't breathe spontaneously)
- increasing partial pressure of arterial oxygen to at least 60 mm Hg and pH greater than 7.2 to avoid cardiac arrhythmias
- aerosolized or I.V. bronchodilators to open constricted airways
- antibiotics to treat pneumonia
- chest tubes to correct pneumothorax
- positive end-expiratory pressure to prevent alveolar collapse
- thrombolytic or anticoagulant therapy for massive pulmonary emboli
- bronchoscopy to remove excessive retained secretions.

Treatment for patients with COPD includes:

- bronchodilators
- oxygen at low flow rates (more oxygen than the person's normal removes the hypoxic drive, further reducing alveolar ventilation)
- corticosteroids
- gradual reduction in $Paco_2$ to baseline to provide sufficient chloride and potassium ions to enhance renal excretion of HCO_3^- (in chronic respiratory acidosis).

Other treatments include:
- drug therapy for such conditions as myasthenia gravis
- dialysis or charcoal to remove toxic drugs
- correction of metabolic alkalosis.

NURSING CONSIDERATIONS
- Be alert for critical changes in the patient's respiratory, CNS, and cardio-vascular functions. Report such changes as well as any variations in ABG levels or electrolyte status immediately. Also, maintain adequate hydration.
- Maintain a patent airway and provide adequate humidification if acidosis requires mechanical ventilation. Perform tracheal suctioning regularly and vigorous chest physiotherapy if ordered. Continuously monitor ventilator settings and respiratory status.
- To prevent respiratory acidosis, closely monitor patients with COPD and chronic CO_2 retention for signs of acidosis. Also, administer oxygen at low flow rates.
- Closely monitor all patients who receive opioids and sedatives. Instruct patients who have received a general anesthetic to turn, cough, and perform deep-breathing exercises frequently to prevent the onset of respiratory acidosis.

Respiratory alkalosis

Respiratory alkalosis is an acid-base disturbance characterized by a partial pressure of arterial carbon dioxide ($PaCO_2$) less than 35 mm Hg and blood pH greater than 7.45; alveolar hyperventilation is the cause. Hypo-capnia (below normal $PaCO_2$) occurs when the lungs eliminate more carbon dioxide (CO_2) than the cells produce.

Respiratory alkalosis is the most common acid-base disturbance in critically ill patients and, when severe, has a poor prognosis.

CAUSES
Causes of respiratory alkalosis fall into two categories:
- nonpulmonary — anxiety, aspirin toxicity, central nervous system (CNS) disease (inflammation or tumor), fever, hepatic failure, metabolic acidosis, pregnancy, and sepsis
- pulmonary — acute asthma, interstitial lung disease, pneumonia, pulmonary vascular disease, and severe hypoxemia.

PATHOPHYSIOLOGY
When pulmonary ventilation increases more than needed to maintain normal CO_2 levels, excessive amounts of CO_2 are exhaled. The consequent hypocapnia leads to a chemical reduction of carbonic acid (H_2CO_3), excretion of hydrogen ions (H^+) and bicarbonate (HCO_3^-), and a rising pH.

In defense against the increasing serum pH, the hydrogen-potassium buffer system pulls H^+ out of the cells and into the blood in exchange for potassium ions. H^+ entering the blood combine with available HCO_3^- to form H_2CO_3, and pH falls.

Hypocapnia stimulates the carotid and aortic bodies as well as the medulla, increasing the heart rate (which hypokalemia can further aggravate) but not the blood pressure. At the same time, hypocapnia causes cerebral vasoconstriction and decreased cerebral blood flow. It also overexcites the medulla, pons, and other parts of the autonomic nervous system. When hypocapnia lasts more than 6 hours, the kidneys secrete more HCO_3^- and less H^+. Full renal adaptation to respiratory alkalosis requires normal volume status and renal function, and it may take several days.

Continued low Pa_{CO_2} and the vasoconstriction it causes increases cerebral and peripheral hypoxia. Severe alkalosis inhibits calcium ionization; as calcium ions become unavailable, nerves and muscles become progressively more excitable. Eventually, alkalosis overwhelms the CNS and heart.

CLINICAL FINDINGS

- Deep, rapid breathing (possibly more than 40 breaths/minute and much like the Kussmaul's respirations that characterize diabetic acidosis) usually causing CNS and neuromuscular disturbances (cardinal sign of respiratory alkalosis)
- Agitation, light-headedness, or dizziness due to decreased cerebral blood flow
- Circumoral and peripheral paresthesia, carpopedal spasms, twitching (possibly progressing to tetany), and muscle weakness due to cellular excitability

Alert *Possible complications of severe respiratory alkalosis include: cardiac arrhythmias that may not respond to conventional treatment as the hemoglobin-oxygen buffer system becomes overwhelmed; hypocalcemic tetany, seizures; and periods of apnea if pH remains high and Pa_{CO_2} remains low.*

TEST RESULTS

- Arterial blood gas (ABG) analysis shows Pa_{CO_2} less than 35 mm Hg; elevated pH in proportion to decrease in Pa_{CO_2} in the acute stage but decreasing toward normal in the chronic stage; normal HCO_3^- in acute stage but less than normal in the chronic stage confirms respiratory alkalosis and rules out respiratory compensation for metabolic acidosis.

- Serum electrolyte studies detect metabolic disorders causing compensatory respiratory alkalosis.
- Electrocardiogram findings may indicate cardiac arrhythmias.
- Low chloride level reveals severe respiratory alkalosis.
- Toxicology screening is done to detect salicylate poisoning.
- Basic urine pH as kidneys excrete HCO_3^- to raise blood pH reveal the disorder.

TREATMENT

- Removal of ingested toxins, such as salicylates, by inducing emesis or using gastric lavage
- Treatment of fever or sepsis
- Oxygen for acute hypoxemia
- Treatment of CNS disease
- Having patient breathe into a paper bag to increase CO_2 and help relieve anxiety (for hyperventilation caused by severe anxiety)
- Adjustment of tidal volume and minute ventilation in patients on mechanical ventilation to prevent hyperventilation (by monitoring ABG analysis results)

NURSING CONSIDERATIONS

- Watch for and report any changes in neurologic, neuromuscular, or cardiovascular functions.
- Monitor ABG and serum electrolyte levels closely, reporting variations immediately.

Sodium imbalance

Sodium is the major cation (90%) in extracellular fluid (ECF); potassium, the major cation in intracellular fluid (ICF). During repolarization, the sodium-potassium pump continuously shifts sodium into the cells and potassium out of the cells; during repolarization, it does the reverse.

Sodium cation functions include maintaining tonicity and concentration of ECF, acid-base balance (reabsorption of sodium ions and excretion of hydrogen ions), nerve conduction and neuromuscular function, glandular secretion, and water balance.

CAUSES

Hypernatremia
● Decreased water intake
● Excess adrenocortical hormones, as in Cushing's syndrome, and antidiuretic hormone (ADH) deficiency (diabetes insipidus)
● Salt intoxication, an uncommon cause, possibly resulting from excessive ingestion of table salt

Hyponatremia
● Burns, surgery (wound drainage), and trauma, which cause sodium to shift into damaged cells, can lead to decreased serum sodium levels, as can adrenal gland insufficiency (Addison's disease), cirrhosis of the liver with ascites, and hypoaldosteronism
● Certain drugs (chlorpropamide [Diabinese] and valproate sodium [Depakene]) may produce a syndrome of inappropriate antidiuretic hormone (SIADH)–like syndrome
● Excessive drinking of water, infusion of I.V. dextrose in water without other solutes, a low-sodium diet, and malnutrition or starvation, usually in combination with one of the other causes
● Excessive GI loss of water and electrolytes due to diarrhea, suctioning, or vomiting; excessive perspiration or fever; potent diuretics; or use of tap-water enemas
● SIADH, resulting from brain tumor, stroke, neoplasm with ectopic ADH production, or pulmonary disease

PATHOPHYSIOLOGY

Sodium is the major cation in ECF, and potassium is the major cation in ICF. Especially in nerves and muscles, communication within and between cells involves changes (repolarization and depolarization) in surface charge on the cell membrane. During repolarization, an active transport mechanism in the cell membrane, called the *sodium-potassium pump,* continuously shifts sodium into and potassium out of cells; during depolarization, the process is reversed.

Physiologic roles of sodium cations include maintaining tonicity of ECF; regulating acid-base balance by renal reabsorption of sodium ion (base) and excretion of hydrogen ion (acid); facilitating nerve conduction and neuromuscular function; facilitating glandular secretion; and maintaining water balance.

In hypernatremia, when severe vomiting and diarrhea can cause water loss that exceeds sodium loss, serum sodium levels rise but overall ECF volume decreases. (See *Fluid movement in hypernatremia.*)

When sodium losses decrease circulating fluid volume, increased secretion of ADH promotes maximum wa-

FLUID MOVEMENT IN HYPERNATREMIA

With hypernatremia, the body tries to maintain balance by shifting fluid from the inside of cells to the outside. This illustration shows fluid movement in hypernatremia.

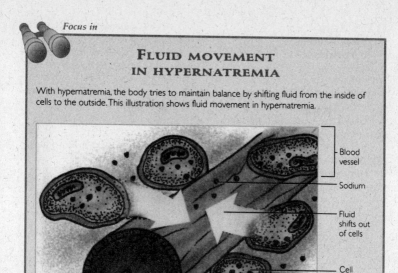

- Blood vessel
- Sodium
- Fluid shifts out of cells
- Cell

ter reabsorption, which further dilutes serum sodium. These factors are especially likely to cause hyponatremia when combined with too much electrolyte-free water intake.

CLINICAL FINDINGS

Hypernatremia
- Agitation, restlessness, fever, and decreased level of consciousness due to altered cellular metabolism
- Hypertension, tachycardia, pitting edema, and excessive weight gain due to water shift from ICF to ECF
- Thirst, increased viscosity of saliva, rough tongue due to fluid shift
- Dyspnea, respiratory arrest, and death from dramatic increase in osmotic pressure

Hyponatremia
- Produces muscle twitching and weakness due to osmotic swelling of cells
- Lethargy, confusion, seizures, coma due to altered neurotransmission
- Hypotension and tachycardia due to decreased extracellular circulating volume
- Nausea, vomiting, and abdominal cramps due to edema affecting receptors in the brain or vomiting center of the brain stem
- Oliguria or anuria due to renal dysfunction

TEST RESULTS
Hypernatremia
● Hypernatremia occurs when the serum sodium level is greater than 145 mEq/L.
● Other supportive test findings include urine sodium level less than 40 mEq/L in 24 hours and high serum osmolality.

Hyponatremia
● Hyponatremia occurs when serum sodium level is less than 135 mEq/L.
● Other supportive test findings include decreased urine specific gravity, decreased serum osmolality level, urine sodium level greater than 100 mEq/24 hours, and increased red blood cell count.

TREATMENT
Hypernatremia
● Primary treatment of hypernatremia, administration of salt-free solutions (such as dextrose in water) to return serum sodium levels to normal, followed by infusion of half-normal saline solution to prevent hyponatremia
● Other measures including a sodium-restricted diet and discontinuation of drugs that promote sodium retention

Hyponatremia
● Restricting electrolyte-free water intake when it results from hemodilution, SIADH, or such conditions as heart failure, cirrhosis of the liver, and renal failure
● In extremely rare instances of severe symptom-producing hyponatremia (when serum sodium level falls below 110 mEq/L) an infusion of 3% or 5% saline solution
 *Alert* *Treatment with saline infusion requires careful monitoring of ve-*

nous pressure to prevent potentially fatal circulatory overload.
● In secondary hyponatremia, correcting the underlying disorder

NURSING CONSIDERATIONS
Hypernatremia
● Measure serum sodium levels every 6 hours or at least daily. Monitor vital signs for changes. Watch for signs of hypervolemia.
● Record fluid intake and output accurately, checking for body fluid loss. Weigh the patient daily.
● Obtain a drug history to check for drugs that promote sodium retention.

Hyponatremia
● Watch for extremely low serum sodium and accompanying serum chloride levels. Monitor urine specific gravity and other laboratory results. Record fluid intake and output accurately, and weigh the patient daily.
● During administration of isosmolar or hyperosmolar saline solution, watch closely for signs of hypervolemia (dyspnea, crackles, engorged jugular veins).

15

GENETICS

Genetics is the study of heredity — the passing of physical, biochemical, and physiologic traits from biological parents to their children. In this transmission, disorders can be transmitted and mistakes or mutations can result in disability or death. Every normal nucleated human cell (except reproductive cells) has 46 chromosomes, 22 paired chromosomes called autosomes, and 2 sex chromosomes (a pair of Xs in females and an X and a Y in males). A representation of a person's individual set of chromosomes is called his karyotype. Deoxyribonucleic acid ultimately controls the formation of essential substances throughout the life of every cell in the body. It does this through genes.

Trait transmission

Germ cells, or gametes (ovum and sperm), are one of two classes of cells in the body; each germ cell contains 23 chromosomes (called the haploid number) in its nucleus. All the other cells in the body are somatic cells, which are diploid, meaning they contain 23 pairs of chromosomes.

When ovum and sperm unite, the corresponding chromosomes pair up so that the fertilized cell and every somatic cell of the new person has 23 pairs of chromosomes in its nucleus.

GERM CELLS
The body produces germ cells through a type of cell division called meiosis. Meiosis occurs only when the body is creating haploid germ cell from their diploid precursors. Each of the 23 pairs of chromosomes in the germ cell separates so that, when the cell then divides, each new cell (ovum or sperm) contains one set of 23 chromosomes. Most of the genes on one chromosome are identical or almost identical to the gene on its mate. (As discussed later in this chapter, each chromosome may carry a different version of the same gene.) The location (or locus) of a gene on a chromosome is specific and doesn't vary from person to person.

DETERMINING GENDER
Only one pair of chromosomes in each cell — pair 23 — is involved in determining a person's gender. These are the sex chromosomes; the other 22 numbered chromosome pairs are called autosomes. Females have two

X chromosomes and males have one X and one Y chromosome. Each gamete produced by a male contains either an X or a Y chromosome. When a sperm with an X chromosome fertilizes an ovum, the offspring is female (two X chromosomes); when a sperm with a Y chromosome fertilizes an ovum, the offspring is male (one X and one Y chromosome). Extremely rare errors in cell division can result in a germ cell that has no sex chromosome or two sex chromosomes. After fertilization, with a gamete that contains a missing or extra sex chromosome, the zygote may have an XO, XXY, XXX, or XYY karyotype and still survive. Most other errors in sex chromosome division are incompatible with life.

MITOSIS

The fertilized ovum—now called a zygote—undergoes a type of cell division called mitosis. Before a cell divides, its chromosomes duplicate. During this process, the double helix of deoxyribonucleic acid (DNA) separates into two chains; each chain serves as a template for constructing a new chain. Individual DNA nucleotides are linked into new strands with bases complementary to those in the originals. In this way, two identical double helices are formed, each containing one of the original strands and a newly formed complementary strand. These double helices are duplicates of the original DNA chain.

Mitotic cell division occurs in five phases: an inactive phase called interphase and four active phases: prophase, metaphase, anaphase, and telophase. (See *Five phases of mitosis*.) The result of every mitotic cell division is two new daughter cells, each genetically identical to the original and to each other. Each of the two resulting cells likewise divides, and so on, eventually forming a many-celled human embryo. Thus, each cell in a person's body (except ovum or sperm) contains an identical set of 46 chromosomes that are unique to that person.

TRAIT PREDOMINANCE

Each parent contributes one set of chromosomes (and therefore one set of genes) so that every offspring has two genes for every locus (location on the chromosome) on the autosomal chromosomes. Some characteristics, or traits, are determined by one gene that may have many variants (alleles), such as the ability to roll the tongue. Others, called polygenic traits, such as eye color, require the interaction of one or more genes. In addition, environmental factors may affect how a gene or genes are expressed. Variations in a particular gene—such as brown, blue, or green eye color—are called alleles. A person who has identical alleles on each chromosome is homozygous for that gene; if the alleles are different, they're said to be heterozygous.

AUTOSOMAL INHERITANCE

For unknown reasons, on autosomal chromosomes, one allele may be more influential than the other in determining a specific trait. The more powerful, or dominant, allele is more likely to be expressed in the offspring than the less influential, or recessive, allele. Offspring will express a dominant allele when one or both chromosomes in a pair carry it. A recessive allele won't be expressed unless both chromosomes carry recessive alleles.

FIVE PHASES OF MITOSIS

In mitosis (used by all cells except gametes), the nuclear contents of a cell reproduce and divide, resulting in the formation of two daughter cells. The five steps, or phases, are illustrated below.

INTERPHASE

During interphase, the protein synthesis and preparation for cell division takes place. The nucleus and nuclear membrane are well defined and the nucleolus is prominent. Chromosomes replicate, each forming a double strand that remains attached at the center of each chromosome by a structure called the centromere; they appear as an indistinguishable matrix within the nucleus. Centrioles (in animal cells only, not plant cells) appear outside the nucleus.

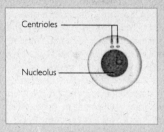

Centrioles

Nucleolus

PROPHASE

In prophase, the nucleolus disappears and chromosomes become distinct. Halves of each duplicated chromosome (chromatids) remain attached by a centromere. Centrioles move to opposite sides of the cell and radiate spindle fibers.

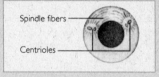

Spindle fibers

Centrioles

METAPHASE

Chromosomes line up randomly in the center of the cell between spindles, along the metaphase plate. The centromere of each chromosome replicates.

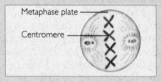

Metaphase plate

Centromere

ANAPHASE

In anaphase, the centromeres move apart, pulling the separate chromatids (now called chromosomes) to opposite ends of the cell. In human cells, each end of the cell now contains 46 chromosomes. The number of chromosomes at each end of the cell equals the original number.

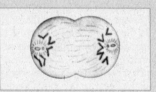

TELOPHASE

In telophase, a nuclear membrane forms around each end of the cell, and spindle fibers disappear. The cytoplasm compresses and divides the cell in half. Each new cell contains the diploid number (46 in humans) of chromosomes.

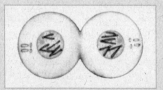

SEX-LINKED INHERITANCE

The X and Y chromosomes aren't literally a pair because the X chromosome is much larger than the Y. The male literally has less genetic material than the female, which means he has only one copy of most genes on the X chromosome. Inheritance of those genes is called X-linked. A man will transmit one copy of each X-linked gene to his daughters and none to his sons. A woman will transmit one copy to each child, male or female.

Inheritance of genes on the X chromosomes is different in another way. Some recessive genes on the X chromosomes act like dominants in males. Due to X-inactivation, one recessive allele will be expressed in some somatic cells and the partner allele, whether dominant or recessive in other somatic cells.

MULTIFACTORIAL INHERITANCE

Some traits require a combination of two or more genes and environmental factors to be expressed. This is called multifactorial inheritance. Height is a classic example of a multifactorial trait. In general, the height of offspring will be in a range between the height of the two parents. However, the combination of multiple genes contributed by each parent, nutritional patterns, health care, and other environmental factors also influence development. The better-nourished, healthier children of two short parents may be taller than either. Common health problems, such as obesity, diabetes, and hypertension, are associated with effects from multiple genes that are modified by environmental and lifestyle factors.

Pathophysiologic changes

Autosomal, sex-linked, and multifactorial disorders originate from damage to genes or chromosomes. Some defects arise spontaneously, whereas others may be caused by environmental mutagens. A permanent change in genetic material is a mutation, which may occur spontaneously or after exposure of a cell to radiation, certain chemicals, or viruses. Mutations can occur anywhere in the genome — the person's entire inventory of genes.

A trait altering mutation usually produces some abnormal protein that makes the cell different from its ancestors. Mutations may have no effect on a gene's protein and have no effect on the gene's associated trait. Some mutations in somatic cells can lead to cancer.

AUTOSOMAL DISORDERS

In single-gene disorders, an error occurs at a single gene site on the deoxyribonucleic acid strand. A mistake may be in the form of additions, deletions, excessive repetitions, or changes in one or more bases. Single-gene disorders are inherited in clearly identifiable patterns that are the same as those seen in inheritance of normal traits. Because every person has 22 pairs of autosomes and only 1 pair of sex chromosomes, most hereditary disorders are caused by autosomal mutations.

Autosomal dominant transmission usually affects male and female offspring equally. If one parent is affected, each child has one chance in two of being affected. If both parents are affected, the offspring may not be affected. An example of this type of inheritance occurs in Marfan syndrome.

Autosomal recessive inheritance also usually affects male and female offspring equally. If both parents are affected, all their offspring will be affected. If both parents are unaffected but are heterozygous for the trait (carriers of the defective gene), each child has one chance in four of being affected. If only one parent is affected, and the other isn't a carrier, none of their offspring will be affected, but all will carry the defective gene. If one parent is affected and the other is a carrier, their offspring will have a 50% chance of being affected. Autosomal recessive disorders may occur without a family history of the disease.

SEX-LINKED DISORDERS

Genetic disorders caused by genes located on the sex chromosomes are termed sex-linked disorders. Most sex-linked disorders are passed on the X chromosome, usually as recessive traits. Because males have only one X chromosome, a single X-linked recessive gene can cause disease to be exhibited in a male. Females receive two X chromosomes, so they can be homozygous for a disease allele, homozygous for a normal allele, or heterozygous (a carrier).

Most people who express X-linked recessive traits are males with unaffected parents. All daughters of an affected male will be carriers. Sons of an affected male will be unaffected, and the unaffected sons aren't carriers. Unaffected male children of a female carrier don't transmit the disorder. In rare cases, the father is affected and the mother is a carrier. Hemophilia is an example of an X-linked inheritance disorder. Characteristics of X-linked dominant inheritance include evidence of the inherited trait in the family history. A person with the abnormal trait usually has one affected parent, except in the case where a new mutation occurred. If the father has an X-linked dominant disorder, all his daughters and none of his sons will be affected. If a mother has an X-linked dominant disorder, each of her children has a 50% chance of being affected.

MULTIFACTORIAL DISORDERS

Most multifactorial disorders result from the effects of several different genes and an environmental component. In polygenic inheritance, each gene has a small additive effect, and the effect of a combination of genetic errors in a person is unpredictable. Multifactorial disorders can result from a less-than-optimum expression of many different genes, not from a specific error.

Some multifactorial disorders are apparent at birth, such as cleft lip, cleft palate, congenital heart disease, anencephaly, clubfoot, and myelomeningocele. Others don't become apparent until later, such as type 2 diabetes mellitus, hypertension, hyperlipidemia, most autoimmune diseases, and many cancers. Multifactorial disorders that develop during adulthood are usually believed to be strongly related to environmental factors, not only in incidence but also in the degree of expression.

ENVIRONMENTAL TERATOGENS

Teratogens are environmental agents that can harm the developing fetus by causing congenital structural or functional defects. Teratogens may also cause spontaneous miscarriage, com-

CHROMOSOMAL DISJUNCTION AND NONDISJUNCTION

The illustrations below show normal disjunction and nondisjunction of an ovum. When disjunction proceeds normally, fertilization with a normal sperm results in a zygote with the correct number of chromosomes. In nondisjunction, the sister chromatids fail to separate; the result is one trisomic cell and one monosomic cell.

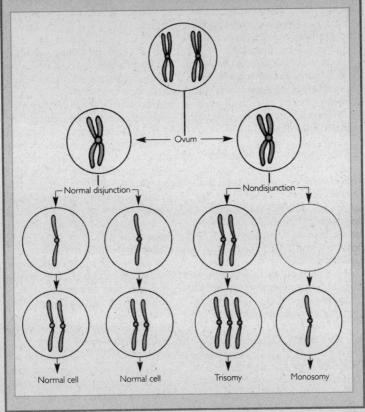

plications during labor and delivery, hidden defects in later development (such as cognitive or behavioral problems), or neoplastic transformations.

Environmental factors of maternal or paternal origin include the use of chemicals (such as drugs, alcohol, or hormones), exposure to radiation, general health, and age. Maternal factors include infections during pregnancy, existing diseases, nutritional factors, exposure to high altitude, maternal-fetal blood incompatibility, and poor prenatal care.

The embryonic period — the first 8 weeks after fertilization — is a vulnerable time when specific organ systems are actively differentiating. Exposure to teratogens usually kills the embryo. During the fetal period, organ systems are formed and continue to mature. Exposure during this time can cause intrauterine growth retardation, cognitive abnormalities, or structural defects.

CHROMOSOME ANOMALIES

Aberrations in chromosome structure or number cause a class of disorders called congenital anomalies, or birth defects. The aberration may be loss, addition, or rearrangement of genetic material. If the remaining genetic material is sufficient to maintain life, an endless variety of clinical manifestations may occur. Most clinically significant chromosome aberrations arise during meiosis. Potential contributing factors include maternal age, radiation, and use of some therapeutic or recreational drugs.

Translocation, the shifting or moving of chromosomal material, occurs when chromosomes split apart and rejoin in an abnormal arrangement. The cells still have a normal amount of genetic material, so commonly there are no visible abnormalities. However, the children of parents with translocated chromosomes may have serious genetic defects, such as monosomies or trisomies. Parental age doesn't seem to be a factor in translocation.

Errors in chromosome number

During both meiosis and mitosis, chromosomes normally separate in a process called disjunction. Failure to separate, called nondisjunction, causes an unequal distribution of chromosomes between the two resulting cells. If nondisjunction occurs during mitosis soon after fertilization, it may affect all the resulting cells. Gain or loss of chromosomes is usually caused by nondisjunction of autosomes or sex chromosomes during meiosis. The incidence of nondisjunction increases with maternal age. The presence of one chromosome less than the normal number is called monosomy; an autosomal monosomy is nonviable. The presence of an extra chromosome is called a trisomy. A mixture of both trisomic and normal cells results in mosaicism, which is the presence of two or more cell lines in the same person. The effect of mosaicism depends on the proportion and anatomic location of abnormal cells. (See *Chromosomal disjunction and nondisjunction.*)

Cleft lip and cleft palate

Cleft lip and cleft palate may occur separately or in combination. They originate in the second month of pregnancy if the front and sides of the face and the palatine shelves fuse imperfectly. Cleft lip with or without cleft palate is twice as common in males as females. Cleft palate without cleft lip is more common in females. Cleft lip deformities can occur unilaterally, bilaterally or rarely, in the midline. Only the lip may be involved, or the defect may extend into the upper jaw or nasal cavity. (See *Types of cleft deformities,* page 488.)

Incidence is highest in children with a family history of cleft defects. Cleft lip with or without cleft palate

TYPES OF CLEFT DEFORMITIES

The following illustrations show variations of cleft lip and cleft palate.

Notch in the vermillion border (junction of the lip and surrounding skin)

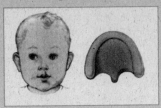

Unilateral cleft lip and palate

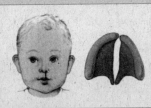

Bilateral cleft lip and palate

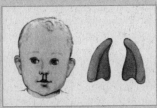

Cleft palate

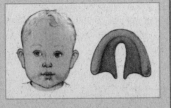

occurs in about 1 in 1,000 births among Whites; the incidence is higher in Asians (1.7 in 1,000) and Native Americans (more than 3.6 in 1,000) but lower in Blacks (1 in 2,500).

CAUSES

- Chromosomal syndrome (cleft defects are associated with more than 300 syndromes)
- Combined genetic and environmental factors (75% of children with isolated cleft)
- Exposure to teratogens during fetal development

PATHOPHYSIOLOGY

During the second month of pregnancy, the front and sides of the face and the palatine shelves develop. Because of a chromosomal abnormality, exposure to teratogens, genetic abnormality, or environmental factors, the lip or palate fuses imperfectly. The deformity may range from a simple notch to a complete cleft. A cleft palate may be partial or complete. A complete cleft includes the soft palate, the bones of the maxilla, and the alveolus on one or both sides of the premaxilla. A double cleft is the most severe of the deformities. The cleft runs from the soft palate forward to either side of the nose. A double cleft separates the maxilla and premaxilla into freely moving segments. The tongue and other muscles can displace the segments, enlarging the cleft.

Alert Isolated cleft palate is more commonly associated with other congenital defects than isolated cleft lip with or without cleft palate. The constellation of U-shaped cleft palate, mandibular hypoplasia, and glossoptosis is known as Pierre Robin syndrome, or Robin's syndrome. Because of the mandibular hypoplasia and glossoptosis, careful evaluation and management of the airway are mandatory for infants with Robin's syndrome.

CLINICAL FINDINGS
- Obvious cleft lip or cleft palate
- Feeding difficulties due to incomplete fusion of the palate

🔔 *Alert* *Complications of cleft lip or cleft palate may include malnutrition, because the abnormal palate affects nutritional intake; hearing impairment, usually due to middle-ear damage or recurrent infections; permanent speech impediment, even after surgical repair.*

TEST RESULTS
- Prenatal targeted ultrasound reveals diagnosis.

TREATMENT
- Surgical correction of cleft lip in the first few days of life to permit sucking, or delayed for 8 to 10 weeks (sometimes as long as 6 to 8 months) to allow the infant to grow and mature, thereby minimizing surgical and anesthesia risks, ruling out associated congenital anomalies, and allowing time for parental bonding
- Orthodontic prosthesis to improve sucking
- Surgical correction of cleft palate at 12 to 18 months, after the infant gains weight and is infection-free
- Speech therapy to correct speech patterns
- Use of a contoured speech bulb attached to the posterior of a denture to occlude the nasopharynx when a wide horseshoe defect makes surgery impossible (to help the child develop intelligible speech)
- Adequate nutrition for normal growth and development
- Use of a large soft nipple with large holes, such as a lamb's nipple, to improve feeding patterns and promote nutrition

🔔 *Alert* *Daily use of folic acid before conception decreases the risk of isolated (not associated with another genetic or congenital malformation) cleft lip or palate by up to 25%. Women of childbearing age should be encouraged to take a daily multivitamin containing folic acid until menopause or until they're no longer fertile.*

NURSING CONSIDERATIONS
🔔 *Alert* *Never place a child with Pierre Robin syndrome on his back because his tongue could fall back and obstruct his airway. Place the infant on his side for sleeping. Most other infants with a cleft palate can sleep on their backs without difficulty.*

- Maintain adequate nutrition to ensure normal growth and development. Experiment with feeding devices. An infant with a cleft palate usually feeds better from a bottle and nipple designed specifically for feeding infants with cleft defects.
- Teach the parents to feed the infant in a near-sitting position, with the flow directed to the side or back of the infant's tongue. Tell them to burp the infant frequently because he tends to swallow a lot of air. Tell them to gently clean the palatal cleft with a cotton-tipped applicator dipped in half-strength hydrogen peroxide or water after each feeding.
- Encourage the mother of an infant with cleft lip to breast-feed if the cleft doesn't prevent effective sucking. Breast-feeding an infant with a cleft palate or one who has just had corrective surgery isn't usually possible. However, if the mother desires, suggest that she use a breast pump to express breast milk and then feed it to her infant from a bottle.

- After surgery, record intake and output and maintain good nutrition.
- To prevent atelectasis and pneumonia, the physician may gently suction the nasopharynx (this may be necessary before surgery, too). Restrain the infant with elbow restraints to prevent him from hurting himself. When necessary, use an infant seat to keep the child in a comfortable sitting position. Hang toys within reach of restrained hands.
- Surgeons sometimes place a curved metal bow over a repaired cleft lip to minimize tension on the suture line. Remove the gauze before feedings, and replace it often. Moisten it with normal saline solution until the sutures are removed as per facility policy.
- Include the parents in the infant's care and provide the instructions, emotional support, and reassurance that the parents will need to take proper care of the child at home.
- Refer them to a social worker who can guide them to community resources, if needed, and to a genetic counselor to determine the recurrence risk.

Cystic fibrosis

In cystic fibrosis, dysfunction of the exocrine glands affects multiple organ systems. The disease affects males as well as females and is the most common fatal genetic disease in white children. Cystic fibrosis is accompanied by many complications and is characterized by chronic airway infection leading to bronchiectasis, bronchiolectasis, exocrine pancreatic insufficiency, intestinal dysfunction, abnormal sweat gland function, and reproductive dysfunction. The incidence of cystic fibrosis varies with ethnic origin. It occurs in 1 of 2,000 births in Whites of North America and northern European descent, 1 in 17,000 births in Blacks, and 1 in 90,000 births in the Asian population in Hawaii.

The responsible gene is on chromosome 7q; it encodes a membrane-associated protein called the cystic fibrosis transmembrane regulator (CFTR). The exact function of CFTR remains unknown, but it appears to help regulate chloride and sodium transport across epithelial membranes.

CAUSES
Causes of cystic fibrosis include:
- abnormal coding found on over 1,000 CFTR alleles
- autosomal recessive inheritance.

PATHOPHYSIOLOGY
The mutation that affects the genetic coding for a single amino acid, results in a protein (the CFTR) that doesn't function properly. This type occurs in 70% of those of Northern European descent; the frequency of certain mutations varies by ethnicity and race. The CFTR resulting from this mutation resembles other transmembrane transport proteins, but it lacks the phenylalanine in the protein produced by normal genes. This regulator interferes with cyclic adenosine monophosphate-regulated chloride channels and transport of other ions by preventing adenosine triphosphate from binding to the protein or by interfering with activation by protein kinase.

The mutation affects volume-absorbing epithelia (in the airways and intestines), salt-absorbing epithelia (in sweat ducts), and volume-secretory epithelia (in the pancreas). The altered chloride channel leads to dehydration, increasing the viscosity of mucous-gland secretions, leading to obstruction of glandular ducts. Cystic fibrosis has a varying effect on electrolyte and water transport.

CLINICAL FINDINGS
- Thick secretions and dehydration due to ionic imbalance
- Chronic airway infections by *Staphylococcus aureus, Pseudomonas aeruginosa,* and *Pseudomonas cepacia,* possibly due to abnormal airway surface fluids and failure of lung defenses
- Dyspnea due to accumulation of thick secretions in bronchioles and alveoli
- Paroxysmal cough due to stimulation of the secretion-removal reflex
- Barrel chest, cyanosis, and clubbing of fingers and toes from chronic hypoxia
- Crackles on auscultation due to thick, airway-occluding secretions
- Wheezes heard on auscultation due to constricted airways
- Retention of bicarbonate and water due to the absence of the CFTR chloride channel in the pancreatic ductile epithelia; limits membrane function and leads to retention of pancreatic enzymes, chronic cholecystitis and cholelithiasis, and ultimate destruction of the pancreas
- Obstruction of the small and large intestine due to inhibited secretion of chloride and water and excessive absorption of liquid
- Fatal shock and arrhythmias due to hyponatremia and hypochloremia from sodium lost in sweat
- Failure to thrive: poor weight gain, poor growth, distended abdomen, thin extremities, and sallow skin with poor turgor due to malabsorption

- Clotting problems, retarded bone growth, and delayed sexual development due to deficiency of fat-soluble vitamins
- Rectal prolapse in infants and children due to malnutrition and wasting of perirectal supporting tissues

Alert Complications of cystic fibrosis may include obstructed glandular ducts (leading to peribronchial thickening) due to increased viscosity of bronchial, pancreatic, and other mucous-gland secretions; atelectasis or emphysema due to respiratory effects; diabetes, pancreatitis, and hepatic failure due to effects on the intestines, pancreas, and liver; malnutrition and malabsorption of fat-soluble vitamins (A, D, E, and K) due to deficiencies of trypsin, amylase, and lipase (from obstructed pancreatic ducts, preventing the conversion and absorption of fat and protein in the intestinal tract); lack of sperm in the semen (azoospermia); secondary amenorrhea and increased mucus in the reproductive tracts, blocking the passage of ova.

TEST RESULTS
The Cystic Fibrosis Foundation has developed criteria for a definitive diagnosis:
- Two sweat tests (to detect elevated sodium chloride levels) using a pilocarpine solution (a sweat inducer) and presence of an obstructive pulmonary disease, confirmed pancreatic insufficiency or failure to thrive, or a family history of cystic fibrosis confirm the disorder.

Alert The sweat test may be inaccurate in very young infants because they may not produce enough sweat for a valid test. The test may need to be repeated.
- Chest X-rays indicate early signs of obstructive lung disease.
- Stool specimen analysis indicates the absence of trypsin, suggesting pancreatic insufficiency.

The following test results may support the diagnosis:

- Deoxyribonucleic acid testing identifies mutations.
- Pulmonary function tests reveal decreased vital capacity, elevated residual volume due to air entrapments, and decreased forced expiratory volume in 1 second. This test is used if pulmonary exacerbation already exists.
- Liver enzyme tests may reveal hepatic insufficiency.
- Sputum culture reveals organisms that patients with cystic fibrosis typically and chronically colonize, such as *Staphylococcus* and *Pseudomonas*.
- Serum albumin measurement helps assess nutritional status.
- Electrolyte analysis assesses hydration status.

TREATMENT

The aim of treatment is to help the child lead as normal a life as possible. The type of treatment depends on the organ system involved. Possible treatments include:

- hypertonic radio-contrast materials delivered by enema to treat acute obstructions due to meconium ileus
- breathing exercises, postural drainage, and chest percussion to clear pulmonary secretions
- antibiotics to treat lung infection, guided by sputum culture results
- drugs to increase mucus clearance
- inhaled beta-adrenergic agonists to control airway constriction
- pancreatic enzyme replacement to maintain adequate nutrition
- sodium-channel blocker to decrease sodium reabsorption from secretions and improve viscosity
- uridine triphosphate to stimulate chloride secretion by a non-CFTR channel
- salt supplements to replace electrolytes lost through sweat
- Dornase alfa (Pulmozyme), a genetically engineered pulmonary enzyme, to help liquefy mucus
- recombinant alpha-antitrypsin to counteract excessive proteolytic activity produced during airway inflammation
- transplantation of heart or lungs in severe organ failure.

NURSING CONSIDERATIONS

- Promote a patent airway and prevent development of complications through maintaining oxygenation, hydration, and adequate nutrition.
- Throughout this illness, teach the patient and his family about the disease and its treatment. The Cystic Fibrosis Foundation can provide educational and support services.

Down syndrome

Down syndrome, or trisomy 21, is a spontaneous chromosome abnormality that causes characteristic facial features, other distinctive physical abnormalities, and mental retardation; 60% of affected persons have cardiac defects. It occurs in 1 of 650 to 700 live births. Improved treatment for heart defects, respiratory and other infections, and acute leukemia has significantly increased life expectancy. Fetal and neonatal mortality remain high, usually resulting from complications of associated heart defects.

CAUSES

- Extra chromosome 21 material due to nondisjunction; higher risk of this in women over age 35

• Monitor vital signs often. Watch for signs of shock, infection, and increased intracranial pressure (ICP), such as projectile vomiting. Frequently assess the infant's fontanels.

• Change the dressing regularly as ordered, and check and report any signs of drainage, wound rupture, and infection.

• Place the infant in the prone position to protect and assess the site.

Provide psychological support and encourage a positive attitude.

• To prevent constipation and bowel obstruction, stress the need for increased fluid intake, a high-bulk diet, exercise, and a stool softener as ordered.

• Urge early recognition of developmental lags (a possible result of hydrocephalus). If present, stress the importance of follow-up assessment to help plan educational goals. Help parents plan activities appropriate to their child's age and abilities. Also refer parents to the Spina Bifida Association of America.

Sickle cell anemia

Sickle cell anemia is a congenital hemolytic anemia resulting from defective hemoglobin (Hb) molecules. One-half of patients with sickle cell anemia live beyond age 50. Sickle cell anemia occurs primarily in people of African and Mediterranean descent, but it also affects other populations. Although most common in tropical Africans and people of African descent, it also occurs in Puerto Rico, Turkey, India, the Middle East, and the Mediterranean.

CAUSES

• Mutation of Hb S gene (heterozygous inheritance results in sickle cell trait, a condition that usually produces no symptoms)

PATHOPHYSIOLOGY

Sickle cell anemia results from substitution of the amino acid valine for glutamic acid in the Hb S gene encoding the beta chain of Hb. Abnormal Hb S, found in the red blood cells (RBCs) of patients, becomes insoluble during hypoxia. As a result, these cells become rigid, rough, and elongated, forming a crescent or sickle shape. (See *Characteristics of sickled cells,* page 498.) The sickling produces hemolysis. The altered cells also pile up in the capillaries and smaller blood vessels, making the blood more viscous. Normal circulation is impaired, causing pain, tissue infarctions, and swelling.

Each patient with sickle cell anemia has a different hypoxic threshold and different factors that trigger a sickle cell crisis. Illness, exposure to cold, stress, acidotic states, or a pathophysiologic process that pulls water out of the sickle cells precipitates a crisis in most patients. (See *Sickle cell crisis,* page 499.) The blockages then cause anoxic changes that lead to further sickling and obstruction.

CLINICAL FINDINGS

Alert *Symptoms of sickle cell anemia don't develop until after age 6 months because fetal Hb protects infants for the first few months after birth.*

• Tachycardia, cardiomegaly, chronic fatigue, unexplained dyspnea, hepatomegaly, joint swelling, aching bones, or chest pain

• Severe pain in the abdomen, thorax, muscle, or bones (characterizes painful crisis)

CHARACTERISTICS OF SICKLED CELLS

Normal red blood cells (RBCs) and sickled cells vary in shape, life span, oxygen-carrying capacity, and the rate at which they're destroyed. The illustrations below show normal and sickled cells and list the major differences.

NORMAL RBCs
◆ 120-day life span
◆ Hemoglobin (Hb) has normal oxygen-carrying capacity
◆ 12 to 14 g/dl of Hb
◆ RBCs destroyed at normal rate

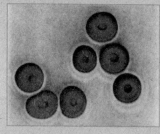

SICKLED CELLS
◆ 10- to 20-day life span
◆ Hb has decreased oxygen-carrying capacity
◆ 6 to 9 g/dl of Hb
◆ RBCs destroyed at accelerated rate

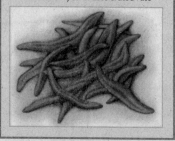

● Jaundice, dark urine, and low-grade fever due to blood vessel obstruction by rigid, tangled, sickle cells (leading to tissue anoxia and possibly necrosis)

● *Streptococcus pneumoniae* sepsis due to autosplenectomy (splenic damage and scarring in patients with long-term disease)

Suspect any of the following crises in a sickle cell anemia patient with pale lips, tongue, palms or nail beds; lethargy; listlessness; sleepiness; irritability; severe pain; and fever:
● aplastic crisis (megaloblastic crisis) due to bone marrow depression (associated with infection, usually viral, and characterized by pallor, lethargy, sleepiness, dyspnea, possible coma, markedly decreased bone marrow activity, and RBC hemolysis)
● acute sequestration crisis (rare; affects infants ages 8 months to 2 years; may cause lethargy, pallor, and hypovolemic shock) due to the sudden massive entrapment of cells in spleen and liver
● hemolytic crisis (rare; usually affects patients who also have glucose-6-phosphate dehydrogenase deficiency; degenerative changes cause liver congestion and enlargement and chronic jaundice worsens).

Alert *Complications of sickle cell anemia may include retinopathy, nephropathy, and cerebral vessel occlusion due to organ infarction; hypovolemic shock and death due to massive entrapment of cells; necrosis; infection; and gangrene.*

TEST RESULTS
● Positive family history and typical clinical features confirm diagnosis.
● Hb electrophoresis shows Hb S.
● Electrophoresis of umbilical cord blood provides screening for all neonates at risk.
● Stained blood smear shows sickle cells.
● Blood studies reveal low RBC counts, elevated white blood cell and platelet counts, decreased erythrocyte

SICKLE CELL CRISIS

Infection, exposure to cold, high altitudes, overexertion, or other situations that cause cellular oxygen deprivation may trigger a sickle cell crisis. The deoxygenated, sickle-shaped red blood cells stick to the capillary wall and each other, blocking blood flow and causing cellular hypoxia. The crisis worsens as tissue hypoxia and acidic waste products cause more sickling and cell damage. With each new crisis, organs and tissues are slowly destroyed, especially the spleen and kidneys.

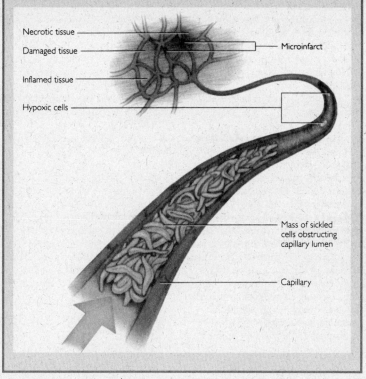

sedimentation rate, increased serum iron levels, decreased RBC survival, and reticulocytosis (Hb levels may be low or normal).

- Lateral chest X-ray shows "Lincoln log" deformity in the vertebrae of many adults and some adolescents.

- Neonatal screening for Hb abnormalities, including sickle cell anemia is mandated in most states.
- Prenatal and preimplantation diagnosis is available, especially if the mutation in the family is known.

TREATMENT

- Packed RBC transfusion to correct hypovolemia (if Hb levels decrease)
- Sedation and analgesics, such as morphine, for pain
- Oxygen administration to correct hypoxia
- Large amounts of oral or I.V. fluids to correct hypovolemia and prevent dehydration and vessel occlusion
- Prophylactic penicillin before age 4 months to prevent infection
- Hydroxyurea to reduce painful episodes by increasing the production of fetal Hb which seems to alleviate symptoms
- Iron and folic acid supplements to prevent anemia

NURSING CONSIDERATIONS

- During a crisis, administer analgesic-antipyretics as ordered and apply warm compresses to painful areas. Encourage bed rest, and place the patient in a sitting position.
- During remissions advise the patient to avoid tight clothing that restricts circulation and conditions that provoke hypoxia, such as strenuous exercise, vasoconstricting medications, cold temperatures (including drinking large amounts of ice water and swimming), unpressurized aircraft, and high altitude.
- Emphasize the need for prompt treatment of infection.
- Tell parents to encourage the child to drink more fluids, especially in the summer.
- Warn women with sickle cell anemia that they may have increased obstetrical risks.
- Adolescents or adult males with sickle cell anemia may develop sudden, painful episodes of priapism. Advise the patient to contact the physician when these episodes occur.
- Provide emotional support to the family and refer them to resource groups as indicated.

16

INFECTION

Infection is the invasion and multiplication of microorganisms in or on body tissue that produce signs and symptoms as well as an immune response. Such reproduction injures the host by causing cell damage from microorganism-produced toxins or from intracellular multiplication, or by competing with host metabolism. Infectious diseases range from relatively mild illnesses to debilitating and lethal conditions. The severity of the infection varies with the pathogenicity and number of the invading microorganisms and the strength of host defenses.

⚘ *Alert* *The very young and very old are at higher risk for infection. The immune system doesn't fully develop until about age 6 months and so an infant exposed to an infectious agent usually develops an infection. Advancing age is associated with a declining immune system, partly as a result of decreasing thymus function. Chronic diseases, such as diabetes and atherosclerosis, can weaken defenses by impairing blood flow and nutrient delivery to body systems.*

A microbe must be present in sufficient quantities to cause a disease in a healthy human. The number needed to cause a disease varies from one microbe to the next and from host to host, and may be affected by the mode of transmission. The severity of an infection depends on several factors, including the microbe's pathogenicity, that is, the likelihood that it will cause pathogenic changes or disease. Factors that affect pathogenicity include the microbe's specificity (host it's attracted to), invasiveness (ability to invade and multiply), quantity, virulence (severity of disease a pathogen can produce), toxigenicity (potential to damage the host), adhesiveness (ability to attach to host tissue), antigenicity (ability of pathogen to induce immune response), and viability (survival outside the host).

Stages of infection

Development of an infection usually proceeds through four stages. The first stage, *incubation,* may be almost instantaneous or last for years. During this time, the pathogen is replicating, and the infected person is contagious and can transmit the disease. The *prodromal* stage (stage two) follows incubation, and the still-contagious host makes vague complaints of feeling unwell. In stage three, *acute illness,* microbes are

Focus in

VIRAL INFECTION OF A HOST CELL

The virion (A) attaches to receptors on the host-cell membrane and releases enzymes (called absorption) (B) that weaken the membrane and enable the virion to penetrate the cell. The virion removes the protein coat that protects its genetic material (C), replicates (D), and matures, and then escapes from the cell by budding from the plasma membrane (E). The infection then can spread to other host cells.

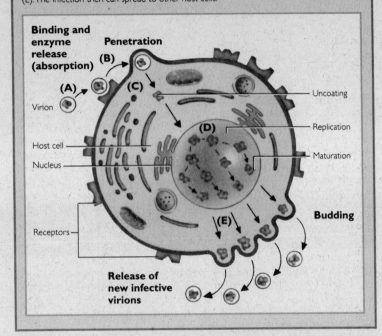

actively destroying host cells and affecting specific host systems. The patient recognizes which area of the body is affected and voices complaints that are more specific. Finally, the *convalescent* stage (stage four) begins when the body's defense mechanisms have confined the microbes and healing of damaged tissue is progressing. Microorganisms that are responsible for infectious diseases include bacteria, viruses, fungi, parasites, mycoplasmas, rickettsia, and chlamydiae.

Bacteria and viruses are the most commonly encountered.

Bacteria damage body tissues by interfering with essential cell function or by releasing exotoxins or endotoxins, which cause cell damage. During bacterial growth, the cells release exotoxins, enzymes that damage the host cell, altering its function or killing it. Enterotoxins are a specific type of exotoxin secreted by bacteria that infect the GI tract; they affect the vomiting center of the brain and cause gastroenteritis. Exotoxins can also cause diffuse reactions in the host, such as inflammation, bleeding, clotting, and fever. Endotoxins are contained in the cell walls of gram-negative bacteria, and they're released during lysis of the bacteria.

Independent of the host cells, viruses can't replicate. Rather, they invade a host cell and stimulate it to participate in forming additional virus particles. Some viruses destroy surrounding tissue and release toxins. (See *Viral infection of a host cell*.) Viruses lack the genes necessary for energy production. They depend on the ribosomes and nutrients of infected host cells for protein production. Most viruses enter the body through the respiratory, GI, and genital tracts. A few, such as human immunodeficiency virus, are transmitted through blood, broken skin, and mucous membranes. Signs and symptoms depend on the host cell's status, the specific virus, and whether the intracellular environment provides good living conditions for the virus.

Pathophysiologic changes

During the prodromal stage, a person will complain of common, nonspecific signs and symptoms, such as fever, muscle aches, headache, and lethargy. In the acute stage, signs and symptoms that are more specific provide evidence of the microbe's target. However, some illnesses don't produce symptoms and are discovered only by laboratory tests.

The inflammatory response is a major reactive defense mechanism in the battle against infective agents. Inflammation may be the result of tissue injury, infection, or allergic reaction. Acute inflammation has two stages: vascular and cellular. In the vascular stage, arterioles at or near the injury's site briefly constrict and then dilate, causing fluid pressure to increase in the capillaries. The consequent movement of plasma into the interstitial space causes edema. At the same time, inflammatory cells release histamine and bradykinin, which further increase capillary permeability. Red blood cells and fluid flow into the interstitial space, contributing to edema. The extra fluid arriving in the inflamed area dilutes microbial toxins.

During the cellular stage of inflammation, white blood cells and platelets move toward the damaged cells. Phagocytosis of the dead cells and microorganisms begins. Platelets control any excess bleeding in the area, and mast cells arriving at the site release heparin to maintain blood flow to the area.

Anthrax

Anthrax is an acute bacterial infection that most commonly occurs in grazing animals, such as cattle, sheep, goats, and horses. It can also affect people who come in contact with contaminated animals or their hides, bones, fur, hair, or wool. It's also used as an agent for bioterrorism and biological warfare. Anthrax occurs worldwide but is most common in developing countries. In humans, anthrax occurs in three forms, depending on the mode of transmission: cutaneous, inhalation, and GI.

HOW BACTERIA DAMAGE TISSUE

Bacteria and other infectious organisms constantly infect the human body. Some, such as the intestinal bacteria that produce vitamins, are beneficial. Others are harmful, causing illnesses ranging from the common cold to life-threatening septic shock.

To infect a host, bacteria must first enter it. They do this by adhering to the mucosal surface and directly invading the host cell or by attaching to epithelial cells and producing toxins, which invade host cells. To survive and multiply within a host, bacteria or their toxins adversely affect biochemical reactions in cells. The result is a disruption of normal cell function or cell death (see illustration below). For example, the diphtheria toxin damages heart muscle by inhibiting protein synthesis. In addition, as some organisms multiply, they extend into deeper tissue and eventually gain access to the bloodstream.

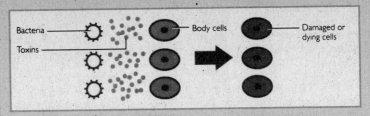

Bacteria — Toxins — Body cells — Damaged or dying cells

CAUSES

● Bacteria *Bacillus anthracis,* which exists in the soil as spores that can live for years

● Exposure to or handling of infected animals or animal products (transmission to humans)

● Not known to spread from person-to-person (see *How bacteria damage tissue*)

PATHOPHYSIOLOGY

B. anthracis is an encapsulated, chain-forming, aerobic, gram-positive rod that forms oval spores; spores are hardy and can survive for years under adverse conditions. *B. anthracis,* an extracellular pathogen, evades phagocytosis, invades the bloodstream, and multiplies rapidly. In cutaneous anthrax, spores enter the body through abraded or broken skin or by biting flies; the spores germinate within

hours, the vegetative cells multiply and anthrax toxin is produced. In inhalation anthrax, spores are deposited directly into the alveoli and phagocytized by macrophages; some are carried to and germinate in mediastinal nodes. This may result in overwhelming bacteremia, hemorrhagic mediastinitis, and secondary pneumonia. In GI anthrax, primary infection can occur in the intestine by organisms that survive passage through the stomach; acute inflammation of the intestinal tract results.

CLINICAL FINDINGS

● Cutaneous anthrax producing a small, elevated, itchy lesion that resembles an insect bite, develops into a vesicle, and finally becomes a small, painless ulcer with a necrotic (black) center due to anthrax toxin

Some toxins cause blood to clot in small blood vessels. The tissues supplied by these vessels may be deprived of blood and damaged (see illustration below).

Other toxins can damage the cell walls of small blood vessels, causing leakage. This fluid loss results in decreased blood pressure, which in turn impairs the heart's ability to pump enough blood to vital organs (see illustration below).

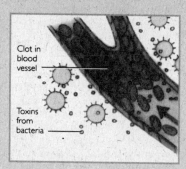

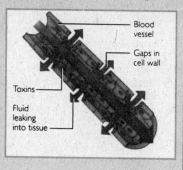

- Enlarged lymph glands due to infectious response
- Inhalational anthrax initially presenting with flulike symptoms, such as malaise, fever, headache, myalgia, and chills; progression to severe respiratory difficulties, such as dyspnea, stridor, chest pain, and cyanosis; onset of shock then occurring
- Intestinal anthrax toxins producing nausea and vomiting, decreased appetite, and fever; progression to abdominal pain, vomiting blood, and severe diarrhea

TEST RESULTS

- Isolation of *B. anthracis* from cultures of the blood, skin lesions, or sputum confirms the diagnosis.
- Specific antibodies may be detected in the blood.

TREATMENT

- Immediately initiated treatment to prevent anthrax infection; only treatment helps to prevent fatality
- Antibiotics including penicillin, ciprofloxacin (Cipro), levofloxacin (Levaquin), and doxycycline (Vibramycin)

NURSING CONSIDERATIONS

- Any case of anthrax in either livestock or a person must be reported to the appropriate public health office.
- Supportive measures are geared toward the type of anthrax exposure.
- An anthrax vaccine is available but, due to limited supplies, it's administered only to U.S. military personnel and isn't for routine civilian use.

Chlamydial infections

Chlamydial infections are the most common sexually transmitted diseases in the United States affecting an estimated 4 million Americans each year, resulting in urethritis in men and urethritis and cervicitis in women. Trachomatis conjunctivitis, a chlamydial infection that occurs rarely in the United States, is a leading cause of blindness in third world countries. Lymphogranuloma venereum, a rare disease in the United States is also caused by *Chlamydia trachomatis*.

Untreated chlamydial infections can lead to such complications as acute epididymitis, salpingitis, pelvic inflammatory disease and, eventually, sterility. Some studies show that chlamydial infections in pregnant women are associated with spontaneous abortion and premature delivery. Other studies haven't confirmed these findings.

CAUSES

- Associated conjunctivitis, otitis media, and pneumonia during passage through the birth canal in children born of mothers who have chlamydial infections
- Rectal or vaginal intercourse or oral-genital contact with an infected person *C. trachomatis*
- Sexual transmission of the organism typically occurring unknowingly due to signs and symptoms commonly appearing late in the course of the disease

PATHOPHYSIOLOGY

Chlamydial infections are transmitted by direct contact (such as sexual) producing local inflammatory action as the result of infection. Endometritis and salpingitis occur as the organism ascends the genitourinary tract.

CLINICAL FINDINGS

Chlamydial infection resulting in:
- cervicitis — producing cervical erosion, dyspareunia, micropurulent discharge, and pelvic pain
- endometritis or salpingitis — producing pain and tenderness of the lower abdomen, cervix, uterus, and lymph nodes; chills, fever; breakthrough bleeding; bleeding after intercourse; and vaginal discharge; dysuria
- urethral syndrome — producing dysuria, pyuria, and urinary frequency
- urethritis — producing dysuria, erythema, tenderness of the urethral meatus; urinary frequency; pruritus and urethral discharge (copious and purulent or scant and clear or mucoid)
- epididymitis — producing painful scrotal swelling; and urethral discharge
- prostatitis — producing low back pain; urinary frequency, nocturia, and dysuria; and painful ejaculation
- proctitis — producing diarrhea; tenesmus; pruritus; bloody or mucopurulent discharge; and diffuse or discrete ulceration in the rectosigmoid colon.

TEST RESULTS

- Swab from site of infection establishes a diagnosis of urethritis, cervicitis, salpingitis, endometritis, or proctitis.
- Culture of aspirated material establishes a diagnosis of epididymitis.
- Antigen-detection methods are the diagnostic tests of choice for identifying chlamydial infection.
- Polymerase chain reaction test is highly sensitive and specific.

TREATMENT

• For adults and adolescents who have a chlamydial infection, drug therapy with oral doxycycline (Vibramycin) for 7 days or oral azithromycin (Zithromax) in a single dose (recommended first-line treatment)

• For pregnant women with a chlamydial infection, azithromycin, in a single dose for both the male and female partners (treatment of choice)

NURSING CONSIDERATIONS

• Make sure that the patient fully understands the dosage requirements of any prescribed medications for this infection.

• If required in your state, report all cases of chlamydial infection to the appropriate local public health authorities, who will then conduct follow-up notification of the patient's sexual contacts.

• Suggest that the patient and his sexual partners receive testing for human immunodeficiency virus.

• Check neonates of infected mothers for signs of chlamydial infection. Obtain appropriate specimens for diagnostic testing.

Gonorrhea

A commonly sexually transmitted disease, gonorrhea is an infection of the genitourinary tract (especially the urethra and cervix) and, occasionally, the rectum, pharynx, and eyes. Untreated gonorrhea can spread through the blood to the joints, tendons, meninges, and endocardium; in females, it can also lead to chronic pelvic inflammatory disease (PID) and sterility.

After adequate treatment, the prognosis in both males and females is excellent, although reinfection is common. Gonorrhea is especially prevalent among young people and people with multiple partners, particularly those between ages 19 and 25.

CAUSES

• Passage through the birth canal (in children born of infected mothers), allowing for contraction of gonococcal ophthalmia neonatorum

• Sexual contact with an infected person causing transmission of *Neisseria gonorrhoeae* (the organism that causes gonorrhea)

• Touching of the eyes with hands contaminated with gonococcal conjunctivitis (in children and adults with gonorrhea)

PATHOPHYSIOLOGY

Gonococci infect mucus-secreting epithelial surfaces and penetrate through or between the cells to the connective tissue. Inflammation and spread of the infection results.

CLINICAL FINDINGS

• Males (may be asymptomatic), or possibly developing urethritis, including dysuria and purulent urethral discharge, with redness and swelling at the site of infection

• Females (may be asymptomatic), or possibly developing inflammation and a greenish yellow discharge from the cervix

• Males or females possibly presenting with pharyngitis or tonsillitis, or rectal burning, itching, and bloody mucopurulent discharge

Clinical features vary according to the site involved:

• Urethra — dysuria, urinary frequency and incontinence, purulent discharge, itching, red and edematous meatus

- Vulva — occasional itching, burning, and pain due to exudate from an adjacent infected area
- Vagina — engorgement, redness, swelling, and profuse purulent discharge
- Liver — right-upper-quadrant pain
- Pelvis — severe pelvic and lower abdominal pain, muscle rigidity, tenderness, and abdominal distention; nausea, vomiting, fever, and tachycardia (may develop in patients with salpingitis or PID

TEST RESULTS
- Culture from the site of infection, grown on a Thayer-Martin or Transgrow medium, establishes the diagnosis by isolating *N. gonorrhoeae*.
- Gram stain shows gram-negative diplococci.
- Complement fixation and immunofluorescent assays of serum reveal antibody titers four times the normal rate.

TREATMENT
- For *N. gonorrhoeae*, ceftriaxone (Rocephin) or azithromycin (Zithromax)
- For concurrent *C. trachomatis* infection, doxycycline (Vibramycin)
- Routine instillation of 1% silver nitrate or erythromycin (Romycin) drops into neonates' eyes (greatly reducing the incidence of gonococcal ophthalmia neonatorum)

NURSING CONSIDERATIONS
- Before treatment, establish whether the patient has any drug sensitivities, and watch closely for adverse effects during therapy.
- Warn the patient that until cultures prove negative, he's still infectious and can transmit gonococcal infection.

- If the patient has gonococcal arthritis, apply moist heat to ease pain in affected joints.
- Urge the patient to inform sexual contacts of his infection so that they can seek treatment, even if cultures are negative. Advise them to avoid sexual intercourse until treatment is complete.

Alert *Report all cases of gonorrhea to local public health authorities for follow-up on sexual contacts. Examine and test all people exposed to gonorrhea as well as neonates of infected mothers.*
- Routinely instill two drops of 1% silver nitrate or erythromycin in the eyes of all neonates immediately after birth. Check neonates of infected mothers for signs of infection. Take specimens for culture from the infant's eyes, pharynx, and rectum.

Alert *Report all cases of gonorrhea in children to child abuse authorities.*

Herpes simplex

A recurrent viral infection, herpes simplex is subclinical in about 85% of cases. The others produce localized lesions and systemic reactions. After the first infection, a patient is a carrier susceptible to recurrent infections, which may be provoked by fever, menses, stress, heat, and cold. In recurrent infections, the patient usually has no constitutional signs and symptoms.

CAUSES
- Herpesvirus hominis (HVH) (widespread infectious agent)
- Primary HVH, the leading cause of gingivostomatitis in children ages 1 to 3 (It causes the most common nonepidemic encephalitis and is the second most common viral infection in preg-

nant women. It can pass to the fetus transplacentally and, in early pregnancy, may cause spontaneous abortion or premature birth.)
● Purulent eye exudates, saliva, skin lesions, stools, and urine (potential sources of infection)
● Type 1 herpes (transmitted by oral and respiratory secretions) affecting skin and mucous membranes and commonly producing cold sores and fever blisters
● Type 2 herpes (primarily affecting the genital area) transmitted by sexual contact; cross-infection possibly resulting from orogenital sex

PATHOPHYSIOLOGY

The virus enters mucosal surfaces or abraded skin sites and initiates replication in cells of the epidermis and dermis. Replication continues to permit infection of sensory or autonomic nerve endings. The virus enters the neuronal cell and is transported intra-axonally to nerve cell bodies in ganglia (where the virus establishes latency) and spreads by the peripheral sensory nerves. (See *Understanding the genital herpes cycle.*)

Herpes is equally common in males and females. It occurs worldwide and is most prevalent among children in lower socioeconomic groups who live in crowded environments.

CLINICAL FINDINGS

● Type 1 infection producing fever; sore, red, swollen throat; and submaxillary lymphadenopathy; increased salivation, halitosis, and anorexia
● Severe mouth pain resulting from edema of the mouth
● Vesicles (on the tongue, gingiva, and cheeks, or anywhere in or around the mouth) on a red base that eventu-

---

UNDERSTANDING THE GENITAL HERPES CYCLE

After a patient is infected with genital herpes, a latency period follows. The virus takes up permanent residence in the nerve cells surrounding the lesions, and intermittent viral shedding may take place.

Repeated outbreaks may develop at any time, again followed by a latent stage during which the lesions heal completely. Outbreaks may recur as often as three to eight times yearly. Although the cycle continues indefinitely, some people remain symptom-free for years.

Initial infection
Highly infectious period marked by fever, aches, adenopathy, pain, and ulcerated skin and mucous membranes.

↓

Latency
Intermittently infectious period marked by viral dormancy or viral shedding and no disease symptoms.

↓

Recurrent infection
Highly infectious period similar to initial infection with milder symptoms that resolve faster.

---

ally rupture, leaving a painful ulcer and then yellow crusting
● Type 2 infection producing tingling in the area involved, malaise, dysuria, dyspareunia (painful intercourse), and leukorrhea (white vaginal discharge containing mucus and pus cells)
● Localized, fluid-filled vesicles found on the cervix, labia, perianal skin, vulva, vagina, glans penis, fore-

BLOCKING INFLAMMATION

Several substances act to control inflammation. The flowchart below shows the progression of inflammation and the points ✻ at which drugs can reduce inflammation and pain.

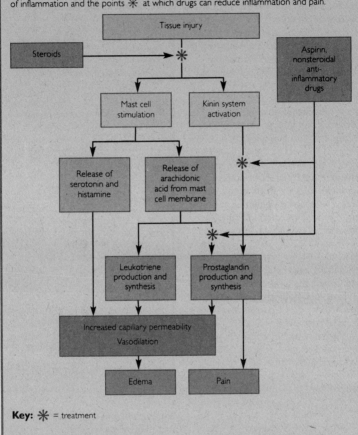

Key: ✻ = treatment

skin, and penile shaft, mouth or anus; inguinal swelling may be present

TEST RESULTS
● Tzanck test shows multinucleated giant cells.

● Herpes simplex virus culture is positive.
● Virus is isolated from local lesions.
● Tissue biopsy aids in diagnosis.
● Elevated antibodies and increased white blood cell count indicate primary infection.

TREATMENT

Treatment of symptoms and supportive therapy are essential.

● Generalized primary infection usually requiring an analgesic-antipyretic to reduce fever and relieve pain (see *Blocking inflammation*)

● Anesthetic mouthwashes, such as viscous lidocaine to treat the pain of gingivostomatitis, enabling the patient to eat and preventing dehydration

● Drying agents, such as calamine lotion, to make labial lesions less painful

● Referring patients with eye infections to an ophthalmologist (Topical corticosteroids are contraindicated in active infection, but trifluridine [Viroptic] is effective.)

● A 5% acyclovir ointment to bring relief to patients with genital herpes or to immunosuppressed patients with HVH skin infections (I.V. acyclovir helps treat more severe infections.)

NURSING CONSIDERATIONS

● Abstain from direct patient care if you have herpetic whitlow.

● Patients with central nervous system infection alone need no isolation.

● Teach patients how to care for themselves (warm compresses or sitz bath to treat genital lesions) during an outbreak of HVH and how to avoid infecting others.

Herpes zoster

Also called *shingles,* herpes zoster is an acute unilateral segmental inflammation of the dorsal root ganglia caused by infection with the herpesvirus varicella-zoster, which also causes chickenpox. It produces localized vesicular skin lesions confined to a dermatome and severe neuralgic pain in peripheral areas innervated by the nerves arising in the inflamed root ganglia.

The prognosis is good unless the infection spreads to the brain. Eventually, most patients recover completely, except for possible scarring and, in corneal damage, vision impairment. Occasionally, neuralgia may persist for months or years. Herpes zoster is found primarily in adults, especially those older than age 50. It seldom recurs.

CAUSES

● Exactly how or why this reactivation occurs isn't clear (Some believe that the virus multiplies as it's reactivated and that it's neutralized by antibodies remaining from the initial infection. However, if effective antibodies aren't present, the virus continues to multiply in the ganglia, destroy the host neuron, and spread down the sensory nerves to the skin.)

● Reactivation of varicella virus that has lain dormant in the cerebral ganglia (extramedullary ganglia of the cranial nerves) or the ganglia of posterior nerve roots since a previous episode of chickenpox

PATHOPHYSIOLOGY

Herpes zoster erupts when the virus reactivates after dormancy in the cerebral ganglia (extramedullary ganglia of the cranial nerves) or the ganglia of posterior nerve roots. The virus may multiply as it reactivates, and antibodies remaining from the initial infection may neutralize it. Without opposition from effective antibodies, the virus continues to multiply in the ganglia, destroys neurons, and spreads down the sensory nerves to the skin.

CLINICAL FINDINGS

- Pain and pruritus within the dermatome affected
- Fever and malaise from the infectious process
- Possible paresthesia or hyperesthesia in the trunk, arms, or legs
- Small, red, nodular skin lesions on painful areas (nerve specific) that change to pus- or fluid-filled vesicles
- Herpes zoster occasionally involving the cranial nerves, especially the trigeminal and geniculate ganglia or the oculomotor nerve (herpes zoster)
- Geniculate zoster possibly causing vesicle formation in the external auditory canal, ipsilateral facial palsy, hearing loss, dizziness, and loss of taste
- Trigeminal ganglion involvement causing eye pain and possibly corneal and scleral damage and impaired vision
- Rarely oculomotor involvement causing conjunctivitis, extraocular weakness, ptosis, and paralytic mydriasis

Alert *In rare cases, herpes zoster leads to generalized central nervous system infection, muscle atrophy, motor paralysis (usually transient), acute transverse myelitis, and ascending myelitis. More commonly, generalized infection causes acute retention of urine and unilateral paralysis of the diaphragm. In postherpetic neuralgia, a complication most common in elderly patients, intractable neuralgic pain may persist for years. Scars may be permanent.*

TEST RESULTS

- Staining antibodies from vesicular fluid and identification under fluorescent light differentiates herpes zoster from localized herpes simplex.
- Examination of vesicular fluid and infected tissue shows eosinophilic intranuclear inclusions and varicella virus.
- Lumbar puncture shows increased pressure; cerebrospinal fluid shows increased protein levels and possibly pleocytosis.

TREATMENT

No specific treatment exists.

- Calamine lotion or another antipruritic to relieve itching
- Aspirin, possibly with codeine or another analgesic, to relieve neuralgic pain
- Collodion or compound benzoin tincture applied to unbroken lesions for itching and pain relief
- If bacteria have infected ruptured vesicles, treatment usually including an appropriate systemic antibiotic
- Instillation of an antiviral ophthalmic agent for trigeminal zoster with corneal involvement
- Corticosteroids to reduce inflammation; tranquilizers, sedatives or tricyclic antidepressants with phenothiazines to treat intractable pain of postherpetic neuralgia
- Acyclovir (Zovirax) to stop progression of the rash and prevent visceral complications (In immunocompromised patients, acyclovir therapy may be administered I.V. to prevent disseminated, life-threatening disease in some patients.)
- Acyclovir and famciclovir (Famvir) to shorten the duration of pain and symptoms in normal adults

NURSING CONSIDERATIONS

- Keep the patient comfortable, maintain hygiene, and prevent infection. During the acute phase, encourage adequate rest.
- Apply calamine lotion liberally to the lesion. If lesions are severe and widespread, apply a wet dressing. If vesicles rupture, apply a cold compress.

- To decrease the pain of oral lesions, tell the patient to use a soft toothbrush, eat a soft diet, and use saline mouthwash.
- To minimize neuralgic pain, never withhold or delay administration of analgesics. Give on schedule.

Lyme disease

Lyme disease is a multisystemic disorder caused by the spirochete *Borrelia burgdorferi*, which is carried by the minute tick Ixodes dammini or another tick in the Ixodidae family. It typically begins in summer, with the classic skin lesion called erythema chronicum migrans (ECM). Weeks or months later, cardiac or neurologic abnormalities sometimes develop, possibly followed by arthritis.

Lyme disease occurs primarily in areas of the United States inhabited by the deer tick, such as in the northeast (from Massachusetts to Maryland), in the Midwest (in Wisconsin and Minnesota), and in the west (California and Oregon).

CAUSES
- Tick (injects spirochete-laden salvia into the bloodstream or deposits fecal matter on the skin)

PATHOPHYSIOLOGY
A tick injects spirochete-laden saliva into the bloodstream or deposits fecal matter on the skin. After incubating for 3 to 32 days, the spirochetes migrate outward on the skin, causing a rash, and disseminate to other skin sites or organs through the bloodstream or lymph system. Spirochetes may survive for years in the joints, or die after triggering an inflammatory response in the host.

CLINICAL FINDINGS
Stage 1
- ECM: red macule or papule, commonly on the site of a tick bite, which may grow to over 20″ (50.8 cm), feels hot and itchy, and resembles a bull's eye or target; after a few days, more lesions erupt and a migratory, ringlike rash appears
- Conjunctivitis
- Diffuse urticaria from inflammatory reaction
- Lesions replaced by small red blotches in 3 to 4 weeks
- Malaise and fatigue, fever, chills, and achiness, regional lymphadenopathy from the infectious process
- Intermittent headache and neck stiffness

Stage 2
- Neurologic abnormalities: fluctuating meningoencephalitis with peripheral and cranial neuropathy; begins weeks to months later
- Facial palsy
- Cardiac abnormalities: brief, fluctuating atrioventricular heart block, left ventricular dysfunction, cardiomegaly

Stage 3
- Arthritis with marked swelling begins weeks or years later
- Neuropsychiatric symptoms such as psychotic behavior, memory loss, dementia, and depression
- Encephalopathic symptoms, such as headache, confusion, and difficulty concentrating
- Ophthalmic manifestations such as iritis, keratitis, renal vasculitis, optic neuritis

HOW CEPHALOSPORINS ATTACK BACTERIA

The antibacterial action of cephalosporins depends on their ability to penetrate the bacterial wall and bind with proteins on the cytoplasmic membrane, as shown here.

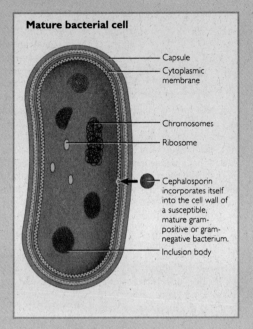

Mature bacterial cell

- Capsule
- Cytoplasmic membrane
- Chromosomes
- Ribosome
- Cephalosporin incorporates itself into the cell wall of a susceptible, mature gram-positive or gram-negative bacterium.
- Inclusion body

TEST RESULTS

- Because *B. burgdorferi* is unusual in humans and indirect immunofluorescent antibody tests are marginally sensitive, diagnosis is usually based on the characteristic ECM lesion and related clinical findings.
- Serology reveals mild anemia and elevated erythrocyte sedimentation rate, white blood cell count, serum immunoglobulin M level, and aspartate aminotransferase.
- Cerebrospinal fluid analysis reveals presence of antibodies to *B. burgdorferi* if the disease has affected the central nervous system.

TREATMENT

- A 3 to 4 week course of antibiotic treatment using doxycycline (Vibramycin) in early disease (generally effective)
- Cefuroxime axetil (Ceftin) and ceftriaxone sodium (Rocephin) (alternatives) (see *How cephalosporins attack bacteria*)
- Oral penicillin (usually prescribed for children)

When given in the early stages, these drugs can minimize later complications. When given during the late stages, high-dose I.V. penicillin or I.V. ceftriaxone may be a successful treat-

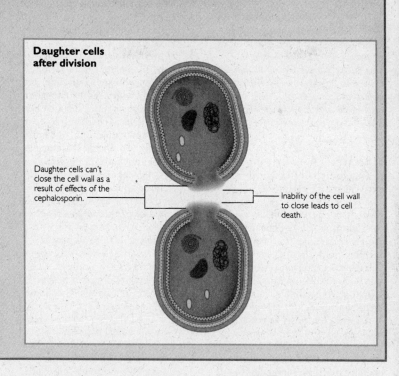

Daughter cells after division

Daughter cells can't close the cell wall as a result of effects of the cephalosporin.

Inability of the cell wall to close leads to cell death.

ment. Neurologic abnormalities are best treated with I.V. ceftriaxone or I.V. penicillin.

NURSING CONSIDERATIONS

● Take a detailed history, asking about travel to endemic areas and exposure to ticks.

● For a patient with arthritis, help with range-of-motion and strengthening exercises, but avoid overexertion.

Alert Monitor for complications. Assess the patient's neurologic function and level of consciousness frequently; watch for signs of increased intracranial pressure and cranial nerve involvement,

such as ptosis, strabismus, and diplopia. Check for cardiac abnormalities, such as arrhythmias and heart block.

Otitis media

Inflammation of the middle ear, otitis media may be suppurative or secretory, acute or chronic. Acute otitis media is common in children; its incidence rises during the winter months, paralleling the seasonal rise in nonbacterial respiratory tract infections.

With prompt treatment, the prognosis for acute otitis media is excellent.

Alert *Prolonged accumulation of fluid within the middle ear cavity causes chronic otitis media, with possible perforation of the tympanic membrane. Chronic suppurative otitis media may lead to scarring, adhesions, and severe structural or functional ear damage; chronic secretory otitis media, with its persistent inflammation and pressure, may cause conductive hearing loss.*

CAUSES
- Results from disruption of eustachian tube patency

Secretory otitis media
- Chronic secretory otitis media following persistent eustachian tube dysfunction from edema (allergic rhinitis, chronic sinus infection), mechanical obstruction (adenoidal tissue overgrowth, tumors), or inadequate treatment of acute suppurative otitis media
- Effusion secondary to eustachian tube dysfunction from viral infection or allergy (It may also follow barotrauma — pressure injury caused by inability to equalize pressures between the environment and the middle ear — as can occur during rapid aircraft descent in a person with an upper respiratory tract infection or during rapid underwater ascent in scuba diving [barotitis media].)
- With secretory otitis media, obstruction of the eustachian tube causing a buildup of negative pressure in the middle ear, promoting transudation of sterile serous fluid from blood vessels in the membrane of the middle ear

Suppurative otitis media
- Chronic suppurative otitis media resulting from inadequate treatment of acute otitis episodes, or from infection by resistant strains of bacteria or, rarely, tuberculosis
- Predisposing factors, including anatomic anomalies; genetic factors such as susceptibility to infection; and the normally wider, shorter, more horizontal eustachian tubes and increased lymphoid tissue in children
- In the suppurative form, respiratory tract infection, allergic reaction, nasotracheal intubation, or positional changes allowing nasopharyngeal flora to reflux through the eustachian tube and colonize the middle ear
- Suppurative otitis media usually resulting from bacterial infection with beta hemolytic streptococci, gram-negative bacteria, *Haemophilus influenzae* (the most common cause in children under age 6), *Moraxella catarrhalis,* pneumococci, or staphylococci (most common in children age 6 or older)

PATHOPHYSIOLOGY
The suppurative form of otitis media results from nasopharyngeal flora reflux through the eustachian tube and colonizing of the middle ear. Respiratory tract infections, allergic reactions, and position changes allow reflux of nasopharyngeal flora through the eustachian tube and colonization in the middle ear. The secretory form of otitis media produces obstruction of the eustachian tube promoting transudation of sterile serous fluid from blood vessels in the middle ear membrane.

CLINICAL FINDINGS
- Ear pain from stimulation of nerve endings and localized edema
- Ear drainage
- Hearing loss from edema

• Fever, lethargy, and irritability from the infectious process
• Vertigo and tinnitus from stimulation of the inner ear
• Signs of upper respiratory tract infection (such as sneezing and coughing)

TEST RESULTS
• Otoscopy reveals obscured or distorted bony landmarks of the tympanic membrane.
• Pneumatoscopy can show decreased tympanic membrane mobility.
• Culture of the ear drainage identifies the causative organism.

TREATMENT
• Antibiotic therapy (if the disease is bacteria in origin)
• Nasal spray, nose drops, oral decongestants, or antihistamines to promote drainage of fluid through the eustachian tube
• Eardrops or analgesics to relieve pain
• Oral corticosteroids to reduce inflammation
• Myringotomy for severe, painful bulging of the tympanic membrane
• Valsalva's maneuver several times per day to inflate the eustachian tube for acute secretory otitis media
• Treatment of underlying cause

NURSING CONSIDERATIONS
• After myringotomy, maintain drainage flow. Don't place cotton or plugs deep in the ear canal; however, sterile cotton may be placed loosely in the external ear to absorb drainage.
• To prevent infection, change the cotton whenever it gets damp, and wash hands before and after giving ear care. Watch for headache, fever, severe pain, or disorientation.

• Encourage the patient to complete the prescribed course of antibiotic therapy. Teach correct instillation of eardrops, if prescribed.

Alert *Most children will have an effusion present at the completion of a 10 to 14 day course of antibiotic therapy. Effusion may last up to 12 weeks before spontaneous clearance can be expected.*
• Apply heat to the ear with a warm cloth or water bottle to relieve pain.

Severe acute respiratory syndrome

Severe acute respiratory syndrome (SARS) is a viral respiratory illness caused by a coronavirus, called the SARS-associated coronavirus (SARS-CoV). SARS was first reported in China, Vietnam, and Hong Kong in February 2003. It had spread to other countries, including the United States until a global outbreak was contained in 2003.

CAUSES
• New type of CoV (suspected cause)
• Possibly spread broadly through the air or by other means
• Spread through contact with contaminated objects (highly contagious)

PATHOPHYSIOLOGY
The SARS Co-V is spread in droplets that are shed from the respiratory secretions of infected persons. Fecal or airborne transmission is less common.

CLINICAL FINDINGS
• Commonly beginning with a fever greater than 100.4°F (38° C), headache, general discomfort and body

aches, and in some patients, mild respiratory symptoms
- After 2 to 7 days, patients possibly developing a dry cough and difficulty breathing; fever mostly associated with other symptoms including chills, rigors, headache, dizziness, malaise, and myalgia

TEST RESULTS

The diagnosis of SARS remains based on clinical and epidemiologic findings. As defined by the World Health Organization, a suspected case is classified as:
- disease in a person with a documented fever with a temperature greater than 100.4° F (38° C)
- lower respiratory tract symptoms
- contact with a person believed to have had SARS or a history of travel to a geographic area where there has been documented transmission of the illness.

Indications of SARS include chest X-ray findings of pneumonia, acute respiratory distress syndrome (ARDS), or an unexplained respiratory illness resulting in death (with autopsy findings consistent with ARDS without an identifiable cause).
- Presently available tests generally can't detect the small amounts of SARS-CoV initially shed. SARS-CoV-specific ribonucleic acid (RNA) can be detected in various clinical specimens, such as blood, stools, respiratory secretions, or body tissues by the polymerase chain reaction.
- During the course of illness, abnormal hematologic values are common. Early studies have shown lymphopenia and thrombocytopenia to be common in SARS patients.
- Common electrolyte and biochemical abnormalities include elevated levels of lactate dehydrogenase, aspartate

and alanine aminotransferases, and creatine kinase; these findings may be associated with tissue damage, such as the extensive lung injury which occurs with SARS.

TREATMENT

Treatment is primarily palliative.
- Ensuring prompt isolation in a properly equipped facility, and management according to strict infection control procedures
- Identifying close contacts of each case and follow-up (including daily health checks and possible voluntary home isolation)
- Assisted ventilation in a noninvasive or invasive form instituted in SARS patients complicated by respiratory failure
- Broad-spectrum antibiotics and supportive care as well as antiviral agents and immunomodulatory therapy
- Antivirals, such as oseltamivir (Tamiflu) and ribavirin (Copegus), and steroids in combination with antivirals
- Ribavirin, a nucleoside analog, as empirical therapy for SARS (because of its broad-spectrum antiviral activity against many deoxyribonucleic acid and RNA viruses; usually used with corticosteroids and has since become the most commonly administered antiviral agent for SARS)
- Interferons (limited to interferon-alfa)
- Corticosteroids

NURSING CONSIDERATIONS

- Report all suspected cases immediately to proper health authorities.
- Provide respiratory and cardiopulmonary support; assist with treatments as indicated and monitor for complications.
- Enforce strict isolation as ordered.

Smallpox

Smallpox, or variola, is an acute, highly contagious infectious disease caused by poxvirus variola. Vaccination for smallpox is being reconsidered in light of potential biological attacks. Variola develops in three major forms: variola major (classic smallpox), which once carried a high mortality; variola minor, a mild form from a less virulent strain; and varioloid, a mild variant that occurred in those with partial immunity.

Alert *Hemorrhagic variola, an uncommon form of variola major, has a much shorter incubation period, making initial recognition as variola unlikely. It's usually fatal and vaccination doesn't provide much protection.*

CAUSES

Variola can affect people of all ages. Before its eradication, incidence was highest during the winter in cold temperature zones; during the hot, dry months in the tropics.

- Direct transmission of respiratory droplets or dried scales of virus-containing lesions or indirect transmission through contact with contaminated linens or other objects
- Exposure through inhalation (in a terrorist attack, most likely to occur)

Alert *Variola major is contagious from onset until after the last scab is shed. Individuals infected with variola minor and varioloid are infectious at the appearance of the first rash and remain contagious until the last variola scab falls off.*

PATHOPHYSIOLOGY

Poxviruses are characterized by a large double-stranded deoxyribonucleic acid (DNA) genome and a brick-shaped morphology. Poxviruses are the only DNA viruses that replicate in cytoplasm. The virus is spread through direct contact or inhalation of respiratory droplets. The incubation period is 7 to 19 days. Illness onset is in 10 to 14 days, with onset of the characteristic rash in 2 to 4 days. Fever and macular rash appear after an average incubation period of 12 days, with a progression to typical vesicular and pustular lesions over 1 or 2 weeks. It's most contagious before the eruptive period and from the time between lesion development and scab disappearance.

CLINICAL FINDINGS

- Abrupt onset of chills (and possible seizures in children), and high fever (above 104° F [40° C]) from inflammatory response
- Headache, backache, severe malaise, vomiting (especially in children), and marked prostration
- Occasionally, violent delirium, stupor, or coma
- Sore throat and cough as well as lesions on the mucous membranes of the mouth, throat, and respiratory tract
- Skin lesions progressing from macular to papular, vesicular, and pustular, with eventual desquamation causing intense pruritus and permanently disfiguring scars
- In fatal cases, death typically resulting from encephalitic manifestations, extensive bleeding from orifices, or secondary bacterial infections

TEST RESULTS

- Most conclusive laboratory test is culture of variola virus isolated from an aspirate of vesicles and pustules.
- Microscopic examination of smears from lesion scrapings and complement fixation detect virus or

antibodies to the virus in the patient's blood.

TREATMENT
- Hospitalization with strict isolation
- Antimicrobial therapy to treat bacterial complications
- Vigorous supportive measures and symptomatic treatment of lesions with antipruritics, starting during the pustular stage
- Anti-inflammatories, codeine, or morphine to relieve pain
- I.V. fluids and gastric tube feedings to provide fluids, electrolytes, and calories because pharyngeal lesions make swallowing difficult

NURSING CONSIDERATIONS
- Report all suspected cases immediately to proper health authorities.
- Provide supportive therapy as ordered (antipyretics, skin care, anti-inflammatories) and monitor response.

Syphilis

A chronic, infectious, sexually transmitted disease, syphilis begins in the mucous membranes and quickly becomes systemic, spreading to nearby lymph nodes and the bloodstream. This disease, when untreated, is characterized by progressive stages; primary, secondary, latent, and late (formerly called tertiary). The primary and secondary stages of syphilis have a high incidence among urban populations, especially in people between ages 15 and 39, drug users, and those infected with the human immunodeficiency virus (HIV). Untreated syphilis leads to crippling or death but the prognosis is excellent with early treatment.

CAUSES
- Infection from the spirochete *Treponema pallidum*
- Possible prenatal transmission occurring from an infected mother to her fetus
- Transmission occurring primarily through sexual contact during the primary, secondary, and early latent stages of infection

PATHOPHYSIOLOGY
The infecting organism penetrates intact mucous membranes or abrasions in the skin, entering lymphatics and blood. Systemic infection and systemic foci precede primary lesion development at the site of inoculation. Organ involvement occurs from dissemination.

CLINICAL FINDINGS
- Primary syphilis — producing chancres (small, fluid-filled lesions) on the anus, fingers, lips, tongue, nipples, tonsils, or eyelids; and regional lymphadenopathy
- Secondary syphilis — producing symmetrical mucocutaneous lesions; general lymphadenopathy; rash may be macular, papular, pustular, or nodular; headache; malaise; anorexia, weight loss, nausea, and vomiting; sore throat and slight fever; alopecia; brittle and pitted nails
- Late syphilis — producing benign gumma lesion found on any bone or organ; gastric pain, tenderness, enlarged spleen; anemia; involvement of the upper respiratory tract; perforation of the nasal septum or palate; destruction of bones and organs; fibrosis of elastic tissue of the aorta; aortic insufficiency; aortic aneurysm; meningitis;

paresis; personality changes; arm and leg weakness

TEST RESULTS
- Dark-field examination of a lesion identifies *T. pallidum.*
- Fluorescent treponemal antibody absorption test identifies antigens of *T. pallidum* in tissue, ocular fluid, cerebrospinal fluid, tracheobronchial secretions, and exudates from lesions.
- Venereal Disease Research Laboratory slide test and rapid plasma reagin test detect nonspecific antibodies.

TREATMENT
- Penicillin I.M. (treatment of choice)
- Oral tetracycline (Sumycin) or doxycycline (Vibramycin) in nonpregnant patients who are allergic to penicillin

  Alert *Tetracycline is contraindicated in pregnant women.*
- Abstinence from sexual contact until the syphilis sores are completely healed

NURSING CONSIDERATIONS
- Stress the importance of completing the course of therapy even after symptoms subside. Instruct those infected to inform their partners that they should be tested and, if necessary, treated.
- In secondary syphilis, keep lesions clean and dry. If they're draining, dispose of contaminated materials properly.
- In late syphilis, provide symptomatic care during prolonged treatment.
- Encourage follow-up to detect possible relapse.
- Report all cases to local public health authorities.

Urinary tract infection

Cystitis and urethritis, the two forms of lower urinary tract infection (UTI), are nearly 10 times more common in women than in men and affect approximately 10% to 20% or all women at least once. Lower UTI is also a prevalent bacterial disease in children, with girls most commonly affected. In men and children, lower UTIs are usually related to anatomic or physiologic abnormalities and therefore require extremely close evaluation. UTIs usually respond readily to treatment, but recurrence and resistant bacterial flare-up during therapy are possible.

CAUSES
- Ascending infection by a single gram-negative enteric bacterium, such as *Enterobacter, Escherichia coli, Klebsiella, Proteus, Pseudomonas,* or *Serratia*
- Breakdown in local defense mechanisms in the bladder that allow bacteria to invade the bladder mucosa and multiply (These bacteria can't be readily eliminated by normal micturition.)
- Cystitis, risk being higher when the bladder or urethra become blocked and urine flow stops; also occurring when instruments are inserted into the urinary tract during procedures such as catheterization or cystoscopy
- During treatment, bacterial flare-up due to the pathogenic organism's resistance to the prescribed antimicrobial therapy
- In a patient with neurogenic bladder, an indwelling urinary catheter, or a fistula between the intestine and bladder, causing lower UTI from si-

multaneous infection with multiple pathogens
- Lack of adequate fluids, bowel incontinence, immobility or decreased mobility, indwelling urinary catheters, and placement in a nursing home

> **Alert** *Elderly individuals are at increased risk for developing UTIs due to incomplete emptying of the bladder; this is associated with conditions such as benign prostatic hyperplasia and prostate and urethral strictures.*

- Recurrent lower UTI usually resulting from reinfection by the same organism or from some new pathogen; in the remaining 1%, recurrence reflecting persistent infection, usually from renal calculi, chronic bacterial prostatitis, or a structurally anomaly that may become a source of infection
- Other risks including diabetes, a history of analgesic or reflux nephropathy, and pregnancy

PATHOPHYSIOLOGY

Local defense mechanisms in the bladder breakdown. Bacteria invade the bladder mucosa and multiply and can't be eliminated by normal urination. The pathogen's resistance to prescribed antimicrobial therapy usually causes bacterial flare-up during treatment. Recurrent lower UTIs result from reinfection by the same organism or a new pathogen.

CLINICAL FINDINGS

- Cystitis producing dysuria, frequency, urgency, and suprapubic pain; cloudy, malodorous, and possibly bloody urine; fever; nausea and vomiting; costovertebral angle tenderness
- Acute pyelonephritis producing fever and shaking chills; nausea, vomiting, and diarrhea; symptoms of cystitis may be present; tachycardia
- Generalized muscle tenderness

- Urethritis producing dysuria, frequency, and pyuria

TEST RESULTS

- Urine culture reveals microorganism.
- Urinary microscopy is positive for pyuria, hematuria, or bacteriuria.

TREATMENT

- Appropriate antimicrobials are the treatment of choice for most initial lower UTIs.
- If the urine isn't sterile after repeat urine cultures are done 3 days after taking antibiotics, bacterial resistance has probably occurred, making the use of a different antimicrobial necessary.
- Recurrent infections due to infected renal calculi, chronic prostatitis, or structural abnormality may necessitate surgery.
- Prostatitis requires long-term antibiotic therapy.

NURSING CONSIDERATIONS

- Watch the patient for GI disturbances from antimicrobial therapy.
- Provide the patient with education on treatment and prevention of UTIs.
- Collect all urine specimens for culture and sensitivity testing carefully and promptly.

SELECTED REFERENCES

INDEX

———◆———

SELECTED REFERENCES

◆

General

ACC Atlas of Pathophysiology, 2nd ed. Philadelphia: Lippincott Williams & Wilkins, 2005.

Copstead-Kirkhorn, L.E.C., and Banasik, J.L. *Pathophysiology,* 3rd ed. Philadelphia: W.B. Saunders Co., 2005.

Handbook of Pathophysiology, 2nd ed. Philadelphia: Lippincott Williams & Wilkins, 2004.

Huether, S.E., and McCance, K.L. *Understanding Pathophysiology,* 3rd ed. St. Louis: Mosby–Year Book, Inc., 2004.

Cardiovascular system

Cardiovascular Care Made Incredibly Easy. Philadelphia: Lippincott Williams & Wilkins, 2004.

Deaton, C., and Grady, K.L. "State of the Science for Cardiovascular Nursing Outcomes: Heart Failure," *Journal of Cardiovascular Nursing* 19(5):329-38, September-October 2004.

Garrett, K., et al. "The Effects of Obesity on the Cardiopulmonary System: Implications for Critical Care Nursing," *Progress in Cardiovascular Nursing* 19(4):155-61, Fall 2004.

Griffin, B.P., and Topol, E.J., eds. *Manual of Cardiovascular Medicine,* 2nd ed. Philadelphia: Lippincott Williams & Wilkins, 2004.

Heger, J.W., et al. *Cardiology,* 5th ed. Philadelphia: Lippincott Williams & Wilkins, 2004.

Respiratory system

Albert, R.K., et al. *Clinical Respiratory Medicine,* 2nd ed. St. Louis: Mosby–Year Book, Inc., 2004.

"Decreasing the Risk of Ventilator-Associated Pneumonia: The Impact of Nursing Care," *Progress in Cardiovascular Nursing* 19(3):123-24, Summer 2004.

Dent, M.R. "Hospital-Acquired Pneumonia: The 'Gift' That Keeps on Taking," *Nursing2004* 34(2):48-51, February 2004.

Goss, C.H., et al. "Incidence of Acute Lung Injury in the United States," *Critical Care Medicine* 31(6):1607-11, June 2003.

Vollman, K.M. "Prone Positioning in the Patient Who has Acute Respiratory Distress Syndrome: The Art and Science," *Critical Care Nursing Clinics of North America* 16(3):319-36, September 2004.

Nervous system

Alspach, G. "Improving the Odds for Avoiding Dementia in Advanced Age," *Critical Care Nurse* 24(5):8, 10, 12, October 2004.

Imke, S. "Parkinson's Disease: More than Meets the Eye," *Advance for Nurse Practitioners* 11(9):42-44, 47-48, 51, September 2003.

McKearnan, K.A., et al. "Pain in Children with Cerebral Palsy: A Review," *Journal of Neuroscience Nursing* 36(5):252-59, October 2004.

Weiner, H.L., et al. *Neurology,* 7th ed. Philadelphia: Lippincott Williams & Wilkins, 2004.

Gastrointestinal system

Carlson, D.S., and Pfaldt, E. "Perforated Peptic Ulcer," *Nursing2004* 34(12):88, December 2004.

Krumberger, J.M. "How to Manage an Acute Upper GI Bleed," *RN* 68(3):34-39, March 2005.

Reiser, D.J. "Neonatal Jaundice: Physiologic Variation or Pathologic Process," *Critical Care Nursing Clinics of North America* 16(2):257-69, June 2004.

Rolstad, B.S., and Erwin-Toth, P.L. "Peristomal Skin Complications: Prevention and Management," *Ostomy/Wound Management* 50(9):68-77, September 2004.

Smith, G. *Gastrointestinal Nursing.* Cambridge, Mass.: Blackwell Scientific Pubs., 2003.

Renal system

Cannon, J.D. "Recognizing Chronic Renal Failure...The Sooner, The Better," *Nursing2004* 34(1):50-53, January 2004.

Knotek, B., and Biel, L. "Peritoneal Dialysis Travel 'Tool Box,'" *Nephrology Nursing Journal* 31(5):549-79, 589, September-October 2004.

Pile, C. "Hemodialysis Vascular Access: How Do Practice Patterns Affect Outcomes?" *Nephrology Nursing Journal* 31(3):305-308, May-June 2004.

Wilcox, C.S. *Handbook of Nephrology and Hypertension,* 5th ed. Philadelphia: Lippincott Williams & Wilkins, 2004.

Endocrine system

Appel, S.J., et al. "Central Obesity and the Metabolic Syndrome: Implications for Primary Care Providers," *Journal of the American Academy of Nurse Practitioners* 16(8):335-42, August 2004.

Camacho, P.M., et al. *Evidence-Based Endocrinology.* Philadelphia: Lippincott Williams & Wilkins, 2003.

DeCoste, K.C., and Scott, L.K. "Diabetes Update: Promoting Effective Disease Management," *AAOHN Journal* 52(8):344-53, August 2004.

Hematologic system

Anderson, S.C., and Poulsen, K.B. *Anderson's Atlas of Hematology.* Philadelphia: Lippincott Williams & Wilkins, 2003.

Kirschman, R.A. "Finding Alternatives to Blood Transfusions," *Nursing2004* 34(6):58-62, June 2004.

Rodgers, G.P., and Young, N.S. *Bethesda Handbook of Clinical Hematology.* Philadelphia: Lippincott Williams & Wilkins, 2004.

Immune system

Abbas, A.K., and Lichtman, A.H. *Basic Immunology: The Functions of the Immune System,* 2nd ed. Philadelphia: W.B. Saunders Co., 2004.

Burns, A. "Anaphylaxis," *Nursing2004* 34(3):88, March 2004.

Capriotti, T. "The 'Alphabet' of Rheumatoid Arthritis Treatment," *Medsurg Nursing* 13(6):420-28, December 2004.

Ochs, H.D., et al., eds. *Primary Immunodeficiency Disease.* New York: Oxford University Press, 2004.

Pullen, R.L., Jr., et al. "Managing Organ-Threatening Systemic Lupus Erythematosus," *Medsurg Nursing* 12(6):368-79, December 2003.

Stevens, C.D. *Clinical Immunology and Serology: A Laboratory Perspective,* 2nd ed. Philadelphia: F.A. Davis Co., 2003.

Trent, J.T., and Kirsner, R.S. "Cutaneous Manifestations of HIV: A Primer," *Advances in Skin and Wound Care* 17(3):116-27, April 2004.

Sensory system

Bess, F.H., and Humes, L.E. *Audiology: The Fundamentals,* 3rd ed. Philadelphia: Lippincott Williams & Wilkins, 2003.

Houde, S.C., and Huff, M.H. "Age-Related Vision Loss in Older Adults. A Challenge for Gerontological Nurses," *Journal of Gerontological Nursing* 29(4):25-33, April 2003.

Integumentary system

Baranoski, S., and Ayello, E.A. *Wound Care Essentials: Practice Principles.* Philadelphia: Lippincott Williams and Wilkins, 2003.

Burns, T., et al., eds. *Rook's Textbook of Dermatology,* 7th ed. Cambridge, Mass.: Blackwell Scientific Pubs., 2004.

Goodheart, H.P. *Goodheart's Photoguide of Common Skin Disorders: Diagnosis and Management,* 2nd ed. Philadelphia: Lippincott Williams & Wilkins, 2003.

Hess, C.T. *Clinical Guide to Wound Care,* 5th ed. Philadelphia: Lippincott Williams & Wilkins, 2004.

Wound Care Made Incredibly Easy. Philadelphia: Lippincott Williams & Wilkins, 2003.

Musculoskeletal system

Blakeley, J.A., and Ribeiro, V.E. "Glucosamine and Osteoarthritis," *AJN* 104(2):54-59, February 2004.

Hohler, S.E. "Looking into Minimally Invasive Total Hip Arthroplasty," *Nursing2005* 35(6):54-57, June 2005.

McLean, K.R. "Osteogenesis Imperfecta," *Neonatal Network* 23(2):7-14, March-April 2004.

Miller, T., and Schweitzer, M. *Diagnostic Musculoskeletal Imaging.* New York: McGraw-Hill Book Co., 2004.

Northrop, D.E. "MS Presents Special Challenges," *Provider* 30(7):43-44, 47-48, July 2004.

Pruitt, W.C., and Jacobs, M. "Interpreting Arterial Blood Gases: Easy as ABC," *Nursing2004* 34(8):50-53, August 2004.

Reproductive system

Bosarge, P.M. "Understanding and Treating PMS/PMDD," *Nursing2003* Suppl. 13-14, 17, November 2003.

Farrell, M. "Improving the Care of Women with Gestational Diabetes," *The American Journal of Maternal Child Nursing* 28(5):301-305, September-October 2003.

Maternal-Neonatal Nursing Made Incredibly Easy. Philadelphia: Lippincott Williams & Wilkins, 2004.

Scott, J.R., et al. *Danforth's Obstetrics and Gynecology,* 9th ed. Philadelphia: Lippincott Williams & Wilkins, 2004.

Sherrod, R.A. "Understanding the Emotional Aspects of Infertility: Implications for Nursing Practice," *Journal of Psychosocial Nursing and Mental Health Services* 42(3):40-47, March 2004.

Cancer

Bourbonniere, M., and Kagan, S.H. "Nursing Intervention and Older Adults Who Have Cancer: Specific Science and Evidence-Based Practice," *Nursing Clinics of North America* 39(3):529-43, September 2004.

Devenney, B., and Erickson, C. "Multiple Myeloma: An Overview," *Clinical Journal of Oncology Nursing* 8(4):401-405, August 2004.

Glajchen, M. "The Emerging Role and Needs of Family Caregivers in Cancer Care," *Journal of Supportive Oncology* 2(2):145-55, March-April 2004.

Hartmuller, V.W., and Desmond, S. "Professional and Patient Perspectives on Nutritional Needs of Patients with Cancer," *Oncology Nursing Forum* 31(5):989-96, September 2004.

Fluids and electrolytes

Alexander, M., and Corrigan, A.M. *Core Curriculum for Infusion Nursing,* 3rd ed. Philadelphia: Lippincott Williams & Wilkins, 2003.

Fluids and Electrolytes: A 2-in-1 Reference for Nurses. Philadelphia: Lippincott Williams & Wilkins, 2005.

Pruitt, W.C., and Jacobs, M. "Interpreting Arterial Blood Gases: Easy as ABC," *Nursing2004* 34(8):50-53, August 2004.

Genetics

Aronson, B.S., and Marquis, M. "Care of the Adult Patient with Cystic Fibrosis," *Medsurg Nursing* 13(3):143-54, June 2004.

D'Arcy, Y. "Managing Sickle-Cell Crisis," *Nursing2004* 34(1):24-25, January 2004.

DeSevo, M.R. "Would You Suspect this Genetic Disorder?" *RN* 68(3):47-50, March 2005.

Miller, K.L. "Factor Products in the Treatment of Hemophilia," *Journal of Pediatric Health Care* 18(3):156-57, May-June 2004.

Prows, C.A., and Prows, D.R. "Medication Selection by Genotype: How Genetics is Changing Drug Prescribing and Efficacy," *AJN* 104(5):60-70, March 2004.

Trent, J.T., and Kirsner, R.S. "Leg Ulcers in Sickle Cell Disease," *Advances in Skin and Wound Care* 17(8):410-16, October 2004.

Infection

Bartlett, J.G. *2004 Pocket Book of Infectious Disease Therapy,* 12th ed. Philadelphia: Lippincott Williams & Wilkins, 2004.

Bielan, B. "What's Your Assessment? Herpes Zoster," *Dermatology Nursing* 16(5):431-32, October 2004.

Mayhall, C.G. *Hospital Epidemiology and Infection Control,* 3rd ed. Philadelphia: Lippincott Williams & Wilkins, 2004.

Purssell, E. "Symptoms in the Host: Infection and Treatment Model," *Journal of Clinical Nursing* 14(5):555-61, May 2005.

Walker, B.W. "Reducing the Risk of Rabies," *Nursing2003* 33(10):20, October 2003.

INDEX

A

Absence seizures, 176
Acid-base balance, 447-450
  buffer systems and, 449
  compensation by kidneys and, 449
  compensation by lungs and, 449-450
  pathophysiologic changes in, 448-450
  tonicity and, 448
Acidemia, 448
Acidosis, 448-449
  metabolic, 465-467
  respiratory, 473-476
Acne, 351-353
  types of, 351
Acquired immunity, 308
Acquired immunodeficiency syndrome, 308-313
  Centers for Disease Control and Prevention classification matrix and, 311
  conditions associated with, 312
  highly active retroviral therapy for, 311
  human immunodeficiency virus infection as cause of, 308-311
  opportunistic infections in, 310t
Actinic keratosis, 444i
Acute angle-closure glaucoma, 339
Acute coronary syndromes, 1-5, 3i, 4t, 5, 6-7i, 8-9. *See also* Myocardial infarction.
  chest pain in, 3-4
Acute idiopathic polyneuritis. *See* Guillain-Barré syndrome.
Acute infective tubulointerstitial nephritis, 228-231
Acute leukemia, 420-423
  risk factors for, 420-421
  types of, 420
  white blood cell proliferation in, 421, 421i

Acute lymphocytic leukemia, 420
Acute myeloblastic leukemia, 420
Acute myeloid leukemia, 420
Acute nonlymphocytic leukemia, 420
Acute poststreptococcal glomerulonephritis, 244, 245
Acute pyelonephritis, 228-231
  preventing, 231
Acute renal failure, 231-236
  phases of, 233-234
  types of, 231, 232-233
Acute respiratory distress syndrome, 84-90
  progression of, 87i
Acute respiratory failure, 90-93
Acute tubular necrosis, 236-238
Acute tubulointerstitial nephritis, 236-238
Addisonian crisis, 262-263, 264, 265-266
Addison's disease, 262-266
Adenovirus infection, 111t
Adrenal crisis, 262-263, 264, 265-266
Adrenal hypofunction, 262-266
Adrenal insufficiency, 262-266
Adrenocortical hormone deficiency, 263
AIDS. *See* Acquired immunodeficiency syndrome.
Alcoholic cirrhosis, 196
Aldosterone deficiency, 264
Alimentary canal, 189
Alkalemia, 449
Alkalosis, 449
  hyperchloremic, 457i
  metabolic, 467-469
  respiratory, 476-477
Allergic granulomatosis angiitis, 334-335t
Allergic rhinitis, 313-315
  triggers for, 313
Alpha-fetoprotein as tumor cell marker, 440t

i refers to an illustration; t refers to a table.

Alzheimer's disease, 129-131
  factors associated with development
    of, 130
Amyotrophic lateral sclerosis, 132-133
Anaphylactic shock, 67, 68-69, 70. *See also*
    Shock.
Anaphylaxis, 315-319
  process of, 315, 316-317i, 318
Anaplasia, 418, 418i
Androgen deficiency, 264
Anemia
  aplastic, 289-292
  Cooley's, 304-306
  erythroblastic, 304-306
  folic acid deficiency, 292-293
  hypoplastic, 289-292
  iron deficiency, 293-295
  pernicious, 296-298
  sickle cell, 497-500
Anencephaly, 494, 495
Aneurysm, intracranial, 155-158
Angina, unstable. *See* Acute coronary
    syndromes.
Ankylosing spondylitis, 319-322
  diagnostic criteria for, 321
Anterior cord syndrome, 179t
Anthrax, 503-505
  forms of, 503, 504-505
Antidiuretic hormone, blood pressure
    regulation and, 52
Antiretroviral drug classes, 311
Antithyroid therapy, 279-280
Aortic arch syndrome, 334-335t
Aortic insufficiency, 78-79t, 80
Aortic stenosis, 78-79t, 80
Aplastic anemias, 289-292
Appendicitis, 189-190
Aqueous humor
  in glaucoma, 339-340
  normal flow of, 340i
ARDS. *See* Acute respiratory distress syn-
    drome.
Arterial blood gas values, interpreting,
    450-451t
Arterial occlusive disease, 9-14
  major sites of, 10i
  predisposing factors for, 9
  types of, 12t
Arteriovenous malformation, 134-135
Arthritic joints, specific care for, 391
Asbestosis, 93-95
Aspiration pneumonia, 110, 112t. *See also*
    Pneumonia.

Asthma, 95-103. *See also* Chronic obstruc-
    tive pulmonary disease.
  averting attack of, 99i
  bronchiole in, 98i
  levels of, 98-100
  progression of, 97i
Asystole, 24-25t
Ataxic cerebral palsy, signs of, 137t. *See also*
    Cerebral palsy.
Atherosclerosis, 11
Athetoid cerebral palsy, signs of, 137t. *See
    also* Cerebral palsy.
Atonic seizures, 176
Atrial fibrillation, 20-21t
Atrial flutter, 20-21t
Atrial septal defect, 14-16
  types of, 14
Autoimmune Addison's disease, 263
Automaticity, altered, 26i
Autonomic dysreflexia as spinal cord injury
    complication, 180
Autonomic hyperreflexia as spinal cord
    injury complication, 180
Autosomal disorders, 484-485
Autosomal dominant polycystic kidney
    disease, 255, 256
Autosomal inheritance, 482
Autosomal recessive polycystic kidney
    disease, 256

B

Bacteria
  cephalosporins' action against, 514-515i
  tissue damage and, 504-505i
Bacterial endocarditis. *See* Endocarditis.
Bacterial pneumonia, 110, 111-112t. *See also*
    Pneumonia.
Ball valving in chronic obstructive pulmo-
    nary disease, 104i
Basal cell carcinoma, 444i
Becker's muscular dystrophy, 387, 388
Bedsores. *See* Pressure ulcers.
Behçet's syndrome, 334-335t
Benign prostatic hyperplasia, 404-408
  prostatic enlargement in, 405i
Benign prostatic hypertrophy. *See* Benign
    prostatic hyperplasia.
Benign pseudohypertrophic muscular
    dystrophy, 387, 388
Beta-thalassemia, 304-306
Biliary tree, gallstone formation and, 195i
Blood, functions of, 289
Blood pressure readings, classifying, 54t

---

i refers to an illustration; t refers to a table.

Blood pressure regulation, mechanisms for, 52
Bone fracture, 370-373
  classifying, 371
Bone marrow failure. *See* Aplastic anemias.
Brain attack. *See* Stroke.
Breast cancer, 423-426
  classifying, 423-424
  risk factors for, 423
Brown-Sèquard syndrome, 179t
Bryant's traction, 379
  caring for child in, 381
Budd-Chiari syndrome, 196, 198i
Buffer systems, 449
Burns, 353-359
  classification of, 355i
  estimating extent of, 356-357i
  first-degree, 353, 354, 355i
  fourth-degree, 354, 355, 355i, 358
  second-degree, 353-355, 355i
  third-degree, 354, 355, 355i, 358

C

Calcium
  controlling balance of, 452-453i
  function of, 450
  imbalance of, 450-451, 454-455
Cancer, 417-446. *See also specific type.*
  cell differentiation in, 417-419, 418i
  grading, 419-420
  metastasis of, 424-425i
  TNM staging in, 419, 420
  treatment of, 420
  tumor classification in, 419-420
  warning signs of, 442
Capillary fluid shift, blood pressure regulation and, 52
Carcinoembryonic antigen as tumor cell marker, 440t
Carcinogenesis, 417
Carcinoma in situ, 426
Cardiac arrhythmias, 16-17, 24
  types of, 18-25t
Cardiac cirrhosis, 196
Cardiac conduction system, 26-27i
Cardiac output, monitoring, 71
Cardiac tamponade, 24-30
  obstructed blood flow in, 27, 28i
Cardiogenic shock, 67, 69, 70. *See also* Shock.
Cardiomyopathy, 30-39
  comparing diagnostic tests in, 36-37t
  comparing types of, 32-33t
Cardiovascular system disorders, 1-83

Carotid artery occlusion, 12t, 13
Carpal tunnel, 374i
Carpal tunnel syndrome, 373-375
Cast care, 377
Cataract, 336-339
  congenital, 337
  developmental stages of, 337
  removal techniques for, 338-339i
Celiac disease, 190-192
Cell cycle, chemotherapy's action in, 436i
Cell differentiation, cancer and, 417-419
Cell-mediated immunity, 308
Central cord syndrome, 179t
Central diabetes insipidus, 270. *See also* Diabetes insipidus.
Central venous pressure, monitoring, 71
Cephalosporins, antibacterial action of, 514-515i
Cerebral aneurysm. *See* Intracranial aneurysm.
Cerebral palsy, 135-138
  assessing signs of, 137t
  types of, 13
Cerebrovascular accident. *See* Stroke.
Cervical cancer, 426-427
  classifying, 426
Cervical intraepithelial neoplasia, 426
Cervicitis, 506-507
Chemical sensitivity dermatitis, 322
Chemotherapy, action of, in cell cycle, 436i
Chickenpox, 111t
Chlamydial infections, 506-507
Chloride
  function of, 455-456
  imbalance of, 455-458
Cholecystitis, 192-196
  gallstone formation and, 194-195i
Chromosomal disjunction, 486i
Chromosomal nondisjunction, 486i
Chromosome anomalies, 487
Chronic autoimmune thyroiditis, 282
Chronic lymphocytic leukemia, 427-429
Chronic lymphocytic thyroiditis, 282
Chronic obstructive pulmonary disease, 103-105. *See also* Asthma.
  air trapping in, 104i
Chronic open-angle glaucoma, 339, 342i
Chronic polyarticular gout, 382
Chronic pyelonephritis, 229
Chronic renal failure, 238-244
  extrarenal consequences of, 239-240
Chronic vasomotor rhinitis, distinguishing, from allergic rhinitis, 314
Churg-Strauss syndrome, 334-335t

i refers to an illustration; t refers to a table.

Cirrhosis, 196-200
   types of, 196
Cleft lip and palate, 487-490
   types of deformities in, 488i
Clubfoot, 376-378
Coarctation of the aorta, 39-41
Colorectal cancer, 429-430
   risk factors for, 429
Common bile duct, gallstone formation
   and, 195i
Common cold, distinguishing, from allergic
   rhinitis, 314
Compartment syndrome, 372
Complete heart block, 22-23t
Compression test, 375
Concussion, 146-147t
Conductive hearing loss, 343
   otosclerosis as cause of, 348-350
Congenital cataracts, 337
Congenital glaucoma, 341
Congenital hearing loss, 342-344
Congenital heart defects. *See specific defect.*
Congenital hip dysplasia. *See* Developmen-
   tal dysplasia of the hip.
Constipation in irritable bowel
   syndrome, 215
Consumption coagulopathy. *See* Dissemi-
   nated intravascular coagulation.
Contact dermatitis, 361t
Continuous arteriovenous hemo-
   filtration, 462
Continuous venovenous hemofiltration, 462
Contusion of the brain, 146-147t
Cooley's anemia, 304-306
COPD. *See* Chronic obstructive pulmonary
   disease.
Cor pulmonale, 105-109
   common pathway of causes of, 107i
   stages of, 107
Cortisol deficiency, 263
Coup/contrecoup injury, 145
Crescentic glomerulonephritis, 244, 246
CREST syndrome, 368
Crohn's disease, 200-202
   bowel changes in, 201i
Cryptogenic cirrhosis, 196
Cushing's disease, 266
Cushing's syndrome, 266-269
Cutaneous anthrax, 504
Cystic fibrosis, 490-492
   diagnostic criteria for, 491
Cystitis, 521-522
Cystometry, 254
Cytomegalovirus infection, 111t

D
Deafness. *See* Hearing loss.
Defibrination syndrome. *See* Disseminated
   intravascular coagulation.
Degenerative joint disease. *See* Osteo-
   arthritis.
Delta hepatitis, 208-209, 211t
Dementia. *See* Alzheimer's disease.
Demyelination, 163i
Dermatitis, 359-362
   types of, 360-362t
Developmental dysplasia of the hip, 378-381
   forms of, 378
   Ortolani's sign of, 379
   Trendelenburg's sign of, 379
Diabetes insipidus, 269-272
   forms of, 370
Diabetes mellitus, 272-276
   classifications of, 272
Dialysis
   aftercare for, 244
   nursing considerations for, 235-236
   preparing patient for, 243-244
Diarrhea in irritable bowel syndrome, 215
Diastolic dysfunction, heart failure and, 46
DIC. *See* Disseminated intravascular
   coagulation.
Diffuse systemic sclerosis. *See* Scleroderma.
Dilated cardiomyopathy, 30, 31, 32t, 34, 35,
   36t, 37-38. *See also* Cardiomyopathy.
Discoid lupus erythematosus, 323
Disseminated intravascular coagulation,
   298-301
   process of, 300i
   treatment of, 300i
Distributive shock, 67, 68-69, 70, 72. *See also*
   Shock.
Diverticular disease, 202-205
   common sites for, 202
   forms of, 202
Diverticulitis, 202, 203
Diverticulosis, 202, 203
Down syndrome, 492-494
Drug-induced hepatitis, 207
Duchenne's muscular dystrophy, 387, 388
Duodenal ulcers. *See* Peptic ulcers.
Dysplastic nevus, 444i

E
Edema, 448
Electrolyte balance, 447. *See also specific*
   electrolyte imbalance.
Electrophysiologic testing, 17
Embolectomy, 11

i refers to an illustration; t refers to a table.

Embolic stroke, 183t
Encephalocele, 494-495, 496
Endemic goiter, 278, 285-286
Endocarditis, 41-44
    degenerative changes in, 42i
    predisposing factors for, 41-42
Endocrine system, 262-288
    components of, 262
Endolymphatic hydrops, 346-348
Endometrial bleeding, abnormal, 402-404
Endometriosis, 408-410
    common sites of, 409i
Endotoxins, 502, 503
Enterotoxins, 502-503
Environmental teratogens, 485-487
Eosinophilia-myalgia syndrome. See
    Scleroderma.
Epidural hematoma, 146-147t
Epilepsy, 174-178
Erectile dysfunction, 411-413
Erythema chronicum migrans, 513
Erythremia, 302-304
Erythroblastic anemia, 304-306
Exchange transfusion, 213-214
Exfoliative dermatitis, 362t
Exotoxins, 502, 503
Extracapillary glomerulonephritis, 244, 246
Extracapsular cataract extraction, 338i
Extracellular fluid, 447

F

Facioscapulohumeral muscular dystrophy,
    387, 388
Femoral artery occlusion, 12t, 14
First-degree atrioventricular block, 20-21t
Fluid
    estimating loss of, 461
    imbalance of, 458-463
    movement of
        in hypernatremia, 479i
        in hyponatremia, 459i
Fluid balance, 447
Focal glomerulosclerosis, 250
Folic acid, 292
    foods high in, 293t
Folic acid deficiency anemia, 292-293
Fractures. See Bone fracture.
Functioning metastatic thyroid
    carcinoma, 277

G

Gallbladder, gallstone formation and, 194i
Gallstone formation, 194-195i
Gas exchange, 84

Gastric cancer, 430-432
    classifying, 431
    predisposing factors for, 430-431
Gastric ulcers. See Peptic ulcers.
Gastroesophageal reflux disease, 205-207
    decreased lower esophageal sphincter
        pressure in, 205, 206i
Gastrointestinal anthrax, 504, 505
Gastrointestinal system disorders, 189-227
Gastrointestinal tract, 189
Gender determination, trait transmission
    and, 481-482
Generalized seizures, 176
Generalized tonic-clonic seizures, 176
Genetics, 481-500
Genital herpes cycle, 509i. See also Herpes
    simplex.
GERD. See Gastroesophageal reflux disease.
Germ cells, trait transmission and, 481
Gestational diabetes, 272, 273, 274
Glaucoma, 339-342
    aqueous humor flow and, 339-340
    congenital, 341
    forms of, 339
    optic disk changes in, 342i
Glomerulonephritis, 244-249
    averting renal failure in, 248i
    lesion characteristics in, 245
Glomerulosclerosis, 239
Glucocorticoid deficiency, 262, 263,
    264, 265
Gluten intolerance. See Celiac disease.
Gonorrhea, 507-508
Goodpasture's syndrome, 244, 246
Gout, 381-383
Gouty arthritis, 381-383
Graft-versus-host disease. See Scleroderma.
Granulomatous colitis. See Crohn's disease.
Graves' disease, 276, 277. See also Hyper-
    thyroidism.
Guillain-Barré syndrome, 138-142
    phases of, 139
    sensorimotor nerve degeneration in, 140i

H

HAART, antiretroviral drugs included in, 311
Hand or foot dermatitis, 361t
Hashimoto's thyroiditis, 282
Hay fever, 313-314
Headache, 142-144
    phases of, 143
Head trauma, 144-150
    categorizing, 145
    types of, 146-149t

---

i refers to an illustration; t refers to a table.

Hearing loss, 342-345. *See also* Otosclerosis.
　types of, 342, 343
Heartburn. *See* Gastroesophageal reflux
　disease.
Heart failure, 44-49
　causes of, 45t
　classifying, 38
　diastolic dysfunction and, 46-47
　left-sided, 45-46, 47
　right-sided, 46, 47-48
　systolic dysfunction and, 46
Hematologic system disorders, 289-307
Hematoma
　epidural, 146-147t
　intracerebral, 148-149t
　subdural, 148-149t
Hematopoiesis, 289
Hemodialysis, nursing considerations for,
　235-236
Hemodynamic monitoring, 71
Hemorrhagic stroke, 183t, 187. *See also*
　Stroke.
Hepatitis
　nonviral, 207-208
　viral, 208-211
　　forms of, 208-209, 210-211t
　　stages of, 209
Herniated disk. *See* Herniated nucleus pul-
　posus.
Herniated intervertebral disk. *See* Herniated
　nucleus pulposus.
Herniated nucleus pulposus, 150-152,
　383-387
　development of, 385i
　progression of, 151
Herpes simplex, 508-511
　genital herpes cycle and, 509i
　types of, 509
Herpes zoster, 511-513
Hip dysplasia. *See* Developmental dysplasia
　of the hip.
Hodgkin's disease, 432-433
Host cell, viral infection of, 502i, 503
Host defenses, 308
Human chorionic gonadotropin as tumor
　cell marker, 440t
Human immunodeficiency virus infection
　as cause of acquired immunodeficiency
　　syndrome, 308-311
　transmission of, 309
Humoral immunity, 308
Hyaline membrane disease, 124-127
Hydrocephalus, 153-155
　risk factors for, 153

Hyperbilirubinemia, 212-214
Hypercalcemia, 450, 451, 454-455
Hyperchloremia, 456, 457
Hyperchloremic alkalosis, 457i
Hyperkalemia, 471, 472, 473
Hypermagnesemia, 463, 464, 465
Hypernatremia, 478, 479, 480
　fluid movement in, 479i
Hyperphosphatemia, 469, 470, 471
Hypersensitivity reaction, type I. *See*
　Anaphylaxis.
Hypersensitivity vasculitis, 334-335t
Hypertension, 50-56
Hypertensive crisis, pathophysiology of, 53i
Hyperthyroidism, 276-282
　forms of, 276, 277
Hypertonic solutions, 448
Hypertrophic cardiomyopathy, 30, 31, 33t,
　　34, 35-36, 36-37t, 38. *See also*
　　Cardiomyopathy.
Hypertrophic obstructive cardiomyopathy.
　See Hypertrophic cardiomyopathy.
Hypervolemia, 458, 460, 461-462, 463
Hypocalcemia, 450-451, 454, 455
Hypochloremia, 456-457
Hypokalemia, 471, 472, 473
Hypomagnesemia, 463-464, 465
Hyponatremia, 478-479, 480
　fluid movement in, 459i
Hypophosphatemia, 469-471
Hypoplastic anemias, 289-292
Hypothyroidism, 282-285
　acquired, clinical findings in, 283
　thyroid test results in, 284t
Hypotonic solutions, 448
Hypovolemia, 458-461, 462-463
Hypovolemic shock, 67, 69, 70-71. *See also*
　Shock.

I

IBS. *See* Irritable bowel syndrome.
Idiopathic thrombocytopenic purpura,
　301-302
Iliac artery occlusion, 12t, 14
Immune system, 308-335
Impotence, 411-413
Infection, 501-522
　pathophysiologic changes in, 503
　stages of, 501-503
　viral replication in, 502i, 503
Infectious hepatitis, 208, 210t
Infectious polyneuritis. *See* Guillain-Barré
　syndrome.

---

i refers to an illustration; t refers to a table.

Infectious rhinitis, distinguishing, from allergic rhinitis, 314
Infective endocarditis. *See* Endocarditis.
Inflammation
  blocking, 510i
  stages of, 503
Inflammatory response, 308, 503
Influenza, 111t
Inhalation anthrax, 504, 505
Innominate artery occlusion, 12t, 13
Insulin-dependent diabetes mellitus. *See* Type 1 diabetes mellitus.
Integumentary system disorders, 351-369
Intracapsular cataract extraction, 339i
Intracellular fluid, 447
Intracerebral hematoma, 148-149t
Intracranial aneurysm, 155-158
  common sites of, 156i
  ruptured, grading, 157
Intrarenal failure, 231, 232
Iron deficiency anemia, 293-295
Irritable bowel syndrome, 214-216
  intestinal function in, 215
Ischemic stroke, 183t, 185. *See also* Stroke.
Isolated systolic hypertension, 50
Isotonic solutions, 448

J
Jones criteria for diagnosing rheumatic fever, 65
Junctional rhythm, 20-21t

K
Kawasaki disease, 334-335t
Kidneys, compensation by, in acid-base balance, 449
Kidney stones. *See* Renal calculi.
Klebsiella pneumonia, 112t

L
Labyrinthine dysfunction. *See* Ménière's disease.
Lacunar stroke, 183t
Läennec's cirrhosis, 196
Landouzy-Dejerine muscular dystrophy, 387, 388
Landry-Guillain-Barré syndrome. *See* Guillain-Barré syndrome.
Lasègue's sign, 385
Latex allergy, 322-323
  individuals at risk for, 322
Left atrial pressure, monitoring, 71
Leriche syndrome, 12t

Leukemia
  acute, 420-423
  chronic lymphocytic, 427-429
Lichen simplex chronicus, 361t
Limb-girdle muscular dystrophy, 387, 388
Lipid nephrosis, 249
Liver, gallstone formation and, 194i
Long-incubation hepatitis, 208, 210t
Lou Gehrig disease, 132-133
Lower esophageal sphincter pressure, decreased, in gastroesophageal reflux disease, 205, 206i
Lumpectomy, 425
Lund-Browder chart for estimating extent of burn, 357i
Lung cancer, 434-435, 437
  classes of, 434
Lungs, compensation by, in acid-base balance, 449
Lupus erythematosus, 323-326
  forms of, 323
Lyme disease, 513-515
  stages of, 513

M
Macular degeneration, 345-346
  risk factors for, 345
  types of, 345
Magnesium
  function of, 464
  imbalance of, 463-465
Malignant conditions, tumor cell markers for, 440t
Malignant lymphoma, 437-438
Malignant melanoma, 443-445, 444i
  risk factors for, 443
Malignant neoplasia. *See* Cancer.
Marie-Strümpell disease. *See* Ankylosing spondylitis.
Mastectomy, 425
Measles, 111t
Meckel's diverticulum, 202
Mediterranean disease, 304-306
Meiosis, 481
Melanoma. *See* Malignant melanoma.
Membranoproliferative glomerulo-nephritis, 250
Membranous glomerulonephritis, 249-250
Ménière's disease, 346-348
Meningeal irritation, signs of, 160
Meningitis, 159-161
Meningocele, 494
Mesenteric artery occlusion, 12t, 13-14

---

i refers to an illustration; t refers to a table.

Metabolic acidosis, 465-467
  arterial blood gas values in, 450-451t
Metabolic alkalosis, 467-469
  arterial blood gas values in, 450-451t
Metastasis, process of, 424-425i
Metyrapone test, 265
Migraine headache. *See* Headache.
Minimal cervical dysplasia, 426
Mitosis, 482
  phases of, 483i
Mitral insufficiency, 78-79t, 80
Mitral stenosis, 78-79t, 80
Mixed cerebral palsy, signs of, 137t. *See also*
  Cerebral palsy.
Mixed hearing loss, 343
Mobitz block I and II, 22-23t
Mosaicism, 487
Mucocutaneous lymph node syndrome,
  334-335t
Multifactorial disorders, 485
Multifactorial inheritance, 484
Multiple sclerosis, 161-165
  demyelination in, 163i
  types of, 162
Muscular dystrophy, 387-389
  types of, 387, 388
Musculoskeletal system disorders, 370-401
Mutations, 484
Myasthenia gravis, 165-168
  neuromuscular transmission in, 167i
Myasthenic crisis, 167, 168
Myelin, function of, 163i
Myelomeningocele, 494
Myelosuppressive treatment, nursing
  considerations for, 304
Myocardial infarction. *See also* Acute
  coronary syndromes.
  electrocardiographic leads for
    pinpointing, 4t
  treating, 6-7i
  zones of, 3i
Myoclonic seizures, 176
Myxedema coma, 282, 283, 285

N

Neonatal jaundice, 212-214
Nephrogenic diabetes insipidus, 270. *See also*
  Diabetes insipidus.
Nephrolithiasis. *See* Renal calculi.
Nephrotic syndrome, 249-251
Nerve entrapment syndrome, 373-375
Nervous system, 129-188
Neural tube defects, 494-497
  forms of, 494

Neuritic plaques, 130
Neurodermatitis, localized, 361t
Neurofibrillary tangles, 130
Neurogenic bladder, 251-255
  types of, 253t
Neurogenic diabetes insipidus, 270. *See also*
  Diabetes insipidus.
Neurogenic shock, 67, 68, 72. *See also*
  Shock.
  as spinal cord injury complication, 180
Neurologic bladder dysfunction. *See* Neuro-
  genic bladder.
Neuromuscular dysfunction of the lower
  urinary tract. *See* Neurogenic bladder.
Neuromuscular transmission, impaired, in
  myasthenia gravis, 167i
Neurons, 129
Neuropathic bladder. *See* Neurogenic
  bladder.
Noise-induced hearing loss, 343, 344
Non-A, non-B hepatitis, 209, 211t
Non-Hodgkin's lymphoma, 437-438
Non–insulin-dependent diabetes mellitus,
  272, 273, 274
Nonmalignant conditions, tumor cell
  markers for, 440t
Nontoxic goiter, 278, 285-287, 286i
Nonviral hepatitis, 207-208
Nummular dermatitis, 360t
Nutritional cirrhosis, 196

O

Obesity, 216-217
Oculogyric crises, 170
Opportunistic infections in acquired
  immunodeficiency syndrome, 310t
Ortolani's sign, 379
Osteitis deformans, 398-400
Osteoarthritis, 389-392
  joint care in, 391
Osteomyelitis, 392-395
  avoiding, 394i
Osteoporosis, 395-398
Osteotomy, 331
Otitis media, 515-517
Otosclerosis, 348-350. *See also* Hearing loss.
Ovarian cancer, 438-441
  types of, 438-439

Pq

Paget's disease, 398-400
Pancreatitis, 218-220
  forms of, 218

i refers to an illustration; t refers to a table.

Parathyroid hormone, phosphorus and, 470i
Parkinson's disease, 169-171
Paroxysmal supraventricular tachycardia, 18-19t
Partial seizures, 176
Patent ductus arteriosus, 56-58
Pathogenicity, factors that affect, 501
Pathologic jaundice, 212
Peptic ulcers, 220-225
    predisposing factors for, 224
    scarring in, 221i
    treating, 222-223i
Perennial allergic rhinitis, 313-314
Pericardial friction rub, 59
Pericarditis, 58-61
Peritoneal dialysis, nursing considerations for, 235
Pernicious anemia, 296-298
Phalen's maneuver, 375
Phantom breast syndrome, 426
Phlebotomy, nursing considerations for, 303-304
Phosphorus
    functions of, 469
    imbalance of, 469-471
    parathyroid hormone and, 470i
Phototherapy, 213
Physiologic jaundice, 212
Pierre Robin syndrome, 488-489
Platelet deficiency. See Idiopathic thrombo-cytopenic purpura.
Pneumoconiosis. See Asbestosis.
Pneumonia, 109-113
    classifying, 109-110
    predisposing factors for, 110
    types of, 111-112t
Pneumothorax, 113-117
    types of, 113, 115i
Polyangiitis overlap syndrome, 334-335t
Polyarteritis nodosa, 334-335t
Polycystic kidney disease, 255-257
    cystic damage in, 255i
    forms of, 255
Polycystic ovarian disease, 413-414
Polycythemia rubra vera, 302-304
Polycythemia vera, 302-304
Popliteal artery occlusion, 12t, 14
Portal cirrhosis, 196
Portal hypertension as cirrhosis complication, 198i
Postmenopausal osteoporosis, 396
Postnecrotic cirrhosis, 196
Postrenal failure, 231-233

Potassium
    function of, 471
    imbalance of, 471-473
Premature ventricular contraction, 22-23t
Prerenal failure, 231, 232
Presbycusis, 343, 344
Pressure sores. See Pressure ulcers.
Pressure ulcers, 363-367
    common locations for, 363
    preventing, 366
    staging, 364-365i
Primary polycythemia, 302-304
Prostate cancer, 441-443
Prostate-specific antigen as tumor cell marker, 440t
Prostatic acid phosphatase as tumor cell marker, 440t
Prostatic enlargement, 405i. See also Benign prostatic hyperplasia.
Prostatism, 405
Prostatitis, 414-416
    classifying, 414
Pruritus, essential, 361t
Pseudohypertrophic muscular dystrophy, 387, 388
Psychogenic diabetes insipidus, 270. See also Diabetes insipidus.
Pulmonary artery pressure, monitoring, 71
Pulmonary artery wedge pressure, monitoring, 71
Pulmonary edema, 117-120
    alveolus in, 118-119i
    predisposing factors for, 117
Pulmonary embolism, 121-123
    predisposing factors for, 121
Pulmonic stenosis, 78-79t, 80
Pyelonephritis
    acute, 228-231
    chronic, 229

R

Rapid corticotropin stimulation test, 265
Rapidly progressive glomerulonephritis, 244, 246
Raynaud's disease, 61-63
Raynaud's phenomenon, 61-62
Reentry, cardiac conduction and, 26-27i
Regional enteritis. See Crohn's disease.
Renal calculi, 257-261
    predisposing factors for, 257-258
    preventing recurrence of, 261
    types of, 258-259, 258i

---

i refers to an illustration; t refers to a table.

Renal failure
  acute, 231-236
  averting, in glomerulonephritis, 248i
  chronic, 238-244
Renal replacement therapy, 462
Renal system
  components of, 228
  disorders of, 228-261
Renin-angiotensin system, blood pressure
     regulation and, 52
Reproductive system disorders, 402-416
Respiratory acidosis, 473-476
  arterial blood gas values in, 450-451t
Respiratory alkalosis, 476-477
  arterial blood gas values in, 450-451t
Respiratory distress syndrome of the
     newborn, 124-127
Respiratory syncytial virus infection, 111t
Respiratory system
  components of, 84
  disorders of, 84-128
Restless leg syndrome, 240
Restrictive cardiomyopathy, 30, 31, 33t, 34,
     36-37, 37t, 39. See also Cardio-
     myopathy.
Reye's syndrome, 171-174
  stages and treatment for, 173-174t
Rhabdomyolysis, 400-401
Rheumatic fever, 63-66
  Jones criteria for diagnosing, 65
Rheumatic heart disease, 63-66
Rheumatoid arthritis, 326-332
  drug therapy for, 328-329i
  stages of, 327
Rheumatoid spondylitis. See Ankylosing
     spondylitis.
Rhinitis medicamentosa, distinguishing,
     from allergic rhinitis, 314
RICE treatment for fracture, 372
Right atrial pressure, monitoring, 71
Right ventricular pressure, monitoring, 71
Robin's syndrome, 488-489
Rubeola, 111t
Rule of Nines for estimating extent of
     burn, 356i
Ruptured disk. See Herniated nucleus
     pulposus.

S
Saddle block occlusion, 12t, 14
SARS. See Severe acute respiratory
     syndrome.
Scleroderma, 367-369
  forms of, 367

Seasonal allergic rhinitis, 313-314
Seborrheic dermatitis, 360t
Second-degree atrioventricular block, types I
     and II, 22-23t
Secretory otitis media, 516
Seizure disorder, 174-178
Seizures, types of, 176
Sensorineural hearing loss, 343
Sensory system disorders, 336-350
Septic shock, 67, 68, 72. See also Shock.
Serum hepatitis, 208, 210t
Severe acute respiratory syndrome, 517-518
Sex-linked disorders, 485
Sex-linked inheritance, 484
Shaking palsy, 169-171
Shingles, 511-513
Shock, 66-73
  stages of, 67-69
  types of, 68-69
Shock lung. See Acute respiratory distress
     syndrome.
Short-incubation hepatitis, 208, 210t
SIADH. See Syndrome of inappropriate
     antidiuretic hormone.
Sickle cell anemia, 497-500
  crises in, 498, 499i
Sickle cell crisis, 498, 499i
Sickled cells, characteristics of, 498i
Silent thyroiditis, 277
Simple goiter, 278, 285-287, 286i
Simple partial seizure, 176
Sinus bradycardia, 18-19t
Sinus tachycardia, 18-19t
Skin cancer, 443-445
  types of, 444i
Skin disorders. See Integumentary system.
Skull fracture, 148-149t
Slipped disk. See Herniated nucleus
     pulposus.
Smallpox, 519-520
Sodium
  function of, 478
  imbalance of, 478-480
Sodium-potassium pump, 478
Spastic cerebral palsy, signs of, 137t. See also
     Cerebral palsy.
Spastic colitis. See Irritable bowel syndrome.
Spastic colon. See Irritable bowel syndrome.
Sphincter electromyelography, 254
Spica cast, caring for child in, 380-381
Spina bifida, 494, 495, 496
Spinal cord injury, 178-181
  complications of, 180
  types of, 179t

i refers to an illustration; t refers to a table.

Spinal shock as spinal cord injury complication, 180
Splenomegalic polycythemia, 302-304
Sporadic goiter, 278, 285, 286
Squamous cell carcinoma, 444i
Staphylococcal pneumonia, 112t
Stasis dermatitis, 362t
Status asthmaticus, 96, 98
Status epilepticus, 176
Stiff lung. See Acute respiratory distress syndrome.
Streptococcal pneumonia, 111t
Stress relaxation, blood pressure regulation and, 52
Stroke, 181-188
    preventing, 188
    risk factors for, 182
    treatment of, 186i
    types of, 183t
Subacute glomerulonephritis, 244, 246
Subacute thyroiditis, 277, 282
Subclavian artery occlusion, 12t, 13
Subdural hematoma, 148-149t
Sucking chest wound. See Pneumothorax.
Sudden deafness, 343, 344
Suppurative otitis media, 516
Sympathetic nervous system, blood pressure regulation and, 52
Syndrome of inappropriate antidiuretic hormone, 287-288
Synovectomy, 331
Syphilis, 520-521
    stages of, 520-521
Systemic lupus erythematosus, 323-326
    diagnostic criteria for, 324
Systemic sclerosis. See Scleroderma.
Systolic dysfunction, heart failure and, 46

T

Takayasu's arteritis, 334-335t
Talipes, 376-378
Temporal arteritis, 334-335t
Tensilon challenge test, 167
Tension headache. See Headache.
Tension pneumothorax, 113-114, 115i. See also Pneumothorax.
Teratogens, environmental, 485-487
Testicular cancer, 445-446
Tetralogy of Fallot, 73-75
Thalassemia, 304-306
    forms of, 304-305
Third-degree atrioventricular block, 22-23t
Thromboendarterectomy, 11

Thrombotic stroke, 183t
    treating, 186i
Thyroid enlargement. See Simple goiter.
Thyroid-stimulating hormone–secreting pituitary tumor, 277
Thyroid storm, 276, 279, 280
Thyrotoxicosis, 276-282
Thyrotoxicosis factitia, 277
Tinel's sign, 375
Tissue damage, bacterial, 504-505i
TNM staging, 419, 420
Tonicity, 448
Toxic adenoma, 277
Toxic oil syndrome. See Scleroderma.
Trachomatis conjunctivitis, 506
Trait predominance, 482
Trait transmission, 481-482, 483i, 484
Transient ischemic attack, treatment of, 185-186
Translocation, 487
Transposition of the great arteries, 75-77
Traumatic brain injury. See Head trauma.
Trendelenburg's sign, 379
Trisomy 21, 492-494
Tuberculosis, 127-128
Tumor cell markers, 440t
Tumors
    benign, 419
    classification of, 419-420
    factors that affect growth of, 418
    grading, 419-420
    malignant, 419
    staging, 420
Type 1 diabetes mellitus, 272-273, 274
    treatment of, 275i
Type 2 diabetes mellitus, 272, 273, 274

U

Ulcerative colitis, 225-227
Urethritis, 506-507, 521-522
Urinary tract infection, 521-522
Urodynamic studies, 254
Uterine bleeding, abnormal, 402-404

V

Valvular heart disease, 77-81
    types of, 78-79t
Vaquez-Osler disease, 302-304
Varicella pneumonia, 111t
Variola, 519-520
Vascular headache. See Headache.
Vasculitis, 332-335
    types of, 334-335t

i refers to an illustration; t refers to a table.

Vasopressin deficiency. *See* Diabetes
insipidus.
Ventricular fibrillation, 24-25t
Ventricular septal defect, 81-83
Ventricular tachycardia, 24-25t
Vertebral artery occlusion, 12t, 13
Vestibular function, normal, 347
Viral hepatitis, 208-211
    forms of, 208-209, 210-211t
    stages of, 209
Viral pneumonia, 110, 111t. *See also*
    Pneumonia.
Vitamin B$_{12}$ deficiency, 296
von Willebrand's disease, 306-307

W

Warning signs of cancer, 442
Wegener's granulomatosis, 334-335t
Wenckebach block, 22-23t
Wet lung. *See* Acute respiratory distress
    syndrome.
White lung. *See* Acute respiratory distress
    syndrome.

Xyz

X-linked inheritance, 484

---

i refers to an illustration; t refers to a table.